CRC HANDBOOK OF Dietary Fiber in Human Nutrition
2nd Edition

Edited by
Gene A. Spiller, D.Sc., Ph.D.
Director
Health Research and Studies Center
SPHERA Foundation
Los Altos, California

CRC Press
Boca Raton   Ann Arbor   London   Tokyo

Library of Congress Cataloging-in-Publication Data

CRC Handbook of dietary fiber in human nutrition / editor, Gene A.
Spiller. -- 2nd ed., updated.
    p. cm.
    Includes bibliographical references and index.
    ISBN 0-8493-4249-X
    1. Fiber in human nutrition--Handbooks, manuals, etc.
I. Spiller, Gene A.   II. Title: Handbook of dietary fiber in human
nutrition.
    [DNLM: 1. Dietary Fiber--handbooks.   2. Nutrition--handbooks. WB
39 C911]
QP141.C773   1992
613.2'8--dc20
DNLM/DLC
for Library of Congress   92-12254
                                                                                                                              CIP

    This book represents information obtained from authentic and highly regarded sources. Reprinted material is quoted with permission, and sources are indicated. A wide variety of references are listed. Every reasonable effort has been made to give reliable data and information, but the author and the publisher cannot assume responsibility for the validity of all materials or for the consequences of their use.

    Neither this book nor any part may be reproduced or transmitted in any form or by any means, electronic or mechanical, including photocopying, microfilming, and recording, or by any information storage and retrieval system, without permission in writing from the publisher.

    All rights reserved. Authorization to photocopy items for internal or personal use, or the personal or internal use of specific clients, is granted by CRC Press, Inc., provided that $.50 per page photocopied is paid directly to Copyright Clearance Center, 27 Congress Street, Salem, MA, 01970 USA. The fee code for users of the Transactional Reporting Service is ISBN 0-8493-4249-X/93 $0.00 + $.50. The fee is subject to change without notice. For organizations that have been granted a photocopy license by the CCC, a separate system of payment has been arranged.

    The copyright owner's consent does not extend to copying for general distribution, for promotion, for creating new works, or for resale. Specific permission must be obtained from CRC Press for such copying.

    Direct all inquiries to CRC Press, Inc. 2000 Corporate Blvd., N.W., Boca Raton, Florida, 33431.

                              © 1993 by CRC Press, Inc.

                International Standard Book Number 0-8493-4249-X

                  Library of Congress Card Number 92-12254

              Printed in the United States of America   2 3 4 5 6 7 8 9 0

                          Printed on acid-free paper

DEDICATION

To Hugh Trowell (1904–1989), who with Dennis Burkitt pioneered a new understanding of the role of plant fibers in human health. He has been to me a teacher of science, medicine, and humility. He should be remembered not only as a pioneer in medicine, but for his selfless and total dedication to the prevention of disease and human suffering.

PREFACE TO THE FIRST EDITION

The *CRC Handbook of Dietary Fiber in Human Nutrition* is proof of the amazing growth in the study of dietary fiber during the 1970s and 1980s. When I first edited a book on dietary fiber, *Fiber in Human Nutrition,* in the mid-1970s, I was happy to find at least a few good investigators who could contribute chapters to it. It would have been impossible to find a large number of scientists that could have made a major contribution to that early book.

However, as work was beginning on this Handbook in 1982 and I was presenting the design at the Symposium on Fiber in Human and Animal Nutrition in New Zealand that year, not only was I able to find all the 50-plus authors I needed, but I had the sad task of omitting some outstanding names.

Interest in what used to be the disregarded cinderella nutrient of the early 20th century has grown at a rate greater than almost any other nutrient. The plant cell wall and the gums and mucilages had found their well-deserved niche in nutrition and medicine.

Even though few people still believe that dietary fiber has not found the *ultimate* proof that makes it a required nutrient, the momentum is with the ones who have found valid uses for it in high fiber foods in treating diseases such as type II diabetes. The momentum is also with the epidemiologists who have found correlations with lower incidence of colorectal cancer, the ones that have found in high fiber foods one of the best ways to prevent excessive fat and food intake. It is a list that can go on and on.

Has the ultimate study on the long range effects of dietary fiber been published? Of course not. It is probably impossible to carry out the ultimate study on the correlation of nutrition to chronic diseases under present conditions: we must accept the pieces of evidence derived from good epidemiology, from controlled human studies and, of course, animal studies. The lifetimes of many of us would be needed to satisfy the purists who hope for the ultimate study, in this or any other field in which we deal with the lifetime of a human being.

There is more to complicate things: dietary fiber polymers are quite elusive, unlike vitamins that can be isolated or synthesized readily. Some of these polymers may change when torn apart from their complex structure in the cell wall. Thus, when we attempt to extract them, too often we isolate something quite different from the original material, perhaps useful, but most certainly different. This bothers many scientists who would like to use the pure form of nutrients for their investigations. There is more: dietary fiber is so interactive that other components of the diet probably vary its effect on humans. All this makes dietary fiber research so challenging and so difficult!

This book is proof that there are many dedicated scientists and clinicians that have given their best efforts to dietary fiber. There are many who could not be included here, as there is a point in an effort of this kind at which the editor must sadly stop asking for contributions and recognize that the book must be a finite number of pages. I owe a very special thanks to all the authors in this book, for after all it is their book.

The book presents a large volume of data. The reader is directed to the Table of Contents which illustrates the design of the book, a design that was conceived to make it as easy as possible to find the needed data. Chemistry, analytical methodologies, physiological and biochemical aspects, clinical and epidemiological studies, and consumption patterns are covered extensively. Tables with the dietary fiber content of various foods analyzed by different methods are given at the end of the book.

Gene A. Spiller
Los Altos, California
February 1985

PREFACE TO THE SECOND EDITION

Dietary fiber research has seen a great deal of progress since the first edition of this Handbook. This new edition is revised and updated by individual authors and, with the exception of a few chapters, such as the Southgate and the crude fiber analytical methods, that are unchanged, new material is added. Some new authors and chapters have been added, including the new method of analysis by Englyst and Hudson (Chapter 3.3) and Bosello, Armellini, and Zamboni's chapter on fiber consumption in Italy. Hugh Trowell passed away in 1989; his chapter has been left untouched. A major addition in the second edition is the inclusion of more extensive tables of data on dietary fiber in foods. They are prepared by various authors to give the reader a chance to compare data from different sources or methods.

This new edition should give researchers, physicians, nutritionists, and other health professionals a useful and ready source of information, as a handbook should. Again, as in the first edition, we could not ask all the experts in this field to contribute, so we decided to stay with the original authors as much as possible. We hope that our efforts will make this work valuable to everyone interested in this topic.

Gene A. Spiller
Health Research and
Studies Center, Inc.
SPHERA Foundation
Los Altos, California
January 1992

THE EDITOR

Gene Alan Spiller, D.Sc., Ph.D. is the director of the Health Research and Studies Center and of the SPHERA Foundation in Los Altos, California. He is the editor of many nutrition-related books.

Dr. Spiller received his doctorate in chemistry from the University of Milan (Italy) in 1949, and a Master's degree (1968) and a Ph.D. (1972) from the University of California at Berkeley. He did additional studies at the Stanford University School of Medicine at Stanford, California from 1980 to 1983.

In the 1970s, he was in charge of the Nutritional Physiology Section of Syntex Research in Palo Alto, California, where he did extensive human and animal research on dietary fiber. He continued his work on fiber in the 1980s, first as an independent consultant and later as the director of the Health Research and Studies Center in Los Altos, California. Many human clinical studies, reviews, and other publications were results of this work. In addition to his research and writings on dietary fiber, Dr. Spiller has carried out clinical studies on the effect of complex whole foods high in fiber and other beneficial nutrients such as monounsaturated fats.

In the early days of dietary fiber research in nutrition and medicine (1970s), Dr. Spiller was responsible for one of the first multiauthor books on this topic when he edited *Fiber in Human Nutrition* (Plenum Press, 1975) which was followed by two other multiauthor books on the same topic, *Topics in Dietary Fiber Research* (1978) and *Medical Aspects of Dietary Fiber* (1980) both published by Plenum Press. In 1986 he edited the first edition of this Handbook. His latest multiauthor nutrition-medical book is *The Mediterranean Diets in Health and Disease* (Van Nostrand, 1991).

In addition, Dr.Spiller has been a lecturer in nutrition in the San Francisco Bay Area at Mills College and Foothill College.

He has a special interest in lesser known nutritional factors that may be beneficial to human health even though not essential to life, especially factors that are present in plant foods and that may work together with dietary fiber in the prevention of degenerative diseases. He continues human studies on dietary fiber, including the investigation of differences between high fiber diets and fiber concentrates.

Dr. Spiller has been responsible for organizing international workshops on dietary fiber, such as the International Nutrition Congress in Brazil in 1978 and in Brighton (U.K.) in 1985, and he has chaired many symposia and sessions on this topic.

CONTRIBUTORS

James W. Anderson, M.D.
Professor of Medicine and Clinical
 Nutrition
Metabolic Research Group
Veterans Administration Medical Center
University of Kentucky
Lexington, Kentucky

Abayomi O. Akanji, M.D., Ph.D.
Department of Chemical Pathology
University College Hospital
Ibadan, Nigeria

Fabio Armellini, M.D.
Istituto di Clinica Medica
Policlinico di Borgo Roma
Università di Verona
Verona, Italy

Nils-Georg Asp, M.D.
Professor
Department of Food Chemistry
Chemical Center
University of Lund
Lund, Sweden

Katrine I. Baghurst, B.Sc., Ph.D.
Senior Principal Research Scientist
Division of Human Nutrition
CSIRO
Adelaide, Australia

Sheila Bingham, Ph.D.
Medical Research Council
Dunn Clinical Nutrition Centre
Cambridge, England

Ottavio Bosello, M.D.
Istituto di Clinica Medica
Policlinico di Borgo Roma
Università di Verona
Verona, Italy

Denis P. Burkitt, M.D.
Hartwell College
Gloucester, England

I. Marylin Buzzard, Ph.D., R.D.
Nutrition Coordinating Center
University of Minnesota
Minneapolis, Minnesota

Beverly M. Calkins, D.H.Sc.
Department of Epidemiology
School of Public Health
University of California
Los Angeles, California

Richard J. Calvert, Ph.D.
Nutrition Division
Federal Drug Administration
Washington, D.C.

Marie M. Cassidy, Ph.D.
Professor
Department of Physiology
George Washington University Medical
 Center
Washington, D.C.

John H. Cummings, M.D.
Medical Research Council
Dunn Clinical Nutrition Centre
Cambridge, England

Hans N. Englyst, Ph.D.
Medical Research Council
Dunn Clinical Nutrition Centre
Cambridge, England

Sharon E. Fleming, Ph.D.
Associate Professor
Department of Nutritional Sciences
University of California
Berkeley, California

Hugh J. Freeman, M.D.
Professor of Medicine and Head,
 Gastroenterology
University Hospital and University of
 British Columbia
Vancouver, British Columbia, Canada

Wenche Frølich, Ph.D.
Matforsk
Norwegian Food Research Institute
Osloveien, Aas, Norway

Ivan Furda, Ph.D.
Advanced Research Programs
General Mills
James Ford Bell Technical Center
Minneapolis, Minnesota

Daniel D. Gallaher, Ph.D.
Assistant Professor;
Department of Food Science and
  Nutrition
University of Minnesota
St. Paul, Minnesota

Sherwood H. Gorbach, M.D.
Department of Community Health
Nutrition/Infection Unit
Tufts University School of Medicine
Boston, Massachusetts

Barbara F. Harland, Ph.D., R.D.
Associate Professor
Department of Nutritional Sciences
College of Allied Health Sciences
Howard University
Washinton, D.C.

Kenneth W. Heaton, M.D.
Reader in Medicine
University Department of Medicine
Bristol Royal Infirmary
Bristol, England

Peter J. Horvath, Ph.D.
Department of Animal Science
Cornell University
Ithaca, New York

Geoffrey J. Hudson, Ph.D.
Medical Research Council
Dunn Clinical Nutrition Centre
Cambridge, England

Alexandra L. Jenkins, B.Sc., R.D.
Department of Nutritional Sciences
Faculty of Medicine
University of Toronto
Toronto, Ontario, Canada

David J. A. Jenkins, M.D., Ph.D.
Professor
Department of Nutritional Sciences
Faculty of Medicine
University of Toronto
Toronto, Ontario, Canada

Joseph L. Jeraci, Ph.D.
Syracuse Research Corp.
Syracuse, New York

Heinrich Kasper, M.D.
Professor of Medicine
Department of Internal Medicine
University of Wurzburg
Wurzburg, Germany

David Kritchevsky, Ph.D.
Institute Professor
The Wistar Institute
Philadelphia, Pennsylvania

Yves Le Quintrec, M.D.
Assistance Publique Hopitaux de Paris
Service de Gastro-enterologie et
  Pathologie Digestive Postoperatoire
Hospital Rothschild
Paris, France

Betty A. Lewis, Ph.D.
Associate Professor
Department of Nutritional Sciences
Cornell University
Ithaca, New York

Ruth McPherson, M.D., Ph.D.
Director, Lipid Research
Division of Endocrinology and
  Metabolism
Royal Victoria Hospital—McGill
  University
Ottawa Heart Institute, Ottawa
Montreal, Quebec, Canada

Bunpei Mori, Ph.D.
Professor
Department of Life Science
Toita Women's College
Tokyo, Japan

Juan M. Munoz, M.D.
Endocrinology Department
Fargo Clinic
Fargo, North Dakota

David G. Oakenfull, Ph.D.
Division of Food Processing
CSIRO
North Ryde, New South Wales, Australia

Donald Oberleas, Ph.D.
Department of Education, Nutrition, and
  Restaurant/Hotel Management
Texas Tech University
Lubbock, Texas

John D. Potter, M.D., Ph.D.
Director, Cancer Prevention Research
 Unit
School of Public Health
University of Minnesota
Minneapolis, Minnesota

Cynthia G. Rainey-Macdonald, B.Sc.
Department of Nutritional Sciences,
  Faculty of Medicine
University of Toronto
Toronto, Ontario, Canada

Sally J. Record, M.A.C.S.
Senior Technical Officer
Division of Human Nutrition
CSIRO
Adelaide, Australia

Bandaru S. Reddy, D.V.M., Ph.D.
Member and Chief
Division of Nutrition and Endocrinology
American Health Foundation
Valhalla, New York

James B. Robertson, Ph.D.
Department of Animal Science
Cornell University
Ithaca, New York

Sally F. Schakel, R.D.
Database Nutritionist
Nutrition Coordinating Center
University of Minnesota
Minneapolis, Minnesota

Barbara O. Schneeman, Ph.D.
Professor
Department of Nutrition
University of California
Davis, California

Zhi-Ping Shen, M.D.
Professor
Institute of Nutrition and Food Hygiene
Chinese Academy of Preventive Medicine
Beijing, China

Yvonne A. Sievert, M.S., R.D.
Nutrition Coordinating Center
University of Minnesota
Minneapolis, Minnesota

David A. T. Southgate, Ph.D.
Former Head
Nutrition, Diet and Health Department
AFRC Institute of Food Research
Norwich, England

Peter J. Spadafora, M.Sc.
Department of Nutritional Sciences
Faculty of Medicine
University of Toronto
Toronto, Ontario, Canada

Gene A. Spiller, D.Sc., Ph.D.
Director
Health Research and Studies Center, Inc.
SPHERA Foundation
Los Altos, California

Ion A. Story, Ph.D.
The Wistar Institute
Philadelphia, Pennsylvania

Clifford Tasman-Jones, M.D.
Head
Section of Gastroenterology
Department of Medicine
University of Auckland
Auckland, New Zealand

Olof Theander, Techn. Dr.
Professor of Organic Chemistry
Department of Chemistry
Swedish University of Agricultural
 Sciences
Uppsala, Sweden

Keisuke Tsuji, M.D., Ph.D.
Chief of Laboratory
The National Institute of Health and
 Nutrition
Tokyo, Japan

Peter J. Van Soest, Ph.D.
Professor
Animal Nutrition, Department of Animal
 Science
Cornell University
Ithaca, New York

Alexander R. P. Walker, D.Sc.
Human Biochemistry Research Unit
The South African Insitute for Medical
 Research
Johannesburg, South Africa

Eric Westerlund, Ph.D.
Associate Professor
Department of Food Science
Swedish University of Agricultural
 Sciences
Uppsala, Sweden

Margaret White
AFRC Institute of Food Research
Norwich, England

J. Scott Whittaker, M.D.
Assistant Professor of Medicine
University of British Columbia
Vancouver, British Columbia, Canada

Thomas M. S. Wolever, B.M., B.Ch., Ph.D.
Associate Professor
Department of Nutritional Sciences,
 Faculty of Medicine and Clinical
 Nutrition and Risk Factor Modification
 Centre, St. Michael's Hospital
University of Toronto
Toronto, Ontario, Canada

Margo N. Woods, D.Sc.
Department of Community Health
Nutrition/Infection Unit
Tufts University School of Medicine
Boston, Massachusetts

Mauro Zamboni, M.D.
Istituto di Clinica Medica
Policlinico di Borgo Roma
Università di Verona
Verona, Italy

Su-Fang Zheng, M.D.
Professor
Institute of Cancer
Chinese Academy of Medical Sciences
Beijing, China

ACKNOWLEDGMENTS

The editor wishes to thank Monica Alton for her extensive assistance in all phases of editing from the original design to the various stages of manuscript assessment and the final proofreading of the first edition of this Handbook.

For the second edition of this Handbook, the editor wishes to thank Rebecca Carr and Monica Alton for their assistance in the editing process.

TABLE OF CONTENTS

Section 1. Dietary Fiber: Overview and Historical Perspectives

Chapter 1.1
Dietary Fiber: From Early Hunter-Gatherers to the 1990s 3
Denis P. Burkitt and Gene A. Spiller

Chapter 1.2
Dietary Fiber — A Perspective 7
Ruth McPherson

Section 2. Definitions and Physico-Chemical Properties of Dietary Fiber

Chapter 2.1
Definition of Dietary Fiber 15
Gene A. Spiller

Chapter 2.2
Dietary Fiber Parts of Food Plants and Algae 19
David A. T. Southgate

Chapter 2.3
Food Components that Behave as Dietary Fiber 21
David A. T. Southgate

Chapter 2.4
Food Components Associated with Dietary Fiber 23
David A. T. Southgate

Chapter 2.5
Polysaccharide Food Additives that Contribute To Dietary Fiber 27
David A. T. Southgate

Chapter 2.6
Glossary of Dietary Fiber Components 29
David A. T. Southgate, Gene A. Spiller, Margaret White, and Ruth McPherson

Section 3. Methods of Analysis for Dietary Fiber

Chapter 3.1
Enzymatic Gravimetric Methods 37
Nils-Georg Asp

Chapter 3.2
Detergent Analysis of Foods 49
James B. Robertson and Peter J. Horvath

Chapter 3.3
Dietary Fiber and Starch: Classification and Measurement 53
Hans N. Englyst and Geoffrey J. Hudson

Chapter 3.4
The Southgate Method of Dietary Fiber Analysis 73
David A. T. Southgate

Chapter 3.5
Determination of Individual Components of Dietary Fiber 77
Olof Theander and Eric Westerlund

Chapter 3.6
The Crude Fiber Method 99
Ivan Furda

Chapter 3.7
Newer Methods for the Analysis of Phytate and Its Hydrolysis Products 101
Barbara F. Harland and Donald Oberleas

Chapter 3.8
Determination of the Saponin Content of Foods 105
David Oakenfull and John D. Potter

Section 4. Effect of Dietary Fiber on Carbohydrate, Lipid, and Protein Metabolism

Chapter 4.1
Effect of Dietary Fiber and Foods on Carbohydrate Metabolism 111
Thomas M. S. Wolever and David J. A. Jenkins

Chapter 4.2
Effect of Dietary Fiber on Intestinal Absorption of Lipids 153
Marie M. Cassidy and Richard J. Calvert

Chapter 4.3
Influence of Dietary Fiber on Cholesterol Metabolism in Experimental
Animals 163
David Kritchevsky and Jon A. Story

Chapter 4.4
Effect of Dietary Fiber on Protein Digestibility and Utilization 179
Daniel D. Gallaher and Barbara O. Schneeman

Section 5. Effect of Dietary Fiber on Vitamin and Mineral Metabolism

Chapter 5.1
Bioavailability of Minerals from Cereals 209
Wenche Frølich

Chapter 5.2
Overview of the Effects of Dietary Fiber on the Utilization of Minerals and
Trace Elements 245
Juan M. Munoz and Barbara F. Harland

Chapter 5.3
Effects of Dietary Fiber on Vitamin Metabolism 253
Heinrich Kasper

Section 6. Effect of Dietary Fiber on Gastrointestinal Function

Chapter 6.1
The Effect of Dietary Fiber on Fecal Weight and Composition........................263
John H. Cummings

Chapter 6.2
Suggestions for a Basis on which to Determine a Desirable Intake of Dietary
Fiber 351
Gene A. Spiller

Chapter 6.3
Effect of Dietary Fiber and Fiber-Rich Foods on Structure of the Upper
Gastrointestinal Tract...355
Clifford Tasman-Jones

Chapter 6.4
Effect of Dietary Fiber on the Structure of the Colon 359
Clifford Tasman-Jones

Chapter 6.5
Influences of Fiber on the Ecology of the Intestinal Flora............................361
Margo N. Woods and Sherwood L. Gorbach

Chapter 6.6
Interaction Between Human Gut Bacteria and Fibrous Substrates 371
Joseph L. Jeraci, Betty A. Lewis, and Peter J. Van Soest

Chapter 6.7
Effects of Dietary Fiber on Digestive Enzymes 377
Barbara O. Schneeman and Daniel Gallaher

Chapter 6.8
Influence of Dietary Fiber on the Production, Absorption, or Excretion of
Short Chain Fatty Acids in Humans...387
Sharon E. Fleming

Chapter 6.9
Effects of Dietary Fiber on Fecal-Luminal Mutagenic Activities 413
Hugh J. Freeman

Section 7. Dietary Fiber in the Prevention and Treatment of Disease

Chapter 7.1
Fiber in the Treatment of Hyperlipidemia 419
**David J. A. Jenkins, Peter J. Spadafora, Alexandra L. Jenkins,
and Cynthia G. Rainey-Macdonald**

Chapter 7.2
Development of the Dietary Fiber Hypothesis of Diabetes Mellitus 439
Hugh C. Trowell

Chapter 7.3
Treatment of Diabetes with High Fiber Diets..443
James W. Anderson and Abayomi O. Akanji

Chapter 7.4
Gallstones 471
Kenneth W. Heaton

Chapter 7.5
Human Epidemiological Studies on Dietary Fiber and Colon Cancer...................477
Hugh J. Freeman

Chapter 7.6
Fiber and Colonic Diverticular Disease...483
Hugh J. Freeman

Chapter 7.7
Fiber and Inflammatory Bowel Disease 487
J. Scott Whittaker and Hugh J. Freeman

Chapter 7.8
Disease Patterns in South Africa as Related to Dietary Fiber..........................491
Alexander R. P. Walker

Chapter 7.9
Disease Patterns in Japan and Changes in Dietary Fiber (1930–1980).................497
Keisuki Tsuji and Bunpei Mori

Chapter 7.10
Modification by Dietary Fiber of Toxic or Carcinogenic Effects 501
Bandaru S. Reddy and Gene A. Spiller

Section 8. Consumption Patterns of Dietary Fiber

Chapter 8.1
Patterns of Dietary Fiber Consumption in Humans 509
Sheila Bingham

Chapter 8.2
The Consumption of Fiber in Vegetarians and Nonvegetarians 525
Beverly M. Calkins

Chapter 8.3
Fiber Consumption in Australian Populations 535
Katrine I. Baghurst, Sally J. Record, and John D. Potter

Chapter 8.4
Consumption of Dietary Fiber-Rich Foods in China....................................543
Zhi-Ping Shen and Su-Fang Zheng

Chapter 8.5
Consumption of Dietary Fiber in France (1850–1981) 547
Yves Le Quintrec

Chapter 8.6
Fiber Consumption in Italy...557
Ottavio Bosello, Fabio Armellini, and Mauro Zamboni

Appendix I: Tables of Dietary Fiber and Associated Substances Content in Foods

Table 1.
Dietary Fiber Values for Common Foods...567
Sally F. Schakel, Yvonne A. Sievert, and I. Marilyn Buzzard

Table 2.
Dry Matter, Ash, Crude Protein, Total Dietary Fiber, Soluble Fiber, Neutral Detergent Residue, Hemicelluloses, Cellulose, and Lignin Content of Selected Foods...595
James B. Robertson

Table 3.
Dietary Fiber Content of Selected Foods by the Southgate Methods....................607
David A. T. Southgate

Table 4.
Dietary Fiber Content of Cereals in Norway 611
Wenche Frølich

Table 5.
Crude Fiber Values of Typical Samples 613
Ivan Furda

Table 6.
Comparison of Analyses of Dietary Fiber and Crude Fiber...........................615
Gene A. Spiller

Table 7.
Phytate Contents of Foods...617
Barbara F. Harland

Table 8.
Plant Foods that Contain Significant Levels of Saponins and Their Estimated Saponin Content..625
David Oakenfull and John D. Potter

Appendix II

Report of the Recommendations on Fiber Classification of the Fiber Supplement Workshop at the XIII International Congress of Nutrition, Brighton, U.K. 627
Gene A. Spiller and David J. A. Jenkins

Appendix III

Beyond Dietary Fiber 633
Gene A. Spiller

Index 639

TABLES

Definitions and Alternative Terms for Dietary Fiber 16

Dietary Fiber Components of Foods 20

Food Components that Behave as Dietary Fiber 22

Food Components Associated with Dietary Fiber 25

Polysaccharide Food Additives Contributing to Dietary Fiber 38

Enzymatic Gravimetric Methods Measuring Both Soluble and Insoluble Fiber 38

Nonstarch Polysaccharides (NSP) in Some Plant Products 56

Digestibility *In Vitro* of Some Carbohydrate-Containing Foods 69

Comparison of Main Steps in Total Dietary Fiber Determination by GLC with the Latest Modifications of the Uppsala Method and the U.K. Method 78

Content of Dietary Fiber (DF) as Determined by the Uppsala Method and Nonstarch Polysaccharides (NSP) as Determined by the U.K. Method and of Resistant Starch (RS) and Klason Lignin (KL) in Some Food Products 79

Distribution of Low Molecular Weight Sugars in 80% Ethanolic Extracts of Carrot 82

Content of DF Polysaccharides and Resistant Starch in Dough and White Bread Fractions 83

Amounts of Neutral Soluble Fiber Polysaccharide Residues not Recovered on Precipitation of Soluble Fiber with 80% Ethanol in Samples Analyzed by the Uppsala Procedure 84

Klason Lignin Values in Heat-Treated Cereals and Potato Samples 90

Content of Ester Substituents in Some High Fiber Products 91

Chemical Characterization of Water-Soluble and Water-Insoluble Dietary Fibers in Various Foods Using Method A 92

Chemical Characterization of Total Dietary Fibers of the Samples in a Collaborative AOAC Study Using Method B 93

Reproducibility of Method C for Dietary Fiber Analysis 94

Content of Different Dietary Fiber Constituents of Sixteen Oats (Whole Grain) with Different Starch Content 95

Effect of Adding Guar Gum (G) Alone, or with Hemicellulose (H) or Pectin (P) on Blood Glucose and Insulin Responses to Single Test Meals 112

Effect of Adding Pectin (P) Alone, or Wheat Bran (B) on Blood Glucose and Insulin Responses to Single Test Meals 113

Effect of Adding Various Gelling Agents on Blood Glucose and Insulin Responses to Single Test Meals 114

Effect of Adding Various Nongelling Fibers on Blood Glucose and Insulin Responses to Single Test Meals 115

Effect of Refining Food (i.e., Removal of Fiber) on Blood Glucose and
Insulin Responses 115

Effect of Dietary Fiber on Fiber-Free Glucose Tolerance Tests 117

Treatment of Diabetes with Guar (G) or Guar plus Wheat Bran (B) 118

Treatment of Diabetes with Miscellaneous Types of Dietary Fiber 120

Glycemic Index Values of Foods Tested in Several Studies 123

Glycemic Index (GI) of Foods Tested Only Once 126

Effect of Fat and Protein on Metabolic Responses to Foods 129

Effect of Grinding on Metabolic Responses 131

Effect of Cooking/Processing on Metabolic Responses 132

Utility of Glycemic Index of Foods in Predicting the Relative Blood Glucose
Responses of Single Mixed Meals 133

Metabolic Effects of High Carbohydrate, Low Fiber Diets 136

Metabolic Effects of Increasing Fiber Intake From Whole Foods with No Change
in Available Carbohydrate 137

Metabolic Effects of High Carbohydrate, High Fiber Diets 138

Long-Term Effects of Low Glycemic Index (GI) Diets 141

Dietary Fiber and Fat Excretion in Humans 154

Effect of Dietary Fiber on Fecal Steroid Excretion in Humans 154

Effect of Fiber Supplements on Fecal Bile Acids and Cholesterol
Absorption in the Rat 155

Binding of Micellar Components by Ion-Exchange Resin and Dietary
Fiber Derivatives 156

Influence of Feeding Fiber Supplements in Defined Diets on the Lymphatic
Absorption of Cholesterol in Fasted Rats 157

Effect of 4-Week Intakes of Fiber Supplements on Cholesterol
Absorption in Fasted Rats 158

Effect of 4-Week Intakes of Fiber Supplements on Oleic Acid
Absorption in Fasted Rats 158

Lipoprotein Distribution of Absorbed Cholesterol and Oleic Acid in the Thoracic
Duct Lymph of Rats Fed Dietary Fiber Supplements 159

Lipid Distribution of Absorbed Oleic Acid in Thoracic Duct Lymph of
Rats Fed Dietary Fiber Supplements 159

Effect of Dietary Fiber on Blood and Liver Cholesterol in Rats 164

Effect of Dietary Fiber on Blood and Liver Cholesterol in Rabbits 168

Effect of Dietary Fiber on Blood and Liver Cholesterol in Chickens 169

Effect of Dietary Fiber on Blood and Liver Cholesterol in Monkeys 169

Effect of Dietary Fiber on Blood and Liver Cholesterol in Pigs 170

Effect of Dietary Fiber on Blood and Liver Cholesterol in Guinea Pigs 170

Bile Acid Adsorption to Dietary Fiber Sources 171

Alteration by Water Holding Capacity of Bile Acid Adsorption by
Sources of Dietary Fiber 171

Adsorption of Cholic and Deoxycholic Acids by Components of Alfalfa
and Wheat Bran 172

Adsorption of Bile Acids by Various Isolated Polysaccharides 173

Steroid Excretion in Experimental Animals in Response to Various
Sources of Dietary Fiber 173

Steroid Excretion in Response to Various Sources of Dietary Fiber 174

Changes in Fecal Bile Acid Spectrum in Rats in Response to Dietary Fiber 174

Modification of Human Fecal Bile Acid Spectrum by Dietary Fiber 175

Effect of Purified Dietary Fibers on Protein Digestibility 180

Effect of Fiber-Rich Sources on Protein Digestibility 186

Effect of Purified Dietary Fibers on Nitrogen Excretion and Balance 190

Effect of Fiber-Rich Sources on Nitrogen Excretion and Balance 195

Effect of Purified Dietary Fibers on Measures of Protein Utilization 197

Effect of Fiber-Rich Sources on Measures of Protein Utilization 202

References to Minerals Studied with Respect to Bioavailability from Cereals 213

Description of Mineral Bioavailability Studies from Cereals 214

Description of Mineral Bioavailability Studies from Cereals
(References after 1984) 224

In Vitro Binding Studies 231

In Vitro Binding Studies (References after 1984) 233

Effect of Addition of Other Foods on Bioavailability of Minerals 235

Average Increase in Fecal Output per Gram Fiber Fed 264

Effect of Wheat Fiber in Various Forms on Fecal Composition 273

Effect of Purified Pectin on Fecal Composition 286

Effect of Cellulose and Cellulose Derivatives on Fecal Composition 291

Effect of Plant Gums, Mucilages, and Other Polysaccharides on
Fecal Composition 296

Effect of Oats and Corn Products on Fecal Composition 301

Effect of Miscellaneous Purified Forms of Fiber on Fecal Composition 305

Effect of Foods Containing Fiber on Fecal Composition 310

Effect of Mixed Sources of Fiber on Fecal Composition 317

Effect of Particle Size on Fecal Composition 320

Effect of Fiber on Fecal Composition in Patients with Diverticular Disease 323

Effect of Cereal Products on Fecal Composition 326

Effect of Legumes on Fecal Composition 331

Effect of Gums and Mucilages and Other Purified Sources on Fecal Composition 333

Effect of Foods and Mixed Diets on Fecal Composition 337

Morphologic Characteristics of Human Intestinal Microflora 362

Fecal Microflora in Different Human Populations 364

Effect of Various Fiber on Fecal Microflora 365

Some of the Predominant Anaerobic Bacterial Species which Have Been Studied in Pure Cultures and Carbohydrates Found in the Human Intestine 372

Concentration of Various Neutral Detergent Fibers Remaining after Being Incubated with Inoculum from Different Human Donors at Various Times in Batch Culture 372

Effect of Inoculum Source on the Fermentation of Neutral Detergent Fibers in Various Substrates 373

Concentration of Batch *In Vitro* Substrates Remaining after Being Incubated with Different Inoculum Sources at Various Times 374

Isolation of Cellulolytic Bacteria from Human Feces from Five Subjects 374

Percent of Control Enzyme Activity *In Vitro* 378

Pancreatic Lipase Inhibition by Cereals, *In Vitro* 379

Decrease in *In Vitro* Casein Digestibility Due to Fiber Addition 379

In Vitro Carbohydrate Hydrolysis of Foods 380

In Vitro Pancreatic Enzyme Activity: Values Expressed as Percentage of Fiber-Free Treated Controls 381

Effect of Fiber Sources on Lipid Digestion and Absorption 382

Small Intestinal Enzyme Activity: Change in Enzyme Activity 383

Reasons for Differences in Enzyme Values 383

Effect of Dietary Fiber on Viscosity of Duodenal Juice (mPa) 383

Influence of the Microflora on Production, Absorption, or Excretion of SCFA 388

Influence of Gender on Production, Absorption, or Excretion of SCFA 390

Influence of the Duration of Feeding on Production, Absorption, or Excretion of SCFA 393

Influence of the Dietary Fiber Concentration on Production, Absorption, or Excretion of SCFA 396

Influence of the Presence or Absence of Fiber on Production, Absorption, or Excretion of SCFA 399

Influence of the Source of Dietary Fiber on SCFA Production 403

Influence of the Source of Dietary Fiber on SCFA Absorption 406

Influence of the Source of Dietary Fiber on Excretion of SCFA in Feces 407

Effect of Lignin and Cellulose on Serum Lipid Concentrations in
Hyperlipidemic Subjects 421

Effect of Soluble, Purified Fibers on Lipid Concentrations in
Hyperlipidemic Subjects 423

Effect of Fiber-Rich Whole Foods and Supplements on Serum Lipids 428

Effect of Legume Protein (± Saponins) on Serum Lipid Concentrations of
Hyperlipidemic Subjects 432

Effect of Dietary Fiber on Glycemic Responses to Single Meals for
Diabetic Subjects 444

Response of Diabetic Subjects to Fiber-Supplemented Diets 449

Response of Diabetic Subjects to High Fiber Diets Developed from
High Fiber Foods 456

Diseases and Metabolic Disturbances Statistically Associated with Gallstones
and Increased Cholesterol Saturation of Bile 472

Case-Control Studies of Dietary Fiber and Gallstones 472

Possible Mechanisms Whereby Bran Reduces the DCA Content of Bile 474

Recent Studies on Fiber in Colon Cancer 479

Variables for Future Fiber Studies 430

Controlled Clinical Trials of Bran in Colonic Diverticular Disease 485

Fiber Intake in Crohn's Disease 488

Fiber Trials in Crohn's Disease 488

Fiber in Ulcerative Colitis 489

Frequencies of Some Diseases of Prosperity in South African Populations 492

Cancer Patterns in South African Populations 492

Frequencies of Noninfective Bowel Disease in South African Populations 492

Dietary Patterns Respecting Fat, Total Carbohydrate, and Fiber Intakes 493

Studies on the Antitoxic Effect of Dietary Fiber or High Fiber Foods and Early
Carcinogenesis Studies in Experimental Animals 502

Studies on the Protective Effect of Dietary Fiber or High Fiber Foods in Chemical
Carcinogenesis Studies 503

Non-Starch Polysaccharide and Fiber Intake 511

Per Capita Dietary Fiber Supply in Europe 1972–1974 513

Dietary Fiber Consumption in Europe: Individual Surveys 514

Sources of Dietary Fiber in 11 Regions of the European
Economic Community 516

Long-Term Trends in Dietary Fiber Consumption in Europe 516

Dietary Fiber Intakes in Africa and India.. 517

Per Capita Dietary Fiber Supply 1972–1974... 518

Dietary Fiber Intakes in Australasia 519

Secular Changes in Major Nutrient Intakes, 1950–1979 in Japan...................... 519

Dietary Fiber Intake in North America 520

Fiber Intake of Vegetarians and Nonvegetarians...................................... 526

Intake of Total Fiber and Fiber Components of Seventh-Day Adventist Vegetarians and Nonvegetarians and the Nonvegetarian General Population............ 530

Mean Daily Fiber and Energy Consumption in Nonrandom Australian Population Samples From 1977–1985 537

Random Surveys of Australian Population Samples from 1983–1990 538

Intakes of Total Dietary Fiber, Insoluble, and Soluble Non-Starch Polysaccharides in the Australian Population 539

Density of Total Dietary Fiber, Insoluble, and Soluble Non-Starch Polysaccharides in the Australian Population by Gender, Age, and Occupation 540

Sources of Dietary Fiber in the Australian Population................................. 541

Consumption Pattern of Fiber-Containing Foods and Crude Fiber Intake in Different Parts of China 544

Contribution of Crude Fiber from Various Foods in North China Peasant Daily Diets... 544

Crude Fiber Contents of Processed Cereal Grains in China........................... 544

Comparison Between Crude Fiber and Neutral Detergent Fiber Contents in Selected Chinese Foods 545

Average Daily Consumption of Dietary Fiber in France Calculated from Dietary Recall 548

Dietary Fiber Content of Bread and Flour from Southgate 548

Total Human Consumption of Cereals in France 549

Average Annual Consumption of Cereal in Flour Equivalent 549

Average Daily Consumption of Wheat and Rice Calculated from Annual Consumption 549

Average Annual At Home Consumption of Cereal Foods 549

Average Annual Consumption of Cereal Foods by Occupation Group................. 550

Total Human Consumption of Fruits and Vegetables 551

Average Annual Consumption of Fruits and Vegetables 551

Average Daily Consumption of Fruits and Vegetables Calculated from Annual Consumption 551

Average Annual At Home Consumption of Fruits and Vegetables..................... 551

Average Consumption of Fruits and Vegetables by Occupation Group 552

Average Daily Fiber Intake 553

Average Daily Fiber Intake by Occupation Groups Calculated from
Southgate's Analyses 554

Changes in Food Consumption from 1954–1978 in Italy 558

Mean Daily Energy, Nutrient, and Dietary Fiber Consumption in an Urban
Northern Italian Population by Sex and Age, in 1989 559

Dietary Fiber Intake from Food in Three Italian Regions, 1963–1965 560

Mean Fiber, Nutrients, and Energy Intake in Italy, 1980–1984 560

Percentage Intake of Fiber, Nutrients, and Energy in Four Geographical Areas,
Compared with the Whole of Italy, 1980–1984 561

Food Preferences in Four Italian Geographical Areas, 1980–1984 562

Mean Fiber, Nutrients, and Energy Intake by Lacto-Ovo-Vegetarians and
Omnivores, Living in a Northern Italian Town, 1989 563

Dietary Fiber Values for Common Foods 567

Dry Matter, Ash, Crude Protein, Total Dietary Fiber, Soluble Fiber,
Neutral Detergent Residue, Hemicelluloses, Cellulose, and Lignin Content of
Selected Foods 595

Dietary Fiber Content of Selected Foods by the Southgate Methods 607

Dietary Fiber Content of Cereals in Norway 611

Crude Fiber Values of Typical Samples 613

Comparison of Analyses of Dietary Fiber and Crude Fiber 615

Phytate Contents of Foods 617

Plant Foods that Contain Significant Levels of Saponins and Their Estimated
Saponin Content 625

Section 1: Dietary Fiber — Overview and Historical Perspectives

Chapter 1.1

DIETARY FIBER: FROM EARLY HUNTER-GATHERERS TO THE 1990s

Denis P. Burkitt and Gene A. Spiller

The decline in plant fiber consumption by humans over tens of thousands of years is shown in Figure 1.[1] According to Kliks, the author of this figure, over the past 20,000 years the human diet has changed from one based on a coarse, plant-based regimen of greens, seeds, stalks, roots, flowers, pollen, and small amounts of animal products, to a more limited, often monotypic diet in which the plant foods are primarily a few cereal grains, tubers, and legumes. Even though the study of specimens of coprolite from lower Pleistoceine humans has proved difficult, this coprolite has been extremely valuable in the study of human diets of civilization dating back about 10,000 years.[1] These specimens of coprolite showed a high consumption of fibrous plant food.

In more recent history, the concept that *coarse foods* of plant origin help to combat constipation goes back to Hippocrates in the 4th century B.C., who commented on the laxative action of outer layers of cereal grains, an observation repeated over 1000 years later (9th century A.D.) by the Persian physician Hakim. Shakespeare referred to the action of cereal bran in his play *Corialanus* in 1610.

In the early 19th century, Graham[2] and Burne[3] in the U.S. and in the late 19th century and at the dawn of the 20th century, Allinson in Britain extolled the virtues of whole grains in improving health by combating constipation.

The history of dietary fiber and health in the first 50 years of the 20th century reveals occasional interest, but very few scientific publications. Fiber was relegated to being the cinderella of nutrients. It may be well to remember that these were the days of major discoveries in vitamins, minerals, and all the other digestible nutrients. Somehow the concept that a group of substances practically undigestible by human GI enzymes could be important to health did not appeal to nutritionists, physiologists, and physicians in those years.

In the 1920s, McCarrison[4] drew attention to the good health of tribesmen in North India, which he attributed to the consumption of whole grains little tampered with by modern technology. In the same decade, John and Harvey Kellogg were extolling the virtues of whole grains in the U.S. The convictions of the latter culminated in the development of the breakfast cereal industry. Cowgill and Anderson in the 1930s published well-controlled research that proved that "fiber" was responsible for the laxative action of wheat bran. At the same time, the British surgeon Albuthnot Lane, whose name is eponymously commemorated in anatomical anomalies and surgical instruments, recognized the "dangers" of stagnant fecal content in the colon. His first reaction was to remove (!) the colon surgically, but fortunately he subsequently appreciated that the administration of bran was altogether simpler, safer, and equally effective. In the late 1930s, Dimmock, a young British physician, reported his careful studies on the effectiveness of wheat bran in treating constipation and, in the last 1940s, Walker of South Africa was one of the first to appreciate the properties of plant fibers and to study it in a truly scientific manner.

In the years that followed, some epidemiological correlations by Cleave in Britain (1956 to 1966) and Trowell in Africa, with his 1960 book, *Non-Infectious Diseases in Africa*,[5] attributed protective effects to unrefined carbohydrates and "bulky" foods.

This, we could say, is the early history of fiber. What followed from the late 1960s to the publication of this Handbook is covered in detail by McPherson in Chapter 1.2, entitled

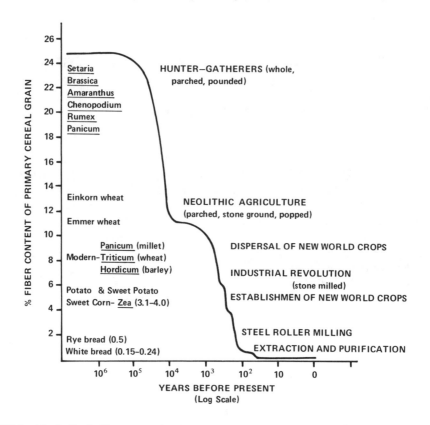

FIGURE 1. The decline in fiber consumption by humans. (From Kliks, M., *Topics in Dietary Fiber Research*, Spiller, G. A. and Amen, R. J. Eds., Plenum Press, New York, 1978, 182. With permission.)

"Dietary Fiber - A Perspective". These are the years of rapid development in dietary fiber research, years that have made dietary fiber the important nutritional entity that it is today. The reader is referred to her presentation for an overview of research in the various aspects of dietary fiber and health.

Other events took place in the 1970s and 1980s: the publication of a series of multiauthor books contributed to the clarification of the role of dietary fiber. As books are key steps in the growth of any field of science and as they become an intrinsic part of the history of science, it is worthwhile to recall some of their titles.

Some of the pioneering books appeared in 1975 to 1976: Burkitt and Trowell published *Refined Carbohydrate Foods and Disease*,[6] Reilly and Kirsner published *Fiber Deficiency and Colonic Disorders*,[7] and Spiller and Amen published *Fiber in Human Nutrition*.[8] They were followed in 1977 by Spiller and Amen, *Topics in Dietary Fiber Research*,[9] in 1978 by Heaton, *Dietary Fiber: Current Developments of Importance to Health*,[10] and in 1979 by Inglett And Falkenag, *Dietary Fibers: Chemistry and Nutrition*.[11] In the 1980s, as dietary fiber had become well established as a topic worthy of extensive research in human nutrition, more books on specific topics began to appear: Spiller and McPherson-Kay published *Medical Aspects of Dietary Fiber*,[12] the Royal College of Physicians wrote *Medical Aspects of Dietary Fiber*,[13] James and Theander wrote *The Analysis of Dietary Fiber in Food*,[14] and Vahouny and Kritchevsky wrote *Dietary Fiber in Health and Disease*,[15] and Trowell and Burkitt wrote *Western Diseases: Their Emergence and Prevention*.[16]

Many more books followed in the late 1980s and early 1990s, too many to list here. The pioneering days were over and *dietary fiber* had become an established, important factor in human nutrition and medicine.

It is interesting to realize that only 4 or 5 years before the publication of the first edition of this Handbook in 1986 it would have been quite difficult to find sufficient scientific and medical data to publish a Handbook such as this. This Handbook is proof of how rapidly the field of dietary fiber research is growing. Fast growth is exciting, but we should also take time to set up proper experiments and to review the literature carefully. In spite of all this growth, there are still conflicting views as to how dietary fiber should be defined (see Chapter 2.1) and there is less than precise use of terms in some publications. The complexity of dietary fiber and its tremendous interactions with other food components make its study a most difficult one indeed!

Since 1978 many major meetings that focused on various aspects of dietary fiber have taken place, meetings that have led to important debates on definition, functions, and health effects of dietary fiber. International congresses of nutrition in Brazil (1978), San Diego (1981), Brighton (U.K., 1985), and others began to include dietary fiber as an integral part of their programs. The National Institutes of Health sponsored a major international meeting in Washington (1977) that appears to us now as a milestone in the history of dietary fiber. The proceedings were published in a special supplement of the *American Journal of Clinical Nutrition*[17] in 1978. In 1981 and 1984 two major symposia were also held in Washington at George Washington University. The Royal Society of New Zealand held a major symposium[18] in Palmerston North in 1982 which was reported in their Bulletin 20. Many other meetings have taken place in recent years, including several in analytical and chemical aspects of dietary fiber.

Notwithstanding all this progress and widespread interest by scientists, physicians, and health professionals on every continent, there are still many controversial aspects that will become evident to the reader of this Handbook, not least the definition of *dietary fiber* and even the term *fiber,* itself.

Since the first edition of this Handbook, the field of fiber research has also suffered the loss of two great pioneers in dietary fiber work. Hugh Trowell passed away in England in 1989, at the age of 85, after a life-long dedication to medicine. During the last 20 years of his life, dietary fiber was the most important topic in his work, work he carred on to his very last days. And George Vahouny, who had developed many animal models for fiber research and who was an author in the first edition of this Handbook, passed away in Washington, D.C.

It is hoped that this review, combined with the "Perspectives" by Ruth McPherson that follow, will be a useful introduction to this Handbook.

REFERENCES

1. **Kliks, M.,** Paleodietetics: a review of the role of dietary fiber in preagricultural human diets, in *Topics in Dietary Fiber Research,* Spiller, G. A. and Amen, R. J., Eds., Plenum Press, New York, 1978, 181.
2. **Graham, S.,** *Lectures on the Science of Human Life,* Capen, Lyon and Webb, Boston, 1829.
3. **Burne, J.,** *Treatise on the Causes and Consequences of Constipation,* Haswell, Barrington and Haswell, New Orleans, LA, 1840.
4. **McCarrison, R.,** *Studies in Deficiency Disease,* Frowde, Hodder and Stoughton, London, 1921.
5. **Trowell, H.,** *Non-Infectious Diseases in Africa,* Edward Arnold, London, 1960.
6. **Brukitt, D. P. and Trowell, H. C.,** *Refined Carbohydrate Foods and Disease,* Academic Press, New York, 1975.

7. **Reilly, W. R. and Kirsner, J. B.**, *Fiber Deficiency and Colonic Disorders*, Plenum Press, New York, 1975.
8. **Spiller, G. A. and Amen, R. J.**, *Fiber in Human Nutrition*, Plenum Press, New York, 1976.
9. **Spiller, G. A. and Amen, R. J.**, *Topics in Dietary Fiber Research*, Plenum Press, New York, 1978.
10. **Heaton, K. W.**, *Dietary Fiber: Current Developments of Importance to Health*, John Libbey, London, 1978.
11. **Inglett, G. E. and Falkehag, S. I.**, *Dietary Fibers: Chemistry and Nutrition*, Academic Press, New York, 1979.
12. **Spiller, G. A. and McPherson-Kay, R.**, *Medical Aspects of Dietary Fiber*, Plenum Press, New York, 1980.
13. Royal College of Physicians, *Medical Aspects of Dietary Fiber*, Pitman Medical, Tunbridge Wells, Kent, 1980.
14. **James, W. P. T. and Theander, O.**, *The Analysis of Dietary Fiber in Food*, Marcel Dekker, New York, 1981.
15. **Vahouny, G. V. and Kritchevsky, D.**, *Dietary Fiber in Health and Disease*, Plenum Press, New York, 1982.
16. **Trowell, H. C. and Burkitt, D. P.**, *Western Diseases: Their Emergence and Prevention*, Harvard University Press, Cambridge, MA, 1981.
17. **Roth, H. P. and Mehlman, M. A., Eds.**, Proceedings: symposium on the role of dietary fiber, *Am. J. Clin. Nutr.*, 31S, 1978.
18. **Wallace, G. and Bell, L., Eds.**, Proceedings: fiber in human and animal nutrition, *R. Soc. N.Z. Bull.*, 1983.

Chapter 1.2

DIETARY FIBER — A PERSPECTIVE

Ruth McPherson

Dietary fiber consists of a complex group of materials of diverse chemical and morphological structure, resistant to the action of human digestive enzymes. The physiological effects of fiber are relevant not only to gastrointestinal function and pathology, but also to lipid and glucose metabolism and trace mineral homeostasis.

Prior to 1965, there was relatively little interest in the role of dietary fiber in human nutrition. Serious proponents of the benefits of fiber, such as Graham in the U.S. (1840) and Allinson in Britain (1905), were often dismissed as cranks. Their claims, at times extravagant, were not put to serious test. In the 1930s, there was a brief period of research on the gastrointestinal role of fiber. Careful studies on the effects of dietary fiber on bowel function were carried out by Cowgill and Anderson and later by Dimmock, but their findings were generally ignored by the medical community. This is perhaps surprising in view of the steady increase in the incidence of constipation and diverticular disease that paralleled the decline in cereal fiber intake with the introduction of roller milling in the 1870s.

The recent surge in dietary fiber research began in the late 1960s and was sparked mainly by epidemiological observations. As a result of their African experience, Burkitt, Trowell, and Walker succeeded in bringing fiber to the forefront by pointing out the great disparity between Europeans and rural Africans in the age-specific incidence of a number of degenerative diseases. They attributed this, in part, to the vast differences between the two populations in dietary fiber consumption. Thus, the "fiber hypothesis" was conceived, launching a period of intense laboratory and clinical research that has continued until today.

The effects of fiber on gastrointestinal physiology were studied intensively by Eastwood, Painter, and later Cummings and Heaton. A need for better quantitative information led to a new emphasis on dietary fiber chemistry and analysis with major contributions from Southgate, Van Soest, and Theander. The question of the relevance of dietary fiber to cholesterol metabolism was addressed by Kritchevsky, Story, Sirtori, Kay, Miettinen, and Spiller, while Jenkins and Anderson launched an important series of studies on fiber and glycemic control. More recently, Cummings, Vahouny, and others have explored the relationship between dietary fiber intake and colonic neoplasia.

CURRENT STATUS OF DIETARY FIBER RESEARCH

Constipation

It is likely that were it not for its desirable effects on stool bulk and motility, dietary fiber might still rest in obscurity. The effect of fiber on stool bulk was initially related to the hydration capacity of the surviving residue and production of osmotically active metabolites. More recently, attention has focused on the effect of fiber on the induction of bacterial growth, since bacterial cells are normally 80% water and represent an important fraction of total stool volume. It is likely that the mechanism by which stool bulk and laxation is promoted will vary for different fibers. Stephen and Cummings demonstrated that 48% of the increase in stool bulk and water content in subjects fed wheat fiber could be accounted for by the water-holding capacity of the hydrated fiber.[1]

Only 36% of the wheat fiber fed was bacterially degraded. By contrast, when an almost completely digestible (92%) fiber (cabbage) was fed, stool bulk and water content also increased, but much of this increase (35%) was due to enhanced bacterial output.[2] Similarly, the reported relationship of fecal weight to intake of pentose-containing polysaccharides may be mediated by their tendency to increase bacterial growth and output.

Although large amounts of fermentable fibers enhance fecal bulk and water content, they are somewhat less effective than less fermentable types. Stasse-Wolthuis and colleagues[3] demonstrated in a carefully controlled study that the mean increase in stool weight was 4.1 g/g of added fiber for coarse wheat brain (fermentation resistant) as compared to 1.9 g/g of added fiber when fruit and vegetables (highly fermentable) were used as a fiber source. The influence of various unprocessed wheat brans on fecal weight is partially dependent on particle size,[4] which affects the water-holding capacity of the fiber matrix. Cooked wheat bran has a reduced stool-bulking capacity — probably due to structural alterations which allow greater bacterial degradation.

Diverticular Disease

Painter and Burkitt[5] proposed that a diet which provides little colonic residue results in a small hard stool that requires vigorous segmentation for propulsion along the colon, eventually culminating in circular muscle hypertrophy, high colonic pressures, and production of diverticula. In contrast, populations ingesting much fiber have bulky stools and low colonic pressure and the disease incidence is low.

Clinical studies have demonstrated that abnormally high intraluminal pressures occur within the sigmoid in diverticular disease, particularly in response to cholinergic stimuli. Cineradiographic techniques showed that this was due to segmental occlusion of the bowel as the circular muscle contracted. However, circular muscle hypertrophy is not a consistent accompaniment of diverticular disease, and many asymptomatic patients do not have abnormally increased intraluminal pressures, suggesting that the pathogenesis of the disease may be more complex.

Available information does indicate that the incidence of diverticular disease is low in populations ingesting much fiber, and emergence of the disease has been attributed to the acquisition of a Western life-style. The presence of symptom-less diverticular disease has been related to the consumption of dietary fiber in vegetarians and nonvegetarians.[6]

Despite incomplete information on the etiology of the disease, the work of many investigators has resulted in a dramatic revision in the medical treatment of diverticular disease in the last decade. Although the concept has been challenged,[7] there is now general clinical consensus that a high fiber diet is the treatment of choice in simple uncomplicated diverticular disease. Whereas large amounts of fruit and vegetables may elicit an undesirable increase in gas production, coarse wheat bran usually results in a gradual amelioration of disease symptoms provided sufficient amounts are given.

Colonic Cancer

Fiber consumption is only one of several dietary variables tentatively implicated in the etiology of large bowel cancer. Certain epidemiological and clinical studies are suggestive of a protective effect, but other data are complex and contradictory. It has been postulated that fiber may act as a protective factor in cancer of the large bowel by shortening transit time, thus reducing the time for the formation and action of carcinogens. In addition, through its stool-bulking effect, fiber may lower the concentration of fecal carcinogens and thereby reduce the amount of carcinogen that comes in contact with the gut wall. Other changes may occur in the physical and chemical environment of the colon, the bacterial flora, or in the interaction between bacteria and potential carcinogens. Most types of fiber do increase stool bulk and dilute the concentration of specific substances in the colon, and the concentration of bacterially modified bile acids in the colon has been implicated in tumor formation.

Animal studies have indicated that stool-bulking fibers are protective against chemical carcinogenesis, although the applicability of this animal model to human colon cancer is not established.

Epidemiological studies have attempted to relate colon cancer to nutritional variables. Consumption of dietary fiber was found to differ in two communities in Denmark and Finland with a fourfold variation in colon cancer; however, the diets also differed in other respects.[8] Bingham et al.[9] reported a significant negative correlation between intake of pentose-containing dietary fiber and colon cancer normality in England.

In summary, there is preliminary evidence that stool bulk-promoting fibers may modify the action of colonic carcinogens or promoters. Other environmental and genetic factors are undoubtedly operative.

Glucose Absorption and Metabolism

Certain types of dietary fiber have a modulating effect on the glucose absorption rate and attendant hormonal responses.

Jenkins and co-workers[10] have suggested that soluble mucilaginous fibers such as guar have the most potent effects on glucose metabolism. Although effective, these substances are of limited palatability. Hence, efforts have been made to treat diabetics with diets containing a predominance of fiber-rich foods. The concept of a "glycemic index" to differentiate between the effect of various carbohydrate-containing food has been well developed by Jenkins and co-workers.[11,12] Improvements in diabetic control and reduction in insulin and sulfonylurea requirements have been reported in both mild and moderate diabetics on high fiber diets containing a normal or high proportion of carbohydrate. In certain studies, reversal of lipid abnormalities also occurred. Further controlled trials are required, but certain fiber-rich foods are a useful adjunct in diabetic therapy.[13]

Hyperlipidemia

Certain types of dietary fiber have been reported to significantly lower plasma cholesterol concentrations. Most effective are the mucilaginous fibers such as guar and oat bran[14,15] as well as various mixtures of fruit and vegetables.[16] In contrast, particulate nonsoluble fibers such as wheat bran are without effect on plasma lipids.[17]

There is a widespread conviction that the effect of dietary fiber on plasma cholesterol concentration may be largely mediated by enhanced fecal excretion of bile acids. Many types of dietary fiber shown to be hypocholesterolemic in man do increase fecal bile acid output. Miettinen and Tarpila[18] reported at least partial compensation of enhanced sterol loss in subjects fed pectin since cholesterol synthesis as assessed by serum concentrations of methyl sterols increased. However, increased fecal bile acid output due to fiber is not always accompanied by a reduction in plasma cholesterol. Recently we have shown that the addition of a mixture of fiber-rich foods to a fat modified diet further reduces plasma total and LDL cholesterol levels by up to 20 mg/dl without altering bile acid output.[19] Hence, the mechanism by which fiber exerts its hypocholesterolemic effect remains an intriguing question.

Many types of dietary fiber modulate glucose absorption, resulting in a reduction in postprandial levels of glucose and insulin. Albrink et al.[20] demonstrated that a reduction in plasma triglycerides and cholesterol in subjects ingesting high fiber diets was associated with a markedly lower insulin response to a representative high fiber meal than a low fiber meal.

Insulin has been reported to increase cholesterol synthesis and hepatic synthesis and secretion of very low density lipoprotein. Inclusion of dietary fiber in a high carbohydrate diet markedly reduces carbohydrate-associated lipemia. Mucilaginous fibers appear to have the greatest effect on plasma total cholesterol concentrations and are of similar importance in their effects on glucose metabolism, suggesting that fiber-induced changes in the ambient insulin concentration may influence lipid metabolism.

SUMMARY

Fiber has certain established therapeutic and homeostatic functions in human nutrition, but gaps remain in our understanding of the relative importance of fiber both in the etiology and treatment of many diseases. Progress is impeded in part by the nature of the material under study. Dietary fiber consists of a diverse group of substances of chemical and morphological complexity. The effects of a particular fiber are likely to depend on its association with other polysaccharides and lignin within the plant wall and on the nutrient composition of the diet of which it is part. Thus, standardization of experimental protocols and interpretation of both clinical and epidemiological findings are indeed difficult.

These problems will continue to evade simple solutions. We have developed the concept that dietary fiber is a polymer matrix with definable physicochemical properties.[21] Determination of the physical and chemical characteristics of fiber and the evolution of these properties during passage along the GI tract are likely to be fundamental to the prediction of the role of various types of dietary fiber in human physiology. There is also a need for more complete and accurate epidemiological information on dietary fiber intake in different populations. Improved analytical methods are now making the collection of such data feasible. Further clinical and metabolic studies remain to be carried out with particular relevance to the mechanism of action of dietary fiber on metabolism, glycemic control, inflammatory bowel disease, and colon carcinogenesis.

REFERENCES

1. **Stephen, A. M. and Cummings, J. H.,** Mechanism of action of dietary fibre in the human colon, *Nature,* 284, 283, 1980.
2. **Cummings, J. H., Southgate, D. A. T., Branch, W., Houston, H., Jenkins, D. J., and James, W. P.,** Colonic response to dietary fiber from carrot, cabbage, apple, bran and guar gum, *Lancet,* 1, 5, 1978.
3. **Stasse-Wolthuis, J. G., Ablers, H. F., Van Jeveson, G., De Jong, J., Hautvast, M. D., Katan, M., Brydon, W. G., and Eastwood, M. A.,** Influence of dietary fibers from vegetables and fruits, bran or citrus pectin on serum lipids, fecal lipids and colonic function, *J. Clin. Nutr.,* 33, 1734, 1980.
4. **Heller, S. M., Hackler, S. R., Rivers, J. M., Van Soest, P. J., Roe, D. A., Lewis, B. A., and Robertson, J.,** Dietary fiber: the effect of particle size of wheat bran on colonic function in young adult men, *J. Clin. Nutr.,* 33, 1734, 1980.
5. **Painter, N. S. and Burkitt, D. P.,** Diverticular disease of the colon: a deficiency disease of Western civilization, *Br. Med. J.,* 2, 450, 1971.
6. **Gear, J. S., Ware, A., Fursdon, P., Mann, J. I., Nolan, D. J., Brodribb, A. J., and Vessey, M. P.,** Symptomless diverticular disease and intake of dietary fiber, *Lancet,* 1, 511, 1979.
7. **Ornstein, M. H., Littlewood, A. R., and McLean-Baird, I.,** Are fibre supplements really necessary in diverticular disease? *Br. Med. J.,* 282, 1353, 1981.
8. IARC, Intestinal microecology group. Dietary fiber, transit time, fecal bacteria, steroids and colon cancer in two Scandinavian populations, *Lancet,* 2, 207, 1977.
9. **Bingham, S., Williams, D. R., Cole, T. J., and James, W. P.,** Dietary fibre and regional large bowel cancer mortality in Britain, *Br. J. Cancer,* 40, 456, 1979.

10. **Jenkins, D. J., Wolever, T. M., Leeds, A. R., Gassull, M. A., Haisman, P., Dilawari, J., Goff, D. V., Metz, J. L., and Alberti, K. G.,** Dietary fibers, fiber analogus and glucose tolerance: importance of viscosity, *Br. Med. J.,* 1, 1392, 1978.
11. **Jenkins, D. J. A., Wolever, T. M. S., Jenkins, A. L., Josse, R. G., and Wong, G. S.,** The glycemic response to carbohydrate foods, *Lancet,* 2, 388, 1984.
12. **Jenkins, D. J. A., Wolever, T. M. S., and Kalmusky, J.,** Low glycemic index diet in hyperlipidemia: use of traditional starchy foods, *Am. J. Clin. Nutr.,* 46, 66, 1987.
13. **Anderson, J. W. and Bryant, C. A.,** Dietary fiber, diabetes and obesity, *Am. J. Gastroenterol.,* 81, 898, 1986.
14. **Spiller, G. A., Farquhar, J. W., Gates, J. E., and Nichols, S. F.,** Guar gum and plasma cholesterol: effect of guar gum and an oat fiber source on plasma lipoproteins and cholesterol in hypercholesterolemic adults, *Arteriosclerosis,* 11, 1201, 1991.
15. **Anderson, J. W. and Gustafson, N. J.,** Hypocholesterolemic effects of oat and bran products, *Am. J. Clin. Nutr.,* 48, 749, 1988.
16. **Lewis, B., Hammett, F., Katan, M., McPherson Kay, R., Merkx, I., Nobels, A., Miller, N., and Swan, A. V.,** Towards an improved lipid lowering diet: additive effects of changes in nutrient intake, *Lancet,* 2, 1310, 1981.
17. **McPherson Kay, R.,** Dietary fiber, *J. Lipid. Res.,* 23, 221, 1982.
18. **Miettinen, T. A. and Tarpila, S.,** Effects of pectin on serum cholesterol, fecal bile acids and biliary lipids in normolipidemic and hyperlipidemic individuals, *Clin. Chim. Acta,* 79, 471, 1977.
19. **McPherson Kay, R., Jacobs, M., Lewis, B., Miller, N., and Katan, M. B.,** Relationship between changes in plasma lipoprotein concentrations and fecal steroid excretion in man during consumption of four experimental diets, *Atherosclerosis,* 55, 15, 1985.
20. **Albrink, M. J., Newman, T., and Davidson, P. C.,** Effects of high and low fiber diets on plasma lipids and insulin, *Am. J. Clin. Nutr.,* 32, 1486, 1979.

Section 2: Definitions and Physicochemical Properties of Dietary Fiber

Chapter 2.1

DEFINITION OF DIETARY FIBER

Gene A. Spiller

CRUDE FIBER AND DIETARY FIBER

Crude fiber is an old term based on a method of analysis that has been criticized by many investigators such as Van Soest and Southgate, because it is based on the harsh extraction of plant material with acid and then alkali (see Chapter 3.5). The method dates back to the first part of the 19th century and there is a consensus that it is defective, using chemical, botanical, or nutritional criteria, and that it should be discontinued.[1] It recovers variable amounts of components of dietary fiber: 50 to 80% of the cellulose, 10 to 50% of the lignin, and only a small fraction of the hemicelluloses. It is, however, at the time of this writing still the legal term used for food labeling in some countries. McCance and Lawrence in the 1920s were instrumental in developing the concept of unavailable carbohydrate; that was a stepping stone to the modern concept of dietary fiber. Hipsley[2] defined dietary fiber in 1953 and later this definition was expanded by other investigators, including Southgate. Trowell[3] in 1974 published a definition of dietary fiber that is based on the *physiological* characteristics of some of the plant cells which are *resistant to hydrolysis by the digestive enzymes of humans*.

NEED FOR AND LIMITATIONS OF ALL-ENCOMPASSING DEFINITIONS

A group of substances that share certain chemical or biological properties have traditionally been gathered under all-encompassing terms in nutrition. While this is useful, we should **never** forget that the substances covered by the general definition may differ considerably from each other in their specific physiological effects; for instance, no one would doubt that it is useful to call a certain group of compounds *vitamins,* but it is also clear that the effects of vitamin A are quite different from those of folic acid. While we need an all-encompassing term for the undigestible portion of plant foods, we must guard ourselves against the temptation of generalizing about the effects of individual purified compounds. Thus, while we must agree on a reasonable all-encompassing term such as dietary fiber or plantix and its definition, we must be sure to use names of specific compounds or types of fiber when the research has been carried out with these specific substances.

IS FIBER A FIBER?

The term *fiber* itself is an unfortunate term since fiber reminds us of long fibrils, which is in agreement with the physical characteristics of some components of dietary fiber, mainly cellulose, but not of others. The term *Plantix* has been suggested as an alternative to dietary fiber (Table 1). Plantix implies that the source is a plant and that matrix formation is one of its characteristics. The matrix referred to is in the plant or in the GI tract of humans. This term, used only sporadically since its introduction in 1977, is now the subject of renewed interest.

TABLE 1
Definitions and Alternative Terms for Dietary Fiber[a]

Term recommended and author	Definition
Dietary fiber (DF) (Trowell)	Plant substances not digested by human digestive enzymes, including plant cell wall substances (cellulose, hemicelluloses, pectin, and lignin) as well as intracellular polysaccharides such as gums and mucilages. Largely identical to undigested (unavailable) carbohydrates plus lignin. The early definition by Trowell of "the remnants of plant cells resistant to hydrolysis by the alimentary enzymes of man" remains as a key definition, even though it may better apply to the dietary fiber complex defined later in this table. A key contribution by Trowell was to emphasize the distinction between dietary fiber and crude fiber.
Dietary fiber complex (Trowell, Spiller)	Same as dietary fiber but defined to include other plant substances that are undigested by human digestive enzymes, such as waxes, cutins, and undigestible cell wall proteins. These are the substances that are normally associated with and concentrated around the plant cell wall.
Dietary fiber (Southgate)	The sum of lignin and the polysaccharides that are not hydrolyzed by the endogenous secretions of the human digestive tract. Southgate considers this as a physiological and philosophical definition, and feels that it is necessary to produce a definition that can be translated into purely analytical terms. This author suggests a chemical definition based on the fact that the sum of lignin and the non-α glucan polysaccharides (nonstarch polysaccharides) are the best index of dietary fiber in the diet.
Dietary fiber (Furda)	Chemical definition: the sum of the plant nonstarch polysaccharides and lignin. Physiological definition: the remnant of plant foods resistant to hydrolysis by the alimentary enzymes of humans.
Plantix (Spiller)	A term designed to represent dietary fiber as defined by Trowell, but that avoids the word fiber, since many of the substances defined may not be strictly speaking of a fibrous nature. In fact, cellulose is the only truly fibrous component of the plant cell wall. It also implies that the material is present in plants only. It includes the plant polysaccharides and lignin that are not digested by human digestive enzymes.
Plantix complex (Spiller)	Suggested to replace dietary fiber complex, again to avoid the word fiber. It includes undigestible parts of the plant cell that are not included in plantix, such as waxes, undigestible proteins, and others.
Purified plant fiber (Spiller)	Any highly purified single polymer derived from plants that is not digested by human digestive enzymes but that may be digested by microorganisms in the human intestinal tract. Examples are purified pectin and purified cellulose. This is a modification of an earlier definition that included more than one substance.
Unavailable carbohydrate (McCance and Lawrence)	A classical term used in nutrition for many years to distinguish between available and nonavailable carbohydrate in humans. As originally defined it included lignin, which is not a carbohydrate. Furthermore, the fact that some of these carbohydrates are digested by bacteria in the human intestine and produce fatty acids that are actually "available" makes the term "unavailable" ambiguous.
Edible fiber (EF) (Trowell, Godding)	An expanded definition of dietary fiber as given above; other groups of undigested (human enzyme-undigested) polysaccharides and related substances are added: (1) animal fibers not digested by human digestive enzymes, e.g., aminopolysaccharides; (2) synthetic or partially synthetic polysaccharides not digested by human digestive enzymes, e.g., methylcelluloses; (3) polysaccharides that are not part of traditional foods and that are not digested by human digestive enzymes. These products may be of pharmaceutical importance.
Neutral detergent residue (NDR) (Van Soest)	A residue after special digestion (see Section 3) with detergents, essentially the sum of cellulose, hemicellulose, and lignin. Often called neutral detergent fiber (NDF).

TABLE 1 (continued)
Definitions and Alternative Terms for Dietary Fiber[a]

Term recommended and author	Definition
Crude fiber	The remnants of plant material after extraction with acid and alkali. The term should not be used with reference to dietary fiber, but many publications and food tables still use this expression (see Chapter 3.5). Crude fiber values include only variable portions of the cellulose, hemicelluloses, and lignin present in dietary fiber.
Nonstarch polysaccharides (NSP) (Englyst)	The carbohydrate plant cell wall material originally called *dietary fiber* less the lignin, analyzed in such a way to eliminate any other plant substance that may appear as fiber in other analytical methods. Methods to determine NSP must be such that any *resistant starch* (see below) is not taken into account.
Resistant starch (RS) (Englyst)	Starch that is not digested by human digestive enzymes and that reaches the colon, often acting in the same way as *fiber*.

[a] These definitions were either supplied directly by these authors for this Handbook or were prepared from the reference list.

CURRENT ALL-ENCOMPASSING DEFINITIONS

Table 1 lists the terms and definitions recommended by various proponents of meaningful terminology in this field. Each definition or term may be recommended by more than one key investigator. These definitions have been prepared from personal communications especially for this Handbook. The definitions given may originate from a *physiological, chemical,* or *botanical* point of view, or a combination of these three.

Some of the terms and definitions of dietary fiber listed have been expanded to include nondigestible proteins, waxes, and other plant compounds (*dietary fiber complex* or *plantix complex*). In Section 3, methods are given to determine dietary fiber as a whole, e.g., the new AOAC method described by Asp (Chapter 3.1) as well as methods for the determination of specific components, e.g., Theander (Chapter 3.5). Methods for specific groups of polymers, groups that some authors such as Asp, Furda, and others have called "water-insoluble fiber" and "water-soluble fiber", are also given. Other terms used to define groups of polymers include the widely used "neutral and acid detergent residue" which is defined by the Van Soest method of determination. The reader is referred to Section 3 for details.

No matter which definition we choose, we must remember that we are dealing with a complex of substances which are often very sensitive to processing such as cooking, type of milling, and fermentation. The methods used in preparation of the food must be stated by dietary fiber investigators and writers and should be carefully considered in the planning of animal or human studies.

REFERENCES

1. **Van Soest, P. J. and Robertson, J. B.,** What is fiber and fiber in food?, *Nutr. Rev.,* 35, 14, 1977.
2. **Hipsley, E. H.,** Dietary fiber and pregnancy toxemia, *Br. Med. Jr.,* 2, 420, 1953.
3. **Trowell, H.,** Definition of fiber, *Lancet,* 1, 503, 1974.
4. **Trowell, H.,** Dietary fiber and coronary heart disease, *Rev. Eur. D'Etud. Clin. Biol.,* 17, 343, 1972.
5. **Trowell, H.,** Crude fiber, dietary fiber and atherosclerosis, *Atherosclerosis,* 16, 138, 1972.
6. **Trowell, H.,** Ischemic heart disease and dietary fiber, *Am. J. Clin. Nutr.,* 25, 926, 1972.

7. **Trowell, H. C.,** Refined carbohydrate foods and fiber, in *Refined Carbohydrate Foods and Disease: Some Implications of Dietary Fiber,* Burkitt, D. P., and Trowell, H. C., Eds., Academic Press, New York, 1975, chap. 3.
8. **Trowell, H., Southgate, D. A. T., Wolever, T. M. S., Leeds, A. R., Gassull, M. A., and Jenkins, D. J. A.,** Dietary fiber redefined, *Lancet,* 1, 967, 1976.
9. **Trowell, H.,** Definition of dietary fiber and hypotheses that it is a protective factor in certain diseases, *Am. J. Clin. Nutr.,* 29, 417, 1976.
10. **Trowell, H.,** The development of the concept of dietary fiber in human nutrition, *Am. J. Clin. Nutr.,* 31, S3, 1978.
11. **Trowell, H., Godding, E., Spiller, G., and Briggs, G.,** Fiber bibliographies and terminologies, *Am. J. Clin. Nutr.,* 31, 1489, 1978.
12. **Spiller, G. A. and Amen, R. J.,** Plant fibers in nutrition: need for better nomenclature, *Am. J. Clin. Nutr.,* 28, 675, 1975.
13. **Spiller, G. A. and Amen, R. J.,** Dietary fiber in human nutrition, *CRC Crit. Rev. Food Sci. Nutr.,* 7, 39, 1975.
14. **Spiller, G. A., Fassett-Corneliums, G., and Briggs, G. M.,** A new term for plant fibers in nutrition, *Am. J. Clin. Nutr.,* 29, 934, 1976.
15. **Spiller, G. A.,** Fiber in the vocabulary of nutrition, *Lancet,* 1, 198, 1977.
16. **Spiller, G. A., Shipley, E. A., and Blake, J. A.,** Recent progress in dietary fiber (plantix) in human nutrition, *CRC Crit. Rev. Food Sci. Nutr.,* 10, 31, 1978.
17. **Southgate, D. A. T.,** The definition and analysis of dietary fiber, *Nutr. Rev.,* 35, 31, 1977.
18. **Heaton, K. W.,** Fiber: new terminology or new concepts?, *Am. J. Clin. Nutr.,* 32, 2373, 1979.
19. **Trowell, H.,** Food and dietary fiber, *Nutr. Rev.,* 35, 6, 1977.
20. **Englyst, H. N. and Hudson, G. J.,** Dietary fiber and starch. In *Handbook of Dietary Fiber in Human Nutrition,* Spiller, G. A., Ed., CRC Press, Boca Raton, FL, 1992, chap. 3.3.

Chapter 2.2

DIETARY FIBER PARTS OF FOOD PLANTS AND ALGAE

David A. T. Southgate

The major portion of dietary fiber in foods is derived from plant cell walls in foods.[1] A wide range of plant organs and types of tissue is consumed in the diet although highly lignified (woody) tissues are often rejected.[2,3] The organization and detailed composition of the plant cell wall varies with the type of tissue, but the essential features are common to virtually all walls. This is a network of cellulose fibrils in a matrix of noncellulosic polysaccharide.[4]

The composition of the matrix varies with the maturity of the plant tissue and is often characteristic of the plant species or group.[3] The matrix polysaccharides include water-soluble polysaccharides which were designated pectic substances in classical cell wall fractionation schemes.[5] In addition to galacturonans corresponding to the *pectins*, the fraction includes arabinogalactans, β-glucans, and arabinoxylans. The water-insoluble but alkali-soluble fraction, the *hemicellulose* fraction, includes a range of xylans, with arabinosyl and 4-*O*-methylglucuronyl substituents, galacto- and glucomannans, and xyloglucans. It is known that the fractions obtained in the classical schemes are arbitrary and that artifacts are produced; Albersheim[5] proposed that the term *noncellulosic polysaccharides* (NCP) should be used.

The alkali-insoluble fraction includes cellulose per se and lignin where present. The noncarbohydrate lignin is covalently linked to the polysaccharides in the wall and by convention is included in dietary fiber (see Trowell et al.[6]).

Plant foods contain a range of water-soluble gums and mucilages. These have analogous structures to many cell wall components and are included in the noncellulosic polysaccharides and the nonstarch polysaccharides (NSP) of Englyst et al.[7]

TABLE 1
Dietary Fiber Components of Foods

Classical nomenclature	Solubility characteristics	Classes of polysaccharide	Nomenclature used in dietary fiber literature
Plant Cell Wall Components			
Pectic substances	Water soluble[a]	Galacturonans Arabinogalactans β-glucans Arabinoxylans	Noncellulosic polysaccharides (NCP)[2,6] Nonstarch polysaccharides (NSP)[7] Dietary fiber[4]
Hemicelluloses	Insoluble in water Soluble in alkali	Arabinoxylans Galactomannans Xyloglucans	
α-Cellulose	Insoluble in alkali	Cellulose (glucan)	Cellulose Nonstarch polysaccharides (NSP)[7] Dietary fiber[6]
Lignin	Insoluble in 12 M H$_2$SO$_4$	Lignin[b] (Klason) Noncarbohydrate	Lignin Dietary fiber[6]
Nonstructural Components			
Gums	Water soluble or	Galactomannans Arabinogalactans	Noncellulosic polysaccharides (NCP)[2,5] Nonstarch polysaccharides (NSP)[7]
Mucilages	Dispersible[c]	Wide range of branched and substituted galactans	Dietary fiber[6]

[a] Solubility depends on pH; in many fractionation schemes chelating agents such as EDTA or ammonium oxalate are used.
[b] Lignin is the name given to a group of complex polymers of phenylpropane.
[c] Hot water is usually necessary and colloidal viscous solutions are produced.

REFERENCES

1. **Southgate, D. A. T.,** Fibre in nutrition, *Bibl. Nutr. Dieta,* 22, 109, 1975.
2. **Southgate, D. A. T.,** The chemistry of dietary fiber, in *Fiber in Human Nutrition,* Spiller, G. A. and Amen, R. J., Eds., Plenum Press, New York, 1976, 31.
3. **Selvendran, R. R.,** The plant cell wall as a source of dietary fiber: chemistry and structure, *Am. J. Clin. Nutr.,* 39, 320, 1984.
4. **Siegel, S. M.,** The biochemistry of the plant cell wall, in *Comprehensive Biochemistry,* Vol. 26A, Florkin, M. and Stotz, E. H., Eds., Elsevier, Amsterdam, 1968, 1.
5. **Albersheim, P.,** Biogenesis of the Cell Wall, in *Plant Biochemistry,* Bonner, J. and Varner, J. E., Eds., Academic Press, New York, 1965, 298.
6. **Trowell, H., Southgate, D. A. T., Wolever, T. M. S., Leeds, A. R., Gassull, M. A., and Jenkins, D. A.,** Dietary fibre redefined, *Lancet,* 1, 967.
7. **Englyst, H., Wiggins, H. S., and Cummings, J. H.,** Determination of the non-starch polysaccharides in plant foods by gas liquid chromatography of constituent sugars as alditol acetates, *Analyst,* 107, 307, 1982.

Chapter 2.3

FOOD COMPONENTS THAT BEHAVE AS DIETARY FIBER

David A. T. Southgate

The characteristic feature of dietary fiber is that it is resistant to hydrolysis in the GI tract by the endogenous secretions of the tract[1,2] and that any degradation which occurs is a consequence of the activities of the intestinal microflora.[3,4]

In most diets, the plant cell wall material in the diet is the major source of dietary fiber; however, the diet contains other substances that share the property of undigestibility with dietary fiber. These include, first, noncarbohydrate materials which are associated with or are integral parts of the plant cell wall structure[1,4] such as cutin, suberin, waxes, protein, and inorganic matter. Some of these components escape digestion, either because they are intrinsically nondigestible or because the cell wall structures inhibit or prevent enzymatic attack.

A second group includes polysaccharides, that are not α-linked glucans, that are present in foods but that are not part of the cell wall structure or are food ingredients or additives. Some exudate gums are used as ingredients in some confectionery and a range of other polysaccharides are used as food additives, usually to control or influence the physical properties of a food.[5]

A third group contains degraded carbohydrates from carbohydrate-protein complexes formed during the processing of foodstuffs. Thus, some starch in baked products is rendered resistant to enzymolysis.[6]

Fourth, other nonassimilable components of foods include some oligosaccharides, sugar alcohols and pigments, hydrocarbon oils, waxes and dyes, degraded connective tissue protein, "chitin" exoskeletons of crustacea and insects, mucopolysaccharides, and hair.[7]

All these substances can be said to behave as dietary fiber in the sense that they are indigestible. It is, however, inappropriate to regard all unassimilable components of food as falling into a total dietary fiber fraction, since these include a heterogeneous collection of materials far removed from the conceptual definition and original use of the term "dietary fiber" which is not synonymous with undigestible or unassimilable components.

TABLE 1
Food Components that Behave as Dietary Fiber

Category	Dietary sources		Frequency of occurrence
Noncarbohydrates associated with or part of plant cell wall	Cutin Suberin Waxes	Associated with epidermal tissues of plants	a See Chap. 2.4
	Protein	Present in all cell walls	a See Chap. 2.4
	Inorganic material (lignin)	Present in all cell walls Present in most plant tissues	a See Chaps. 2.2 and 2.4
Non-α glucan polysaccharides	Gums Mucilages Polysaccharide Food additives	Present in many fruits and seeds and some other tissues. Some used as food ingredients. Present in many processed foods	a See Chap. 2.2 a See Chap. 2.2 a See Chap. 2.5
Degradation products	Modified carbohydrates Protein-carbohydrate complexes	Mainly arising in foods which have been thermally treated	a
Other nonassimilable components	Oligosaccharides	Tri- and tetrasaccharides in many vegetables	b
	Sugar alcohols	Used in food additives or diabetic and low-calorie or sugar-free confectionery	b
	Hydrocarbon waxes Hydrocarbon oils	Contaminants from food processing and some dried fruits	c
	Dyes	Processed foods	b
	Pigments	Naturally occurring	
	Degraded connective tissue proteins	Animal products	c
	Chitin exoskeletons	Insects and crustacea	c
	Mucopolysaccharides	Animal connective tissues	b
	Hair	Animal products	c

Note: a, Present in most if not all diets, usually at low levels. b, Depends on choice of foods — present in many diets at low levels. c, Very infrequently present in Western diets; low levels in other diets.

REFERENCES

1. **Trowell, H.,** Ischemic heart disease and dietary fiber, *Am. J. Clin. Nutr.,* 25, 926, 1972.
2. **Southgate, D. A. T.,** The chemistry of dietary fiber, in *Fiber in Human Nutrition,* Spiller, G. A. and Amen, R. J., Eds., Plenum Press, New York, 1976, 31.
3. **Bacon, J. S. D.,** Plant Cell Wall Digestibility and Chemical Structure, No. 35, Report of Rowett Research Institute, Bucksburn, Aberdeen, U.K., 1979, p. 99.
4. **Stephen, A. M. and Cummings, J. H.,** Mechanism of action of dietary fibre in the human colon, *Nature (London),* 284, 283, 1980.
5. **Glicksman, M.,** *Gum Technology in the Food Industry,* Academic Press, New York, 1969.
6. **Englyst, H., Wiggins, H. S., and Cummings, J. H.,** Determination of the non-starch polysaccharides in plant foods by gas-liquid chromatography of constituent sugars as alditol acetates, *Analyst,* 107, 307, 1982.
7. **Southgate, D. A. T.,** Non-assimilable components of foods, in *Nutritional Problems in a Changing World,* Hollingsworth, D. F. and Russell, M., Eds., Applied Science Publishers, London, 1973, 199.

Chapter 2.4

FOOD COMPONENTS ASSOCIATED WITH DIETARY FIBER

David A. T. Southgate

INTRODUCTION

The plant cell wall contains or is associated with a range of noncarbohydrate substances.[1] Some are integral parts of the cell wall structure whereas others appear to be chance inclusions, and others are closely associated with the walls at the exterior surfaces of the plant. These noncarbohydrate constituents are usually quantitatively minor components of the wall; nevertheless, they modify the physical and chemical properties of the wall polysaccharides and thereby can be expected to modify the physiological properties of dietary fiber when eaten.[2]

LIGNIN

Although many authors consider the lignins[3] (for a wide range of structures are found in foods) as part of dietary fiber (Chapter 2.2) in a formal sense, it is appropriate to consider it as an associated component since it is only by the convention of common usage that it is so regarded.

Lignin is the name applied to a complex group of essentially aromatic polymers formed by the condensation of the aromatic alcohols, cinnamyl, guaiacyl, and syringyl alcohol. Lignification of the wall is an infiltration process of the matrix and the cell wall expands in volume as it occurs.

In many food plants, the lignification is limited to spiral and annular bands in the xylem-conducting vessels. More intensively lignified xylem elements are present in mature tissues but heavily lignified woody tissues are not frequently consumed.[4]

Lignified seeds are commonly present in the diet and some fruits (especially the pear) contain heavily lignified clumps of cells within their fleshy tissues.

The external cell walls of cereal grain coats are also lignified.

Lignification produces a hydrophobic region in the wall and lignin is highly resistant to enzymatic and bacterial attack. Lignified tissues are therefore recoverable virtually unaltered from fecal material.

Analytical procedures for lignin are often nonspecific and depend on the resistance of the material to chemical attack — thus, insolubility in 12 M H_2SO_4 is the basis of the measurement of Klason lignin; however, in the Van Soest and Wine[5] method, the susceptibility of lignin to permanganate oxidation is the basis of the determination.

PROTEIN

Protein is found in virtually all cell walls and may form up to 10% of the wall in immature walls. The proportion falls as the wall matures and proportionately more polysaccharides are deposited in the wall. The cell wall proteins appear to play an important structural role and are, in some tissues, characteristically rich in hydroxy-proline;[6] the majority are covalently linked to glycosaccharide side chains, i.e., they are glycoproteins.[7]

The cell wall proteins in some tissues appear to have a lower apparent digestibility[8] and some authors believe that the intrinsically lower digestibility implies that the protein in cell walls should be regarded as part of the dietary fiber complex.

CUTIN, SUBERIN, AND PLANT WAXES

These substances are complex lipid materials present in many plant tissues.[1]

Cutin

Many external surfaces of plants, especially leaves and fruits, are covered with a waxy layer which includes a range of complex substances which contain long-chain hydroxy aliphatic acids which form internal esters. The material is highly hydrophobic and intimately associated with the cell wall at the surface. Cutinized tissues are resistant to hydrolysis and degradation in the intestine and can frequently be recovered from fecal material. In some analytical systems, cutin is analyzed with lignin unless the material has been extracted with a lipid solvent. Extension of the detergent fiber procedures of Van Soest[9] provides methods for the separate measurement of cutin.

Suberin

A range of similar complex materials which includes phenolic components, long-chain alcohols, and acids can be isolated from suberinized tissues. Suberin is deposited in layers below the epidermis in many plant tissues, particularly in underground organs, but also in the skins of some fruits. Suberinized tissues are also hydrophobic and resistant to degradation in the intestine and usually analyze with lignin.

Waxes

Complex hydrocarbon waxes are found in many plants (in very minor amounts). The waxes are usually very complex mixtures and include ketones, esters, phenolic esters, and alcohols. The waxes coat external surfaces with a hydrophobic layer.

Although the materials are hydrolyzed by lipases in the presence of bile salts (*in vitro*), degradation in the intestine appears to be limited.

INORGANIC MATERIALS

Most plant cell walls contain inorganic material. In some plants, the inorganic inclusions in the wall appear to have structural significance, this being especially true of silica.[10] Other inclusions appear to be deposits of potassium, calcium, and magnesium salts of organic acids.

While the major part of the inorganic materials would be expected to contribute to the inorganic pool in the intestine, insolubility and possibly steric hindrance to diffusion in the wall renders a proportion of the material undigested.

EDITOR'S NOTE

Saponins and phytates are also commonly associated with dietary fiber in plant foods. Diets high in dietary fiber may include saponins and phytates in concentrations that can have physiological effects.

TABLE 1
Food Components Associated with Dietary Fiber

Component	Source	Main structural features
Lignins	Found in all vascular plants; major component of wood tissues and some seeds	Complex aromatic polymers formed by the condensation of cinnamyl, guaiacyl, and syrngyl alcohols
Protein	Present in all cell walls	May be rich in hydroxyproline; glycoproteins are very common
Cutin	Cutinized surfaces of plants	Polymeric material containing C_{16}, C_{18} family of hydroxyaliphatic acids
Suberin	Suberinized tissues (subepidermal) of many plants	Polymeric material long-chain C_{20}, C_{26} acids and alcohols with substantial amounts of phenolics and dicarboxylic acids
Plant waxes	External surfaces and some internal tissues	Complex mixtures of long-chain hydrocarbons, ketones, ketols, etc.
Inorganic constituents	Virtually all walls	Ca, K, Mg, and Si are common

REFERENCES

1. **Bonner, J. and Varner, J. E., Eds.**, *Plant Biochemistry,* Academic Press, New York, 1977.
2. **Van Soest, P. J.**, The uniformity and nutritive availability of cellulose, *Fed. Proc. Fed. Am. Soc. Exp. Biol.,* 32, 1804, 1973.
3. **Freudenberg, K.**, *The Formation of Wood in Forest Trees,* Zimmermann, M. H., Ed., Academic Press, New York, 1964, 203.
4. **Cutting, E. G.**, *Plant Anatomy Experiment and Interpretation,* Part 2, Edward Arnold, London, 1971.
5. **Van Soest, P. J. and Wine, R. H.**, Determination of lignin and cellulose in acid-detergent fiber with permanganate, *J. Assoc. Off. Analyst. Chem.,* 51, 780, 1968.
6. **Lamport, D. T. A.**, Cell wall metabolism, *Annu. Rev. Plant Physiol.,* 21, 235, 1970.
7. **Selvendran, R. R. and O'Neill, M. A.**, Plant glycoproteins, in *Plant Carbohydrates J.,* Loewus, F. A. and Tanner, W., Eds., Springer-Verlag, Basel, 1982, 575.
8. **Saunders, R. M. and Betschart, A. A.**, The significance of protein as a component of dietary fiber, *Am. J. Clin. Nutr.,* 33, 960, 1980.
9. **Goering, H. K. and Van Soest, P. J.**, Forage Fiber Analyses (Apparatus, Reagents, Procedures and some Applications), Agriculture Handbook No. 379, U.S. Department of Agriculture, Washington, D.C., 1970.
10. **Jones, L. H. P.**, Mineral components of plant cell walls, *Am. J. Clin. Nutr.,* 31, 594, 1978.

Chapter 2.5

POLYSACCHARIDE FOOD ADDITIVES THAT CONTRIBUTE TO DIETARY FIBER

David A. T. Southgate

A variety of polysaccharides are added to processed foods.[1] While none of them is synthetic in the true sense, many of them have been chemically modified in some way to enhance specific properties or to reduce undesirable characteristics. A few are prepared biosynthetically using microorganisms, but the majority are derived from plant polysaccharides and many from cell wall components. The polysaccharides all share the common structural feature in that they *do not contain α-glucosidic* links and are therefore not hydrolyzed by mammalian digestive enzymes. They therefore fall within the definition of dietary fiber and many have been used as models for cell wall components of dietary fiber in experimental studies.

Many of the polysaccharides used are water soluble or water dispersible and hydrolyze in dilute acid. In the analysis of dietary fiber, they form part of the noncellulosic polysaccharide fraction.

Table 1 includes the major types of polysaccharide that are in use. In most food the concentration of the polysaccharide additive is less than 1% v/v and usually less than 0.5% v/v; however, some exudate gums[1,2] are used as ingredients at much higher levels.

These materials make a minor contribution to total dietary fiber intake,[2] but have been fed at higher levels in some experimental studies as models in the study of the mode of action of dietary fiber.

TABLE 1
Polysaccharide Food Additives Contributing to Dietary Fiber

Polysaccharide	Major sources	Principal types in use	Main structural features
Pectin	Citrus and apple cellular residues	High methoxyl	Galacturonans with few side chains — methoxyl varies according to source
		Low methoxyl	
		Amidated	Amidated for special uses
Galactomannan gums	Endosperm of specific leguminous plants	Guar Locust (Carob)	D-mannopyranosides with D-galactosyl side chains
Algal polysaccharides	Cell wall of algae (principally Phaeophyceae)	Agar	Agarose-linear alternating (1-4) 3,6-anhydro-L-galactose, (1 → 3)-D-galactose, and agaropectin-agarose components plus ester sulfate and D-glucuronic acid
		Alginates	Copolymer of D-mannuronic and L-guluronic acids
		Carrageenans	(1-3)D-galactose-4-sulfate and (1-4) 3,6 anhydro-D-galactose
			(1-4)D-galactose 2,6-sulfate, (1-3)D-galactose, or (1-3) D-galactose
			(1-3)-D-galactose-4-sulfate and (1-4) 3,6-anhydro-D-galactose-2-sulfate
Modified celluloses	Cellulose from delignified woody tissues	Cellulose ethers	Methyl cellulose — cellulose with variable degree of methylation
		Cellulose esters	Carboxymethyl and carboxyethyl cellulose
			Cellulose ester
Bacterial gums	Biosynthetically produced gums	Xanthan	Glucose mannose and glucuronic acid in a linear chain with mannose side chains with pyruvate as a side chain

REFERENCES

1. **Glicksman, M.,** *Gum Technology in the Food Industry,* Academic Press, New York, 1969.
2. **Wirths, W.,** Aufnahme an pflanzlichen Hydrokolloiden in der Bundesrepublik Deutschland, *Pflanzenfasern-Ballaststoffe in der menschlichen Ernahrung,* Rottka, H., Ed., George Thieme Verlag, Stuttgart, 1980, 76.

Chapter 2.6

GLOSSARY OF DIETARY FIBER COMPONENTS*

David A. T. Southgate, Gene A. Spiller, Margaret White, and Ruth McPherson

Acid detergent fiber (ADF) — The cellulose plus lignin in a sample; it is measured as the residue after extracting the food with a hot dilute sulfuric acid solution of the detergent, cetyl trimethylammonium bromide (CTAB). See Chapter 3.1.

Agar — A mixture of polysaccharides occurring as the cell wall constituents of certain red marine algae Rhodophytaceae, e.g., *Gelidium* sp., from which it can be extracted with hot water. It gels on cooling at a concentration as low as 0.5%. Agarose, the main constituent, is a neutral polysaccharide containing 3,6-anhydro-L-galactose and D-galactose as the repetitive unit. Agaropectin is a minor constituent polysaccharide and contains carboxyl and sulfate groups. It is not hydrolyzed by mammalian digestive enzymes and is, therefore, part of dietary fiber when used as a thickening agent in foods; it is a laxative. The chief use, however, is as a solid medium for cultivating microorganisms, since it is undigested by almost all of them.

Algal polysaccharides — The extract from the tissues of algae, divided into two groups: (1) reserve polysaccharides which are water soluble and (2) structural polysaccharides which are not. They are not hydrolyzed by the mammalian digestive enzymes and are therefore part of dietary fiber.

Alginates — Algal polysaccharides not hydrolyzed by mammalian digestive enzymes and, therefore, part of dietary fiber. Commercial algin is sodium alginate: it is slowly soluble in water, forming an extremely viscous solution. It is used as a stabilizer for ice cream and other food products.

Alginic acid — Water-insoluble algal polysaccharide, polymannuronic acid, which can be extracted from certain dried seaweeds, as a water-soluble alginate with aqueous alkali metal hydroxides or carbonates, and precipitated by the addition of an acid. Alginic acid is not hydrolyzed by mammalian digestive enzymes and is, therefore, part of dietary fiber.

Arabinans — Polysaccharides that give L-arabinose on hydrolysis. They are present in wood cellulose, are associated with pectin, and have been isolated from the pectic substances of mustard seed and sugar beet.

Arabinogalactans — Substituted galactans that form part of the hemicellulose complex in many tissues. Although most emphasis has been given to arabinogalactans from woody tissues, polymers of this type are widely distributed. The water-soluble arabinogalactan of larch has received considerable study.

Arabinoxylans — Have a main chain composed of $(1 \rightarrow 4)$ β-D-xylopyranosyl units with an occasional branching in some preparations. The arabinose is present as single- or double-residue side chains. Arabinoxylans are widely distributed in the cell walls of many materials, although they are uncommon in woody tissues; they have been isolated from the husks of many grains.

Carrageenan — An algal polysaccharide chiefly composed of polymerized sulfated D-galactopyranose units, but with other residues also present. It is the dried extract from certain red marine algae Rhodophytaceae, and often from the species *Chrondus crispus* (carrageenan, Irish moss). The ability of carrageenan to react with milk protein has led to its widespread

---

* Adapted from Southgate, D. A. T., *Medical Aspects of Dietary Fiber*, Spiller, G. A. and Kay, R. M., Eds., Plenum Press, New York, 1980. With permission.

use in preparations containing milk and chocolate. It has been shown to be a potent cholesterol-lowering agent but, unlike almost any other plant polysaccharide, has an adverse effect on the gut. Ulceration of the cecum of both rats and guinea pigs has been demonstrated when carrageenan was added to the diet.

Cellulose — Best known, most widely distributed, and only truly fibrous component of the plant cell wall. It is a polymer of glucose and the glucoside linkage is β. The β-linkages in cellulose are not hydrolyzed by the enzymes present in man; cellulose is therefore part of dietary fiber. Cellulose also has the property of taking up water (0.4 g water per gram of cellulose) and this explains its ability to increase fecal weight when added to the diet.

Crude fiber — Residue left after boiling the defatted food in dilute alkali and then in dilute acid. The method recovers 50 to 80% of cellulose, 10 to 50% of lignin, and 20% of hemicellulose. Inconsistent results are obtained and it should not be used as a method for the determination of dietary fiber.

Cutin — A complex polymer of mono-, di-, tri-, and polyhydroxy fatty acids, it is a lipid component of the waterproof covering and cuticle on the outer cellulose wall of plants. Cuticular substances are extremely resistant to digestion and in turn are thought to impair the digestibility of the other cell wall constituents. Their resistance to digestion means they appear in the feces, and may constitute a large proportion of the fecal fat. Cutins may account for a substantial part of the increased fecal fat seen in subjects on a high cereal-fiber diet.

Dietary fiber — Includes all the polymers of plants that cannot be digested by the endogenous secretions of the human digestive tract, i.e., cellulose, pectins, hemicellulose, gums, mucilages, and lignin; see also Chapter 2.1.

Galactans — Polysaccharides which, on hydrolysis, give galactose. They occur in wood and in many algae. The most important galactan is agar.

Galactomannans — Polysaccharides that have both galactose and mannose in the chain, in varying proportions. Guar gum (guaram) is a representative example. Galactomannans are part of the hemicellulose fraction of the plant cell wall.

Glucofructans — Linear polymers with both fructose and glucose in the chain. They are found in the hemicellulose section of the cell wall and form the storage polysaccharides in many temperate-climate grasses.

Glucomannans — Appear to be linear polymers with both mannose and glucose in the chain. The ratio of mannose to glucose is between 1:1 and 2.4:1. Hardwood glucomannans appear to contain no galactose and are relatively insoluble, but the glucomannans from gymnosperms have galactose side chains and a higher mannose to glucose ratio (3:1). The presence of side chains tends to make these polysaccharides more soluble in water, possibly because the side chains prevent the formation of intermolecular hydrogen bonding. Glucomannans are part of the hemicellulose fraction of the plant cell wall.

Glucoronoxylans — Have a main "backbone" chain of $(1 \rightarrow 4)$ linked β-D-xylopyranosyl residues, containing side chains of 4-O-methyl-α-D-glucopyranosyluronic acid and in some annual plants, unmethylated D-glucuronic acid. Glucuronoxylans are found in the hemicellulose fraction of all land plants and most plant organs.

Glycan — Generic name for a polysaccharide; from glycose, a simple sugar and the ending -an signifying a polymer.

Glycuronans — Generic name for the polymers of uronic acids, e.g., galacturonan is a polymer of galacturonic acid, and is therefore a glycuronan.

Guar gum (guaran) — A neutral polysaccharide, a D-galacto-D-mannan, that is isolated from the ground endosperm of guar seed, a leguminous vegetable cultivated in India for animal feeds. In small amounts it finds widespread use in the food industry and pharmaceutical industries as a thickener and stabilizer in, for example, salad dressing and ice cream, as well as in nonfood items such as toothpaste.

Gum (exudates and seed gums) — Complex polysaccharides, each containing several different sugar molecules and uronic acid groups. The true plant gums, gum acacia and gum tragacanth, are the dried exudates from various plants obtained when the bark is cut or the plant is otherwise injured. They are soluble in water to give very viscous colloidal solutions, sometimes called mucilages, and are insoluble in organic solvents. These are not part of the cell wall structure but are generally indigestible and are thus considered a part of dietary fiber. Guar and locust bean gums are examples of gums derived from seeds.

Hemicelluloses — A wide variety of polysaccharide polymers, at least 250 of which are known. The largest group consists of pentosans such as the xylans and arabinoxylans; a second group consists of hexose polymers such as the galactans. The acidic hemicelluloses which contain galacturonic acid or glucuronic acid form a third group of hemicelluloses. Hemicelluloses are those polymers extractable from plants by cold aqueous alkali. They are not precursors of cellulose and have no part in cellulose biosynthesis but represent a distinct and separate group of plant polysaccharides. Together with pectin, the hemicelluloses form the matrix of the plant cell wall in which are enmeshed cellulose fibers. The hemicelluloses are not digested in the small intestine but are broken down by microorganisms in the colon more readily than cellulose.

Heteroglycans — Polysaccharides that hydrolyze to two, three, or more monosaccharides. They have prefixes of di- , tri- , and so on to indicate the number of different types of sugar residues.

Hexoses — Monosaccharides with each molecule containing six carbon atoms. Glucose, fructose, galactose, and mannose are all hexoses.

Homoglycan — Polysaccharide containing only one type of sugar unit and hence on hydrolysis giving only one monosaccharide type. The most abundant polysaccharides are of this type, e.g., starch and cellulose.

Lignin — An aromatic polymer of molecular weight of about 10,000 based on coniferyl and sinapyl alcohols; it occurs in woody plant tissues. Since it is virtually indigestible, lignin is usually classified as part of dietary fiber. It is a commercial source of vanillin and other aromatic chemicals.

Mannans — Polysaccharides made up of mannose units, found in the hemicellulose fraction from many cell walls. They seem to be storage polysaccharides.

Middle lamella — Develops from the cell plate that forms between the daughter nuclei of the plant cell wall and extends to meet the existing wall, and therefore is the structure between adjacent cell walls. It appears to be rich in galacturonans, which are characteristically part of the pectic substances.

Mucilages — Polysaccharides usually containing galactose, galacturonic acid residues, and often xylose and arabinose. Structurally, they resemble the hemicelluloses and are water soluble, being obtained as slimy, colloidal solutions. They are found mixed with the endosperm or storage polysaccharides or in special cells in the seedcoat. They retain water and so protect the seed against desiccation.

Neutral detergent fiber (NDF) — That part of food remaining after extraction with a hot neutral solution of the detergent sodium lauryl sulfate. It is a measure of the cell wall constituents of vegetable foodstuffs. The method for determining NDF was designed to divide the dry matter of feeds very nearly into those constituents which are nutritionally available for the normal digestive process and those which depend on microbial fermentation for their availability. See Chapter 3.1.

Noncellulosic polysaccharides — Another term for hemicelluloses, which includes all the matrix polysaccharides from the cell wall, other than cellulose.

Nonstarch polysaccharides (NSP) — A term suggested by Englyst and co-workers for the carbohydrate plant cell wall material originally called *dietary fiber* less the lignin; considered by the authors to be a better definition than *fiber*.

Oligosaccharides — Collective term for di- , tri- , and tetrasaccharides; processed foods may contain oligosaccharides with up to 9 residue.

Pectic substances — Mixtures of acidic and neutral polysaccharides that can be extracted with water from plant tissues. They are characteristically rich in galacturonic acid and are galacturonans with a variable degree of methyl esterification.

Pectin — General term designating those water-soluble pectinic acids of varying methyl ester content and degree of neutralization which are capable of forming gels with water and acid under suitable conditions. Pectin is found in the primary cell wall and intracellular layer. It changes from an insoluble material in the unripe fruit to a much more water-soluble substance in the ripe fruit. Its ability to form gels and its ion binding capacity may be important in human nutrition. Also see pectic substances.

Pectinic acid — Groups of pectins in which only a portion of the acidic groupings are methylated.

Pentoses — Monosaccharides with each molecule containing five carbon atoms. Pentose sugars most commonly present in human foods are L-arabinose and D-xylose, which are widely distributed in the polysaccharides in plants. Pentoses are present in small amounts in all cell walls whether animal, plant, or bacterial. Dietetically, the five-carbon sugars are of little importance as a source of energy for the body.

Plantix — A term coined from "plant" and "matrix" to replace dietary fiber to avoid the uncertain and diversified meaning of the term fiber. It includes the same polymers found in dietary fiber from plants.

Primary plant cell wall — The cellulose fibers of the primary cell wall are laid down in a random network on the middle lamella. The fibrils are surrounded by an amorphous matrix of hemicellulose.

Protopectin — Term applied to the water-insoluble parent pectic substance which occurs in plants, and which upon hydrolysis yields pectinic acid.

Resistant starch — Starch that is not digested by human digestive enzymes and that reaches the colon, often acting in the same way as *fiber*.

Sclerenchyma — Tissue forming the hard parts of plants such as nutshell or seedcoat.

Secondary cell wall — Polysaccharide in nature and apparently amorphous. It is formed after the cell has reached maturity and is laid down inside the primary cell wall either as a continuous layer or as localized thickenings or bands.

Silica — Deposited in the plant cell wall, usually in the aerial part of the plant. The amount varies according to the species, the silica content of the soil, and the maturity of the plant. The ash content of the cell wall, particularly of wheat, may be as high as 10%; of this, the principal element present is often silicon. Silica has the capacity to impair the digestibility of cell wall materials.

Suberin — A cutin-like substance found in cork. It is a plant lipid that cannot be extracted with a simple solvent but needs saponification before extraction.

Uronic acids — Present in the pectic substances and the hemicellulose portion of the plant cell wall. They are found in about half the known plant polysaccharides, the most common being D-galacturonic and D-glucuronic acids. Uronic acids are derived from sugars by oxidation of the terminal $-CH_2OH$ to $-COOH$ and, when present as glycosides, behave like simple hydrocarboxylic acids, forming metal salts, amides, and alkyl and methyl esters.

Water-holding capacity — Amount of water that can be taken up by unit weight of dry fiber to the point at which no free water remains. A close relationship exists between acid detergent fiber content of vegetable dietary fiber and water-holding capacity, but there is no such relationship between lignin content and water-holding capacity.

Water-soluble fraction — Fraction of dietary fiber soluble in water; it includes pectic substances, gums, mucilages, and some polysaccharide food additives.

Xylans — Groups of polymers having a main chain of (1 → 4) β-D-xylopyranosyl residues; arabinose and 4-O-methyl glucuronic acid are the most usual substituents. A few D-xylans are neutral molecules containing D-xylose residues only. Xylans are found in the hemicellulose portion of the plant cell wall in all land plants and in most plant organs.

Xylem — Water-conducting elements of plant tissues, usually made up of cells with lignified walls. In mature woody tissues, the walls of xylem vessels are completely lignified; in less mature tissues, the lignification is partial and localized.

REFERENCES

1. **Southgate, D. A. T., White, M., Spiller, G. A., and Kay, R. M.**, Glossary, in *Medical Aspects of Dietary Fiber*, Spiller, G. A. and Kay, R. M., Eds., Plenum Press, New York, 1980.
2. **Smith, F. and Montgomery, R., Eds.**, *The Chemistry of Plant Gums and Mucilages and Some Related Polysaccharides*, Reinhold, New York, 1959.
3. **Butler, G. W. and Bailey, R. W.**, *Chemistry and Biochemistry of Herbage*, Vol. 1, Academic Press, New York, 1973.
4. **Windholz, M., Budavari, S., Stroumtsos, L. Y., and Fertig, M. N., Eds.**, *The Merck Index*, 9th ed., Merck, Rahway, N.J., 1976.

Section 3: Methods of Analysis for Dietary Fiber

Chapter 3.1

ENZYMATIC GRAVIMETRIC METHODS

Nils-Georg Asp

INTRODUCTION

Enzymatic gravimetric methods date back to the 19th century. In the 1930s, McCance et al.[1] measured total unavailable carbohydrates in fruits, nuts, and vegetables by determining the residue insoluble in 80% ethanol. This was corrected for starch measured after enzymatic hydrolysis with takadiastase and for protein. Similar procedures have been used more recently.[2,3] The main limitation of this approach is that the protein correction gives an unacceptable error in samples with low dietary fiber and high protein content.

METHODS MEASURING INSOLUBLE DIETARY FIBER

Methods employing both amylolytic and proteolytic treatment and separation of an insoluble undigestible residue are listed in Table 1. Weinstock and Benham[4] used the enzyme preparation Rhozyme S with high amylase activity. Thus, starch was removed efficiently, whereas a considerable protein residue remained associated with the fiber.[5,6] Thomas[7] improved the method by adding a pancreatin step. Later on, Elchazly and Thomas[8] omitted the crude Rhozyme preparation and used amyloglucosidase or takadiastase and trypsin or pancreatin. These authors also introduced special centrifugation tubes with fritted glass filters for separation of the insoluble fiber from the enzyme digest.

Hellendoorn et al.[9] used only physiological enzymes, pepsin plus pancreatin. This analytical method is therefore related to a physiological dietary fiber definition.[10,11] The residues of protein and starch associated with the dietary fiber after enzymatic treatment[6,12] were even considered an advantage, representing *in vivo* undigestible material.[13] Saunders and Betschart[14] also suggested that indigestible protein could play a significant role in the physiological effects of dietary fiber. However, the protein and starch residues are dependent upon the choice of enzymes and the conditions for enzymatic digestion,[12–14] and it is impossible to define exactly the degree of hydrolysis obtained *in vivo*. This fact has led most workers to prefer a more "chemical" definition of dietary fiber, i.e., the sum of undigestible polysaccharides and lignin.[15] However, in practice the delimitation is always related to a method involving enzymatic degradation of starch *in vitro*, which may be more or less related to *in vivo* conditions.

METHODS MEASURING INSOLUBLE AND SOLUBLE DIETARY FIBER

Soluble dietary fiber components constitute a considerable fraction of the total dietary fiber in mixed diets[5,6] and include polysaccharides such as pectins and gums with important physiological effects. It is generally agreed that soluble components should be included in the definition and determination of dietary fiber.[15–18] Table 2 lists developments of enzymatic methods also measuring soluble dietary fiber components.

Furda[19,20] used *Bacillus subtilis* amylase and protease in a single overnight incubation at neutral pH. Soluble dietary fiber components were recovered by precipitation with 4 vol

TABLE 1
Enzymatic Gravimetric Methods Measuring Insoluble Fiber

Agents for protein and starch solubilization	Incubation time (h)	Ref.
Rhozyme S	24	4
Pancreatin	5	7
Rhozyme or other amylase	18	
Amyloglucosidase or takadiastase	3 18	8
Trypsin or pancreatin	18	
Pepsin	18	9
Pancreatin	1	

TABLE 2
Enzymatic Gravimetric Methods Measuring Both Soluble and Insoluble Fiber

Agents for protein and starch solubilization	Incubation time	Ref.
B. subtilis amylase and protease	16–18 h	19, 20
Pepsin	20 h	21
Pancreatin + glucoamylase	18 h	
Pepsin	18 h	6
Pancreatin	1 h	
Termamyl	15 min	12
Pepsin	1 h	
Pancreatin	1 h	
Amyloglucosidase	3 h	22
Pancreatin/trypsin	15–18 h	
Termamyl	15–30 min	23
B. subtilis protease	30 min	
Amyloglucosidase	30 min	

of 95% (v/v) ethanol. Both insoluble and precipitated soluble fiber were separated by filtration in crucibles with glass wool as a filtering aid.

The methods of Schweizer and Würsch[21] and Asp et al.[6,12] are developments of Hellendoorn et al.[9] using the physiological enzymes pepsin and pancreatin. Soluble dietary fiber is precipitated with ethanol. Two of these methods[6,21] employ long (19- to 38-h) incubation times and repeated centrifugations to recover the dietary fiber fractions. In the more recent modification of Asp et al.,[12] enzyme incubation time was reduced to 2 h, and separation of both insoluble and precipitated soluble fiber — either separately or together — was carried out by filtration using Celite as a filtering aid. The main steps of this method are shown in Figure 1.

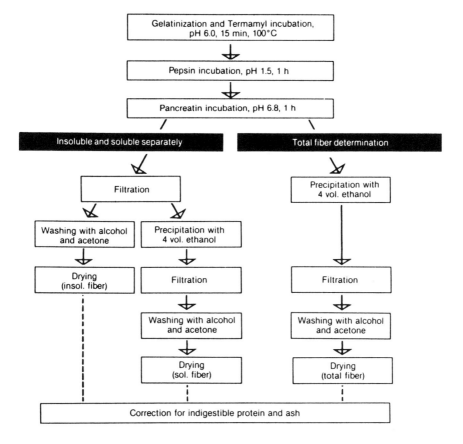

FIGURE 1. Flow diagram of the method of Asp et al.[12]

Meuser et al.[22] developed a method based on the enzymatic method of Elchazly and Thomas,[8] using membrane ultrafiltration to separate the soluble dietary fiber components from the enzyme digest.

The AOAC method[23-26] is based on the common experience of three groups that have developed enzymatic gravimetric methods for the assay of total dietary fiber.[12,20,21] The main steps are shown in Figure 2, and a detailed step-by-step description is given at the end of this chapter. This method employs the short technique, incubation times, and filtration introduced by Asp et al.[12] but with other enzymes. A modification of the AOAC method with further simplifications has recently been tested collaboratively by Lee et al.[27] and approved.

The separate determination of soluble and insoluble dietary fiber was suggested in the different enzymatic gravimetric methods[6,12,19-22] (Figure 1) and has been tested collaboratively for the AOAC method.[25,27] The solubility of the dietary fiber polysaccharides is method dependent, and the experimental conditions giving a solubility most close to that in the intestinal content have not yet been defined. Furthermore, physiological effects on plasma lipid levels and postprandial glucose and hormone response, attributed to soluble fiber, seem to be related to the properties of the soluble fiber, especially the viscosity.

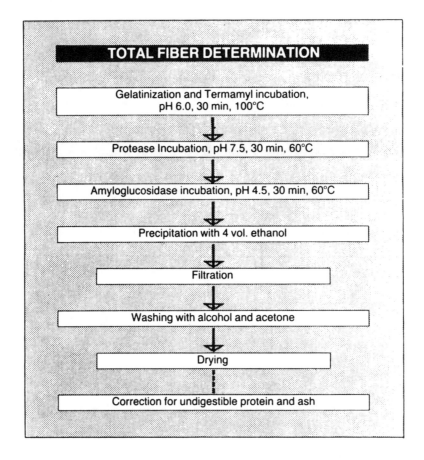

FIGURE 2. Flow diagram of the AOAC method for total dietary fiber.[23-27]

DISCUSSION OF VARIOUS STEPS IN ENZYMATIC GRAVIMETRIC METHODS

Sample Preparation

Milling to small particles is essential for proper enzyme action. Usually, milling to pass a 0.3- to 0.5-mm screen is recommended, but it is recognized that milling to such a small particle size may present difficulties with some materials.

Defatting is usually recommended and may be necessary for proper milling. In the AOAC method,[23,31,32] simple defatting with petroleum ether at room temperature is recommended whenever the fat content exceeds 10%. It should be noted, however, that Asp et al. were able to analyze dietary fiber with their method[12] in samples with 20% fat without defatting. Probably much of the fat melts at the high temperature during the starch gelatinization step, and any fat residue will be dissolved by the alcohol and acetone washing of the dietary fiber residue after filtration.

Starch Gelatinization and Hydrolysis

Whereas some authors[21,22] employ autoclaving for starch gelatinization, Asp et al.[12] demonstrated that a 15-min heating in a boiling waterbath in the presence of the thermostable α-amylase Termamyl gave sufficient gelatinization and prehydrolysis of the starch. Even in starchy materials, such as wheat flour and potatoes, which are recognized as difficult in this respect, only a small amount of starch available to glucoamylase remained in the dietary fiber residue.[12,28]

"Resistant Starch", i.e., starch available to glucoamylase only after solubilization with 2 M KOH, remained associated with the dietary fiber in bread,[26] similarly as found with a gas-chromatographic method[30] using 1-h boiling for starch gelatinization. The total starch remaining in the dietary fiber residue prepared with an enzymatic gravimetric method can be differentiated into one fraction available to glucoamylase without alkali solubilization ("residual starch") and another fraction available only after solubilization in 2 M KOH or dimethylsulfoxide, DMSO ("resistant starch").[31]

The resistant starch in the fiber residue is mainly retrograded amylose.[32] This fraction is resistant to degradation also in the small intestine of both rat[33] and man.[34]

Recently it has been suggested that the term resistant starch be used in a broader sense, representing all the starch escaping digestion and absorption in the human small intestine.[35]

Different methods employ either only α-amylases[6,9,12] or only glucoamylase,[19,20] or a combination of both types of amylase.[21-27] An advantage with glucoamylase is that it degrades the starch to free glucose, which can easily be analyzed in the filtrate to measure starch.

It is essential that all enzyme preparations used are free from contaminating activities hydrolyzing dietary fiber. This can be checked most conveniently by running samples of known polysaccharide preparations through the whole procedure.[23] The reason why the crude Termamyl preparation can be used is the high temperature employed, inactivating contaminating activities. Thus, heating should be performed immediately after Termamyl addition to avoid hydrolysis of dietary fiber components.

Protein Hydrolysis

At very acid pH (around 1) as originally used by Hellendoorn et al.,[9] acid-labile groups of dietary fiber polysaccharides, such as arabinose residues in cereal pentosans, may be hydrolyzed. By increasing the pH to 1.5 and reducing the incubation time to 1 h, Asp et al.[12] were able to use pepsin without measurable loss of dietary fiber constituents. The AOAC method[23-27] employs the *B. subtilis* protease originally used by Furda[19,20] at neutral pH.

To be consistent with the definition of dietary fiber as the sum of undigestible polysaccharides and lignin, values obtained with enzymatic gravimetric methods need to be corrected for undigestible protein associated with the fiber. This can be done by analyzing the dietary fiber residue for nitrogen with the Kjeldahl method.[12,23-27] The universal protein conversion factor 6.25 should be used, since the true correct factor of the undigestible protein is not known. It may differ from that in the original protein.

Recovery of Soluble Dietary Fiber Constituents

Most methods employ precipitation with 78 to 80% (v/v) ethanol to separate soluble fiber components from the enzyme digest. The precipitate is recovered by centrifugation[21] or filtration using glass wool[19,20] or Celite[12,23-27] as a filtering aid. Procedures using ultrafiltration[22] or dialysis have not been documented to be more selective. The 80% ethanol precipitation is an arbitrary delimitation between polysaccharides included in dietary fiber and oligosaccharides not included. Polysaccharides with DP (degree of polymerization) >10 are usually precipitated, but in some cases larger polysaccharides will stay in solution, especially if highly branched. This has been demonstrated for arabinans and pectic substances in sugar beet fiber.[37]

Coprecipitation of minerals may be a problem when using alcohol precipitation.[38,39] Although correction for ash is recommended,[12,23-27] the buffer strength of the incubation medium should be kept low enough to avoid excessive ash precipitation and thus an unnecessary source of variability between samples.

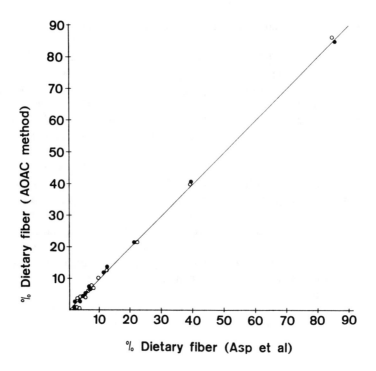

FIGURE 3. Comparison of the methods of Asp et al.[12] and Prosky et al.[23] using different enzymes on samples in the first interlaboratory study of the AOAC method. The different symbols denote two different laboratories.

INTERLABORATORY STUDIES

Enzymatic gravimetric methods have been compared and evaluated vs. other methods. In the EEC/IARC study conducted in 1978, three groups participated with enzymatic methods. Although incompletely developed at that time, the enzymatic methods gave comparatively consistent results and good agreement with gas chromatographic methods.[40]

Raw and processed wheat and potato products were analyzed in another interlaboratory study.[28] Enzymatic methods showed good agreement with each other and with gas chromatographic methods. The AOAC method[23] and the method of Asp et al.[12] showed good agreement on these samples and also on the samples analyzed in the first AOAC collaborative study (Figure 3). Similar results have also been obtained when comparing the component analysis methods of Theander et al. and the enzymatic gravimetric method of Asp et al. for both processed and unprocessed cereals and vegetables.[37] The lower values obtained with the Englyst method can generally be explained by the fact that this method does not include lignin and resistant starch.

The first interlaboratory study with the AOAC method for total dietary fiber (TDF)[23] was the biggest collaborative effort reported so far. It identified a number of problems that were corrected in the second study, after which the method was approved by the AOAC.[24] A Swiss collaborative study with a slightly modified TDF method[26] reported the best precision measures obtained so far. These modifications were introduced and approved in the third AOAC study.[25] Insoluble fiber determination also showed satisfactory results in that study, and soluble fiber determination was approved as the difference between total and insoluble fiber. Later on, direct determination of soluble fiber was approved as well.[27]

All the collaborative studies reported so far — both with enzymatic gravimetric methods and with the method of Englyst et al. — have recently been calculated in the same way and compared.[41] The gravimetric AOAC method has been tested on a wider range of foods with more variable dietary fiber content and has generally shown as good as or better reproducibility values than the Englyst method.

The AOAC method has been officially approved in Switzerland, Germany, Denmark, Finland, Iceland, Norway, Sweden, and the Netherlands. It is recommended in several other countries. Gravimetric dietary fiber values, both with and without correction for protein, have recently been introduced in the Japanese food tables.[42]

CONCLUSION

Enzymatic gravimetric methods using alcohol precipitation of soluble dietary fiber components are suitable for assay of total dietary fiber or insoluble and soluble fiber separately. Correction for undigestible protein and ash associated especially with the soluble fiber should be made to conform with currently accepted definitions of dietary fiber. Once a protein correction is accepted, a somewhat higher protein residue obtained at the very short incubation time in the protease step(s) can be accepted, as well as some variation in the residue due to choice of enzymes.

Alcohol precipitation is the most rapid way to separate soluble dietary fiber components from the enzyme digest. Ultrafiltration and especially dialysis are much slower processes and have not been documented to be more selective and complete.

Filtration in glass filter crucibles can be used to recover both insoluble and alcohol-precipitated soluble components if a filtering aid such as Celite is used. Centrifugation is an alternative, especially to recover very viscous types of fiber that can give filtration problems.

Enzymatic methods are useful as preparatory steps before detailed analysis of dietary fiber composition. The enzymatic treatment removes material that might interfere in later steps, and the total fiber value obtained in the gravimetric assay can serve as a control of the standardization of detailed analyses. The efficiency of starch removal and presence of resistant starch can be checked by analyzing the dietary fiber residue.

THE DETERMINATION OF TOTAL DIETARY FIBER IN FOODS AND FOOD PRODUCTS: APPROVED AOAC METHOD OF PROSKY ET AL.[24,25]

Procedure

Duplicate samples of dried foods, fat extracted if containing more than 10% fat, are gelatinized with Termamyl (heat stable α-amylase), then enzymatically digested with protease and amyloglucosidase to remove the protein and starch present. Then 4 vol of 95% ethanol (v/v) is added to precipitate the soluble dietary fiber. The total residue is filtered, washed with 78% ethanol, 95% ethanol, and acetone. After drying, the residue is weighed. One of the duplicates is analyzed for protein, and the other is incinerated at 525°C and the ash determined. Total dietary fiber is the weight of the residue less the weight of the protein and ash present.

Apparatus

1. Balance, analytical, capable of weighing to 0.1 mg.
2. Fritted crucible, porosity #2. Clean thoroughly, ash at 525°C, soak in distilled water, and rinse in same. Add approximately 0.5 g of Celite 545 to dried crucibles before drying to obtain constant weight. Dry at 130°C for 1 h, cool, and store in desiccator until used. The fritted crucible is a Pyrex 32940, Course ASTM 40 to 60 μm, and

may be purchased from Scientific Products Co., C-8525-1; V. W. R. Scientific Co., 23863-040; Fisher Scientific Co., 08237-1A; Sargent Welch Co., F-243-90-B or F-243-90-C, depending on size needed.

    Crucibles indicated in the procedure may not be available in Europe. Porosity #2 in Europe signifies pores of 40 to 90 μm, whereas it means 40 to 60 μm in the U.S. Several collaborators have reported breakage of crucibles when the temperature was raised to 525°C and have recommended Corning No. 36060 Buchner, fritted disk, Pyrex, 60-ml ASTM 40 to 60, which seems to have less breakage and gives the same results.

3. Vacuum source: a vacuum pump or aspirator equipped with an inline double vacuum flask should be used to prevent contamination in case of water backup.
4. Vacuum oven at 70°C and desiccator; alternatively, an air oven capable of operating at 105°C can be used.
5. Boiling water bath.
6. Constant-temperature water bath adjustable to 60°C and equipped to provide constant agitation of the digestion flasks during enzymatic hydrolysis. This can be accomplished with either a multistation shaker or multistation magnetic stirrer.
7. Vortex mixer.
8. Beaker (tall form) 400 ml.

Reagents

1. Distilled water (DW).
2. 95% ethanol (v/v) — technical grade.
3. 78% ethanol: mix one volume of distilled water with four volumes of 95% ethanol.
4. Acetone — reagent grade.
5. Phosphate buffer 0.08 M pH 6.0: dissolve to 1.400 g of sodium phosphate dibasic anhydrous (or 1.753 g of the dihydrate) and 9.68 g sodium phosphate monobasic monohydrate (or 10.99 g of the dihydrate) in approximately 700 ml of DW. Dilute to 1 l with DW. Check pH.
6. Termamyl (heat-stable α-amylase) solution: 120 L (Novo Laboratories Inc.). Store the enzyme solution in refrigerator after each use.
7. Protease P-3910 (Sigma Chemical Co.): refrigerate the dry enzyme after each use.
8. Amyloglucosidase A-9913 (Sigma Chemical Co.): keep refrigerated when not in use.
9. Sodium hydroxide solution (0.275 N): dissolve 11.00 g sodium hydroxide AR in approximately 700 ml DW in 1-l volumetric flask. Dilute to volume with DW.
10. Hydrochloric acid solution (0.350 N): dilute a stock solution with known titer, e.g., 350 ml of 1 M HCl to 1 l with distilled water. Dilute to volume with DW.
11. Celite 545 (Fisher Scientific Co.). Acid washed. Equivalent to Celite C-211.

Determination

1. Run a blank through the entire procedure along with the samples to measure any contribution from reagents to the residue.
2. Weigh, in duplicate, 1 g of sample accurate to 0.1 mg (sample weight should not differ by more than 20 mg) into 400-ml tall form beakers. Add 50 ml of pH 6.0 phosphate buffer to each beaker. Check pH. Adjust to pH 6.0 ± 0.2 with 0.275 N NaOH if necessary.
3. Add 100 μl Termamyl solution.

4. Cover beaker with aluminum foil and place in boiling waterbath for 15 min. Shake gently at 5-min intervals. Increase the length of incubation time when the number of beakers added to the boiling waterbath makes it difficult for the beaker contents to reach an internal temperature of 100°C; 30 min should be sufficient.
5. Cool. Adjust to pH 7.5 ± 0.1 by adding 10 ml of 0.275 N NaOH solution.
6. Add 5 mg of protease. Since protease sticks to the spatula, it may be preferable to make an enzyme solution just prior to use with a small amount of (about 100 µl) phosphate buffer and pipette the required amount.
7. Cover with aluminum foil. Incubate at 60° for 30 min with continuous agitation.
8. Cool. Add 10 ml of 0.350 M hydrochloric acid solution to adjust pH to 4.0 to 4.6.
9. Add 0.3 ml of amyloglucosidase solution.
10. Cover with aluminum foil. Incubate at 60°C for 30 min with continuous agitation.
11. Add 280 ml of 95% ethanol preheated to 60°C. Measure volume after heating.
12. Allow precipitate to form at room temperature for 60 min.
13. Tare crucible containing Celite to nearest 0.1 mg. After taring the crucible containing the Celite, redistribute the bed of Celite in the crucible using a stream of 78% ethanol from a wash bottle. Suction is then applied to the crucible to draw the Celite onto the fritted glass as an even mat. When the fiber is filtered, i.e., Step 14, the Celite effectively separates the fiber from the fritted glass of the crucible, allowing for easy removal of the crucible contents.
14. Filter enzyme digest from Step 12 through crucible.
15. Wash residue successively with three 20-ml portions of 78% ethanol, two 10-ml portions of 95% ethanol, and two 10-ml portions of acetone. With some samples a gum is formed, trapping the liquid. If the surface film that develops after the addition of the sample to the Celite is broken with a spatula, filtration is improved. Long filtration times can be avoided by careful intermittent suction throughout the filtration. Normal suction can be applied at washing. Back-bubbling of air is another way of speeding up filtrations, if available.
16. Dry crucible containing residue overnight in a 70°C vacuum oven or a 105°C air oven.
17. Cool in desiccator and weigh crucible, Celite, and residue to nearest 0.1 mg.
18. Analyze the residue from one sample of the set of duplicates for protein. Protein is probably most easily analyzed by carefully scraping the Celite and the fiber mat onto a suitable piece of filter paper which can then be folded shut and analyzed for protein. A piece of filter paper should be analyzed to assure that it will not affect the protein value obtained. Collaborators should use the Kjeldahl analysis as specified in "Official Methods of Analysis" of the AOAC. Use 6.25 for the protein factor.
19. Incinerate second sample of the duplicate for 5 h at 525°C.
20. Cool in desiccator. Weigh crucible containing Celite and ash to nearest 0.1 mg (See flow diagram in Figure 4 and formula for calculating "total dietary fiber" from the data in Figure 5.)

Sample preparation (10g), dry, pulverized and if more than 10% lipids
extracted with 25 mL petroleum ether to remove the lipids.

↓

Repeat extraction 2 times with 25 mL petroleum ether.
Weighing of duplicate samples, 1g.
Addition of 50 mL 0.08 M phosphate buffer, pH 6.0.
Addition of Termamyl for gelatinization, 100 μl.

↓

Incubation, boiling water bath, 15–30 min, shaking at 5 min intervals
Adjustment to pH 7.5 with 0.275 N NaOH.
Addition of Protease, 5 mg.

↓

Incubation, 60° C, 30 min, continuous agitation.
Adjustment to pH 4.5 with 10 mL 0.350 M hydrochloric acid.
Addition of Amyloglucosidase, 0.3 mL.
Incubation, 60 °C, 30 min, continuous agitation.
Addition of 280 mL, 95% ethanol, preheated to 60°C.

↓

Formation of precipitate, 60 min.

Filtration through bed containing
0.5 g Celite 545. Washing with three 20 mL
portions of 78% ethanol, two 10 mL portions of 95%
ethanol and two 10 mL portions of acetone.

↓

Drying of crucibles, 70°C vacuum oven or 105°C air oven, overnight.

Cooling and weighing of crucibles.

↙   ↘

Protein determination,   Ash determination
use entire crucible   525°C, 5 hrs.,
contents, Factor = 6.25   cool and weigh

Calculation of Total Dietary Fiber
TDF = weight of residue, minus weight of protein,
minus weight of ash, minus weight of blank

FIGURE 4. Sequences in the analysis of total dietary fiber by the official AOAC method.[24,25]

$$\% \text{ TDF} = \frac{\frac{R_1 + R_2}{2} - P - A - B}{\frac{M_1 + M_2}{2}} \times 100$$

TDF = Total Dietary Fiber
R_1 and R_2 = Residue weights (mg)
P = protein, A = ash, B = blank corrections (mg)
M_1 and M_2 = sample weights (mg)

FIGURE 5. Calculation of percentage dietary fiber from data obtained by official AOAC method.[24,25]

REFERENCES

1. **McCance, R. A., Widdowson, E. M., and Shackleton, L. R. B.**, The nutritive value of fruits, vegetables and nuts, *Med. Res. Counc. (G.B.) Spec. Rep. Serv.*, 213, 32, 1936.
2. **Katan, M. B. and van de Bovenkamp, P.**, Determination of total dietary fiber by difference and of pectin by colorimetry of copper titration, in *The Analysis of Dietary Fiber in Food*, James, W. P. T. and Theander, O., Eds., Marcel Dekker, New York, 1981, 217.
3. **Sandberg, A.-S., Hallgren, B., and Hasselblad, C.**, Analytical problems in the determination of dietary fibre, *Näringsforskning*, 4, 132, 1981.
4. **Weinstock, A. and Benham, G. H.**, The use of enzyme preparations in the crude fibre determination, *Cereal Chem.*, 28, 490, 1951.
5. **Asp, N.-G.**, Critical evaluation of some suggested methods for assay of dietary fibre, in *Dietary Fibre: Current Developments of Importance ot Health*, Heaton, K. W., Ed., John Libbey, London, 1978, 21.
6. **Asp, N.-G. and Johansson, C.-G.**, Techniques for measuring dietary fiber: principal aims of methods and a comparison of results obtained by different techniques, in *The Analysis of Dietary Fiber in Food*, James, W. P. T. and Theander, O., Eds., Marcel Dekker, New York, 1981, 173.
7. **Thomas, B.**, Enzymatische Rohfaserbestimmung in Getreideprodukten, *Getr. Mehl Brot.*, 29, 115, 1975.
8. **Elchazly, M. and Thomas, B.**, Über eine biochemische Methode zum Bestimmen der Ballaststoffe und ihrer Komponenten in pflanzlichen Lebensmitteln, *Z. Lebensm. Unters. Forsch.*, 162, 329, 1976.
9. **Hellendoorn, W., Noordhoff, M. G., and Slagman, J.**, Enzymatic determination of the indigestible residue of human food, *J. Sci. Food Agric.*, 26, 1461, 1975.
10. **Trowell, H. C.**, Crude fibre, dietary fibre and atherosclerosis, *Atherosclerosis*, 16, 138, 1972.
11. **Trowell, H. C.**, Definitions of fibre, *Lancet*, 1, 503, 1974.
12. **Asp, N-G., Johansson, C.-G., Hallmer, H., and Siljeström, M.**, Rapid enzymatic assay of insoluble and soluble dietary fiber, *J. Agric. Food Chem.*, 31, 476, 1983.
13. **Hellendoorn, E. W.**, Some critical observations in relation to 'dietary fibre', the methods for its determination and the current hypotheses for the explanation of its physiological action, *Voeding*, 39, 230, 1978.
14. **Saunders, R. M. and Betschart, A. A.**, The significance of protein as a component of dietary fiber, *Am. J. Clin. Nutr.*, 33, 965, 1980.
15. **Trowell, H., Southgate, D. A. T., Wolever, T. M. S., Leeds, A. R., Gassull, M. A., and Jenkins, D. A.**, Dietary fibre redefined, *Lancet*, 1, 967, 1976.
16. **Southgate, D. A. T., Hudson, G. J., and Englyst, H.**, The analysis of dietary fibre — the choices for the analyst, *J. Sci. Food Agric.*, 29, 979, 1978.
17. **Theander, O. and Åman, P.**, Studies on dietary fibres, *Swed. J. Agric. Res.*, 9, 97, 1979.
18. **Cummings, J. H.**, What is fiber?, in *Fiber in Human Nutrition*, Spiller, G. A. and Amen, R. J., Eds., Plenum Press, New York, 1976, 5.
19. **Furda, I.**, Fractionation and examination of biopolymers from dietary fiber, *Cereal Foods World*, 22, 252, 1977.

20. **Furda, I.**, Simultaneous analysis of soluble and insoluble dietary fiber, in *The Analysis of Dietary Fiber in Food*, James, W. P. T. and Theander, O., Eds., Marcell Dekker, 1981, 163.
21. **Schweizer, T. F. and Würsch, P.**, Analysis of dietary fibre, *J. Sci. Food Agric.*, 30, 613, 1979.
22. **Meuser, F., Suckow, P., and Kulikowski, W.**, Analytische Bestimmung von Ballaststoffen in Brot, Obst und Gemuse, *Getreide Mehl Brot.*, 37, 380, 1983.
23. **Prosky, L., Asp, N.-G., Furda, I., DeVries, J., Schweizer, T. F., and Harland, B.**, Determination of total dietary fiber in foods, food products and total diets: interlaboratory study, *J. Assoc. Off. Anal. Chem.*, 67, 1044, 1984.
24. **Prosky, L., Asp, N.-G., Furda, I., DeVries, J. W., Schweizer, T., and Harland, B.**, Determination of total dietary fiber in foods and food products: collaborative study, *J. Assoc. Off. Anal. Chem.*, 68, 677, 1985.
25. **Prosky, L., Asp, N.-G., Schweizer, T. F., DeVries, J. W., and Furda, I.**, Determination of insoluble soluble and total dietary fiber in foods and food products: interlaboratory study, *J. Assoc. Off. Anal. Chem.*, 71, 1017, 1988.
26. **Schweizer, T. F., Walter, E., and Venetz, P.**, Collaborative study for the enzymatic, gravimetric determination of total dietary fibre in foods, *Mitt. Geb. Lebensmittelunters. Hyg.*, 79, 57, 1988.
27. **Lee, S., Prosky, L., and DeVries, J.**, Determination of total, soluble, and insoluble dietary fiber in foods. Enzymatic-gravimetric method, MES-TRIS buffer: collaborative study, *J. Assoc. Off. Anal. Chem.*, 75, 395, 1992.
28. **Varo, P., Laine, R., and Koivistoinen, P.**, Effect of heat treatment on dietary fiber: interlaboratory study, *J. Assoc. Off. Agric. Chem.*, 66, 933, 1983.
29. **Johansson, C.-G., Siljeström, M., and Asp, N.-G.**, Dietary fibre in bread and corresponding flours — formation of resistant starch during baking, *Z. Lebensm. Unters. Forsch.*, 179, 24, 1984.
30. **Englyst, H. N., Anderson, V., and Cummings, J. H.**, Starch and non-starch polysaccharides in some cereal foods, *J. Sci. Food Agric.*, 34, 1434, 1983.
31. **Siljeström, M. and Asp, N.-G.**, Resistant starch formation during baking — effect of baking time and temperature and variations in the recipe, *Z. Lebensm. Unters. Forsch.*, 181, 4, 1985.
32. **Siljeström, M., Eliasson, A. C., and Björck, I.**, Characterization of resistant starch from autoclaved wheat starch, *Starch/Staerke*, 41, 147, 1989.
33. **Björck, I., Nyman, M., Pedersen, B., Siljeström, M., Asp, N.-G., and Eggum, B.**, On the digestibility of starch in wheat bread, *J. Cereal Sci.*, 4, 1, 1986.
34. **Schweizer, T. F., Andersson, H., Langkilde, A. M., Reimann, S., and Torsdottir, I.**, Nutrients excreted in ileostomy effluents after consumption of mixed diets with beans or potatoes. II. Starch, dietary fibre and sugars, *Eur. J. Clin. Nutr.*, 44, 567, 1990.
35. **Englyst, H. N. and Kingman, S. M.**, Dietary fiber and resistant starch. A nutritional classification of plant polysaccharides, in *Dietary Fiber*, Kritchevsky, D., Bonfield, C., and Anderson, J. W., Eds., Plenum, New York, 1990, 49.
36. **Jeraci, J. L., Lewis, B. A., Van Soest, R. J., and Robertsson, J. B.**, Urea enzymatic dialysis procedure for determination of total dietary fiber, *J. Assoc. Off. Anal. Chem.*, 72, 677, 1989.
37. **Asp, N.-G.**, Delimitation problems in definition and analysis of dietary fiber, in Furda, I. and Brine, C. J., Eds., *New Developments in Dietary Fiber*, Plenum Press, New York, 1990, 227.
38. **Schweizer, T. F., Frølich, W., DeVedovo, S., and Besson, R.**, Minerals and phytate in the analysis of dietary fiber from cereals. I, *Cereal Chem.*, 61, 116, 1984.
39. **Frølich, W., Asp, N.-G., and Schweizer, T. F.**, Minerals and phytate in the analysis of dietary fiber from cereals. II, *Cereal Chem.*, 61, 357, 1984.
40. **James, W. P. T. and Theander, O.**, Eds., *The Analysis of Dietary Fiber in Food*, Marcel Dekker, New York, 1981.
41. **Asp, N.-G., Schweizer, T. F., Southgate, D. A. T., and Theander, O.**, Dietary fiber analysis, in *Dietary Fibre — A Component of Food — Nutritional Function in Health and Disease*, Eastwood, M., Edwards, C., Mauron, J., and Schweizer, T., Eds., Springer, London, 1992, 57.
42. **Nishimune, T., Sumimoto, T., Yakusiji, T., Kunita, N., Ichikawa, T., Doguchi, M., and Nakahara, S.**, Determination of total dietary fiber in Japanese foods. *J. Assoc. Off. Anal. Chem.*, 74, 350, 1991.

Chapter 3.2

DETERGENT ANALYSIS OF FOODS

James B. Robertson and Peter J. Horvath

The use of detergents to isolate plant cell walls of low nitrogen content from forages was proposed in 1963. The detergent systems are neutral solutions of sodium lauryl sulfate[1] for cell wall analysis and an acidic medium containing cetyltrimethylammonium bromide for isolation of the less fermentable fraction of low hemicellulose content from forages.[2,3] Thus, the detergent system has a nutritional basis for the fractionation of food components.[4] The neutral detergent (ND) system has undergone many changes from its inception for use with ruminant forages to human foods. A major advantage of the ND procedure for dietary fiber analysis is that microbial material is soluble.[5] Fecal analysis by the detergent system is not complicated by microbial mass produced during colonic fermentation.[6] The primary drawback of ND is that soluble dietary fiber, primarily pectic substances and soluble hemicelluloses, is not recovered. However, they are normally totally digested.[7]

The original acid detergent (AD) system has not changed much for human food analysis. Baker[8] suggested buffering the AD (pH 1.5 to 2.0) to reduce cellulose loss. This buffered AD system recovered more material. However, some of this additional residue was hemicellulose[9] and pectic substances.[10] ADF has usually been used as a starting material for lignin determination; so hemicellulose should be removed to avoid the production of artifact lignin.[11] Pectin can also undergo Maillard reactions. Because of these problems, a preliminary extraction with ND before refluxing with AD has been suggested.[12,13] ADF has also been used to predict cell wall digestibility, and for this purpose removal of the insoluble hemicellulose and recovery of the AD-soluble cellulose may not be desirable.[14] These "celluloses" are easily fermentable and the linear hemicelluloses are of low fermentability.[15] The decision to obtain an ADF of low fermentability or an ADF composed of cellulose and lignin, free from hemicellulose, depends on how the ADF will be used.

A complex system of detergent extractions and subsequent hydrolysis and oxidation has been developed for a gravimetric component analysis of insoluble dietary fiber.[16] Figure 1 shows a flow diagram for this system. The classification of fiber components and how they can be determined is displayed in the center of Figure 1. Typically, the detergent system has been used as a gravimetric method. Sugar analysis of the NDF and ADF has been progressing.[17-19] One problem with a gravimetric method is that small samples or components in low concentration are difficult to weigh accurately. A semimicro method has been developed for samples of 0.2 g.[20] For very small samples, a sugar component analysis may be useful. Lignin is usually present in low amounts and can be assayed in other ways.

Other problems with the detergent systems include difficulty in starch removal, lipid and protein interference, and difficulty in filtration. Starch in low concentrations is solubilized in the ND, but certain types (modified or retrograded) and high concentrations can lead to filtration problems and an overestimation of dietary fiber (as currently defined). The problem of starch removal has been explored by many workers. In most cases treatment during ND extraction with an amylase from *Bacillus subtilis* is adequate.[6,21] Other procedures have been compared by Mascarenhas-Ferreira et al.[22] Some studies suggested a mammalian or fungal enzyme and a protease, but Marlett and Lee[23] found little difference in results from these methods. They found that temperature, not the length of incubation, is most important. Heat-stable bacterial amylase might be the fastest and easiest.[24,25]

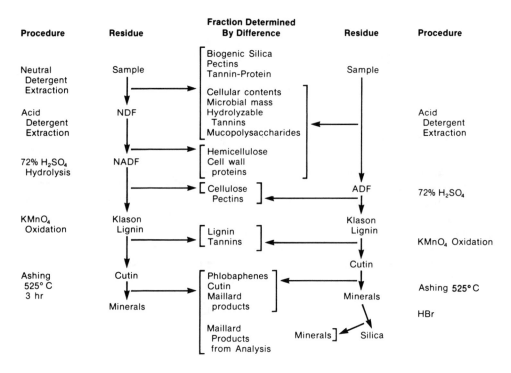

FIGURE 1. Flow diagram for fiber analysis by the detergent system. (The quantity of each fraction is measured as either the amount of residue or the weight loss after each procedure. The materials measured by weight loss are shown in brackets.)

Difficulty with filtration can also occur when other polysaccharides such as β-glucan are present. β-Glucanase has been used to remove these glucans.[26] This may not be desirable because β-glucans are included in the dietary fiber complex as water-soluble unavailable carbohydrates.

Lipids and proteins interfere when in amounts that exceed the capacity of the reagents. The limits are about 10% of dry matter for lipid and 30% for protein. Preextraction with ethanol or ether will remove lipids. Detergent-stable proteases are available to hydrolyze protein for removal.

The sample is usually dried before it is ground. Both drying and particle size can affect the values. Heller et al.[27] found that as particle size was decreased, NDF decreased with other fractions varying nonuniformly. Drying above 60°C or in a microwave oven can increase NDF, ADF, and lignin values.[28,29] Freeze-drying may be the optimum way to dry the sample for grinding.

The reagents used for detergent extractions have undergone important changes since 1970.[14] Cellosolve (2-ethoxy ethanol) is an eye and mucous membrane irritant and could adversely affect the kidneys, liver, and central nervous system. It has the potential to cause adverse reproductive effects in males and females and embryotoxic effects including teratogenesis in the offspring of the exposed, pregnant female. *Consequently, 2-ethoxy ethanol should no longer be used in the neutral detergent solution.* Since cellosolve was included in the original reagent because it facilitates the solution of starch, it can be omitted if only forages are being analyzed. However, in starch containing feeds and foods, a volume for volume substitution of cellosolve with triethylene glycol produces identical analytical values. Decalin has been omitted from both detergent solutions to eliminate filtering problems and the consequent high fiber values. Sulfite, which was used to reduce the nitrogen content of the NDF, has been shown to cause a significant loss of lignin[21] and should be omitted in sequential analysis. The permanganate solution is essentially unchanged.[3] If a detailed analysis of the ADF is done, it is recommended that hydrolysis with 72% H_2SO_4 without the use of asbestos[30] be carried out before lignin oxidation. Cutin can be determined as the residue lost upon ashing.[14]

Detailed instructions and procedures are described in Robertson and Van Soest[16] and Van Soest et al.[25] A summary of total dietary fiber and detergent values is given in Table 2 of the Appendix.

REFERENCES

1. **Van Soest, P. J.**, Use of detergents in the analysis of fibrous feeds. I. Preparation of fiber residues of low nitrogen content, *J. Assoc. Off. Agric. Chem.*, 46, 825, 1963.
2. **Van Soest, P. J.**, Use of detergents in the analysis of fibrous feeds. II. A rapid method for the determination of fiber and lignin, *J. Assoc. Off. Agric. Chem.*, 46, 829, 1963.
3. **Van Soest, P. J. and Wine, R. H.**, Use of detergents in the analysis of fibrous feed. IV. Determination of plant cell-wall constituents, *J. Assoc. Off. Anal. Chem.*, 50, 50, 1967.
4. **Robertson, J. B.**, The detergent system of fiber analysis, in *Topics in Dietary Fiber Research*, Spiller, G. A. and Amen, R., Eds., Plenum Press, New York, 1978, 1.
5. **Mason, V. C.**, Some observations on the distribution and origin of nitrogen in sheep feces, *J. Agric. Sci. Camb.*, 73, 99, 1969.
6. **McQueen, R. E. and Nicholson, J. W. G.**, Modification of the neutral-detergent fiber procedure for cereals and vegetables by using alpha-amylase, *J. Assoc. Off. Anal. Chem.*, 62, 676, 1979.
7. **Cummings, J. H., Southgate, D. A. T., Branch, W. J., Wiggins, H. S., Houston, D. J. A., and Jenkins, D.**, Digestion of pectin in the human gut and its effect on calcium absorption and large bowel function, *Br. J. Nutr.*, 41, 477, 1979.
8. **Baker, D.**, Determining fiber in cereals, *Cereal Chem.*, 54, 360, 1977.
9. **Morrison, I. M.**, Hemicellulose contamination of acid detergent residues and their replacement by cellulose residues in cell wall analysis, *J. Sci. Food Agric.*, 31, 639, 1980.
10. **Belo, P. S., Jr. and De Lumen, B. O.**, Pectic substance content of detergent-extracted dietary fibers, *J. Agric. Food Chem.*, 29, 370, 1981.
11. **Goering, H. K., Van Soest, P. J., and Hemken, R. W.**, Relative susceptibility of forages to heat damage as affected by moisture temperature and pH, *J. Dairy Sci.*, 56, 137, 1973.
12. **Bailey, R. W. and Ulyatt, M. J.**, Pasture quality and ruminant nutrition. II. Carbohydrate and lignin composition of detergent-extracted residues from pasture grasses and legumes, *N.Z. J. Agric. Res.*, 13, 591, 1970.
13. **Testolin, G., Bossi, E., Vercesi, P., Porrini, M., Simonetti, P., and Ciappellano, S.**, A rapid method for the analysis of alimentary fiber, *Nutr. Rep. Int.*, 25, 859, 1982.
14. **Goering, H. K. and Van Soest, P. J.**, Forage fiber analysis (apparatus, reagents, procedures and some applications), Agricultural Handbook 379, U.S. Department of Agriculture, Washington, D.C., 1970.
15. **Gaillard, B. D. E.**, The relationship between the cell-wall constituents of roughages and the digestibility of the organic matter, *J. Agric. Sci. Camb.*, 59, 369, 1962.
16. **Robertson, J. B. and Van Soest, P. J.**, The detergent system of analysis and its application to human foods, in *The Analysis of Dietary Fiber in Foods*, James, W. P. T. and Theander, O., Eds., Marcel Dekker, New York, 1981, 123.
17. **Bittner, A. S. and Street, J. C.**, Monosaccharide composition of alcohol- and detergent-insoluble residues in maturing reed canary grass leaves, *J. Agric. Food Chem.*, 31, 7, 1983.
18. **Slavin, J. L. and Marlett, J. A.**, Evaluation of high-performance liquid chromatography for measurement of the neutral saccharides in neutral-detergent fiber, *J. Agric. Food Chem.*, 31, 467, 1983.
19. **Windham, W. R., Barton, F. E., and Himmelsbach, D. S.**, High pressure liquid chromatographic analysis of component sugars in neutral-detergent fiber for representative warm- and cool-season grasses, *J. Agric. Food Chem.*, 31, 471, 1983.
20. **Sills, V. E. and Wallace, G. M.**, A semi-micro neutral-detergent fiber method for cereal products, in *Fiber in Human and Animal Nutrition*, Bulletin 10, Royal Society of New Zealand, Wellington, N.Z., 1983, 116.

21. **Robertson, J. B. and Van Soest, P. J.,** Dietary fiber estimation in concentrated feedstuffs, *J. Anim. Sci.,* 45(Suppl. 1), 254 (Abstr.), 1977.
22. **Mascarenhas-Ferreira, A., Kerstens, J., and Gasp, C. H.,** The study of several modifications of the neutral-detergent fibre procedure, *Anim. Feed Sci. Technol.,* 9, 19, 1983.
23. **Marlett, J. A. and Lee, S. C.,** Dietary fiber, lignocellulose and hemicellulose contents of selected foods determined by modified and unmodified Van Soest procedures, *J. Food Sci.,* 45, 1688, 1980.
24. **Jeraci, J. L., Hernandez, T. H., Lewis, B. A., Robertson, J. B., and Van Soest, P. J.,** New and improved procedure for neutral-detergent fiber, *J. Anim. Sci.,* 66(Suppl. 1), 351 (Abstr.), 1988.
25. **Van Soest, P. J., Robertson, J. B., and Lewis, B. A.,** Methods for dietary fiber, neutral detergent fiber, and nonstarch polysaccharides in relation to animal nutrition, *J. Dairy Sci.,* 74, 3583, 1991.
26. **Roth, N. J. L., Watts, G. H., and Newman, C. W.,** Beta-glucanase as an aid in measuring neutral-detergent fiber in barley kernels, *Cereal Chem.,* 58, 245, 1981.
27. **Heller, S. N., Rivers, J. M., and Hackler, L. R.,** Dietary fiber: effect of particle size and pH on its measurement, *J. Food Sci.,* 42, 436, 1977.
28. **Van Soest, P. J.,** Use of detergents in analysis of fibrous feeds. III. Study of effects of heating and drying on yield of fiber and lignin in forages, *J. Assoc. Off. Agric. Chem.,* 48, 785, 1965.
29. **Darrah, C. H., Van Soest, P. J., and Fick, G. W.,** Microwave treatment and heat damage artifacts in forages, *Agron. J.,* 69, 120, 1977.
30. **Van Soest, P. J.,** Collaborative study of acid-detergent fiber and lignin, *J. Assoc. Off. Anal. Chem.,* 56, 781, 1973.

Chapter 3.3

DIETARY FIBER AND STARCH: CLASSIFICATION AND MEASUREMENT

Hans N. Englyst and Geoffrey J. Hudson

INTRODUCTION

A wide variety of beneficial effects to health have been attributed to a diet rich in unrefined plant foods. Some of these effects are related to dietary fiber and some are related to starch or to the interaction between these components. Dietary fiber was used as a shorthand term for the plant cell-wall material removed during refining. The principal constituents (approximately 90%) are polysaccharides that do not contain alpha-glucosidic linkages and can therefore be measured as nonstarch polysaccharides (NSP). In contrast, the storage polysaccharide starch is an alpha-linked glucan. Dietary fiber and starch are chemically distinct compounds, have very different physiological roles, and should always be measured separately. This is in agreement with the original concept of dietary fiber. In 1985 Trowell stated in his comment on definitions that "Derived from plant cell walls and not digested by human alimentary enzymes, starch was excluded from all these definitions and was never named at that time or subsequently as a constituent of dietary fiber", and he concluded,[1] "At the present time there is considerable international agreement concerning the principal constituents of dietary fiber. They are all polysaccharides, mainly cellulose, hemicelluloses and pectic substances, conveniently designated non-starch polysaccharides."

Definitions intended for the measurement of cell-wall polysaccharides, however, have been widely misinterpreted, which has led to the development of methods that include a wide range of noncell-wall components as dietary fiber. Some methods, such as the AOAC Prosky technique,[2] include retrograded starch and other substances formed during food processing. However, the starch included as dietary fiber in these methods does not reflect the amount of starch resisting digestion in the small intestine of man.[3]

It is, to a large extent, in the hands of the food industry to control the formation of retrograded starch and other substances measured as dietary fiber by the Prosky procedure. It is, in fact, possible to produce a "high-fiber" food that contains no cell-wall material.

It is not surprising that there is growing unease with the term dietary fiber. The British Nutrition Foundation recommend that scientists stop using the term and replace it with NSP.[4] WHO recommendations for dietary intakes are expressed as NSP,[5] and the word fiber is no longer used in the U.S. Department of Health and Human Services dietary guidelines.[6]

In this chapter, analytical procedures are given for the measurement of dietary fiber as nonstarch polysaccharides. Starch resisting digestion in the small intestine of man is not part of dietary fiber, but it is an important food component. On the basis of a series of studies in man we have proposed a classification of starch into three broad categories for nutritional purposes: rapidly digestible starch (RDS); slowly digestible starch (SDS); and resistant starch (RS), where RS includes all the starch resisting digestion in the small intestiine of man.

DIETARY FIBER

The Choice of Method

Any method intended to measure dietary fiber should, for the reasons already discussed, be a good index of plant cell-wall material. Two main methods for the determination of

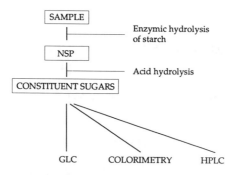

FIGURE 1. The flow diagram illustrates the analytical pathway followed in the Englyst procedure for the measurement of NSP.

dietary fiber have emerged; they adopt contrasting approaches and include different components of the diet. The enzymic chemical method of Englyst et al.[3,7] measures NSP. The enzymic gravimetric method of Prosky et al.[2] measures the weight of the residue remaining after treatment with various enzymes. Neither of the two methods measures all the components of the cell-wall material or attempts to do so. The question then is which method represents the best index of cell-wall material.

Values obtained by the gravimetric procedure are, in general, higher than those obtained by the Englyst procedure. The main reasons are that the gravimetric technique includes some retrograded starch and other substances formed during food processing (see later). The inclusion of such materials means that the values obtained by the gravimetric procedure are not suitable as an index of cell-wall material, especially in processed foods. The measurement of NSP, however, is independent of food processing and therefore represents a good index of cell-wall material in both raw and processed foods. In 1987 it was proposed by Englyst, Trowell, Southgate, and Cummings that dietary fiber should be defined for the purpose of food labeling as NSP.[8]

Measurement of Dietary Fiber as Nonstarch Polysaccharides (NSP)

Principle and Application

The Englyst procedure (Figure 1) measures dietary fiber as NSP, using enzymic chemical methods, —and has evolved from the principles laid down by Southgate in 1969.[9,10]

In the Englyst procedure, starch is completely removed enzymically and NSP measured as the sum of the constituent sugars released by acid hydrolysis. The sugars may be measured by gas liquid chromatography (GLC), giving values for individual monosaccharides or, more rapidly, by colorimetry.[3,7] A value is obtained for total and, if required, for soluble and insoluble NSP. A small modification allows cellulose to be measured separately.

The procedure allows measurement of NSP within an 8-h working day by the colorimetric version and within 1.5 d with the GLC version. It is virtually a single tube procedure and no special skill or equipment, other than a colorimeter or spectrophotometer, is needed for the colorimetric version.

The methods have been used successfully for the analysis of a very wide range of foods.[11,12] The information obtained by the GLC procedure (Table 1) is valuable for interpreting the results of physiological and epidemiological studies where disease may be related to the type of dietary fiber. When detailed information is not required, however, values for NSP can be obtained by colorimetry. In a comparative study of a wide range of food products, good agreement was found between the GLC and colorimetric versions of the Englyst procedure.[13] Recently, we have shown that the constituent sugars of NSP can be measured by high pressure liquid chromatography (HPLC).[14]

ENGLYST PROCEDURE FOR MEASUREMENT OF DIETARY FIBER AS NSP

The procedure as described here provides the following options:

1. GLC procedure. Measure NSP as the sum of neutral sugars obtained by GLC and uronic acids measured separately. Follow Steps 1 through 8.
2. Colorimetric procedure. Measure NSP as reducing sugars. Follow Steps 1 through 5, and Step 9.
3. Colorimetric procedure with separate measurement of uronic acids. Measure NSP as reducing sugars and correct for uronic acids measured separately. Follow Steps 1 through 5, and Steps 7, 9, and 10.

REAGENTS

High-purity reagents should be used throughout the method. Use distilled water or water of equivalent purity.

Reagents Common to the GLC and Colorimetric Procedures

- *Dimethylphenol solution.*
  Dissolve 0.1 g of 3,5-dimethylphenol, $(CH_3)_2C_6H_3OH$, in 100 ml of glacial acetic acid.
- *Sodium acetate buffer (0.1 M, pH 5.2).*
  Dissolve 13.6 g of sodium acetate trihydrate, $CH_3COONa \cdot 3H_2O$, and make to a final volume of 1 l with water. Adjust to pH 5.2 with 0.1 M acetic acid. To stabilize and activate enzymes, add 4 ml of 1 M calcium chloride to 1 l of buffer.
- *Sulfuric acid (12 M).*
  Accurately measure 280 ml of water into a 2-l beaker of good quality. Place the beaker into a bowl of ice water in a fume-cupboard and slowly add 390 ml of concentrated sulfuric acid, with stirring. N.B. Caution should be taken in making this reagent.
- *Enzyme solution I.*
  Take 2.5 ml of Termamyl (Novo Industri, Copenhagen, Denmark), make to 200 ml with the preequilibrated sodium acetate buffer, mix, and keep it in a 50°C water bath.
- *Enzyme solution II.*
  Take 1.2 g of pancreatin (Paynes and Byrne Ltd., Greenford, Middlesex, U.K.) into a 50-ml tube, add 12 ml of water, vortex mix initially, and then mix for 10 min with a magnetic stirrer. Vortex mix again, then centrifuge for 10 min. Take 10 ml of the (cloudy) supernatant, add 2.5 ml of pullulanase (Novo Industri, Copenhagen, Denmark), and vortex mix. Prepare the solution immediately before use and keep it at room temperature. (When using the option of overnight incubation, either 2.5 ml of pullulanase from Boehringer (catalog number 108944) diluted 1:100 or 2.5 ml of pullulanase from Novo Industri diluted 1:25 is used.)

TABLE 1
Nonstarch Polysaccharides (NSP) in Some Plant Products

		Total (g/100 g fresh weight)	Total (g/100 g dry weight)	Composition (g/100 g dry weight)								
				Cellulose	Noncellulosic polysaccharides							
					Rha	Fuc	Ara	Xyl	Man	Gal	Glu	U.Ac.
Plain white flour	Soluble NSP	1.6	18.	—	t	t	0.6	0.7	t	0.2	0.3	t
	Insoluble NSP	1.6	1.8	0.1	t	t	0.6	0.8	0.1	t	0.2	t
	Total NSP	3.2	3.6	0.1	t	t	1.2	1.5	0.1	0.2	0.5	t
Wheat flour, whole	Soluble NSP	2.5	2.8	—	t	t	0.8	1.3	0.1	0.2	0.3	0.1
	Insoluble NSP	7.2	8.1	1.6	t	t	2.3	3.3	t	0.1	0.6	0.2
	Total NSP	9.7	10.9	1.6	t	t	3.1	4.6	0.1	0.3	0.9	0.3
Rye flour, whole	Soluble NSP	3.9	4.5	—	t	t	1.4	2.1	0.1	0.1	0.7	0.1
	Insoluble NSP	7.8	9.0	1.4	t	t	2.2	3.6	0.2	0.2	1.3	0.1
	Total NSP	11.7	13.5	1.4	t	t	3.6	5.7	0.3	0.3	2.0	0.2
Porridge oats	Soluble NSP	3.6	4.0	—	t	t	0.2	0.2	t	0.1	3.4	0.1
	Insoluble NSP	2.8	3.1	0.3	t	t	0.7	1.0	0.1	0.1	0.8	0.1
	Total NSP	6.4	7.1	0.3	t	t	0.9	1.2	0.1	0.2	4.2	0.2
Cornflakes, Kellogg's	Soluble NSP	0.4	0.4	—	t	t	t	t	t	t	0.1	0.1
	Insoluble NSP	0.5	0.5	0.3	t	t	0.1	0.2	t	t	t	t
	Total NSP	0.9	0.9	0.3	t	t	0.1	0.3	t	t	0.1	0.1
Rice, white	Soluble NSP	—	t	—	t	t	t	t	t	t	t	t
	Insoluble NSP	0.4	0.5	0.2	t	t	0.1	0.1	t	t	0.1	t
	Total NSP	0.4	0.5	0.2	t	t	0.1	0.1	t	t	0.1	t
Apples, Cox	Soluble NSP	0.9	5.8	—	0.2	0.1	1.2	0.1	t	0.3	0.1	3.8
	Insoluble NSP	1.1	7.5	4.4	0.1	0.1	0.9	0.7	0.3	0.6	0.1	0.3
	Total NSP	2.0	13.3	4.4	0.3	0.2	2.1	0.8	0.3	0.9	0.2	4.1

						Rha	Fuc	Ara	Xyl	Man	Gal	Glu	U.Ac
Oranges	Soluble NSP	1.4	9.8	—	0.3	t	1.9	0.1	0.1	1.4	0.1	5.9
	Insoluble NSP	0.7	5.2	3.4	t	t	0.3	0.5	0.3	0.4	t	0.3
	Total NSP	2.1	15.0	3.4	0.3	t	2.2	0.6	0.4	1.8	0.1	6.2
Beans, French, cooked	Soluble NSP	1.3	12.7	—	0.2	t	1.1	0.2	0.1	2.6	0.1	8.3
	Insoluble NSP	1.8	17.7	11.1	0.1	t	1.2	1.5	1.2	1.5	0.5	0.6
	Total NSP	3.1	30.4	11.1	0.3	t	2.3	1.7	1.4	4.1	0.6	8.9
Beans, Haricot, cooked	Soluble NSP	3.7	9.1	—	0.2	0.4	4.3	0.8	0.2	0.8	0.4	2.0
	Insoluble NSP	4.6	11.2	5.1	0.1	t	3.1	1.4	0.1	0.3	t	1.1
	Total NSP	8.3	20.3	5.1	0.3	0.4	7.4	2.2	0.3	1.1	0.4	3.1
Cabbage, Winter	Soluble NSP	0.9	15.8	—	1.1	0.2	3.2	t	0.1	2.2	t	9.0
	Insoluble NSP	1.1	18.5	12.5	0.1	t	1.3	1.6	0.7	1.5	0.2	0.6
	Total NSP	2.0	34.3	12.5	1.2	0.2	4.5	1.6	0.8	3.7	0.2	9.6
Carrots, raw	Soluble NSP	1.4	11.4	—	0.7	t	1.7	t	0.1	3.0	t	5.9
	Insoluble NSP	1.0	8.1	6.4	t	t	0.3	0.3	0.3	0.4	0.1	0.3
	Total NSP	2.4	19.5	6.4	0.7	t	2.0	0.3	0.4	3.4	0.1	6.2

Note: Rha = Rhamnose; Fuc = Fucose; Ara = Arabinose; Xyl = Xylose; Man = Mannose; Gal = Galactose; Glu = Glucose; U.Ac. = Uronic acid.

Reagents Used Only in the GLC Procedure

- *Ammonium hydroxide/sodium borohydride solution.*
  A solution of 2 M ammonium hydroxide, containing 200 mg of sodium borohydride, $NaBH_4$, per ml. Prepare immediately before use.
- *Bromophenol blue solution, 0.04% (w/v).*
- *GLC Internal standard solution, 1 mg/ml.*
  Weigh 500 mg of allose (dried to constant weight under reduced pressure with phosphorus pentoxide) to the nearest 0.1 mg. Make to 500 ml with 50% saturated benzoic acid to give a 1 mg/ml solution. Stable for several months at room temperature.
- *Stock sugar mixture for calibration for GLC.*
  Accurately weigh, to the nearest 0.1 mg, 520 mg of rhamnose, 480 mg of fucose, 4750 mg of arabinose, 4450 mg of xylose, 2300 mg of mannose, 2820 mg of galactose, 9400 mg of glucose, and 2790 mg of galacturonic acid. Place them in a 1-l volumetric flask, dissolve them in, and make to the mark with 50% saturated benzoic acid.

Reagents Used Only in the Colorimetric Procedure

- *Stock sugar solution for colorimetry.*
  Make a stock sugar solution as follows. Accurately weigh 13.72 g of arabinose, 6.86 g of glucose, and 2.94 g of galacturonic acid, and transfer them to a 1-l volumetric flask. Dissolve the sugars in and make to the mark with 50% saturated benzoic acid.
- *Color reagent.*
  Dissolve 10 g of 3,5-dinitrosalicylic acid, 16 g of sodium hydroxide, and 300 g of sodium/potassium tartrate in water and make to a final volume of 1 l. Store in a well-capped dark bottle, and keep for 2 days before use. Stable at room temperature for at least 6 months.

THE PROCEDURE

Step 1. Sample Preparation

All samples should be finely divided so that representative subsamples may be taken. Foods with a low water content (<10%) may be milled, and foods with a higher water content may be homogenized wet or milled after freeze-drying. Two portions, (a) and (b), of each sample are required to obtain separate values for total, insoluble, and soluble NSP. Portion (a) is used to measure total NSP; portion (b) is used to measure insoluble NSP. Soluble NSP is determined as the difference. The two portions are treated identically throughout the procedure, except for their separate treatment in Steps 3 and 4.

Step 1.1

Sample weight. Weigh, to the nearest 0.1 mg, between 50 and 1000 mg depending on the water and NSP content of the sample (to give not more than 300 mg of dry matter, e.g., 300 mg is adequate for most dried foods) into 50- to 60-ml screw-top glass tubes. Add 300 (+/−20) mg of sand (low in iron, about 40- to 100-mesh; BDH, Poole, Dorset) and a magnetic stirrer to each. If the sample is dry (85 to 100% dry matter) and contains less than 5% fat, proceed to Step 2; otherwise, go to Step 1.2

Step 1.2

Add 40 ml of acetone, cap the tubes, and mix for 30 min using a magnetic stirrer. Centrifuge at 1000 g to obtain a clear supernatant liquid (5 to 10 min) and remove by aspiration as much of the supernatant liquid as possible without disturbing the residue. Place the tube in a beaker of water at 80°C on a hotplate-stirrer and mix the residue until dry. Either use a fume-cupboard or the beaker may be covered and the acetone vapor removed with a water pump.

Step 2. Dispersion and Enzymic Hydrolysis
Step 2.1

Add 2 ml of dimethyl sulfoxide (DMSO) to the dry sample, cap the tube, and *immediately* mix the contents using a vortex mixer. It is essential that all the sample is wetted and no material is encapsulated or adhering to the tube wall before proceeding. Vortex mix 3 or 4 times during a 5-min period.

Vortex mix and immdiately place 2 tubes in a boiling water bath. Remove after 20 s, vortex mix, and immediately replace the tubes in the bath. Repeat this for subsequent pairs of tubes until all the tubes have been placed in the bath; leave them for 30 min. During this period, prepare enzyme solutions I and II (the volumes given are suitable for 24 samples) if you wish to proceed with the 50-min incubation or enzyme solution II only if you prefer the overnight incubation (see below). Proceed to the 50-min incubation (Step 2.2) or the overnight incubation (Step 2.3).

Step 2.2

The 50 min incubation. Remove *one tube at a time,* vortex mix, uncap, and *immediately* add 8 ml of enzyme solution I (kept at 50°C), cap the tube, vortex mix thoroughly, ensuring that no material adheres to the tube wall, and replace in the boiling water bath. Leave the tubes there for 10 min, timed from the last addition of enzyme.

Transfer the rack of tubes to the 50°C water bath. After 3 min, add 0.5 ml of enzyme solution II to each tube and mix the contents thoroughly to aid distribution of the enzyme throughout the sample. Replace the tubes in the 50°C water bath and leave them there for 30 min. Mix the contents of each tube continuously or after 10 min, 20 min, and 30 min. Transfer the rack of tubes to the boiling water bath and leave them there for 10 min. Cool the samples by placing in water at room temperature.

Step 2.3

The overnight incubation. Remove one tube at a time from the boiling water bath, vortex mix, uncap, and *immediately* add 8 ml of sodium acetate buffer (preequilibrated at 50°C). Cap the tube, vortex mix thoroughly, ensuring that no material adheres to the tube wall. Place the tubes in a water bath at 42 ± 2°C for 3 min, and then add 0.5 ml of enzyme solution II. Vortex mix and incubate at 42 ± 2°C (water bath or oven) for 16 to 18 h. Mix the contents of each tube continuously or after 15 and 30 min as a minimum.

Step 3. Precipitation and Washing of the Residue for Measurement of Total NSP
Only sample portion (a) is given this treatment.

Step 3.1

Add 40 ml of absolute ethanol and mix well by repeated inversion, then leave in ice water for 30 min. Centrifuge at 1500 g for 10 min to obtain a clear supernatant liquid. Remove by aspiration as much of the supernatant liquid as possible, without disturbing the residue, and discard it.

Step 3.2

Add approximately 10 ml of 85% (v/v) ethanol and vortex mix. Make to 50 ml with 85% ethanol, mix by inversion, then use a magnetic stirrer to form a suspension of the residue. Centrifuge and remove the supernatant liquid as above. Repeat this stage using 50 ml of absolute ethanol.

Step 3.3

Add 20 ml of acetone to the residue and vortex mix, then use a magnetic stirrer to form a suspension. Centrifuge and remove the supernatant liquid as above.

Step 3.4

Place the tube in a beaker of water at 80°C on a hotplate-stirrer and mix the residue until dry. (It is essential that the residue and tube are completely free of acetone.) Either use a fume-cupboard, or the beaker may be covered and the acetone vapor removed with a water pump (If aggregation occurs during drying, disperse the sample using a vortex mixer. This is best done before the sample is completely dry.)

Step 4. Extraction and Washing of the Residue for Measurement of Insoluble NSP
Only sample portion (b) is given this treatment.

Step 4.1

After the treatment with enzyme in Step 2, add 40 ml of 0.2 M sodium phosphate buffer pH7. Place the capped tubes in a boiling water bath for 30 min. Mix continuously or 3 times during this period. Remove the tubes to water at room temperature and leave for 10 min. Centrifuge and remove the supernatant liquid as described in Step 3.1.

Step 4.2

Add approximately 10 ml of water and vortex mix. Make to 50 ml with water, mix by inversion, then use a magnetic stirrer to form a suspension of the residue. Centrifuge and remove the supernatant liquid as above. Repeat this stage using 50 ml of absolute ethanol. Proceed as described for Steps 3.3 and 3.4

Step 5. Acid Hydrolysis of the Residue from Enzymic Digestion
Step 5.1

Add 5 ml of 12 M sulfuric acid to the dry residue and immediately vortex mix. It is essential to ensure that all the material is wetted. Leave the tubes at 35°C for 1 h with occasional or continuous mixing to disperse the cellulose.

Add 25 ml of water rapidly and vortex mix. Place into a boiling water bath and leave for 1 h, timed from when boiling recommences; stir continuously or once after 10 min. Cool the tubes in tap water.

The sugars in the hydrolysate may be measured as individual monosaccharides by GLC and separate measurement of uronic acids or as total reducing sugars by colorimetry. Details of the GLC and colorimetric measurements are given here. The measurement of neutral sugars and uronic acids by HPLC is described in detail elsewhere.[14]

Step 5.2

Modification allowing separate measurement of cellulose and noncellulosic polysaccharides (NCP). Weigh a third portion, (c), of sample in Step 1.1 and treat it as described for portion (a) in Steps 1 through 4. Add 30 ml of 2 M sulfuric acid and mix. Place in a boiling water bath and leave for 1 h, timed from when boiling recommences, stirring continuously or after 10 min.

A value for cellulose may be obtained as the difference between glucose (measured by GLC or by glucose oxidase) for sample portions (a) and (c). NCP is calculated as the difference between total NSP and cellulose.

Now go to Steps 6 and 7 for the measurement of the individual NSP constituents or to Step 9 for the colorimetric measurement of NSP constituents as reducing sugars.

Step 6. Measurement of Neutral NSP Constituents by GLC (Figure 2)

Step 6.1

Standard sugar mixture. Mix 2000 µl of the stock sugar solution and 10 ml of 2.4 M sulfuric acid. Treat 3 ml of this standard sugar mixture for calibration of GLC in parallel with the samples in Step 6.2.

Step 6.2

Prepare the alditol acetate derivatives for chromatography as follows. Add 1000 µl of internal standard (1 mg allose/ml) to 3000 µl of the cooled hydrolysates from Step 5 and to 3000 µl of the standard sugar mixture from Step 6.1; vortex mix.

Place the tubes in ice water, add 1 ml of 12.5 M ammonium hydroxide, and vortex mix. Test that the solution is alkaline (add a little more ammonium hydroxide if necessary), then add approximately 5 µl of the antifoam agent octan-2-ol and 0.2 ml of the ammonium hydroxide/sodium borohydride solution; vortex mix.

Leave the tubes in a heating block or in a water bath at 40°C for 30 min then remove and add 0.4 ml of glacial acetic acid; mix again. Remove 0.5 ml to a 30-ml glass tube and add 0.5 ml of 1-methylimidazole and 5 ml of acetic anhydride. Vortex mix then leave for 10 min.

Add 0.9 ml of absolute ethanol, vortex mix, and leave for 5 min. Add 10 ml of water, vortex mix, and leave for 5 min. Add 0.5 ml of bromophenol blue solution. Place the tubes in ice water and add 5 ml of 7.5 M potassium hydroxide; a few minutes later add a further 5 ml of 7.5 M potassium hydroxide, cap the tubes, and mix by inversion.

Leave until the separation into two phases is complete (10 to 15 min) or centrifuge for a few minutes. Draw the upper phase into the tip of an automatic pipette; if any of the blue phase is included, allow it to separate then run it out of the tip before transferring the upper phase alone to a small (auto-injector) vial.

Step 6.3

Carry out conventional GLC measurement of the neutral sugars. Inject 0.5 to 1 µl of the alditol acetate derivatives prepared in Step 6.2.

GLC conditions

Injector temperature	275°C
Column temperature	220°C
Detector temperature	275°C
Carrier gas	Helium, 8 ml/min

Under these conditions, a GLC chromatograph fitted with a flame ionization detector and, preferably, an auto-injector and computing integrator, using a Supelco SP-2330 wide-bore capillary column (30 m × 0.75 mm: Supelco lot no. 2-3751), will allow accurate determination of the individual sugars in the standard sugar mixture within 8 min. For calibration, use the following ratio for the combination of the standard sugar mixture and internal standard (see Step 6.2):

DETERMINATION OF TOTAL, SOLUBLE AND INSOLUBLE DIETARY FIBRE BY THE ENGLYST GLC PROCEDURE

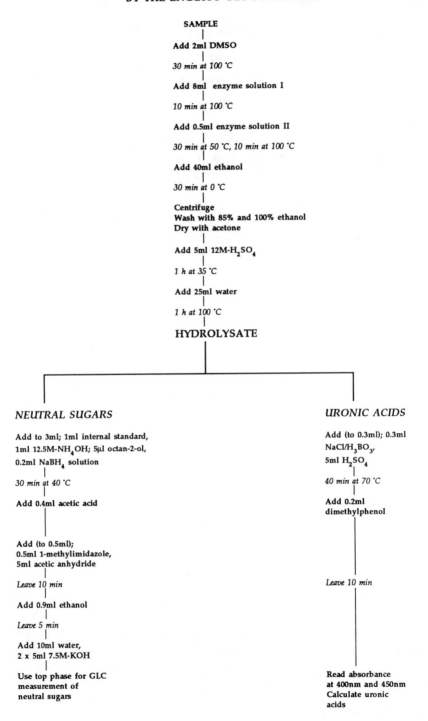

FIGURE 2. Total DF = neutral sugars + uronic acids. Soluble DF = total DF − insoluble DF. For measurement of insoluble dietary fiber, replace the 40 ml of ethanol with 40 ml of pH 7 buffer and extract for 0.5 h at 100°C.

	Sugar mixture (mg/l)	Recovery (%)	Calibration ratio[a]
Rhamnose	520	52	2
Fucose	480	96	1
Arabinose	4750	95	10
Xylose	4450	89	10
Mannose	2300	92	5
Galactose	2820	94	6
Galacturonic acid	2790	93	
Internal standard			
Allose	0	—	4

[a] By using these values, corrections are made for incomplete recovery of NSP constituents.

Step 6.4

Calculation of neutral sugars. The amount of individual sugars (in g/100 g of sample) is calculated as:

$$\frac{A_T \times W_I \times 100 \times R_F}{A_I \times W_T} \times 0.89$$

where A_T and A_I are the peak areas of the sample and the internal standard, respectively; W_T is the weight (in mg) of the sample; W_I is the weight (in mg; here 10 mg) of the internal standard; R_F is the response factor for individual sugars obtained from the calibration run with the sugar mixture treated in parallel with the samples; and 0.89 is a scale factor for converting the experimentally determined values for monosaccharides to polysaccharides.

Step. 7. Measurement of Uronic Acids (Figure 2)

Step 7.1

Make the standard solutions as follows. The standard sugar mixture in 2 M sulfuric acid prepared as described in Step 6.1 contains, for the purpose of calibration, 500 µg of galacturonic acid/ml.

To prepare the uronic acid standard solutions, take 0.5 ml, 2.0 ml, and 3.0 ml of the sugar solution into separate tubes and make to 10 ml with 2 M sulfuric acid to give standards of 25, 100, and 150 µg of galacturonic acid/ml.

Only the 100 µg/ml standard is required for routine analysis, and it may be kept at 5°C for several weeks.

Step 7.2

Measurement. Place into separate tubes (40 to 50 ml capacity) 0.3 ml of blank solution (2 M sulfuric acid), 0.3 ml of each of the standard solutions, and 0.3 ml of the sample hydrolysates, diluted if necessary (with 2 M sulfuric acid) to contain no more than 150 µg of uronic acids/ml (e.g., no dilution for flour, 1:2 for bran, 1:5 for most fruits and vegetables). Add 0.3 ml of 2% (w/v) sodium chloride, 3% (w/v) boric acid, and mix. Add 5 ml of concentrated sulfuric acid and vortex mix. Place the tubes in a heating block at 70°C and leave for 40 min. Remove the tubes and cool to room temperature in water (the tubes may be kept in the water for up to 1 h). Add 0.2 ml of dimethylphenol solution (0.1% (w/v), in glacial acetic acid) and vortex mix immediately. Between 10 and 15 min later, measure the absorbance at 400 nm and at 450 nm in the spectrophotometer against the blank solution. Subtract the reading at 400 nm from that at 450 nm, to correct for interference from hexoses. A straight line should be obtained if the differences for the standards are plotted against concentration.

Step 7.3
Calculation of uronic acids. The amount of uronic acid (in g/100 g of sample) is calculated as:

$$\frac{A_T \times V_T \times D \times 10}{A_S \times W_T} \times 0.89$$

where A_T is the difference in absorbance of the sample solution; V_T is the total volume of sample solution (here 30 ml); D is the dilution of the sample solution; A_S is the difference in absorbance of the 100 µg/ml standard; W_T is the weight (in mg) of the sample; and 0.89 is a scale factor for converting the experimentally determined values for monosaccharides to polysaccharides.

Step 8. Calculation of Total, Soluble, and Insoluble NSP Based on Measurement of Individual Constituent Sugars

The amount of total, soluble, and insoluble NSP, in g/100 g of sample, is calculated as:

Total NSP	= Neutral sugars calculated for portion (a)	(Step 6.4)
	+ Uronic acids calculated for portion (a)	(Step 7.3)
Insoluble NSP	= Neutral sugars calculated for portion (b)	(Step 6.4)
	+ Uronic acids calculated for portion (b)	(Step 7.3)
Soluble NSP	= Total NSP − Insoluble NSP	

BREAKS IN THE GLC PROCEDURE

The procedure may be halted at any of the following stages:

- After precipitation, washing, and drying the starch-free residue in Steps 3 and 4. The residue may be stored for long periods.
- After the hydrolysis with 2 *M* sulfuric acid in Step 5. The hydrolysate may be kept at 5°C for 24 h.
- After acidification of the reduced samples in Step 6. The samples may be stored at room temperature for 2 or 3 days.
- After acetylation and transfer to small vials in Step 6. The samples may be kept at room temperature for 2 to 3 days before analysis by GLC.
- The acid hydrolysate in Step 5 may be kept at 5°C for several weeks before the measurement of uronic acids.

TROUBLESHOOTING FOR THE GLC PROCEDURE

Symptom	Likely cause	Cure/Prevention
1. Extra peaks on the chromatogram	Incomplete reduction of monosaccharides in Step 6.2	Ensure alkaline pH before adding $NaBH_4$; replace old $NaBH_4$; do not compensate for loss of activity by adding more $NaBH_4$
2. Large variation between replicate analyses	Inaccurate pipetting of the internal standard	Test/calibrate dispensers by weighing 1-ml replicates of water
3. Response factors not reproducible	Inaccurate pipetting of the sugar mixture in Step 6	Test/calibrate dispensers by weighing 2-ml replicates of water

Symptom	Likely cause	Cure/Prevention
4. Values for glucose too high and variable for replicates	Incomplete wetting of samples with DMSO in Step 2.1	Vortex mix vigorously after adding DMSO
5. Values for glucose too low and variable for replicates	Incomplete wetting of sample with sulfuric acid in Step 5	Vortex mix vigorously before and after addition of sulfuric acid and at intervals during the incubation

Step 9. Measurement of NSP Constituents by Colorimetry (Figure 3)

Step 9.1

Make the working standards as follows. Take 1000 µl of the stock sugar mixture into a glass tube, add 5000 µl of 2.4 M sulfuric acid and mix to give 6 ml of 4 mg sugars per ml standard solution in 2 M sulfuric acid. (This value of 4 mg sugars per ml is based on a content of 14 mg of arabinose, 7 mg of glucose, and 3 mg of galacturonic acid per 6 ml of the stock sugar mixture as diluted here. The actual amount of each sugar is 2% less, to account for losses during the hydrolysis in Step 5).

Further standards of 2 mg sugars per ml and of 1 mg sugars per ml may be prepared by double dilution of the 4 mg sugars per ml standard and used for the construction of a standard curve to test for linearity of response. For routine analysis, however, a single standard with a concentration close to that expected for the analytical sample may be used.

Step 9.2

Measurement of total reducing sugars. Place into separate tubes 1 ml of blank solution (2 M sulfuric acid), 1 ml of each of the standard sugar solutions, and 1 ml of the hydrolysate from Step 5. Samples with more than about 40 g NSP per 100 g dry matter should be diluted with 2 M sulfuric acid. Add 0.1 ml of glucose solution (1 mg/ml) and 1 ml of 4 M sodium hydroxide to each tube and vortex mix.

Add 2 ml of the color reagent solution to each tube and vortex mix. Place the tubes, *all at the same time,* into a briskly boiling water bath for 15 min. Cool in water to room temperature. Add 25 ml of water and mix well by inversion.

Measure the absorbance in a spectrophotometer at 530 nm. A straight line should be obtained if the absorbance values for the standards are plotted against concentration. The colorimetric reaction is suitable for automation.[13]

Step 9.3

No sample blank is required if the hydrolysate is clear and colorless. If the hydrolysate is colored, however, measure the absorbance of the undiluted hydrolysate and divide the value by 29.1 (final dilution during the colorimetry is 1/29.1).

Step 9.4

Calculation. The amount of total NSP (portion (a)) and of insoluble NSP (portion (b)), in g/100 g of sample, is calculated as:

$$\frac{A_T \times V_T \times D \times F \times C \times 100}{A_S \times W_T} \times 0.89$$

where A_T is the absorbance of the sample solution (subtract the absorbance of the sample blank as appropriate); V_T is the total volume of the sample solution (here, 30 ml); D is the dilution of the sample solution; D = 1 if no dilution in Step 9.2; A_S is the absorbance of the standard used; C is the concentration (in mg sugars per ml) of the standard used; W_T is the weight (in mg) of sample taken for analysis; and F is the factor correcting the difference between the composition of monosaccharides in the standard sugar mixture and that in NSP of various types of plant foods.

ENGLYST PROCEDURE FOR RAPID DETERMINATION OF
TOTAL, SOLUBLE AND INSOLUBLE DIETARY FIBRE
BY COLORIMETRY

SAMPLE
|
Add 2ml DMSO
|
30 min at 100 °C
|
Add 8ml enzyme solution I
|
10 min at 100 °C
|
Add 0.5ml enzyme solution II
|
30 min at 50 °C / 10 min at 100 °C
|
Add 40ml ethanol
|
0.5 h at 0 °C
|
Centrifuge
Wash with ethanol, 85 and 100%
Dry with acetone
|
Add 5ml 12M-H_2SO_4
|
1 h at 35 °C
|
Add 25ml water
|
1 h at 100 °C
|
Add to 1ml:
  0.1ml glucose solution
  1ml 4M-NaOH
  2ml colour reagent
|
15min at 100 °C
|
Add 25ml water
|
Read the absorbance at 530nm
Calculate total NSP

FIGURE 3. Soluble DF = total DF − insoluble DF. For measurement of insoluble dietary fiber, replace the 40 ml of ethanol with 40 ml of pH 7 buffer and extract for 0.5 h at 100°C.

For the calculation of total NSP: cereals, F = 0.97; fruit and nonstarchy vegetables, F = 1.03; starchy vegetables and unknown samples, F = 1. For the calculation of insoluble NSP: F = 1 except for cereals, where F = 0.97; 0.89 is the factor for converting the experimentally determined monosaccharides to polysaccharides.

The amount of soluble NSP is calculated as the difference between total and insoluble NSP.

Step. 10. Calculation of NSP Based on Measurement of Total Reducing Sugars and Separate Measurement of Uronic Acids

The values for NSP obtained in Step 9.4 of the colorimetric procedure are adequate for most purposes. However, more accurate values may be obtained for some types of purified

NSP preparations, such as pectin, if uronic acids are measured separately. Values for NSP may be calculated as X + Y, where X is the value for NSP calculated in Step 9.4 of the colorimetric procedure (using F = 1), and Y is given by:

$$Y = \frac{0.17X}{100} \times \left[\frac{100Z}{X} - 12.5\right] + 0.08Z$$

$$= 0.25Z - 0.021X$$

where 0.17 is the percentage (divided by 100) underestimation of NSP that would be obtained in Step 9.4 of the colorimetric procedure for a polysaccharide consisting of only uronic acids (using F = 1); Z is the value for uronic acids obtained here; 0.08 is the percentage (divided by 100) underestimation of NSP due to incomplete hydrolysis of uronic acid polymers; and 12.5 is the percentage of uronic acid in the standard sugar mixture.

Note: Y may be positive or negative, accounting for the underestimation or overestimation of NSP when the sample has a high or low content of uronic acids, respectively.

TROUBLESHOOTING FOR THE COLORIMETRIC PROCEDURE

Symptom	Likely cause	Cure/Prevention
1. Large variation between replicate analyses	(a) Inaccurate pipetting of the sugar mixture in Step 9.1 (b) Incomplete removal of acetone in Step 3.4	(a) Test/calibrate dispensers by weighing 2 ml replicates of water (b) Ensure an acetone-free powder
2. Values too high and variable for replicates	Incomplete wetting of sample with DMSO in Step 2.1	Mix vigorously immediately after addition
3. Values too low and variable for replicates	Incomplete wetting of sample with sulfuric acid in Step 5	Vortex mix vigorously both before and immediately after the addition of sulfuric acid, and at intervals during the incubation
4. No color produced for standards and/or samples	Error in preparation of sulfuric acid or sodium hydroxide solutions	Make new reagents; test that the solution is neutral/alkaline before adding color reagent solution

STARCH

Resistant Starch

Englyst et al.[15] isolated a fraction from processed starchy foods that was resistant to dispersion in boiling water and to hydrolysis *in vitro* with pancreatic amylase. This fraction, consisting mainly of retrograded amylose, was called resistant starch (RS), and it is part of this fraction that is included as dietary fiber by the AOAC Prosky procedure. However, from studies in man it became clear that retrograded amylose represents only a small proportion of the starch resisting digestion in the small intestine.[16-18] As a result, at the June 1990 meeting of EURESTA (European Concerted Action on Resistant Starch) the definition of RS was broadened to include "any starch which escapes digestion in the small intestine", and it was agreed that RS "had to be defined by a specific *in vitro* technique, which gives an index of the potential of dietary starch to escape digestion in the small intestine".

Classification and Measurement of Nutritionally Important Starch Fractions

Dietary starch is separated into three main groups of different physiological importance, on the basis of physical and chemical properties:

Type of starch	Example of occurrence	Probable digestion in small intestine
Rapidly digestible starch (RDS)	Freshly cooked starchy foods	Rapid and complete
Slowly digestible starch (SDS)	Most raw cereals	Slow but complete
Resistant starch (RS)		
1. Physically inaccessible	Partly milled grains/seeds	Resistant
2. Resistant starch granules	Raw potato and banana	Resistant
3. Retrograded starch	Cooled cooked potato, bread, and corn flakes	Resistant

The digestion of starch is influenced by a number of factors. Apart from the identity of the food, these include the extent of chewing, the transit time of food along the small intestine, the amount of amylase available for breakdown of the starch, the amount of starch consumed, and the presence of other food components that may inhibit enzymic hydrolysis. The rate and extent of digestion of starch may therefore be variable. However, the values obtained for RDS, SDS, and RS by the proposed method represent a reproducible measurement by which starchy foods can be classified and compared according to their potential digestibility in man.

The various types of starch are quantified by controlled enzymic hydrolysis and measurement of the released glucose. Total starch (TS) is measured as the glucose released by enzymic hydrolysis of starch following gelatinization and treatment with potassium hydroxide to disperse retrograded amylose. RDS and SDS are measured after incubation with pancreatic amylase and amyloglucosidase at 37°C. A value of RDS is obtained as the glucose released after 20 min and SDS as the glucose released after a further 100-min incubation. RS is the starch not hydrolyzed after 120 min of incubation. Separate values may be obtained for RS in the form of physically inaccessible starch, resistant starch granules, and retrograded amylose.[19,20]

A measure of the relative rate of starch digestion is given by the starch digestion index (SDI), where SDI = (RDS/TS) × 100. The values given in Table 2 for a range of foods illustrate that the digestibility of starch is dependent on the identity of the food, and the treatment and processing of that food. In a separate study with 62 starchy foods, it was shown that the SDI was highly correlated with the glycemic index.[21]

DISCUSSION

Lignin

Lignin is not a carbohydrate and its physiological significance (in animal studies) is very different from that of NSP. Lignin should therefore not be measured with NSP and it is not included in the analytical definition of dietary fiber.[8] Lignin is quantitatively insignificant in the human diet and it is difficult to determine.[22] None of the present dietary fiber methods that include lignin can justify the values on strict chemical grounds. These methods simply isolate a collection of materials including Maillard reaction products, which are better referred to as substances measuring as lignin. If it is shown in the future that lignin is an important food component, a case must be made for its separate measurement. Values for NSP and lignin should never be grouped together, since this will invalidate both measurements.

TABLE 2
Digestibility *in vitro* of Some Carbohydrate-Containing Foods

	D.M. (%)	Type of starch (g/100 g D.M.)				SDI
		RDS	SDS	RS	TS	
White wheat flour	89.7	40	39	2	81	49
White bread	54.5	69	7	1	77	90
Whole meal bread	52.0	55	4	1	60	92
Corn flakes	95.8	73	2	3	78	94
Porridge oats	90.7	57	6	2	65	88
Ryvita crispbread	94.3	52	6	3	61	85
Pearl barley (boiled 1 h, cold)	23.3	34	30	9	73	47
Potato starch (raw)	81.8	6	19	74	99	6
Potato biscuit (50% wheat)	94.9	23	17	15	55	42
Boiled potato (hot)	22.8	64	5	5	74	87
Boiled potato (cold)	23.8	54	11	10	75	71
Banana flour	99.1	3	15	57	75	4
High amylose maize starch	95.2	70	11	17	98	71
Spaghetti (freshly cooked)	28.3	41	33	5	79	52
Spaghetti (cooled)	34.7	33	41	4	78	42
Peas (frozen, boiled 5 min)	18.3	13	2	5	20	60
Lentils (boiled 20 min, cold)	28.3	23	22	9	54	44
Haricot beans (boiled 40 min)	41.4	8	19	18	45	18

Note: D.M., dry matter.

The Use of Food Table Values for Dietary Fiber

If retrograded starch and other substances formed during food processing and cooking are included as dietary fiber, as in the AOAC Prosky procedure,[2] a single food yields a range of dietary fiber values depending on the treatment it has received before analysis. This makes the meaningful construction of food tables and calculation of the dietary fiber content of mixed dishes difficult if not impossible. Values obtained for NSP are not affected by food processing, so the amount of dietary fiber in all foods or mixed diets can be calculated simply by using the recipe and food table values for the NSP content of raw foods.

Collaborative Trial

A recent international collaborative study[23] of the Prosky procedure and the Englyst procedures, in which 12 samples were analyzed in duplicate, showed that the mean total value obtained by the Prosky procedure was 21% higher than that obtained by the Englyst GLC procedure. The main reason for this is the inclusion in the Prosky procedure of retrograded starch and other substances formed during food processing.

The mean value for the soluble fiber by the Prosky procedure was only two thirds of that measured by the Englyst procedure. This is because more of the cell-wall polysaccharides are extracted at the physiological pH 7 used in the Englyst procedure than at pH 5 as used in the Prosky procedure.

The precision of the methods was judged by values for reproducibility (R-95) for the variation between laboratories, where R-95 is calculated as standard deviation × 2.8. Outliers by the Grubb's test at the $p < 0.01$ level were excluded from the calculation of the mean and the precision data, but for all the methods, less than 5% of the results were excluded. The precision data obtained with the Englyst procedure are superior, with R-95 being 2.67 for the Englyst GLC procedure, 3.56 for the Englyst colorimetric procedure, and 5.34 for the Prosky procedure.

Labeling and Enforcement

Different values for dietary fiber may be obtained by the Prosky procedure if samples are heated, cooled, frozen, or dried. At least one of these treatments is always used before analysis by the gravimetric method. Therefore, dietary fiber values obtained by the Prosky method do not reflect the retrograded starch content of food as eaten but include that produced by storage and pretreatment of the sample. Such values are impossible to defend.

Conclusions

If the term dietary fiber is going to survive, a precise chemical definition must be agreed. NSP is the best index of the cell-wall material originally thought of as dietary fiber. An analytical definition of dietary fiber as NSP, as already proposed for the purposes of food labeling,[8] gives the analyst a clear objective and is in keeping with the original concept of dietary fiber.

The U.K. Ministry of Agriculture Fisheries and Food have made recommendations to the EEC community and issued guidelines on dietary fiber labeling following a series of large, multicenter collaborative trials of methods for measurement of dietary fiber.[22-25] The Ministry recommend that dietary fiber should be defined for the purposes of food labeling as nonstarch polysaccharides.

The physiological importance of dietary fiber, including its effects on blood sugar and insulin response, is, to a large extent, linked to dietary fiber being an integral part of the plant tissue. The consumption of vegetables, fruit, and grain products is therefore encouraged, and the use of fiber supplements discouraged in the U.S. and other dietary guidelines.

The beneficial effect ascribed to "fiber" seems to be mediated partly through changes in starch digestion. The digestibility of starchy foods and its potential control by food processing may develop to a new and interesting concept, which could be of great benefit to the food industry and to the public. Starch and dietary fiber must be measured separately in order to avoid future confusion regarding the chemical identity and physiological properties of plant polysaccharides. Combining the measurement of any starch with dietary fiber, as in the Prosky procedure, is confusing and it would be detrimental to future developments in this new area.

REFERENCES

1. **Trowell, H., Burkitt, D., and Heaton, K., Eds.,** *Dietary Fibre, Fibre-depleted Foods and Disease,* Academic Press, London, 1985.
2. **Prosky, L., Asp, N.-G., Furda, I., Devries, J. W., Schweizer, T. F., and Harland, B. F.,** Determination of total dietary fiber in foods and food products: collaborative study, *J. Assoc. Off. Anal. Chem.,* 68, 677, 1985.
3. **Englyst, H. N. and Cummings, J. H.,** Non-starch polysaccharides (dietary fibre) and resistant starch, in *New Developments in Dietary Fibre,* Furda, I. and Brine, C. J., Eds., Plenum Press, New York, 1990, 205.
4. **British Nutrition Foundation Task Force,** *Complex Carbohydrates in Foods,* Chapman and Hall, London, 1990.
5. **WHO,** *Diet, Nutrition and the Prevention of Chronic Diseases,* Tech Rep. Ser. 797, World Health Organization, Geneva.
6. **U.S. Department of Agriculture and U.S. Department of Health and Human Services,** *Nutrition and Your Health: Dietary Guidelines for Americans* (Home and Garden Bull. 232), 3rd ed., U.S. Government Printing Office, Washington, D.C., 1990.
7. **Englyst, H. N. and Cummings, J. H.,** Improved method for measurement of dietary fiber and non-starch polysaccharides in plant foods, *J. Assoc. Off. Anal. Chem.,* 71, 808, 1988.

8. **Englyst, H. N., Trowell, H. W., Southgate, D. A. T., and Cummings, J. H.,** Dietary fiber and resistant starch, *Am. J. Clin. Nutr.,* 46, 873, 1987.
9. **Southgate, D. A. T.,** Determination of carbohydrates in foods. II. Unavailable carbohydrates, *J. Sci. Food Agric.,* 20, 331, 1969.
10. **Southgate, D. A. T. and Englyst, H. N.,** The chemistry and physical properties of dietary fibre and the amounts in food, in *Dietary Fibre, Fibre-depleted Foods and Disease,* Trowell, H. W., Burkitt, D., and Heaton, K. W., Eds., Academic Press, London, 31.
11. **Englyst, H. N., Bingham, S. A., Runswick, S. A., Collinson, E., and Cummings, J. H.,** Dietary fibre (non-starch polysaccharides) in fruit, vegetables and nuts, *J. Hum. Nutr. Dietet.,* 1, 247, 1988.
12. **Englyst, H. N., Bingham, S. A., Runswick, S. A., Collinson, E., and Cummings, J. H.,** Dietary fibre (non-starch polysaccharides) in cereal products, *J. Hum. Nutr. Dietet.,* 2, 253, 1989.
13. **Englyst, H. N. and Hudson, G. J.,** Colorimetric method for routine measurement of dietary fibre as non-starch polysaccharides. A comparison with gas-liquid chromatography, *Food Chem.,* 24, 63, 1987.
14. **Quigley, M. and Englyst, H. N.,** Measurement of neutral sugars and uronic acids by high-pressure liquid chromatography with pulsed amperometric detection, *Analyst,* in press.
15. **Englyst, H. N., Wiggins, H. S., and Cummings, J. H.,** Determination of the non-starch polysaccharides in plant foods by gas-liquid chromatography of constituent sugars as alditol acetates, *Analyst,* 107, 307, 1982.
16. **Englyst, H. N. and Cummings, J. H.,** Digestion of the polysaccharides of some cereal foods in the human small intestine, *Am. J. Clin. Nutr.,* 42, 778, 1985.
17. **Englyst, H. N. and Cummings, J. H.,** Digestion of the carbohydrates of banana (*Musa paradisiaca sapientum*) in the human small intestine, *Am. J. Clin. Nutr.,* 44, 42, 1986.
18. **Englyst, H. N. and Cummings, J. H.,** Digestion of polysaccharides of potato in the small intestine of man, *Am. J. Clin. Nutr.,* 45, 423, 1987.
19. **Englyst, H. N. and Kingman, S. M.,** Dietary fibre and resistant starch. A nutritional classification of plant polysaccharides, in *Dietary Fiber,* Kritchevsky, D., Bonfield, G., and Anderson, J. W., Eds., Plenum Press, New York, 1990.
20. **Englyst, H. N., Kingman, S. M., and Cummings, J. H.,** Classification and measurement of nutritionally important starch fractions, *Eur. J. Clin. Nutr.,* in press.
21. **Veenstra, J. and Englyst, H. N.,** The relationship between the digestibility of starch and the glycaemic index of a range of starchy foods, in preparation.
22. **Cummings, J. H., Englyst, H. N., and Wood, R.,** Determination of dietary fibre in cereals and cereal products — collaborative trials. I. Initial trial, *J. Assoc. Publ. Analysts,* 23, 1, 1985.
23. **Wood, R., Englyst, H. N., Southgate, D. A. T., and Cummings, J. H.,** Determination of dietary fibre in foods — collaborative trials. IV. Comparison of Englyst GLC and colorimetric measurement with the Prosky procedure, *J. Assoc. Off. Anal. Chem.,* in press.
24. **Englyst, H. N., Cummings, J. H., and Wood, R.,** Determination of dietary fibre in cereals and cereal products — collaborative trials. II. Study of a modified Englyst procedure, *J. Assoc. Publ. Analysts,* 25, 59, 1987.
25. **Englyst, H. N., Cummings, J. H., and Wood, R.,** Determination of dietary fibre in cereals and cereal products — collaborative trials. III. Study of further simplified procedures, *J. Assoc. Publ. Analysts,* 25, 73, 1987.

Chapter 3.4

THE SOUTHGATE METHOD OF DIETARY FIBER ANALYSIS

David A. T. Southgate

INTRODUCTION

The Southgate method was developed in the late 1950s for the analysis of unavailable carbohydrates (dietary fiber) in mixed diets and was part of a procedure for measuring the various classes of carbohydrates in mixed diets (and foods.)[1-4]

The procedure was developed conceptually from the method for unavailable carbohydrate of McCance et al.[5] and aimed to measure the polysaccharide components in the alcohol-insoluble residue directly.

STAGES IN THE METHOD

Preparation of Alcohol-Insoluble Residue

The sample is extracted in aqueous alcohol (originally 85% v/v methanol and in the modified version 80% v/v ethanol). The extracted free sugars can be measured in this extract.

Enzymatic Digestion of Starch

The starch is gelatinized thoroughly in a boiling waterbath; on cooling the pH is adjusted with acetate buffer and amyloglucosidase enzyme is added. The mixture is incubated at 37°C overnight (18 h). The unaltered polysaccharides are precipitated by the addition of ethanol (4 vol) and the mixture is centrifuged (or filtered). The precipitate is washed by resuspension in 80% v/v ethanol and recentrifuged (3 × 10 ml). Starch can be measured as glucose in the extract.

Dilute Acid Hydrolysis

The residue is suspended in 10 ml 1 M H_2SO_4 and heated in a boiling waterbath for $2^1/_2$ h (45 min is permissible when colorimetric methods are used). Ethanol (10 ml) is added and the mixture is centrifuged. The supernatant is decanted off and the residue is washed by resuspension in 50% v/v ethanol (3 × 10 ml). The supernatants are combined and made to volume (100 ml). Hexose, pentose, and uronic acids are measured colorimetrically.

Strong Acid Hydrolysis

The residue is dried by suspending it in ethanol, centrifuging, and then washing the separated residue with diethyl ether; the solvent is finally allowed to evaporate; 72% v/v H_2SO_4 is then added to the residue and the mixture is left overnight. It is then filtered through a sintered glass filter and washed thoroughly with water (70 ml). The filtrate is diluted to volume (100 ml) and hexose, pentose, and uronic acid are measured colorimetrically.

Residual Lignin

The residue on the filter is washed with ethanol and diethyl ether, dried at 103°C for 10 min, cooled, and weighed. The weight of residue is taken as lignin.

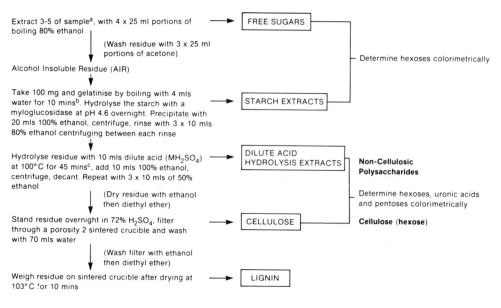

FIGURE 1. Flow diagrams to show the procedure used for the determination of dietary fiber by the modified Southgate Method.

EXPRESSION OF RESULTS

The values for hexose, pentose, and uronic acids in the dilute acid hydrolysate are derived from the *noncellulosic polysaccharides*. The values should be corrected for mutual interference according to the principles of Hudson and Bailey.[6] The values for hexose in the strong acid hydrolysate are taken as cellulose; the values for pentose and uronic acid after suitable correction are added to the noncellulosic polysaccharides from the dilute acid hydrolysate. The values are expressed as monosaccharides and, thus, values quoted in the Southgate procedure customarily expressed are approximately 10% higher than values expressed as polysaccharides.[7]

REFERENCES

1. **Southgate, D. A. T.**, The availability of nutrients in diets containing differing quantities of unavailable carbohydrate: a study of young and elderly men and women. II. Nitrogen, fat, carbohydrates and some inorganic constituents, *Proc. Nutr. Soc.*, 20, iii, 1961.
2. **Southgate, D. A. T.**, Determination of carbohydrates in foods. I. Available carbohydrates, *J. Sci. Food Agric.*, 20, 326, 1969.
3. **Southgate, D. A. T.**, Determination of carbohydrates in foods. II. Unavailable carbohydrates, *J. Sci. Food Agric.*, 20, 331, 1969.
4. **Southgate, D. A. T. and Durnin, J. V. G. A.**, Calorie conversion factors. An experimental reassessment of the factors used in the calculation of the energy value of human diets, *Br. J. Nutr.*, 24, 517, 1970.
5. **McCance, R. A., Widdowson, E. M., and Schackleton, L. R. B.**, The Nutritive Value of Fruits, Vegetables and Nuts, Spec. Rep. Ser. Med. Res. Counc. London No. 213, HMSO, London, 1936.

6. **Hudson, G. J. and Bailey, B. S.,** Mutual interference effects in the colorimetric methods used to determine the sugar composition of dietary fibre, *Food Chem.,* 5, 201, 1980.
7. **Southgate, D. A. T. and White, M. A.,** Commentary on results obtained by the different laboratories using the Southgate Method, in *The Analysis of Dietary Fiber in Food,* James, W. P. T. and Theander, O., Eds., Marcel Dekker, New York, 1981.

Chapter 3.5

DETERMINATION OF INDIVIDUAL COMPONENTS OF DIETARY FIBER

Olof Theander and Eric Westerlund

INTRODUCTION

Our understanding of the chemical composition of dietary fiber (DF) in foods was to a large extent pioneered by Southgate, whose studies are based on the fractionation and colorimetric assay of the hexose, pentose, and uronic acid constituents.[1] This method has, however, some shortcomings since, despite its complexity, it is still not specific in regards to individual sugars; also, starch is incompletely removed. This was demonstrated at the meeting on DF analysis in Cambridge, U.K., in 1978,[2] where results from analyses of different types of food samples by Southgate's and other methods were presented. A large variability of the method between different laboratories was shown, although the agreement within laboratories seemed to be good.[3,4] In the Cambridge study, which initiated several new collaborative studies and further developments in the field of DF analysis, rapid gravimetric methods, as well as more comprehensive, informative ones, were also explored. These included two fractionation methods for soluble and insoluble fibers devised by Englyst[5] and Theander and Åman.[6,7] In both methods starch is removed enzymatically, but with different systems, and a direct gas liquid chromatographic (GLC) assay is used for the neutral sugar constituents of the fiber fractions. The Englyst method has undergone a number of modifications[8–10] including a colorimetric procedure.[11] The original method of Theander and Åman[6] (method A) was later developed into two modifications[12,13] for analysis of total DF (methods B and C). The main differences between the present method[14] for total DF, developed by the Uppsala group and that of the U.K. method of Englyst,[9] are shown in Table 1.

The main reason for the U.K. group to use extraction with dimethylsulfoxide (DMSO) in combination with enzymatic treatments was to remove not only the enzymatically available starch but also the so-called resistant starch (RS). We, as well as the scientists who have developed the enzymatic gravimetric AOAC method for analysis of DF, consider such enzymatically nonavailable starch as part of the DF complex.[15]

On the other hand, as indicated in a recent comparison[14] between the U.K. and Uppsala methods, there was a rather good agreement in total DF if one adds the values for RS and Klason lignin, obtained by the Uppsala method, to the values for nonstarch polysaccharides found by the U.K. method (Table 2). There was, however, a trend that these sums were lower by the latter method. One possible explanation for this may be that the presence of DMSO partly hampers the precipitation of soluble DF polysaccharides (see Reference 16).

Marlett's group has made extensive studies on measurement of DF using a modification of method A of the Uppsala methodology (see Reference 17 and references therein). Another recent method, which is related to the Uppsala methodology but which uses DMSO for solubilization of starch, is that of Faulks and Timms.[18] A group that has been actively engaged in studies of individual fiber components, in particular, the preparation of cell wall materials, is that of Selvendran.[19,20] Their method involves extensive ball-milling, gelatinization at pH 7 and 85 to 90°C, enzymatic treatments with α-amylase and pullulanase, GLC determination of sugar constituents, and colorimetric uronic acid determination. Selvendran has also published a recent review of methods for DF analysis which is recommended for further reading[21] as well as the previously cited book by James and Theander.[2]

TABLE 1
Comparison of Main Steps in Total Dietary Fiber Determination by GLC with the Latest Modifications of the Uppsala Method[14] and the U.K. Method[9]

Procedure	Uppsala method	U.K. method
Sample size (dry matter)	250–500 mg	50–300 mg
Fat removal	Extraction with petroleum ether when content exeeds 5%	Extraction with acetone when content exceeds 5%
Starch removal	1. Termamyl (0.5 h, 96°C) in acetate buffer (0.1 M, pH 5) 2. Amyloglucosidase (16 h, 60°C)	1. Dimethylsulfoxide (DMSO) (0.5 h, boiling waterbath) 2. Termamyl (10 min, boiling waterbath) in acetate buffer (0.08 M, pH 5.2) 3. Pancreatin and pullulanase (0.5 h, 50°C + 10 min, boiling waterbath)
Precipitation of soluble fiber	80% (v/v) ethanol (1h, 4°C)	80% (v/v) ethanol (0.5 h, ice water)
Analysis of neutral sugars	1. 12 M H$_2$SO$_4$ (1 h, 30°C) 2. Addition of internal standard myo-inositol 3. 0.4 M H$_2$SO$_4$ (1 h, 125°C) 4. Alditol acetate preparation by sodium borhydride reduction and 1-methylimidazole/acetic anhydride 5. Individual correction factor regularly determined for each sugar	1. 12 M H$_2$SO$_4$ (1 h, 35°C) 2. 2 M H$_2$SO$_4$ (1 h, 100°C) 3. Addition of internal standard (allose) 4. Alditol acetate preparation by sodium borhydride reduction and 1-methylimidazole/acetic anhydride 5. Individual standard correction factor for each sugar
Analysis of uronic acids	Stoichometric decarboxylation or colorimetry with 3,5-dimethylphenol (Scott, 1979)	Scott procedure with 3,5-dimethylphenol
Lignin	Gravimetrically as Klason (sulfuric acid) lignin including ashing	Not determined

In the following, a more detailed description of the Uppsala methodology is given, including a critical discussion of the various steps and of alternative methods.

THE UPPSALA METHODOLOGY FOR ANALYSIS OF DIETARY FIBER

In connection with the EEC study, we developed the modification called method A (Figure 1) for the analysis of water-soluble and water-insoluble DF.[6,7] For several polysaccharides, there is generally no sharp distinction between water-soluble (or removable) and water-insoluble fractions; the ratio between them is dependent on the choice of conditions during the pretreatment and solubilization procedure. These conditions are, however, never identical with *in vivo* conditions. Polysaccharides such as arabinoxylans, mixed-linked β-glucans, and pectins (including associated neutral polysaccharides) are found both as water-soluble and water-insoluble components in several plant materials. The yield of these components can vary considerably with the fractionation conditions used (physical pretreatment, enzymatic treatment, temperature, time, and so on). Thus, recent studies[22,23] have shown that the yield and composition of soluble fibers were very dependent on extraction conditions

TABLE 2
Content of Dietary Fiber (DF) as Determined by the Uppsala Method and Nonstarch Polysaccharides (NSP) as Determined by the U.K. Method and of Resistant Starch (RS) and Klason Lignin (KL) in Some Food Products[a]

Product	Uppsala method			U.K. method	NSP +KL +RS
	DF	KL	RS	NSP	
Corn flakes	2.7	0.3	1.5	0.8	2.6
Bread crust	3.7	0.3	0.5	2.7	3.5
Bread crumb	3.8	0.3	0.8	2.7	3.8
Rye crisp	23.2	2.1	0.2	20.0	22.3
Green peas	14.5	0.3	0.3	12.8	13.4
Soybean	16.8	0.8	nd	15.1	15.9
Deskinned onion	20.1	1.0	nd	19.2	20.2
Sugar-beet fiber	64.7	1.3	nd	67.0	68.3

[a] Expressed as percentages on a dry matter basis. nd: not detected. See References 9 and 14 for details.

used. The use of DMSO in the U.K. method can be expected to increase the solubility of DF since the reagent is an excellent solvent for hemicellulose polysaccharides.[16]

After removal of 80% ethanolic extractives and of starch enzymatically in method A (Figure 1), the soluble fiber fraction was isolated by dialysis and the insoluble one by centrifugation. The content of neutral DF polysaccharides is then determined by GLC, after acid hydrolysis and preparation of alditol acetates. Uronic acids are determined on a sample of the residues isolated by a decarboxylation procedure.[6] The lignin content is measured gravimetrically as Klason (sulfuric acid) lignin, obtained after acid treatment and ashing of the insoluble residue. Method A has been used in two collaborative studies so far.[7,24]

The group has also published another rapid modification (method B) which can be very suitable when dealing with samples with low contents of starch (Figure 1). It is based on removal of 80% ethanol extractives followed by direct analysis of the DF constituents in the manner described above. The DF glucan content is obtained as the difference between the total glucan content (determined by GLC) and the starch content which is analyzed enzymatically. This modification has, for example, been used in a collaborative study.[25]

For starch-rich samples with low DF contents, such as flours, the subtraction of a high starch value (determined enzymatically) from a high glucan value (determined by GLC) may lower the accuracy. We therefore developed a procedure for total DF (method C) for such types of samples; in this, starch is first removed and the water-insoluble polymers are recovered by ethanol precipitation together with the water-soluble polymers.

Recently a rapid method, the Uppsala method for routine analysis of total DF,[14] was developed. This method (Figure 2) which is based on the previously[13] developed method C was evaluated on various types of fiber sources (cereals, vegetables, and fruits) during 1991-92 in a collaborative AOAC study, in which O. Theander was an associated referee.

The Uppsala method has been applied to a number of divergent samples, including foods, feeds, digesta, and feces and has proven to be rugged, reproducible, adaptable, and accurate. A skilled analyst can run over 40 samples per week by this improved procedure.

Method B and the Uppsala method are not much more time-consuming than the gravimetric enzymatic method[25] in which protein in the residue must be analyzed.

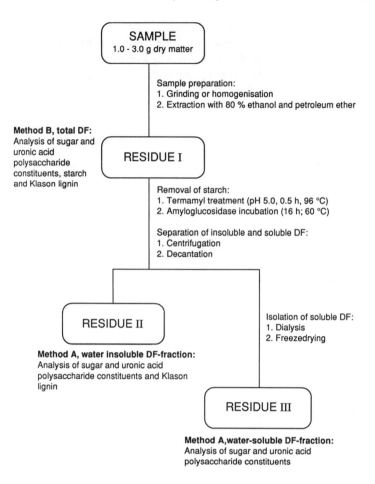

FIGURE 1. Fractionation scheme for methods A, B, and C for dietary fiber (DF).

CRITICAL DISCUSSION OF VARIOUS STEPS IN DETERMINATION OF DIETARY FIBER

Removal of Free Sugars and Lipids

It is important that the samples are representative and homogeneous. Foods with low water content (less than 15%) are ground in a Cyclotec Mill (Tecator, AB, Höganäs, Sweden) fitted with a 0.5-mm screen. Materials with high water content are generally freeze-dried, but for samples which also have a high sugar content, like fruits and vegetables, extraction with 80% aqueous ethanol is preferable. Before analyzing DF, it is important to efficiently remove low-molecular weight sugars and sugar alcohols which otherwise may interfere. For a sugar-rich sample like carrot, this is made in methods A and B by homogenization for 5 min in 80% ethanol (briefly adjusted for the water content of the sample), followed by ultrasonic extraction for 15 min. After centrifugation and decantation, the insoluble residue is extracted likewise twice with ethanol. This extraction procedure was sufficient for removing most (98%) of the free sugars in carrot (Table 3). It can be mentioned that when technical wheat starch was extracted by reflux or ultrasonication and the starch content determined, on average a slightly higher starch value was obtained by ultrasonication

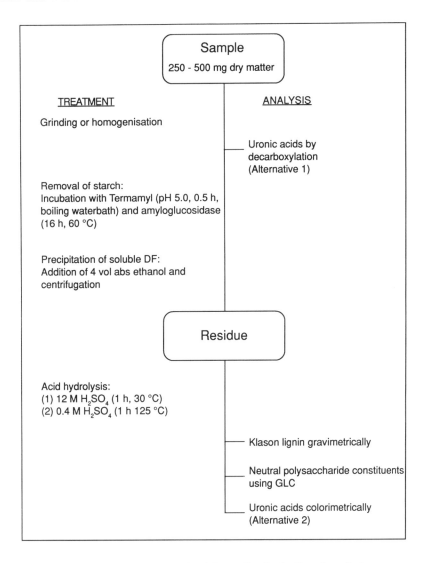

FIGURE 2. Rapid analysis of dietary fiber by the Uppsala method.

(94.7 ± 0.5%) than by reflux (92.1 ± 0.7%). Compare also with Selvendran et al.[20] If the lipid content of the sample exceeds 5%, extraction with petroleum ether is recommended for removing most of the lipids.

Removal of Starch and/or Analysis

Enzymatic removal of starch is a crucial operation in methods A, C, and the Uppsala method in order not to overestimate the DF glucans. Starch is removed by incubations with a thermostable α-amylase (Termamyl) and amyloglucosidase. This enzyme system has proved to be very effective for various types of starch-containing fiber sources and products. The powerful Termamyl-enzyme causes simultaneous gelatinization and hydrolysis of starch. A correct enzymatic starch analysis is also important in method B, which is based on the difference between the total glucan and starch contents. In the present procedure, the sample with Termamyl is treated for 30 min in a boiling waterbath. For practical reasons, the incubation with amyloglucosidase is then left to stand overnight, although complete hydrolysis to glucose is reached after about 6 h.[26] We usually quantify the glucose by a glucose

TABLE 3
Distribution of Low Molecular Weight Sugars in 80% Ethanolic Extracts of Carrot[a]

Extraction no.	Content of low molecular weight sugars (%)			
	fructose	glucose	sucrose	sum
1	10.4	12.3	19.5	42.2
2	3.0	3.4	5.1	11.5
3	0.8	1.1	1.7	3.6
4	0.3	0.3	0.5	1.1

[a] The results are expressed as percentages of the original sample (dry matter). See Reference 13 for details.

oxidase reagent (Mercotest 3395), although similar results are achieved with gas chromatography. Under the conditions used, we have found that neither of the enzymes liberate detectable amounts of sugars from purified barley seed β-glucan, barley straw arabinoxylan, or cotton cellulose.[6] The specificity of the Termamyl enzyme is probably explained by a rapid inactivation, at the high temperature used, of any nonstarch-degrading enzymes present. It is imperative that the enzymes used are free from fiber-degrading activity. Unfortunately it would appear that some commercial amyloglucosidase preparations at present have, for example, β-glucanase activity and will thus give low values for the fiber contents in, for instance, cereal samples. All enzyme preparations and batches should therefore be checked for such activities.

A brief description of the method of starch analysis was given in connection with an interlaboratory study on heat-treated foods.[24] For a detailed description see References 27 and 28. A similar procedure using α-amylase at 85°C after a gelatinization at 100°C has been reported by Baur and Alexander.[29] Dintzis and Harris[30] compared thermophilic enzymatic methods with conventional optical rotation methods in samples of wheat brans and got lower starch values with the latter methods. More recently, Batey[31] reported that the gelatinization and solubilization of starch with a thermostable α-amylase prior to amyloglucosidase treatment resulted in higher starch values than those obtained after 8 M hydrochloric acid dimethyl sulfoxide or potassium hydroxide treatments. He pointed out that the good reproducibility of the analytical values using thermostable α-amylases — which is also our experience from various types of food products — is due to the rapid degradation of starch to lower molecular oligomers which eliminates the phenomenon of retrogradation. The main advantage of using such enzymes — both for removal of starch in the DF determination and for direct starch analysis — is that autoclaving is not needed.

Holm et al.[32] have studied *in vitro* and *in vivo* enzymatic digestibility of amylose-lipid complexes and found *inter alia* that the use of Termamyl in combination with pancreatin almost completely hydrolyzed the complex. The complexed amylose was also hydrolyzed and absorbed to the same extent as free amylose *in vivo* (in rats) but somewhat slower.

The possibility that starch may be underestimated (or incompletely removed by the DF analysis) as a result of the ethanol treatment under reflux conditions has been discussed above. A number of other reactions and modifications of starch are, however, conceivable during various normal heat treatments of food such as extrusion cooking, autoclaving, baking, frying, and so on. The two main routes whereby the amount of enzymatically available starch may decrease (and the DF glucan consequently increase) are (1) retrogradation and (2) chemical modification of the starch structure.

TABLE 4
Content of DF Polysaccharides and Resistant Starch in Dough and White Bread Fractions[a]

	Baking conditions: 210°C for 35 min			
	Dough	Crumb	Inner crust	Outer crust
Fraction yield	100	44	44	12
Soluble DF glucans	0.11	0.08	0.10	0.21
Insoluble DF glucans[b]	0.49	0.60	0.65	0.65
Soluble arabinoxylans	0.72	0.58	0.64	0.86
Insoluble arabinoxylans	1.20	1.09	1.03	0.70
Resistant starch	0.09	1.02	0.62	0.30

[a] Values are expressed as g/100g fraction (dry basis). See Reference 36 for details.
[b] Resistant starch is not included.

It is well established that, after heat treatment, part of the starch in foods may be resistant to α-amylase hydrolysis and that a solution of gelatinized starch may retrograde on cooling and drying (see References 20 and 8). In connection with DF analysis, Englyst et al.[8] solubilized this retrograded enzyme-resistant starch with 2 M potassium hydroxide solution or DMSO[10] before hydrolysis with amyloglucosidase to glucose. They have applied this technique on a large series of cereal foods and report values of RS in the range of 0.1 to 1.2% (except for one breakfast cereal having 3.1%).[33] We, as well as several others working in this field, regard this enzymatically nondegradable starch as a DF constituent.

We have found that starch under food-technical conditions can also to some extent be modified nonreversibly via fragmentation to saccharides with 1,6-anhydroglucose end units, which can further via transglucosidation form enzyme-resistant, branched polysaccharide structures.[34,35] These modifications are dependent on the extent of heat treatment, the moisture content, and other factors. In the cited interlaboratory Helsinki study,[24] we found a slight but significant increase for the DF glucan values of extruded wheat flour and whole meal samples as well as for various heat-treated potato samples. The other type of contribution to the DF increase is from the Maillard reaction, which will be discussed below under the lignin determination.

A recent study[36] in our laboratory has shown that the formation of RS decreased in order from crumb to outer crust during baking (Table 4). This progressive decrease was probably due to water and temperature gradients formed in the bread during heating. The total content of dietary fiber glucans (RS is not included), on the other hand, increased in the order crumb to outer crust, mainly as a result of increasing contents of water-soluble glucans. This observation strongly suggested that formation of nonstarch glucans had, at least in part, occurred via fragmentation of starch and subsequent reactions of the fragments.

The content of insoluble arabinoxylans decreased during baking, particularly in outer crust. This decrease was partly accompanied by an increase in the content of water-soluble arabinoxylans. The total dietary fiber content was higher in the bread fractions than in the dough, mainly due to the formation of RS.

ANALYSIS OF DIETARY FIBER FRACTIONS

In previous studies[37,38] on rapeseed flour, we found that some polysaccharides may remain in solution after precipitation with 80% ethanol. In the Uppsala method it is therefore a key point to reach as complete a recovery as possible of soluble fiber on their precipitation in 80% (v/v) ethanol. We have previously shown[13] that such precipitation losses did not

TABLE 5
Amounts of Neutral Soluble Fiber Polysaccharide Residues Not Recovered on Precipitation of Soluble Fiber with 80% Ethanol in Samples Analyzed by the Uppsala Procedure[a]

Sample	Soluble fiber residues not covered (% of total fiber content)						
	Rhamnose	Arabinose	Xylose	Mannose	Galactose	Glucose	Total
Cornflakes	0.2	0.2	0.2	0.5	0.5	1.0	2.6
Bread crust	0.2	0.2	0.2	0.7	0.5	3.8	5.6
Bread crumb	0.2	0.2	0.2	1.1	0.2	1.9	3.8
Rye crisp	0.1	0.1	0.1	0.3	0.1	1.1	1.8
Green peas	0.1	0.1	0.1	0.1	traces	0.3	0.7
Soybean	0.2	0.1	0.2	0.3	0.3	0.4	1.5
Deskinned onion	0.5	0.1	0.1	0.3	0.2	1.1	1.9
Sugar-beet fiber	0.1	0.5	0.1	0.1	0.1	0.1	1.0

[a] Theander et al., unpublished results.

exceed 3% of the total DF polysaccharides for samples of wheat flour, raw potato, carrot, and wheat bran. Recently in a detailed study using gelfiltration of the ethanolic supernatant,[14] the polysaccharide fraction (DP > 10) escaping precipitation was analyzed in various foods. The amounts of soluble fiber polysaccharides not recovered were marginal (Table 5). Thus losses (1 to 6%) of the total fiber content of the original sample were observed, with the highest values found for the severest heat-treated sample (bread crust). This indicates that the solubility of DF polysaccharides may be changed by thermal treatment, probably by depolymerization.[36]

Determination of Neutral Polysaccharide Constituents

Treatment with 72% (= 12 M) sulfuric acid, in order to effect dissolution of cellulose, followed by a secondary hydrolysis in dilute acid as originally developed by Hägglund et al. (for a summary of the procedure see Reference 39), is a widely used procedure — including later modifications (see for instance, Saeman et al.[40]) — for hydrolysis of lignocellulosic materials in combination with Klason lignin determination (see below). Such a method is used for the hydrolysis of the polysaccharides in the water-insoluble or total DF fractions, namely pretreatment with 12 M sulfuric acid at room temperature for 2 h, dilution to 0.4 M, and hydrolysis for 6 h under reflux[6] or to gain time[13] at 125°C and 1 h (in an autoclave, essentially according to Sloneker[41]). For the hydrolysis of the water-soluble fraction in method A, we use 1 M trifluoroacetic acid (TFA) in a boiling waterbath for 16 h or autoclaving at 125°C for 1 h.[13,42] It is important that the posthydrolysis step with dilute sulfuric acid is sufficient to hydrolyze sulfate ester groups introduced in the first step. Figures 3 and 4, from an investigation made at the Swedish Forest Research Laboratories on the polysaccharide analysis, show an example of the sugar yield and rate of sulfate ester removal after different times of xylose and glucose.[43] They illustrate the well-known higher rates of degradation with acids for pentoses (in particular xylose) and also why we choose 6 h for the posthydrolysis step to avoid surviving sulfate ester groups (also 1 h at 125°C is enough). In a preparative experiment in which the cellulose was hydrolyzed for only 4 h, we isolated part of the original cellulose as glucose-6-sulfate.[44] It is significant that Neilson and Marlett,[45] when comparing a modified neutral detergent fiber method with our method A but using only 3 h in the posthydrolysis step, found (by HPLC) appreciable amounts of cellobiose (around 10% of total sugars). Using the autoclaving conditions, the amounts of cellobiose or other oligosaccharides in our hydrolyzed fractions are negligible. The efficiency of our

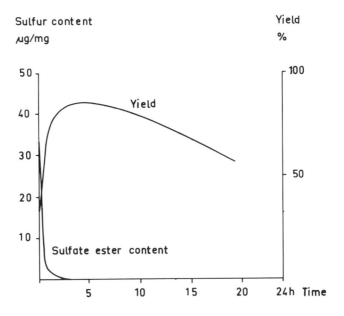

FIGURE 3. Yield and sulfate ester decomposition of xylose by reflux in 0.4 M sulfuric acid hydrolysis after pretreatment (30°C, 1 h) with 12 M sulfuric acid.[43]

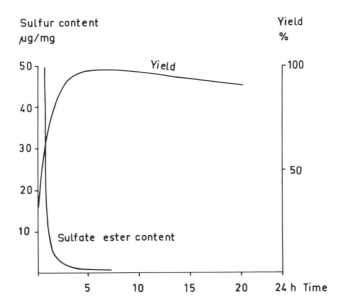

FIGURE 4. Yield and sulfate ester decomposition of glucose by reflux in 0.4 M sulfuric acid hydrolysis after pretreatment (30°C, 1 h) with 12 M sulfuric acid.[43]

conditions for hydrolysis of crystalline cellulose has been demonstrated by eight totally independent analyses of purified cotton linter. On average a cellulose content of 99.0% (SD 1.3) and a xylan content of 0.25% was found.[14] The effect of particle size and different prehydrolysis conditions to achieve optimum hydrolysis yield has recently been investigated.[46]

We have not, as have certain other workers in the field, attempted to estimate the noncellulose component of the insoluble DF separately from the cellulose by using an extra heterogeneous hydrolysis step with dilute sulfuric acid, since varying amounts of noncrystalline cellulose (depending on the source of the sample) may also be hydrolyzed under these conditions. Further, part of the hemicellulose fraction may be difficult to get into solution. It has been reported that for materials such as carrot, cabbage, and soybean, part of the xylose- and mannose-containing polymers need pretreatment with strong sulfuric acid to be completely hydrolyzed with the dilute acid.[8] The so-called β-glucans (containing β-1,4-linked glucose units interdispersed with β-1,3-linkages) are important components of some oat and barley products and can be determined by separate methods.[47] If the contribution due to such β-glucans and the strongly retrograded or chemically modified starch as in heat-treated products can be neglected, in certain sources the glucan content of the DF (determined after complete acid hydrolysis) will mainly represent the cellulose fraction.

GLC, particularly on capillary columns, is the method of choice for an efficient separation and accurate determination of the sugar constituents from the hydrolysates. The sugars are first converted to the volatile alditol acetate derivatives,[6] essentially as described by Sloneker.[48] Hydrolysates containing appreciable amounts of uronic acids must be carefully neutralized and the pH adjusted to the slightly alkaline side with, for instance, dilute ammonium hydroxide (without causing any epimerization of sugars) in order to open any uronolactones, which would otherwise be reduced with borohydride to alditols in the subsequent reduction step. The reduction is left to stand at 40°C for 1 h, but most sugars are probably transformed into alditols much quicker. We have, however, not found any epimerization of hexoses or pentoses under the conditions used. In the original procedure (see, e.g., References 6, 43, and 48), the borate from the borohydride, after acidification, has usually been removed as the volatile trimethylborate by repeated evaporation with methanol. This is essential since borate forms complexes with the alditols and interferes with the subsequent acetylation with acetic anhydride and the commonly used catalyst pyridine. Connors and Pandit[49] introduced the use of 1-methylimidazole as an effective catalyst for rapid acetylation of polyhydroxy compounds, and later Blakeney et al.[50] reported the use of this catalyst for the quantitative and rapid acetylation of alditols in the presence of borate (at room temperature for 10 min). This technique, which we now generally use, facilitates and shortens the derivatization step considerably. Recently a procedure for direct acetylation of aldoses in the acidic hydrolysate (without previous reduction) was developed in our laboratory.[51] So far this procedure has been tested on a limited number of samples but the agreement is good compared with the Uppsala method.

In the GLC separation, myoinositol is added before the hydrolysis step with dilute sulfuric acid. Figure 5 shows a typical GLC separation of alditol acetates derived from a reference mixture, and Figure 6 shows the corresponding separation from a wheat bran sample (the peak preceding number 2 is a phthalate impurity peak). Correction factors for hydrolysis losses, derivatization yields, and GLC responses for the individual sugars have been applied. As the ratio between the different sugars may influence these factors, reference sugar mixtures, typical for the DF composition of the food sample in question, are also analyzed concomitantly. Examples of these combined correction factors (which must be regularly checked because of influence by the type and age of column and hydrolysis conditions) to be used for multiplying the areas of the respective alditol acetates when using myoinositol as an internal standard are given in Table 6. In these values are also included the factors 0.88 and 0.90 used to convert the pentose/deoxyhexose and hexose contents, respectively, to polysaccharides. Capillary column chromatography has been a key factor in the separation of these complex mixtures, and the so-called bonded phase (BP) columns, in which the liquid phase is covalently bonded to the column, imparting good thermal stability and prolonged life, will introduce a further degree of efficiency into the chromatographic operations.

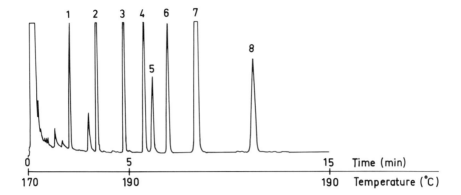

FIGURE 5. GLC-analysis of a monosaccharide reference mixture as alditol acetates. Capillary fused silica column (8 m × 0.25 mm; helium flow ~ 1 m/sec) coated with OV 275. Peak 1, rhamnitol; 2, arabinitol; 3, xylitol; 4, allitol; 5, mannitol; 6, galactitol; 7, glucitol; and 8, myoinositol.

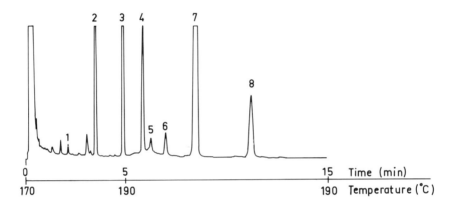

FIGURE 6. GLC-analysis of the monosaccharides in a hydrolysate of wheat bran as alditol acetates. Conditions and peak numbering as in Figure 5.

TABLE 6
Correction Factors for GLC Determination of Polysaccharide Sugar Constituents[a]

Analysis number	Sugars (the relative composition in % is given in brackets)					
	Glucose (40)	Galactose (10)	Mannose (5)	Xylose (20)	Arabinose (20)	Rhamnose (5)
1	0.98	1.06	1.03	1.07	0.97	0.89
2	0.97	1.03	1.02	1.14	1.00	0.94
3	1.03	1.08	1.05	1.18	1.04	1.02
4	0.99	1.05	1.02	1.15	1.02	0.94
5	1.01	1.09	1.03	1.16	1.02	1.01
6	1.02	1.05	1.03	1.09	0.97	1.03
Mean value	1.00	1.06	1.03	1.13	1.00	0.97
SD	0.02	0.02	0.01	0.04	0.03	0.06

[a] The factors are determined by GLC of alditol acitates at 210°C on an OV-225 glass capillary column after treatment of the respective sugars and myoinositol with 12 M H_2SO_4 at 30°C, 1 h and 0.4 M H_2SO_4 at 125°C, 1 h and subsequent neutralization and derivatization.[13]

High performance liquid chromatography (HPLC) offers an alternative procedure for analyzing aldoses in polysaccharide hydrolysates, but has not so far proved to be as powerful a technique as GLC. The choice of method is, however, governed by the requirements of the investigation. An advantage of HPLC is that the preparation of derivatives is obviated, although derivatization has, in fact, often been used in HPLC in order to enhance resolution and detection of the components and to shorten the analysis time. Comprehensive reviews[52-54] on HPLC with various applications in the carbohydrate field have been published including the use of amperometric determination[55] of monosaccharides which seems promising. Automated procedures using ion-exchange resins have also been successfully employed for the separation of monosaccharides.[56,57]

Determination of Uronic Acid in DF Polysaccharides

The determination of uronic acid constituents in DF by GLC presents a greater problem than in the case of the sugar constituents. Although free, low molecular uronic acids may be readily analyzed by GLC in the presence of neutral sugars,[58] the release of these acids in acceptable yields from the polymers is complicated by the high stability of glycosyl uronic acid linkages towards acid hydrolysis — resulting in the formation of aldobiouronic acids. Further, the monomeric uronic acids when released are degraded to noncarbohydrate products more rapidly than the neutral sugars. A useful technique for the separation and analysis of individual monomeric uronic acids by partition chromatography of ion-exchange resins — unmodified[59] (including oligomeric acids) or after reduction to aldonic acids[60] — has been developed.

Most workers in the DF field have used colorimetric assays and, in particular, the modified carbazole method according to Bitter and Muir.[61] A common disadvantage with colorimetric methods is the sensitivity to reaction conditions and the interference from absorbing compounds resulting from neutral sugars, proteins, phenols, and other components present and the inability to distinguish between individual uronic acids. The introduction of 3-phenylphenol by Blumenkrantz and Asboe-Hansen[62] and later 3,5-dimethylphenol by Scott,[63] who also compared the use of different phenol derivatives for colorimetric determination of uronic acids in plant materials, offers certain advantages. The rate of formation of 5-formyl-2-furancarboxylic acid, on which the colorimetric determination is based, was shown by Scott[63] to be faster for galacturonic than for glucuronic acids. The Uppsala group uses galacturonic acid for calibration because of this and the fact that galacturonic acid is more predominant in most DF samples (pectins) compared to glucuronic acid. These phenol reagents seem to suffer less interference from hexoses and have a greater sensitivity than the carbazole reaction. In the Cambridge study, Katan and Van de Bovenkamp[64] used a copper-binding method for determining the uronide content. They also calculated the methyl ester content from the binding of copper to the sample before and after saponification. Methanol released by such a treatment can also be determined by GLC.

The decarboxylation method for uronic acid determination does not suffer from the interference problems which are incurred with the colorimetric methods. We have established that the decarboxylation method developed by Bylund and Donetzhuber[65] for woods and pulps also affords a rapid, accurate, and reproducible method for DF samples, even those with low uronic acid contents.[6,7,12] The sample, containing 1 to 20 mg uronic acid, is refluxed for 30 min with hydroiodic acid under nitrogen. The carbon dioxide released is trapped in a cell containing dilute sodium hydroxide, and the conductivity changes are registered by means of a potentiometric recorder. Several food science laboratories have recently started to use the method and the complete equipment is now also commercially available (Billeruds AB, Technology & Development Centre, S-661 00 Säffle, Sweden; Dr. A. Donetzhuber). Figure 7 shows the decarboxylation curve for the water-insoluble fraction of rye biscuit.[6]

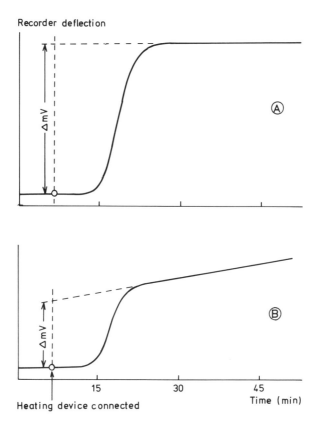

FIGURE 7. Decarboxylation curves of galacturonic acid (A) and the water-insoluble DF fraction of rye biscuit (B).[6]

We have found that the uronic acid determination gives essentially the same result whether it is performed before or after the extraction with organic solvent and starch removal.[13] Different types of uronic acids, such as D-galacturonic acid, D-glucuronolactone, the aldobiouronic acid 2-*O*-(4-*O*-methyl-*a*-D-glucopyranosyluronic acid)-D-xylose, and pectic acid give the same change in conductivity per mole of hexuronic acid.[6] The calibration diagram (we use D-galacturonic acid monohydrate) has to be checked regularly to ensure that the electrode distance within the cell or other parameters in the system have not changed. This method, like the colorimetric methods, does not estimate the amount of individual uronic acid constituents, but only the sum of uronic acids. If the uronide content mainly comprises pectin, acidic xylan constituents, or alginate, paper electrophoresis of the polysaccharide hydrolysate from the sugar analysis (even though the uronides are not completely hydrolyzed) affords a rapid, rough estimate of the ratio between the corresponding galacturonic, glucuronic (or its 4-*O*-methyl ether), and mannuronic acids.[66]

Determination of Lignin

There is no specific method for the determination of lignin, the complex polymer of phenylpropane units — at least, if one wishes to avoid laborious and time-consuming procedures. We have applied an oxidation/methylation technique to determine the lignin contents of different light- and dark-colored turnip rapeseed cultivars without interference from condensed tannins.[67] The acetyl bromide method, originally introduced by Johnson et al.[68] for wood and wood products, has been further developed and applied to forage crops

TABLE 7
Klason Lignin Values in Heat-Treated Cereals and Potato Samples[a]

Sample	Klason lignin (%)	Crude protein (N × 6.25) Percentage of original protein recovered in the Klason lignin
Wheat flour		
Untreated	0.2	0.3
Extruded at 168°C	0.4	2.3
Wheat whole meal		
Untreated	1.4	4.7
Extruded at 180°C	2.8	11.0
Potato		
Raw	0.4	—
Boiled	1.2	—
Pressure cooked	2.6	—

[a] See References 24 and 34 for details.

by Morrison.[69] This method has the advantage of being rapid and requires only about 50 mg of material. The sample is extracted with water and organic solvents, and the lignin content is measured by dissolving the residue in 25% acetyl bromide in acetic acid and measuring the absorption at 280 nm. Eastwood et al., however, consider the method inappropriate and not directly applicable to foods.[70,71] More recently, Selvendran et al.[21] has pointed out that the acetyl bromide procedure can only be used to compare the lignin contents of different organs from the same plant or samples from similar species, since different species require different conversion factors.

We have, like many others working with lignified plant materials, chosen the sulfuric acid method, which was first applied by Klason[72] at the beginning of this century, but which has since been further modified.[73] Essentially, it involves removal of extractives and polysaccharides and the gravimetric determination of the residue as lignin after washing and drying. In the present Uppsala method, an ashing step is included. It is conveniently combined with the determination of the neutral polysaccharide constituents of the DF.[6,14] When applied to human foods, however, the values in most cases represent not only native lignin but also tannins, cutin, and some proteinaceous products. From heat-treated foods, the residue may also contain products of the Maillard reaction and caramelization reactions. These constituents of the Klason lignin residue most likely represent food components, which, like lignin, are unavailable to human enzymes. We therefore propose that *the Klason lignin value will be designated the "noncarbohydrate" part of the DF.*

The lignin content determined according to Goering and Van Soest[74] by $KMnO_4$ oxidation of the ADF (acid detergent fiber) residue is probably generally closer to the amount of native lignin. Van Soest has demonstrated for some forages and feeds that high temperature treatment increases the amount of crude protein and Klason lignin of the ADF residue.[75] We have found a similar increase of the Klason lignin residues and their crude protein contents with the extent of heat treatment for potato and cereals[24,34] (see Table 7 for some examples). A brown water-insoluble polymer was obtained (together with low molecular weight furans, phenols, pyrroles, pyridines, carboxylic acids, and lactones) by refluxing a slightly acidic aqueous solution of glucose and glycine.[76] It analyzed as 90% Klason lignin with a recovery

TABLE 8
Content of Ester Substituents in Some High Fiber
Products (% of dry matter)[a]

Product	Dietary fiber	Coumaroyl groups	Feruloyl groups	Acetyl groups
Maize bran	76.4	0.2	2.4	1.5
Wheat bran	37.2	trace	0.2	0.3
Potato fiber	71.9	trace	trace	0.7
Sugar beet fiber	70.8	trace	0.5	1.6

[a] See Reference 14 for details.

of 84% of the original nitrogen.[77] The crude protein contents which one finds in the Klason lignin residue from heat-treated foods might originate besides from such Maillard reaction products, also from protein-tannin complexes, cell-wall protein, and other nitrogen-containing components. In residues from unprocessed foods, however, we do not find more than 1 to 5% of the nitrogen of the original food. For brans, which represent a very lignin-rich food ingredient, this corresponds to not more than about 10% of the Klason lignin residue, when calculated as crude protein (N × 6.25).

For further reading on the chemistry of DF polysaccharides, lignin, and other nondigestible substances associated with plant cell walls, which may be included in a broader definition of the term dietary fiber, see References 78 to 80. Cell-wall proteins, cutin, waxes, polyphenols other than lignin, phytic acid, silica, and compounds such as acetic acid and phenolic acids, which are present as ester-linked substituents to DF polysaccharides and/or lignin, may be included in this group. So far, the importance of such plant fiber substituents as well as lignin has mainly been discussed in connection with digestion of plant materials by the rumen microflora. It is very likely, however, that phenolic acids, lignin, and other phenolic compounds may also play an important role relative to the microbial fermentation in the human gut, although generally present in only small amounts in human food. For references to the presence of acetyl and phenolic acid substituents in grasses and for suitable GLC methods for their analysis, see Reference 81. Markwalder and Neukom[82] have isolated diferulic acid from wheat flour, where it is thought to be a possible cross-link in pentosans. Hartley and Haverkamp[83] reported the presence of 0.02% p-coumaric acid and 0.66% ferulic acid in wheat bran, as determined by HPLC after removal by alkali. Recently, the contents of these components were determined[14] in some high fiber products (Table 8). The acetyl constituents were quantified as 1-acetylpyrrolidin by GLC[84] and phenolic acids, after release by alkaline treatment by HPLC.[85]

APPLICATIONS

The application of method A on a series of fiber-rich foodstuffs, namely wheat bran, rye bran, whole potato, carrot, pea, white cabbage, lettuce, and apple is presented in Table 9.[6] The figures based on dry matter are in the range of 1 to 4% for water-soluble DF and 8 to 34% for insoluble DF. On a fresh weight basis, the brans are particularly rich fiber sources. The great differences in chemical composition among the different foods are notable, and one would therefore also expect great differences among the physical, biological, and nutritional properties of the different DF sources. The analyses thus indicate that brans have the highest Klason lignin values and are rich in arabinoxylans and cellulose but have a low proportion of uronic acid constituents. The other sources have higher cellulose contents and

TABLE 9
Chemical Characterization of Water-Soluble and Water-Insoluble Dietary Fibers in Various Foods Using Method A[a]

Component	Wheat bran	Rye bran	Potato (whole)	Carrot	Pea	White cabbage	Lettuce	Apple
Water-soluble fraction								
Neutral polysaccharide components	2.1	2.3	3.1	0.9	0.6	0.9	0.3	0.5
Uronic acid polysaccharide components	0.2	0.2	1.2	2.0	0.5	1.9	0.5	2.3
Relative composition of neutral sugar constituents								
Glucose	41.8	36.9	45.9	14.0	24.1	tr	8.9	10.8
Galactose	3.4	8.3	45.3	40.1	17.4	38.9	40.0	26.2
Mannose	tr	tr	tr	tr	tr	tr	5.0	tr
Xylose	20.8	30.3	tr	1.9	3.7	8.3	10.3	tr
Arabinose	34.0	24.5	5.8	28.2	51.9	40.9	34.3	58.2
Rhamnose	tr	tr	2.0	15.8	2.8	11.9	1.5	4.8
Fucose	—	—	1.0	—	—	—	—	—
Water-insoluble fraction								
Neutral polysaccharide components	28.3	21.1	6.2	15.1	15.9	14.3	8.6	11.1
Uronic acid polysaccharide components	1.2	0.6	0.4	5.5	1.7	2.7	4.5	2.3
Klason lignin	4.7	3.9	0.9	1.5	2.6	0.9	2.3	1.3
Relative composition of neutral sugar constituents								
Glucose	31.3	28.2	46.1	60.5	69.0	62.8	63.5	46.0
Galactose	3.7	1.8	34.5	12.5	1.0	9.1	9.7	9.5
Mannose	1.3	tr	1.5	5.4	tr	4.3	4.2	2.8
Xylose	39.2	39.5	6.3	6.3	5.7	9.6	9.1	10.9
Arabinose	24.5	30.5	10.0	11.3	23.3	9.6	9.0	27.5
Rhamnose	tr	tr	1.4	3.8	1.0	3.4	4.5	1.6
Fucose	tr	tr	0.2	0.2	tr	1.2	tr	1.7
Total DF content	36.5	28.1	11.8	25.0	21.3	20.7	16.2	17.5

[a] All figures, except composition of neutral sugars, given as percent of the dry matter of the original material; tr = traces. See Reference 6.

also more of pectic and associated substances (galacturonic acid, rhamnose, arabinose, and galactose being typical constituents) than brans. Typical for potato is the high galactan content.

Our application[13] of the more rapid method B for total DF with the analysis of individual DF components on the samples used in the large collaborative AOAC study[25] (where our values were presented graphically as total DF only) is shown in Table 10. The reproducibility of the analytical methods is exemplified by the application of method C on samples of whole wheat flour, wheat bran, and carrots given in Table 11, indicating a good reproducibility for the methods used for determination of the individual components of dietary fiber.[13] Method C has, for example, been used to study the variation in the content and composition of DF for Swedish oats[86] (Table 12). As mentioned above, the present Uppsala method (an improved method C) will be applied worldwide in an extensive collaborative AOAC study during 1991-92.

TABLE 10
Chemical Characterization of Total Dietary Fibers of the Samples in a Collaborative AOAC Study Using Method B[a,b]

Sample	Anhydro sugar constituents						Anhydro uronic acids	Klason lignin	Total DF
	Rhamnose	Arabinose	Xylose	Mannose	Galactose	Glucose			
Corn bran	0.1	14.6	28.5	0.5	4.2	19.5	5.2	3.8	76.4
Iceburg lettuce	0.7	1.2	1.3	0.7	1.6	8.1	9.1	2.6	25.3
Oat product	tr	1.0	1.2	0.3	0.4	3.0	0.4	3.9	10.2
Potato product	0.2	0.3	0.2	0.2	1.7	5.2	1.3	0.4	9.5
Raisins, seedless	0.1	0.3	0.2	0.1	0.2	1.0	1.0	2.0	4.9
Rice, enriched	tr	0.3	0.3	0.1	0.1	1.1	tr	0.7	2.6
Rye bread	tr	1.0	1.2	0.4	0.3	4.1	tr	0.9	7.9
Soy isolate	0.1	0.2	0.1	0.9	0.3	0.4	0.5	3.2	5.7
Wheat bran	tr	7.7	13.7	0.4	0.9	9.1	1.6	3.8	37.2
Whole wheat flour	tr	2.4	3.7	0.3	0.6	0.6	0.6	2.2	10.4
White wheat flour[b]	—	0.6	0.8	0.3	0.2	0.8	0.2	0.3	3.2
Nonvegetarian mixed diet	0.1	0.9	0.8	0.4	0.8	2.0	0.8	1.1	6.9
Lacto-ovo vegetarian mixed diet	0.1	1.0	0.8	0.3	0.6	1.8	0.9	0.7	6.2

[a] All figures given as percent of the dry matter of the original material; tr = traces; see Reference 25.
[b] Determined by method C.

TABLE 11
Reproducibility of Method C for Dietary Fiber Analysis[a]

Sample (and analysis no.)	Anhydro sugar constituents						Anhydro uronic acids	Klason lignin	Total DF
	Rhamnose	Arabinose	Xylose	Mannose	Galactose	Glucose			
Whole wheat flour									
1	tr	2.5	4.3	0.3	0.4	3.0	0.8	1.2	12.5
2	tr	2.4	4.2	0.3	0.4	3.0	0.8	1.2	12.3
3	tr	2.4	4.3	0.3	0.4	3.0	0.8	1.2	12.4
4	tr	2.3	4.1	0.3	0.4	3.0	0.9	1.2	12.2
5	tr	2.4	4.2	0.3	0.4	3.1	0.7	1.4	12.5
Mean value		*2.4*	*4.2*	*0.3*	*0.4*	*3.0*	*0.8*	*1.2*	*12.4*
SD		*±0.1*	*±0.1*	*±0.0*	*±0.0*	*±0.0*	*±0.1*	*±0.1*	*±0.1*
Wheat bran									
1	0.1	7.6	15.0	0.4	0.8	11.0	1.6	4.9	41.4
2	0.1	7.9	15.8	0.4	0.8	11.5	1.7	4.4	42.6
3	0.1	7.6	15.1	0.4	0.7	9.7	1.7	4.6	39.9
4	0.1	7.6	15.6	0.4	0.7	11.8	1.5	4.9	42.6
5	0.1	7.6	14.7	0.4	0.8	11.6	1.6	4.2	41.0
Mean value	*0.1*	*7.7*	*15.2*	*0.4*	*0.8*	*11.1*	*1.6*	*4.6*	*41.5*
SD	*±0.0*	*±0.1*	*±0.5*	*±0.0*	*±0.0*	*±0.8*	*±0.1*	*±0.3*	*±0.1*
Carrot									
1	0.7	2.0	0.5	0.8	3.5	8.5	13.1	0.1	29.2
2	0.6	1.7	0.4	0.7	2.9	7.4	13.1	0.4	27.2
3	0.6	1.7	0.4	0.8	3.0	7.6	12.6	0.4	27.2
4	0.6	1.9	0.4	0.8	3.1	8.3	13.6	0.1	28.8
5	0.6	1.8	0.4	0.8	3.1	7.9	12.9	0.5	28.0
Mean value	*0.6*	*1.8*	*0.4*	*0.8*	*3.1*	*7.9*	*13.1*	*0.3*	*28.1*
SD	*±0.0*	*±0.1*	*±0.0*	*±0.0*	*±0.2*	*±0.5*	*±0.4*	*±0.2*	*±0.9*

[a] All figures given as % of the dry matter of the original material; see Reference 13; tr = traces.

TABLE 12
Content of Different Dietary Fiber Constituents of Sixteen Oats (Whole Grain) with Different Starch Content[a]

Component	Mean value	Range of values
Starch	47.3	38.8–54.7
Dietary fiber	29.6	19.8–38.7
Arabinose residues	1.5	1.1–2.0
Xylose residues	5.4	2.4–10.6
Mannose residues	0.3	0.2–0.4
Galactose residues	0.7	0.6–0.9
Glucose residues	12.2	9.6–15.7
Uronic acid residues	1.1	0.7–1.9
Klason lignin	8.4	5.4–12.8
β-Glucans[b]	3.2	2.7–3.6
Arabinoxylans[c]	8.0	4.1–14.5
Cellulose[d]	9.1	6.0–12.9

[a] Expressed as percentages of dry matter. See Reference 86 for details.
[b] Determined by enzymic analysis according to Reference 47.
[c] The sum of xylose, arabinose, and uronic acid residues of nonstarch polysaccharides.
[d] Glucose residues of nonstarch polysaccharides minus β-glucans.

REFERENCES

1. **Southgate, D. A. T.**, Determination of carbohydrates in foods. II. Unavailable carbohydrates, *J. Sci. Food Agric.*, 20, 331, 1969.
2. **James, W. P. T. and Theander, O., Eds.**, *The Analysis of Dietary Fiber in Food*, Marcel Dekker, New York, 1981.
3. **Southgate, D. A. T. and White, M. A.**, Commentary on results obtained by the different laboratories using the Southgate method, in *The Analysis of Dietary Fiber in Food*, James, W. P. T. and Theander, O., Eds., Marcel Dekker, New York, 1981, chap. 4.
4. **Theander, O.**, A review of the different analytical methods and remaining problems, in *The Analysis of Dietary Fiber in Food*, James, W. P. T. and Theander, O., Eds., Marcel Dekker, New York, 1981, chap. 16.
5. **Englyst, H.**, Determination of carbohydrate and its composition in plant materials, in *The Analysis of Dietary Fiber in Food*, James, W. P. T. and Theander, O., Eds., Marcel Dekker, New York, 1981, chap. 6.
6. **Theander, O. and Åman, P.**, Studies on dietary fibres. I. Analysis and chemical characterization of water-soluble and water-insoluble dietary fibres, *Swedish J. Agric. Res.*, 9, 97, 1979.
7. **Theander, O. and Åman, P.**, Analysis of dietary fibers and their main constituents, in *The Analysis of Dietary Fiber in Food*, James, W. P. T. and Theander, O., Eds., Marcel Dekker, New York, 1981, chap. 5.
8. **Englyst, H., Wiggins, H. S., and Cummings, J. H.**, Determination of the non-starch polysaccharides in plant foods by gas-liquid chromatography of constituent sugars as alditol acetates, *Analyst*, 107, 307, 1982.
9. **Englyst, H. N. and Cummings, J. H.**, An improved method for the measurement of dietary fibre as non-starch polysaccharides in plant foods, *J. Assoc. Off. Anal. Chem.*, 71, 808, 1988.

10. **Englyst, H. N. and Cummings, J. H.**, Non-starch polysaccharides (dietary fiber) and resistant starch, in *New Developments in Dietary Fiber*, Furda, I. and Brine, C. J., Eds., Plenum Press, New York, 1990, 205.
11. **Englyst, H. N. and Hudson, G. J.**, Colorimetric method for routine measurement of dietary fibre as non-starch polysaccharides. A comparison with gas-liquid chromatography, *Food Chem.*, 24, 63, 1987.
12. **Theander, O. and Åman, P.**, Studies on dietary fibre. A method for the analysis and chemical characterisation of total dietary fibre, *J. Sci. Food Agric.*, 33, 340, 1982.
13. **Theander, O. and Westerlund, E.**, Studies on dietary fiber. III. Improved procedures for analysis of dietary fiber, *J. Agric. Food. Chem.*, 34, 330, 1986.
14. **Theander, O., Åman, P., Westerlund, E., and Graham, H.**, The Uppsala method for rapid analysis of total dietary fiber, in *New Developments in Dietary Fiber*, Furda, I. and Brine, C. J., Eds., Plenum Press, New York, 1990, 273.
15. **Asp, N.-G., Furda, I., Schweizer, T. F., and Prosky, L.**, Dietary fiber definition and analysis, *Am. J. Clin. Nutr.*, 48, 688, 1988.
16. **Hägglund, E., Lindberg, B., and McPhersson, J.**, Dimethylsulphoxide, a solvent for hemicelluloses, *Acta Chem. Scand.*, 10, 1160, 1956.
17. **Marlett, J. A.**, Measuring dietary fiber, *J. Anim. Feed Sci. Technol.*, 23, 1, 1989.
18. **Faulks, R. M. and Timms, S. B.**, A rapid method for determining the carbohydrate component of dietary fibre, *Food Chem.*, 17, 273, 1985.
19. **Selvendran, R. R. and Du Pont, M. S.**, Simplified methods for the preparation and analysis of dietary fibre, *J. Sci. Food Agric.*, 31, 1173, 1980.
20. **Selvedran, R. R., Ring, S. G., and Du Pont, M. S.**, Determination of the dietary fiber content of the EEC samples and a discussion of the various methods of analysis, in *The Analysis of Dietary Fiber in Food*, James, W. P. T. and Theander, O., Eds., Marcel Dekker, New York, 1981, chap. 7.
21. **Selvendran, R. R., Verne, A. V. F. V., and Faulks, R. M.**, Methods for analysis of dietary fibre, in *Plant Fibers. Modern Methods of Plant Analysis*, Linskens, H. F. and Jackson, J. F., Eds., Springer Verlag, Berlin, 1989, Vol. 10, 234.
22. **Graham, H., Grön Rydberg, M.-B., and Åman, P.**, Extraction of soluble dietary fiber, *J. Agric. Food Chem.*, 36, 494, 1988.
23. **Marlett, J. A., Chesters, J. G., Longaere, M. J., and Bogdanske, J. J.**, Recovery of soluble dietary fiber is dependent on the method of analysis, *Am. J. Clin. Nutr.*, 50, 479, 1989.
24. **Varo, P., Laine, R., and Koivistonen, P.**, Effect of heat treatment on dietary fiber: interlaboratory study, *J. Assoc. Off. Anal. Chem.*, 66, 933, 1983.
25. **Prosky, L., Asp, N.-G., Furda, I., Devries, J. W., Schweizer, T., and Harland, B. F.**, Determination of total dietary fiber in foods, food products and ingredients: collaborative study, *J. Assoc. Off. Anal. Chem.*, 67, 1044, 1984.
26. **Åman, P. and Hesselman, K.**, Analysis of starch and other main constituents of cereal grains, *Swed. J. Agric. Res.*, 14, 135, 1984.
27. **Salomonsson, A.-C., Theander, O., and Westerlund, E.**, Chemical characterization of Swedish whole meal and bran fractions, *Swed. J. Agric. Res.*, 14, 111, 1984.
28. **Åman, P., Westerlund, E., and Theander, O.**, Determination of starch using a thermostable α-amylase, in *Methods in Carbohydrate Chemistry*, Vol. XI, John Wiley & Sons, New York, in press, 1993.
29. **Baur, M. C. and Alexander, R. J.**, Enzymatic procedure for determination of starch in cereal products, *Cereal Chem.*, 56, 364, 1979.
30. **Dintzis, F. R. and Harris, C. C.**, Starch determination in some dietary fiber sources, *Cereal Chem.*, 58, 467, 1981.
31. **Batey, I. L.**, Starch analysis using thermostable alfa-amylases, *Stärke*, 34, 125, 1982.
32. **Holm, J., Björck, I., Ostrowska, S., Eliasson, A-C., Asp, N.-G., Larsson, K., and Lundquist, I.**, Digestibility of amylose-lipid complexes in-vitro and in-vivo, *Stärke*, 35, 294, 1983.
33. **Englyst, H. N., Andersson, V., and Cummings, J. H.**, Starch and non-starch polysaccharides in some cereal foods, *J. Sci. Food Agric.*, 34, 1434, 1983.
34. **Theander, O. and Westerlund, E.**, Studies on chemical modifications in heat-processed starch and wheat flour, *Stärke*, 39, 88, 1987.
35. **Siljeström, M., Björck, I., and Westerlund, E.**, Transglycosidation reactions following heat treatment of starch. Effects on enzymic digestibility, *Stärke*, 41, 95, 1989.
36. **Westerlund, E., Theander, O., Andersson, R., and Åman, P.**, Effects of baking on polysaccharides in white bread fractions, *J. Cereal Sci.*, 10, 149, 1989.
37. **Larm, O., Theander, O., and Åman, P.**, Structural studies on a water-soluble arabinan isolated from rapeseed *(Brassica napus)*, *Acta Chem. Scand. B.*, 29, 1011, 1975.

38. **Larm, O., Theander, O., and Åman, P.**, Structural studies on a water-soluble arabinogalactan isolated from rapeseed *(Brassica napus)*, *Acta Chem. Scand. B*, 30, 627, 1976.
39. **Hägglund, E.**, *Chemistry of Wood*, Academic Press, New York, 1951, 326.
40. **Saeman, J. F., Moore, W. E., and Millet, M. A.**, Sugar units present. Hydrolysis and quantitative paper chromatography, in *Methods in Carbohydrate Chemistry*, Vol. 3, Whistler, R. L., Ed., Academic Press, New York, 1963, chap. 12.
41. **Sloneker, J. H.**, Determination of cellulose and apparent hemicellulose in plant tissue by gas-liquid chromatography, *Anal. Biochem.*, 43, 539, 1971.
42. **Albersheim, P., Nevins, D. J., English, P. D., and Karr, A.**, A method for the analysis of sugars in plant cell-wall polysaccharides by gas-liquid chromatography, *Carbohydr. Res.*, 5, 340, 1967.
43. **Bethge, P. O., Rådeström, R., and Theander, O.**, Kvantitativ kolhydratbestämning — en detaljstudie, Communication No. 63B from the Swedish Forest Products Laboratory, Stockholm, 1971, in Swedish.
44. **Hardell, H.-L. and Theander, O.**, Quantitative determination of carbohydrates in cellulosic materials — losses as sulphates, *Svensk Papperstidn.*, 73, 291, 1970.
45. **Neilson, M. J. and Marlett, J. A.**, A comparison between detergent and non-detergent analyses of dietary fiber in human foodstuffs, using high-performance liquid chromatography to measure neutral sugar composition, *J. Agric. Food Chem.*, 31, 1342, 1983.
46. **Hoebler, C., Barry, J. L., David, A., and Delort-Laval, J.**, Rapid acid hydrolysis of plant cell wall polysaccharides and simplified quantitative determination of their neutral monosaccharides by gas-liquid chromatography, *J. Agric. Food Chem.*, 37, 360, 1989.
47. **Åman, P. and Graham, H.**, Analysis of total and insoluble mixed-linked (-3), (1-4)-beta-D-glukans in barley and oats, *J. Agric. Food Chem.*, 35, 704, 1987.
48. **Sloneker, J. H.**, Gas-liquid chromatography of alditol acetates, in *Methods in Carbohydrate Chemistry*, Vol. 6, Whistler, R. L. and BeMiller, J. N., Eds., Academic Press, New York, 1972, chap. 4.
49. **Connors, K. A. and Pandit, N. K.**, N-Methylimidazole as a catalyst for analytical acetylations of hydroxy compounds, *Anal. Chem.*, 50, 1542, 1978.
50. **Blakeney, A. B., Harris, P. J., Henry, R. J., and Stone, B. A.**, A simple and rapid preparation of alditol acetates for monosaccharide analysis, *Carbohydr. Res.*, 113, 291, 1983.
51. **Hämäläinen, M., Theander, O., Nordkvist, E., and Ternrud, I.**, Multivariate calibration in the determination of acetylated aldoses by g.l.c., *Carbohydrate Res.*, 207, 167, 1990.
52. **Verhaar, L. A. T. and Kuster, B. F. M.**, Liquid chromatography of sugars on silica-based stationary phases, *J. Chromatogr.*, 220, 313, 1981.
53. **Honda, S.**, High-performance liquid chromatography of mono- and oligosaccharides, *Anal. Biochem.*, 140, 1, 1984.
54. **Hicks, K. B.**, High-performance liquid chromatography of carbohydrates, *Adv. Carbohydr. Chem. Biochem.*, 46, 17, 1988.
55. **Lee, Y. C.**, High-performance anion-exchange chromatography for carbohydrate analysis, *Anal. Biochem.*, 189, 151, 1990.
56. **Samuelson, O.**, Partition chromatography on ion-exchange resins, in *Methods in Carbohydrate Chemistry*, Vol. 6, Whistler, R. L. and BeMiller, J. N., Eds., Academic Press, New York, 1972, chap. 9.
57. **Mopper, K.**, Improved chromatographic separations on anion-exchange resins. I. Partition chromatography of sugars in ethanol, *Anal. Biochem.*, 85, 528, 1978.
58. **Lehrfeld, J.**, Differential gas-liquid chromatography method for determination of uronic acids in carbohydrate mixtures, *Anal. Biochem.*, 115, 410, 1981.
59. **Johnson, S. and Samuelson, O.**, Automated chromatography of uronic acids on anion-exchange resins, *Anal. Chim. Acta*, 36, 1, 1966.
60. **Samuelson, O. and Thede, L.**, Automated ion exchange chromatography of organic acids in acetate media, *J. Chromatogr.*, 30, 556, 1967.
61. **Bitter, T. and Muir, H. M.**, A modified uronic acid carbazole reaction, *Anal. Biochem.*, 4, 330, 1962.
62. **Blumenkrantz, N. and Asboe-Hansen, G.**, New method for quantitative determination of uronic acids, *Anal. Biochem.*, 54, 484, 1973.
63. **Scott, R. W.**, Colorimetric determination of hexuronic acids in plant materials, *Anal. Chem.*, 51, 936, 1979.
64. **Katan, M. B. and Van de Bovenkamp, P.**, Determination of total dietary fiber by difference and of pectin by colorimetry or copper titration, in *The Analysis of Dietary Fiber in Food*, James, W. P. T. and Theander, O., Eds., Marcel Dekker, New York, 1981, chap. 14.
65. **Bylund, M. and Donetzhuber, A.**, Semimicro determination of uronic acids, *Svensk Papperstidn.*, 15, 505, 1968.
66. **Carlsson, B., Samuelsson, O., Popoff, T., and Theander, O.**, Isomerisation of D-glucuronic acid in neutral aqueous solution, *Acta Chem. Scand.*, 23, 261, 1969.

67. **Theander, O., Åman, P., Miksche, G. E., and Yasuda, S.,** Carbohydrates, polyphenols, and lignin in seed hulls of different colors from turnip rapeseed, *J. Agric. Food Chem.,* 25, 270, 1977.
68. **Johnson, D. B., Moore, W. E., and Zank, L. C.,** The spectrophotometric determination of lignin in small wood samples, *TAPPI,* 44, 793, 1961.
69. **Morrison, I. M.,** A semi-micro method for the determination of lignin and its use in predicting the digestibility of forage crops, *J. Sci. Food Agric.,* 23, 455, 1972.
70. **McConnell, A. A. and Eastwood, M. A.,** A comparison of methods of measuring "fibre" in vegetable material, *J. Sci. Food Agric.,* 25, 1451, 1974.
71. **Robertson, J. A., Eastwood, M. A., and Yeoman, M. M.,** An investigation of lignin extraction from dietary fibre using acetyl bromide, *J. Sci. Food Agric.,* 30, 1039, 1979.
72. **Klason, P.,** Die Verfahren der Holzzellstoff-Fabrikation. Aussprache, in *Verein der Zellstoff und Papier-Chemiker und Ingenieure, Hauptversammlung,* Berlin, 1908, 52.
73. **Browning, B. L.,** Determination of lignin, in *Methods of Wood Chemistry,* Vol. 2, Interscience, New York, 1967, chap. 34.
74. **Goering, H. K. and Van Soest, P. J.,** Forage fiber analyses, U.S. Dept. Agric. Agricultural Handbook No. 379, U.S. Government Printing Office, Washington, D.C., 1970.
75. **Van Soest, P. J.,** Use of detergents in analysis of fibrous feeds. III. Study of effects of heating and drying on yield of fiber and lignin in forages, *J. Assoc. Off. Anal. Chem.,* 48, 785, 1965.
76. **Olsson, K., Pernemalm, P.-Å., and Theander, O.,** Formation of aromatic compounds from carbohydrates. VII. Reaction of D-glucose and glycine in slightly acidic, aqueous solution, *Acta Chem. Scand. B,* 32, 249, 1978.
77. **Theander, O.,** Advances in the chemical characterisation and analytical determination of dietary fibre components, in *Dietary Fibre,* Birch, G. G. and Parker, K. J., Eds., Applied Science, London, 1983, chap. 6.
78. **Theander, O. and Åman, P.,** The chemistry, morphology, and analysis of dietary fiber components, in *Dietary Fibers: Chemistry and Nutrition,* Inglett, G. E. and Falkehag, S. I., Eds., Academic Press, New York, 1979, chap. 15.
79. **Theander, O.,** The chemistry of dietary fibres in different sources, in *Nahrungsfasern Dietary Fibres,* Amado, R. and Schweizer, T., Eds., Academic Press, London, 1986, 13.
80. **Selvendran, R. R.,** in *Dietary Fibre,* Birch, G. G. and Parker, K. J., Eds., Applied Science Publishers, London, 1983, 95.
81. **Theander, O., Udén, P., and Åman, P.,** Acetyl and phenolic acid substituents in timothy of different maturity and after digestion with rumen microorganisms or a commercial cellulase, *Agric. Environ.,* 6, 127, 1981.
82. **Markwalder, H. V. and Neukom, H.,** Diferulic acid as a possible crosslink in hemicelluloses from wheat germ, *Phytochemistry,* 15, 836, 1976.
83. **Hartley, R. D. and Haverkamp, J.,** Pyrolysis-mass spectrometry of the phenolic constituents of plant cell walls, *J. Sci. Food Agric.,* 35, 14, 1984.
84. **Månsson, P. and Samuelsson, B.,** Quantitative determination of O-acetyl and other O-acetyl groups in cellulosic material, *Svensk Papperstidn.,* 84, R15, 1981.
85. **Ternrud, I. E., Lindberg, J. E., and Theander, O.,** Continuous changes in straw carbohydrate digestion and composition along the gastro-intestinal tract in ruminants, *J. Sci. Food Agric.,* 41, 315, 1987.
86. **Åman, P.,** The variation in chemical composition of Swedish oats, *Acta Agric. Scand.,* 37, 347, 1987.

Chapter 3.6

THE CRUDE FIBER METHOD[1]

Ivan Furda

Crude fiber is the loss of ignition of dried residue remaining after digestion of sample with 1.25% sulfuric acid and 1.25% sodium hydroxide solutions under specific conditions. The principle of the method is that a finely ground air-dried sample of the food is extracted with ether to remove lipids and that this dry sample is then extracted successively with boiling acid and alkali. The residue is filtered off and washed. After drying and weighing, the residue is ashed and residual inorganic matter is measured. The method is applicable to grains, cereals, flours, feeds, and any fiber-bearing material from which fat can be extracted to leave workable residue.

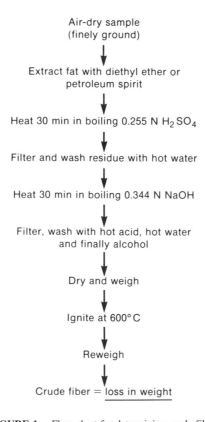

FIGURE 1. Flow chart for determining crude fiber.

REFERENCE

1. **Horwitz, W., Ed.**, *Official Methods of Analysis of the Association of Official Analytical Chemists*, 13th ed., AOAC, Washington, D.C., 1980, 132.

Chapter 3.7

NEWER METHODS FOR THE ANALYSIS OF PHYTATE AND ITS HYDROLYSIS PRODUCTS*

Barbara F. Harland and Donald Oberleas

INTRODUCTION

Since the original anion-exchange method received official AOAC approval in January 1988,[1,2] it has remained valid and in continuous use. The authors discovered that it is possible to reduce the sample size by half (1g), and thus the HCl in half (20 ml instead of 40 ml). Also, the shaking time may be reduced to 3 h without compromising results. The American Association of Cereal Chemists' wheat bran still serves as an internal standard, and the St. Paul, MN 55121 address remains valid.

During the intervening years a number of newer methods have been developed, not only for phytate (myoinositol hexakis dihydrogen phosphate [IP6]), but for the hydrolysis products of phytate: pentakis dihydrogen phosphate (IP5), tetrakis dihydrogen phosphate (IP4), tris dihydrogen phosphate (IP3), and bis dihydrogen phosphate (IP2). Although the lower inositol phosphates have been shown to bind minerals less effectively than the hexakis form, they do contribute to overall binding, particularly the IP5 fraction.[3]

With the ability to measure phytic acid and its hydrolysis products more quickly and accurately has come a greater intensity of research effort to find just what impact the presence of phytate has on the bioavailability of minerals.

Newer methods for the analysis of phytate fractions or modifications thereof are ^{31}P-Fourier transform nuclear magnetic resonance (NMR),[4] near-infrared reflectance spectroscopy,[5] and supercritical fluid chromatography.[6]

For nutrition-related studies of phytic acid and inositol phosphates, the following methods are useful:

1. Ion pair chromatography which is compatible with isocratic elution and refractive index detection, such as methods developed by Lee and Abendroth,[7] Sandberg et al.,[8] Lehrfeld,[9] Sulpice et al.,[10] and Shayman and Barcelon[11]
2. Indirect photometric ion chromatography method by Matsunaga et al.[12]
3. Some modification of the HPLC-post column reaction method developed by Phillippy and Bland[13]

ABSTRACT

Phytates are displaced from the sample with dilute hydrochloric acid, as phytic acid. Any proteins or metal ions that may bind with the phytic acid are complexed with NaEDTA solution at pH 6. Phytic acid is separated from the mixture of complexes and any phosphate with an anion exchange column. The separated phytic acid is converted to phosphate on digestion with a mixture of concentrated sulfuric and nitric acids. Finally, the phosphate, equivalent to the phytic acid in the samples, produces color with a molybdate-sulfonic acid reagent and can be estimated using a spectrophotometer.

---

* A method for the determination of phytate is included here because phytates are often closely associated with dietary fiber. Phytate may be present in a high enough concentration to have a physiological effect when certain high fiber foods are consumed.

PURPOSE

The purpose of this method is to determine the concentration of phytate (myoinositol hexaphosphate) in fat-free, air-dried samples of foods and feedstuffs.

Apparatus

1. Glass barrel columns (0.7 × 15 cm) equipped with a valve (Econo-columns, Biorad Laboratories, Richmond, CA, or equivalent).
2. Anion exchange resin, AGI-X4, 100 to 200 mesh, chloride form (Biorad Laboratories).
3. Micro-Kjeldahl flasks or 25 × 200-mm digestion tubes.
4. Spectrophotometer.

Reagents

1. Hydrochloric acid 2.4% (54 ml conc. HCl per liter).
2. Sodium chloride solutions: 0.1 and 0.7 M.
3. Phosphate standard solutions:
   a. Stock solution (80 μg/ml): weigh 0.350 g of dried, dessicated potassium acid phosphate (primary standard) into a 1-l volumetric flask; add approximately 500 ml of distilled water, add 10 ml of 10 N sulfuric acid, and dilute to mark.
   b. Working solution (16 μg P per milliliter): dilute 20 ml of stock solution to 100 ml with distilled water. Prepare fresh weekly.
4. Molybdate solution: 2.5% ammonium molybdate in 1 N sulfuric acid. Dissolve 12.5 g of ammonium molybdate in 200 ml distilled water. Transfer this to a 500-ml volumetric flask, add 50 ml of 10 N sulfuric acid, make to volume with water. Mix well. Stable.
5. Sulfonic acid reagent: dissolve 0.16-g 1-amino-2-napthol-4-sulfonic acid, 1.92-g sodium sulfite, and 9.60-g sodium bisulfite in 90 ml of water. Quantitatively transfer to a 100-ml volumentric flask. Heat to dissolve if necessary, cool to room temperature, and make to volume. Store in a brown bottle in refrigerator. Prepare fresh weekly.
6. Sodium EDTA/sodium hydroxide reagent: in a 250-ml flask, stir 10.23 g disodium ethylenediaminetetraacetate (EDTA) (0.11 M) and 7.5 g NaOH (0.75 M). Bring to volume with distilled water. Stable.

Procedure

1. Add 0.5 of resin to each column and wash with distilled water.
2. Wash column with 5 ml 0.7 M NaCl.
3. Wash column with 15 ml distilled water.
4. Place 2 g of sample into a 125-ml Erlenmeyer flask.
5. Add 40 ml 2.4% HCl_3 (20:1 ratio).
6. Stopper and shake for 3 h at room temperature.
7. Filter with vacuum through Whatman #1 or equivalent filter paper. (Stable for at least 1 week when stored in a refrigerator.)
8. Pipette 1.0 ml of filtrate into a 25-ml graduated beaker or similar vessel.
9. Add 1.0 ml of NaEDTA/NaOH mixture.
10. Bring to 25 ml with distilled water.
11. Mix contents and pour quantitatively onto column; discard eluate.

12. Elute with 15 ml of 0.1 M NaCl solution; discard eluate.
13. Elute with 15 ml of 0.7 M NaCl; collect eluate into digestion tube or flask.
14. Add 0.5 ml concentrated sulfuric acid and 3.0 ml concentrated nitric acid into each digestion vessel.
15. Add 3 glass beads.
16. Digest on medium heat under a hood until active boiling ceases, and a cloud of thick yellow vapors appears at the neck of the flask or tube. Heat contents for 5 more min on medium heat, then 5 min on low heat; remove and allow to cool.
17. When cool, add 10 ml of distilled water; swirl to dissolve salt; apply low heat if necessary.
18. Heat flasks or tubes in a boiling water bath for 15 min.
19. Quantitatively transfer sample to 50-ml volumetric flask.
20. Add 2.0 ml molybdate solution; mix well.
21. Add 1.0 ml sulfonic acid reagent; mix well.
22. Make to volume and read at 640 nm after an appropriate reaction time.

Note: Before reading results, adjust instrument with a reagent blank. The blank is prepared by mixing 1 ml 2.4% HCl with 1 ml NaEDTA/NaOH, diluting to 25 ml with distilled water, pouring this mixture quantitatively onto column, and proceeding as outlined in steps 11 to 22 above.

Note: Whenever food samples are analyzed, Am. Assoc. Cereal Chem. Certified Food Grade Wheat Bran (St. Paul, MN, approx. 3% phytate) is run simultaneously as an internal standard.

Calculation of Phytate Concentration in Food or Feed

1. Read absorbance or optical density.
2. Multiply by K to obtain micrograms of phosphorus per sample or dilution. (K is derived by dividing concentration of phosphorus in a standard by the absorbance obtained for that standard.) It represents the calculated concentration per unit absorbance for each concentration of standard. The mean K obtained from several standards is comparable to a more precise estimate of the midpoint on the best straight line of a standard curve.
3. Multiply by 20 to obtain micrograms of phosphorus per gram of sample. (20 is a dilution factor derived as follows: 40/2 = 20, where 40 is ml of extraction acid, 2.0 is the weight of sample in grams, and 1 ml of the extract is placed on the column.)
4. Divide by 1000 to get milligrams of phosphorus per gram of sample.
5. Divide by 0.282 to convert milligrams of phosphorus per gram of sample to milligrams of phytate equivalents per gram of sample. (The phytate molecule is 28.2% phosphorus.)
6. Multiply the result of step 5 by 100 to get milligrams of phytate per 100 g of sample.

REFERENCES

1. **Harland, B. F. and Oberleas, D.**, Phytate in foods. In changes in methods, *J. Assoc. Off. Anal. Chem.*, 69(2), 356, 1986.
2. **Harland, B. F. and Oberleas, D.**, Analysis of Phytate with an anion-exchange method, *J. Assoc. Off. Anal. Chem.*, 69(7), 667, 1986. (Official, Jan. 1988).
3. **Tao, S-H., Fox, M. R. S., Phillippy, B. Q., Fry, B. E., Johnson, M. L., and Johnston, M. R.**, Effects of inositol phosphates on mineral utilization, *Fed. Proc.*, 45, 819, 1986.

4. **Ersoz, A., Akgun, H., and Aras, N. K.,** Determination of phytate in Turkish diet by phosphorus-31 Fourier Transform nuclear magnetic resonance spectroscopy, *J. Agric. Food Chem.*, 38, 733, 1990.
5. **Parrish, F. W., Madacsi, J. P., Phillippy, B. Q., Wilfred, A. G., and Buco, S. M.,** Determination of phytic acid in cottonseed by near-infrared reflectance spectroscopy, *J. Agric. Food Chem.*, 38, 407, 1990.
6. **Chester, T. L.,** Phytic acid, inositol triphosphate: supercritical fluid separations, *J. Chromat. Sci.*, 27, 622, 1989.
7. **Lee, K. and Abendroth, J. A.,** High-performance liquid chromatographic determination of phytic acid in foods, *J. Food Sci.*, 48, 1344, 1983.
8. **Sandberg, A.-S., Anderson, H., Carlsson, N. G., and Sandstrom, B.,** Degradation products of bran phytate formed during digestion in the human small intestine: effect of extrusion cooking on digestibility, *J. Nutr.*, 117, 2061, 1987.
9. **Lehrfeld, J.,** High-performance liquid chromatography analysis of phytic acid on a pH-stable, macroporous polymer column, *Cereal Chem.*, 66, 510, 1989.
10. **Sulpice, J. S., Gascard, P., Journet, E., Rendu, F., Renard, D., Poggioli, J., and Giraud, F.,** The separation of (^{32}P) inositol phosphates by ion-pair chromatography: optimization of the method and biological applications, *Anal. Biochem.*, 179, 90, 1989.
11. **Shayman, J. A. and Barcelon, F. S.,** Ion-pair chromatography of inositol polyphosphates with N-methylimipramine, *J. Chromat.*, 528, 142, 1990.
12. **Matsunaga, A., Yamamoto, A., and Mizukami, E.,** Determination of phytic acid in various foods by indirect photometric ion chromatography, *J. Chromat. Sci.*, 29, 408, 1988.
13. **Phillippy, B. Q. and Bland, J. M.,** Gradient ion chromatography of inositol phosphates, *Anal. Biochem.*, 175, 162, 1988.

Chapter 3.8

DETERMINATION OF THE SAPONIN CONTENT OF FOODS

David Oakenfull and John D. Potter

INTRODUCTION

Saponins are present in many fiber-rich foods, particularly legumes. Their presence is relevant to human nutrition because they have been shown to increase fecal excretion of bile acids, in human[1,2] and animal[3-5] studies, and have been shown to lower plasma cholesterol in a number of animal species.[3-5] In particular, yucca saponins[1] and saponin-rich alfalfa seeds[6] have been shown to lower plasma cholesterol in humans.

Saponins are a structurally diverse group of triterpene or steroid glycosides.[7,8] The molecules are amphiphilic, the triterpene or steroid part being hydrophobic and the sugar part hydrophilic. This gives saponins their characteristic surface-activity from which the name is derived. The structure of a typical saponin, one of those present in soybeans, is shown in Figure 1. Saponins have been identified in many hundreds of plant species, but only a few of these are used as food by man (see Table 8 of the Appendix).

There appear to be two mechanisms by which saponins can affect cholesterol metabolism:

1. Some saponins, with particular defined structural characteristics, form insoluble complexes with cholesterol (e.g., the well known precipitation of cholesterol by digitonin). Complexation in the gut then inhibits cholesterol absorption.[9]
2. Saponins can interfere with the enterohepatic circulation of bile acids by forming mixed micelles. These can have molecular weights of several millions[10] and the reabsorption of bile acids from the terminal ileum is effectively blocked.[11]

EXTRACTION PROCEDURE

The dried plant material is first extracted with acetone or hexane, preferably using a Soxhlet extractor, to remove lipids, pigments, etc. The residue is then further extracted with methanol which removes the saponins, along with many other compounds such as simple sugars, oligosaccharides, and flavonoids.

METHODS OF ANALYSIS

Saponins have proved very difficult to assay and many of the results in the literature are, at best, only approximations. For this reason, the majority of the values given in Table 8 of the Appendix are quoted as a range — there are often major discrepancies between results from different techniques and different laboratories. The major methods used are thin-layer chromatography (TLC)[12,13] and high-performance liquid chromatography (HPLC).[14,15]

TLC

The essence of the technique is to spot a TLC plate with a crude saponin extract, develop the plate with a suitable solvent system, and use one of a number of methods for estimating the quantity of saponin on the plate. Suitable solvent systems are *n*-butanol:ethanol:concentrated ammonia (7:2:5) or chloroform:methanol:water (13:7:2). Spots

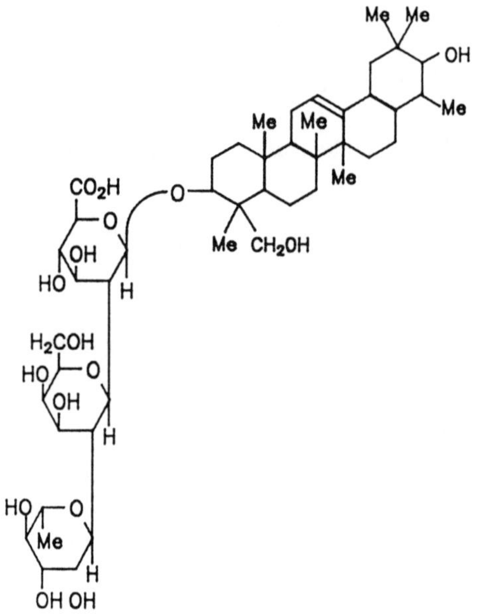

FIGURE 1. Structure of one of the saponins from soybeans.

can be visualized by spraying with 10% H_2SO_4 in ethanol and estimated by densitometry. The method is open to criticism in that spots may be wrongly identified as saponins or may be overlayed by other compounds (such as oligosaccharides).

HPLC

This technique has been used for the separation and analysis of both aglycones (the steroid or triterpene part of the molecule) and intact saponins. A rapid method for soybean saponins has been described[15] in which defatted soy flour is boiled under reflux with 1.5 M H_2SO_4 in dioxane-water (1:3). This hydrolyzes the saponins and the sapogenins can then be extracted with ethyl acetate. HPLC is carried out with a commercial silica column, eluting with light petroleum-ethanol with a gradient technique. The saponin content can be estimated by assuming that the carbohydrate to sapogenin ratio is 1:1 (by weight).

REFERENCES

1. **Bingham, R., Harris, D. H., and Laga, T.,** Yucca plant saponin in the treatment of hypertension and hypercholesterolemia, *J. Appl. Nutr.*, 30, 127.
2. **Potter, J. D., Illman, R. J., Calvert, G. D., Oakenfull, D. G., and Topping, D. L.,** Soya saponins, plasma lipids, lipoproteins and fecal bile acids: a double-blind cross-over study, *Nutr. Rep. Int.*, 22, 521, 1980.
3. **Malinow, M. R., McLaughlin, P., Kohler, G. O., and Livingston, A. L.,** Prevention of elevated cholesterolemia in monkeys by alfalfa saponins, *Steroids*, 29, 105, 1977.
4. **Oakenfull, D. G., Fenwick, D. E., Topping, D. L., Illman, R. J., and Storer, G. B.,** Effects of saponins on bile acids and plasma lipids in the rat, *Br. J. Nutr.*, 42, 209, 1979.
5. **Topping, D. L., Storer, G. B., Calvert, G. D., Illman, R. J., Oakenfull, D. G., and Weller, R. A.,** Effect of dietary saponins on fecal bile acids and neutral sterols, plasma lipids and lipoprotein turnover in the pig, *Am. J. Clin. Nutr.*, 33, 783, 1980.

6. **Molgaard, J., von Schenk, H., and Olsson, A. G.,** Alfalfa seeds lower low density lipoprotein cholesterol and apoprotein B concentrations in patients with type II hyperlipoproteinemia, *Atherosclerosis,* 65, 173, 1987.
7. **Oakenfull, D. G. and Sidhu, G. S.,** Could saponins be a useful treatment for hypercholesterolaemia?, *Eur. J. Clin. Nutr.,* 44, 79, 1990.
8. **Oakenfull, D. G. and Sidhu, G. S.,** Saponins, in *Toxicants of Plant Origin,* Vol. 2, Cheeke, P., Ed., CRC Press, Boca Raton, FL, 1989.
9. **Gestetner, B., Assa, Y., Henis, Y., Tencer, Y., Royman, M., Birk, Y., and Bondi, A.,** Interaction of lucerne saponins with sterols, *Biochim. Biophys. Acta,* 270, 181, 1972.
10. **Oakenfull, D.,** Aggregation of saponins and bile acids in aqueous solution, *Aust. J. Chem.,* 39, 1671, 1986.
11. **Oakenfull, D. G. and Sidhu, G. S.,** A physico-chemical explanation for the effects of dietary saponins on cholesterol and bile salt metabolism, *Nutr. Rep. Int.,* 27, 1253, 1983.
12. **Fenwick, D. E. and Oakenfull, D. G.,** Saponin content of soya beans and some commercial soya products, *J. Sci. Food Agric.,* 32, 273, 1981.
13. **Price, K. R., Curl, C. L., and Fenwick, G. R.,** The saponin content and sapogenol composition of the seed of thirteen varieties of legume, *J. Sci. Food Agric.,* 37, 115, 1986.
14. **Kitagawa, I., Yoshikawa, M., Hayashi, T., and Taniyama, T.,** Quantitative determination of soya-saponins in soybeans of various origins and soybean products by high performance liquid chromatography, *Yakugaku Zasshi,* 104, 275, 1984.
15. **Ireland, P. A. and Dziedzic, S. Z.,** High performance liquid chromatography on silica phase with evaporative light scattering detection, *J. Chromatogr.,* 361, 410, 1986.

Section 4: Effects of Dietary Fiber on Carbohydrate, Lipid, and Protein Metabolism
---

Chapter 4.1

EFFECT OF DIETARY FIBER AND FOODS ON CARBOHYDRATE METABOLISM

Thomas M. S. Wolever and David J. A. Jenkins

INTRODUCTION

This chapter will review the relationship between gastrointestinal events and carbohydrate metabolism in the short and long term, beginning with the effects of dietary fiber and including the extension of this to more recent work on the glycemic index of foods where both fiber, food form, and the so-called "antinutrients" all combine to produce the glycemic response typical of the whole food.

ADDITION OF FIBER TO SINGLE TEST MEALS

There is evidence that the viscosity of purified dietary fiber is directly related to its effect on glucose tolerance.[1,16] Guar, pectin, psyllium, and other viscous fibers have been shown to flatten postprandial blood glucose and insulin responses more consistently than wheat bran and other nonviscous fibers which have little or no acute effect (Tables 1 through 4, Figure 1). In 24 groups of subjects in 15 studies, when guar gum was adequately mixed with a test meal, the blood glucose response was reduced by an average of 44% ($p < 0.001$). The addition of pectin or hemicellulose did not enhance the effect of guar alone (Table 1). By contrast, pectin reduced the glucose response by an average of 29% (n = 10, $p < 0.01$, Table 2), psyllium by 29% (n = 13, $p < 0.001$, Table 3), 6 other gelling agents by 23% (n = 8, $p < 0.01$, Table 3), wheat bran by 27% (n = 6, $p < 0.01$, Table 2), and 7 other nongelling fibers by only 17% (n = 10, ns, Table 4). The degree of flattening of the glycemic response does not appear to be related to the dose of guar or pectin, possibly due to differences in experimental design, but a linear dose-response relationship is seen with psyllium (Figure 2; Table 3).

Necessity of Adequate Mixing of Fiber with Food

To be effective, guar and other viscous fibers must be mixed with the carbohydrate in a hydrated form. Thus, when guar (4 studies, Table 1) or psyllium (1 study, Table 3) were sprinkled dry onto foods or taken before the main carbohydrate portion of the test meal there was no effect on blood glucose responses. The necessity of adequate mixing of fiber with carbohydrate for effectiveness is important because the mechanism of action of viscous fiber is related to its ability to reduce the rate of diffusion of nutrients from the lumen of the small intestine,[14,213–215] although delayed gastric emptying may also play a role.[26,30,77,216] Nevertheless, viscous fiber has not been demonstrated to cause carbohydrate malabsorption.[16,30]

Effect of Food Refining on Postprandial Glucose Responses

Removal of cereal fiber from foods by refining has no effect on the postprandial glucose and insulin responses (Table 5). This is consistent with the lack of effect of cereal fiber when added to carbohydrate test meals (Table 2). On the other hand, the consumption of fruit juice as opposed to whole fruit is associated with a somewhat greater blood glucose response and markedly enhanced peripheral insulin levels.[50–52] In these cases, disruption of food form, rather than removal of, fiber per se may be important.

TABLE 1
Effect of Adding Guar Gum (G) Alone, or with Hemicellulose (H) or Pectin (P) on Blood Glucose and Insulin Responses to Single Test Meals

Fiber (g)	Available carbohydrate (g) Source	Sub[b]	% Change with fiber[a] Glucose	% Change with fiber[a] Insulin	Ref.
G 2.5	50 Glucose	N	−24% ns	−64% ***	1
G 2.5	50 Glucose	N	−34%*	−65% **	2
G 5	50 Glucose	N	0% ns	−44% +	3
G 5	50 Glucose	N		−66% **	4
G 5	49 Guar bread and soup	N	−41% +++	−37% +++	5
G 5	49 Bread and guar soup	N	−54% ***	−50% ***	5
G10	85 Cornflakes, sucrose, milk, bread, and jam (guar sprinkled on cereal)	D	−2% ns	−20% ns	6
G 8	58 Biscuits	D	−53%		7
G15	100 Glucose	N	−36% ++	−37% **	8
G15	100 Glucose	GD	−32% *	−68% ns	8
G 7	42 Bread and cheese	D	−49%		9
G 7	42 Bread and soybeans	D	−58%		9
G 9	50 Glucose	N	−23% *		3
G10	52 Soup, bread, egg, and butter	N	−48% **	−48% **	10
G10	52 Soup, bread, egg, and butter	D	−58% **		10
G10	47 Soup and bread	N,D	−78% *	−59% **	10
G10	46 Guar bread and guar soup	N	−68% ***	−65% ***	5
G 5	23 Mashed potato (guar mixed with meal)	D	−42% **	−40% ns	11
G 5	23 Mashed potato (guar taken before meal)	D	−5% ns	0% ns	11
G16	66 Guar pasta, butter, cheese	N,D	−9% *		12
G20	83 Guar pasta, egg, cheese, butter, ham	N	−80% **	−45% **	12
G23	80 Sucrose	N	−29% ns	−55% +++	13
G14.5	50 Glucose	N	−50% **	−54% **	2
G14.5	50 Glucose	N	−38% **	−60% **	14
G14.5	50 Glucose (mixed with guar)	N	−27% *		15
G14.5	50 Glucose (taken after guar)	N	0% ns		15
G14.5	50 Glucose	N	−68% **	−58% ***	16
G15	50 Glucose (taken after guar)	N	−2% ns	+28% ns	17
G10	20 Oatmeal porridge	D	−61% *		18
G 5,P 5	72 Bread, butter, honey, egg, and milk	N	−60% *	−6% ns	19
G 5,P 5	72 Bread, butter, honey, egg, and milk	D	−41% *	−16% ns	19
G 5,P 5	72 Bread, butter, honey, egg, and milk	AN	−2% ns	0% ns	19
G16,P10	102 Bread, margarine, jam, and milk	N,D	−23%	−51%	20
G16,P10	106 Bread, butter, jam, and milk	D	−51% **	−50% **	21
G15,P10	50 Glucose (after fiber)	N	−7% ns	−1% ns	17
G 4,H 4	25 Bread	D	−22%	−71%	22

[a] % Change in area under the curve (or peak rise) of blood glucose and insulin (lack of a figure means that the data is not available). * = $p < 0.05$; + = $p < 0.025$; ** = $p < 0.01$; ++ = $p < 0.005$; +++ = $p < 0.002$; *** = $p < 0.001$; ns = not significant.

[b] Subjects: N = normal, D = diabetic, GD = gestational diabetes, AN = diabetes with autonomic neuropathy.

LONGER TERM EFFECTS OF DIETARY FIBER SUPPLEMENTS

Normal Volunteers

Nonviscous fibers have been added to the diets of normal individuals more often than viscous fibers (Table 6). These studies show, paradoxically, that nonviscous fibers have more effect than viscous fibers in improving fiber-free glucose tolerance tests given after a period of fiber supplementation (Table 6).

TABLE 2
Effect of Adding Pectin (P) Alone, or Wheat Bran (B) on Blood Glucose and Insulin Responses to Single Test Meals

Fiber (g)	Available carbohydrate (g) Source	Sub[b]	% Change with fiber[a] Glucose	Insulin	Ref.
P10	100 Glucose and beef	N	−59% **	−22% ns	23
P10	100 Glucose	N	+4% ns	+11% ns	23
P10	85 Cornflakes, sucrose, milk, bread, and jam (pectin sprinkled on cereal)	N	−23% ns	−18% ns	6
P 7	60 Bread, cheese, rice, meat, and peach	D	−12% *	−35% *	24
P15	105 Bread and jam	D	−44%		25
P10.5	75 Glucose	PGS	−23% **	−56% +	26
P10	50 Glucose (after pectin)	N	+5% ns	+6% ns	17
P 9	45 Glucose[c]	IGT	−25% +	−11% ns	27
P14.5	50 Glucose	N	−11% ns	−2% ns	16
P14.5	50 Glucose	PGS	−20% **		28
P14.5	50 Glucose	PGS	−40% ***	−76% ***	29
P14.5	50 Glucose	N	−55% +		30
B10	50 Glucose (after bran)	N	+7% ns	+11% ns	17
B0.2g/kg	1 g/kg Glucose	N	−37% **		31
B20	90 Beef, bread, rice, corn, tomato	D	−11% ns	+6% ns[d]	32
B36	50 Glucose, beef, lactulose	N	−54% ns	−16% ns	33
B41.5	50 Glucose	N	−27% ns	−8% ns	16
B50	50 Glucose	D/D	−13% ns	−34% ++	34
B50	50 Glucose	D/O	−21% +	0% ns	34

[a] % Change in area under the curve (or peak rise) of blood glucose and insulin (lack of a figure means that the data is not available). * = $p < 0.05$; + = $p < 0.025$; ** = $p < 0.01$; ++ = $p < 0.005$; +++ = $p < 0.002$; *** = $p < 0.001$; ns = not significant.

[b] Subjects: N = normal; D = diabetic; PGS = postgastric surgery: IGT = impaired glucose tolerance with reactive hypoglycemia; D/D = diabetic on diet alone; D/O = diabetic on oral agents.

[c] Grams pectin and glucose are per square meter of body surface.

[d] Represents change in insulin requirements of Type 1 diabetics on an artificial pancreas.

Treatment of Diabetes

There have been over 20 studies using guar gum or other viscous fibers to treat diabetes and about half that number using various nonviscous fibers (Tables 7 and 8). The improvements in diabetic control after the addition of viscous fibers were larger and more consistent than after the addition of nonviscous fibers (Figure 3). In 18 studies where urinary glucose was measured, losses were reduced by 41% after guar ($p < 0.001$), but in seven studies with nonviscous fibers, there was a mean increase of 34% (ns). Fasting blood glucose was reduced by a mean of 11% after guar ($p < 0.001$) and 3.8% after nonviscous fibers ($p < 0.02$). Glycosylated hemoglobin fell by a mean of 5.0% after guar ($p < 0.01$) and 3.4% (ns) after nonviscous fibers. Insulin doses tended to be reduced on guar (-11%, $p < 0.05$) but not after nonviscous fibers ($+1\%$, ns). Serum cholesterol fell by 11% after guar ($p < 0.001$) but not after nonviscous fibers (-1%, ns).

Summary — Long-Term Effects of Dietary Fiber Supplements

Those types of fiber with the most marked short-term effects also appear to have the greatest ability in the longer term to improve diabetic control. Viscous forms of dietary fiber such as guar gum are most able to alter events occurring within the gastrointestinal tract, such as the rate of absorption of glucose. These fibers are associated with short- and long-term beneficial changes in carbohydrate metabolism.

TABLE 3
Effect of Adding Various Gelling Agents on Blood Glucose and Insulin Responses to Single Test Meals

Fiber[a] (g)	Available carbohydrate (g) Source	Sub[c]	% Change with fiber[b] Glucose	Insulin	Ref.
T14.5	50 Glucose	N	−34% **	−10% ns	16
M14.5	50 Glucose	N	−29% *	−18% ns	16
L2.5	50 Glucose	N	−29% ns	−19% ns	1
L10	85 Cornflakes, sucrose, milk, bread, jam	D	−15% ns	+11% ns	6
X2.5	50 Glucose	N	−41% *	−37% **	1
X/L2.5	50 Glucose	N	−28% ns	−64% **	1
A10	85 Cornflakes, sucrose, milk, bread, jam	D	−7% ns	+17% ns	6
K5	80 Glucose	N	0% ns	−28% *	35
S3.5	50 Glucose (psyllium as Fibogel)	N	−33% ns	−39% ns	2
S3.6	Bread, butter, cheese, meat, milk	D	−33% *	−19% *[d]	36
S6.6	50 Bread, butter, cheese	D	−29%		37
S7	50 Glucose (psyllium as Fibogel)	N	−12% ns	−28% ns	2
S7	50 Glucose (psyllium as Fibogel)	D	−17% ns	−13% ns	2
S7	50 Glucose (psyllium as Metamucil)	N	0% ns		2
S3.9	50 Psyllium-enriched flaked bran cereal	N	−12% ns		38
S8.1	50 Psyllium-enriched flaked bran cereal	N	−24% ns		38
S12.7	50 Psyllium-enriched flaked bran cereal	N	−20% ns		38
S16.8	50 Psyllium-enriched flaked bran cereal	N	−46% **		38
S15.7	50 Psyllium-enriched flaked bran cereal	N	−46% **		38
S15.7	50 Psyllium-enriched flaked bran cereal	D	−51% *		38
S16.2	50 Psyllium sprinkled on bran flakes	N	−56% **		38
S16.2	50 Psyllium taken just before bran flakes	N	−4% ns		38

[a] T = Gum tragacanth; M = Methyl cellulose; L = Locust bean gum; A = agar; S = psyllium; K = Konjac mannan.
[b] % change in area under the curve (or peak rise) of blood glucose and insulin (lack of a figure means that the data is not available). * = $p < 0.05$; + = $p < 0.025$; ** = $p < 0.01$; ++ = $p < 0.005$; +++ = $p < 0.002$; *** = $p < 0.001$; ns = not significant.
[c] Subjects: N = normal; D = diabetic.
[d] This figure represents the percent reduction of GIP response.

BLOOD GLUCOSE RESPONSE TO FOODS

In whole foods, many factors in addition to dietary fiber may alter digestion and absorption of nutrients and hence the glycemic response. Among these are antinutrients such as phytate,[105,217] lectins,[218] tannins,[219] and enzyme inhibitors,[220,221] macronutrient interactions such as protein-starch[222] and lipid-starch,[223] the nature of the starch (amylose vs. amylopectin),[224,225] gastric emptying rate[226] food form (e.g., bread as opposed to spaghetti), cooking, and particle size. It therefore becomes important in any discussion of glycemic response to be able to assess the collective interaction of all these factors in terms of the glycemic response to the whole food, and also to compare the full range of foods, so that the relative importance of each of the factors can be determined, again in the context of the whole food.

The Glycemic Index of Foods

The glycemic index (GI) of foods is an expression which permits the blood glucose response to different foods to be compared directly and so allows the relevance of their constituents (e.g., fiber) to be assessed. It is defined as the incremental blood glucose response following consumption of a 50 g available carbohydrate portion of a food expressed

TABLE 4
Effect of Adding Various Nongelling Fibers on Blood Glucose and Insulin Responses to Single Test Meals

Fiber[a] (g)	Available carbohydrate (g) Source	Sub[c]	% Change with fiber[b] Glucose	Insulin	Ref.
Q14.5	50 Glucose	N	−26% ns	−24% ns	16
B15	105 Bread and jam	D	−6%		25
C 9	45 Glucose	IGT	−22% ns	0% ns	27
C 0.2g/kg	1 g/kg Glucose	N	+16% ns		31
G 0.2g/kg	1 g/kg Glucose	N	+24% ns		31
S20	86 50 g sucrose, 45 g flour	N	−14% ns	0% ns	39
S22	50 Glucose, beef, lactulose	N	−65% *	−24% ns	33
F30	50 Glucose, beef, lactulose	N	−39% ns	−19% ns	33
P10	58 Noodles, egg, milk, juice, margarine	DO	−21%	0% ns	40
P10	67,35 Liquid formula diet	D	−18% ns	−7% ns	41

[a] Q = cholestyramine; B = barley bran; C = cellulose; G = bagasse; S = sugar beet fiber; P = soy polysaccharide; F = pea fiber.
[b] % change in area under the curve (or peak rise) of blood glucose and insulin (lack of a figure means that the data is not available). * = $p < 0.05$; + = $p < 0.025$; ** = $p < 0.01$; ++ = $p < 0.005$; +++ = $p < 0.002$; *** = $p < 0.001$; ns = not significant.
[c] Subjects: N = normal; D = diabetic; IGT = impaired glucose tolerance; DO = obese diabetic.

TABLE 5
Effect of Refining Food (i.e., Removal of Fiber) on Blood Glucose and Insulin Responses

Food	Test meal contents (g) Available carbohydrate	Dietary fiber Whole	Refined	Sub[b]	Change with refining[a] Glucose	Insulin	Ref.
Wheat bread	50	10.2	2.8	N	−6% ns		42
Wheat bread	50	10.2	2.8	D	−2% ns		43
Wheat bread	58 and 60			N	−14% ns	−18% ns	44
Wheat bread	50			N	−5% ns		45
Wheat bread	25			D	+7% ns		46
Rice	50	3.5	1.4	N	+11% ns		42
Rice	75			D	+6% ns	+14% ns	47
Spaghetti	50	7.3	2.0	N	+11% ns		42
Maize meal	50			N	+4% ns		48
Potato	50			N	+14% ns		49
Oranges	50			N	+15% ns		49
Oranges	50	16.0	0.0	N	ns	+50% +++	50
Oranges	30	8.0	0.2	N	+6% ns		51
Grapes	60	4.6	0.0	N	+28% *	+32% +	50
Apples	60			N	ns	+51% **	52

[a] % change in area under the curve (or peak rise) of blood glucose and insulin (lack of a figure means that the data is not available). * = $p < 0.05$; + = $p < 0.025$; ** = $p < 0.01$; ++ = $p < 0.005$; +++ = $p < 0.002$; *** = $p < 0.001$; ns = not significant.
[b] Subjects: N = normal; D = diabetic.

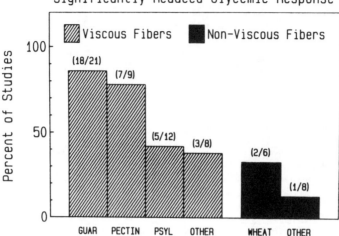

FIGURE 1. Effect of various types of purified dietary fiber on acute glycemic responses: proportion of studies with a statistically significant reduction (data from Tables 1 through 4).

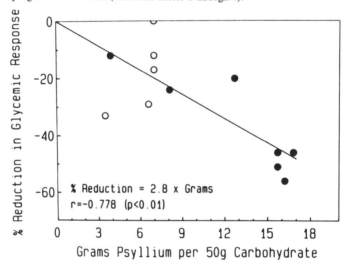

FIGURE 2. Effect of psyllium dose on acute glycaemic responses (data from Table 3).

as a percent of the response after a standard 50 g available carbohydrate portion of white bread taken by the same individual. The methods used to determine the glycemic response and calculate the area under the curve can have a major influence on the results obtained;[227] exact GI methods are given elsewhere.[158]

$$\text{Glycemic Index} = \frac{\text{Area under the glucose curve after a food} \times 100\%}{\text{Area under the glucose curve after white bread}}$$

In this way, the GI makes it possible to compare the blood glucose responses of foods tested in different groups of subjects. Tables 9 and 10 show the wide range of GI values for different foods. The legumes, as a class, have the lowest GI of all starchy foods. Table 9 shows the mean GI values for foods tested in different groups of subjects and by different investigators. In general there is reasonable agreement between the values derived in different centers.

TABLE 6
Effect of Dietary Fiber on Fiber-Free Glucose Tolerance Tests[a]

Fiber dose (g/day)	Study[b] Length	Diet Constituents				Change after fiber[c]		Ref.
		CHO	PRO	FAT	Comments	Glucose	Insulin	
Gum arabic, 25	21 D	39	15	42	FRD, all fiber in morning	+100% ns	ns	53
Pectin, 36	6 W				MD	+18% ns	+11% ns	54
Wheat bran, 12	4 W	47	14	36	FRD	ns	ns	55
Wheat bran, 20	7 W				MD	−32% *	+36% +	56
Wheat bran, 24	6 M				FRD	−15% **		45
Wheat bran, 26	30 D				MD	−17%	ns	57
Wheat bran, 26	30 D				MD	+24%	ns	57
Corn bran, 26	30 D				MD	−56% *	ns	57
Soy hulls, 21	3 W	40	19	40	FRD undried DF	+5% ns	+10% ns	58
Soy hulls, 21	3 W	42	19	37	FRD dried DF	+59% *	−7% ns	58
Soy hulls, 26	30 D				MD	−72% *	ns	57
Apple/carrot, 26	30 D				MD	−28% *	ns	57
Xanthan gum, 12	6 W				FRD	−25% ns[d]		59
Xanthan gum, 12	6 W(D)				FRD	−31% *	−6% ns	59
Guar gum, 15	2 W				FRD	−5% ns	−4% ns	60
Guar gum, 15	2 W(D)				FRD	−4% ns	+13% ns	60

[a] Subjects are normal except where indicated after study length (i.e., (D) = diabetic).
[b] Study length: D = days; W = weeks; M = months.
[c] % change in area under the curve (or peak rise) of blood glucose and insulin (lack of a figure means that the data is not available). * = $p < 0.05$; + = $p < 0.025$; ** = $p < 0.01$; ++ = $p < 0.005$; +++ $p < 0.002$; *** = $p < 0.001$; ns = not significant.
[d] 2-h postglucose blood glucose values.

For 27 foods tested by 3 or more groups of subjects, the mean SD of the mean GI values is 12 (Table 9), regardless of whether the subjects tested were normal or diabetic.

Insulin-dependent diabetic subjects (IDDM) tend to show slightly higher GI values than subjects with noninsulin dependent diabetes.[111] This may be a reflection of the high degree of within-individual variability of blood glucose responses in IDDM to the same meal rather than to true differences between foods tested in these individuals.[111] In a recent study 12 subjects with diabetes, including individuals with IDDM and NIDDM, tested 3 different foods 4 times each. Most of the variability in GI values was due to day-to-day variability within subjects with no significant difference in GI values between the different individuals. In all 12 subjects, the mean glycemic response to bread was greater than that to rice, which, in turn, was greater than that to spaghetti.[228]

The GI values of foods relate strongly to the rate of digestion of foods *in vitro*,[99,106,229–234] but only weakly to total fiber content, and not significantly to soluble fiber.[235] However, in one study, increasing the soluble fiber content of a meal with no change in its GI resulted in a major reduction of the postprandial glycemic response in subjects with NIDDM.[236] Surprisingly, the strongest correlation between food GI and components of fiber was with cellulose and the uronic acid fraction of insoluble fiber, major components of the cell wall (Figure 4). The lack of relationship between food GI and soluble fiber is probably due to the fact that many other factors in foods influence digestibility, and that soluble fibers have differing viscosities and hence variable effects in impeding glucose absorption.

The GI values of foods are related to their fat and protein contents.[49] Fat delays gastric emptying[237] and enhances GIP responses.[123,126] However, only in large amounts (45 to 65%

TABLE 7
Treatment of Diabetes with Guar (G) or Guar plus Wheat Bran (B)

Dose (g)	Length	Subjects[a]	Comments[b] Diet	Form	% Change after fiber treatment[c] FBG	HbA1c	UG Loss	Insulin[d]	CHOL	TG	Ref.
G25	5D	6I,1N	MD	CB	−22%**		−50%**				61
G23	5D	6I,3N	MD	BI	−20%*		−38%++				62
G10	7D	2I,6N	FRD		−7%		−32%				7
G24	7D	12I	HD								63
G 9.2	2W	5I	FRD	BI	−8%ns	−11%ns	−80%**				7
G 9.2	2W	5N	FRD	BI	−18%**	−3%*	−62%**				7
G20	3W	6I,11N	FRD	GR	−10%*				−14%*		64
G15−25	4W	10N	FRD	GR	+13%ns		−51%**		−14%**		65
G.45g/kg	4W	10I,Child	FRD	BR			−8%				66
G20−25	4W	6I	FRD	SW	ns		−49%ns	−4%ns	−9%		67
G15	4W	41N,SU	FRD	MT			−50%*		−9%*	−12%*	68
G15	4W	38N,In	FRD	MT			−14%*	0%	−10%*	−2%ns	68
G15	4W	18N	FRD	GR	−11%*	−10%*			−10%*	+13%ns	69
G20	4W	9I	FRD	GR		+2%ns			−21%+	−25%ns	70
G15	4W	9N,O,PC	FRD	GR	−25%*	−7%ns	−10%ns	−5%+	−8%ns	0%ns	71
G8	6W	14N	FRD	BR	ns	ns			ns	ns	72
G12−19	6W	22I,Child	FRD	VF	−3%ns	−9%***	−15%***	−3%ns	−11%+		73
G10	8W	20N	FRD	GR	−24%**	−9%***	−32%ns		0%ns	+5%ns	74
G10−15	8W	2I,3N	MD	P	−16%ns	−7%ns	−66%+		−16%*	−17%*	12
G15	8W	8N,ND,O	LOW	GR	0%ns	+2%ns			−2%ns	+8%ns	75
G15	8W	29N,EC	FRD	MT	−39%+				−10%***		76
G20,B10	8W	12N,O,PC	FRD	GR	−17%+		−73%*		−30%+	−40%ns	77
G21	3M	9N	FRD	GR	−19%ns	−3%ns	−60%	−14%+	+11%ns		78
G22	3M	10I,B	FRD	R	0%ns				−18%**		79
G15	3M	6N,O,NC	FRD	CAP	−10%ns	−5%ns	−7%ns	−28%***	−9%***	−4%ns	80
G15	3M	20N,O,PC	FRD	GR	+4%ns		−44%*	−26%***	−10%*	+8%ns	81
G14−26	6M	8I,3N	FRD	CB							82
G14−26	12M	6I,2N	FRD	CB							82

a Subjects: I = insulin-dependent; N = noninsulin-dependent; Child = chidren; SU = controlled on sulfonylureas; In = controlled on insulin; O = obese; PC = poorly controlled; ND = newly diagnosed; EC = excellent control; B = brittle; NC = poorly compliant.
b Diets: MD = metabolic diet; FRD = free-range diet; HD = hospital diet; LOW = weight reducing, low calorie (results for guar compared to a separate control group on a low calorie diet not given guar). Form = type of guar formulation; CB = crispbread; BI = biscuits; P = pasta; GR = granulate; BR = bread; SW = snacks and sweets; MT = minitablets; FP = flavored powder taken in water before meals; VF = guar incorporated into various foods (bread, gelly, jam, fruit bar); R = rusks; CAP = capsules.
c FBG = fasting blood glucose; HbA1c = glycoylated hemoglobin; UG = urinary glucose; Insulin = daily insulin dose; CHOL = serum cholesterol; TG = serum triglycerides. * = $p < 0.05$; + = $p < 0.025$; ** = $p < 0.01$; ++ = $p < 0.002$; *** = $p < 0.001$.
d Represents fall in fasting serum insulin. In this study, guar increasd peripheral insulin sensitivity by 70% ($p < 0.025$), insulin binding to monocytes by 28% ($p < 0.025$), and insulin receptor number by 50% ($p < 0.05$).

TABLE 8
Treatment of Diabetes with Miscellaneous Types of Dietary Fiber

Nonviscous Fibers

Dose (g)	Length	Subjects[a]	Comments[b] Diet	Form	% Change after fiber treatment[c] FBG	HbA1c	UG Loss	Insulin	CHOL	TG	Ref.
Apple Fiber											
26	4W	10N	FRD		−2%ns	+2%ns	+49%ns		−5%ns	+5%ns	83
52	4W	10N	FRD		−2%ns	+3%ns	+119%ns		+6%*	+2%ns	83
15	7W	12N	FRD		−8%*	−8%**			−5%ns	0%ns	84
Corn Bran											
26	4W	10N	FRD		−6%ns	−2%ns	+26%ns		−2%ns	+1%ns	83
52	4W	10N	FRD		+2%ns	−8%*	+67%ns		+1%ns	−4%ns	83
Soy Hulls											
26	4W	10N	FRD		−10%ns	−2%ns	+5%ns		0%ns	+9%ns	83
52	4W	10N	FRD		−1%ns	−1%ns	+7%ns		+3%ns	+3%ns	83
Wheat Bran											
14	10–15D	17I	MD	BR	0%ns	−13%ns	−36%**	+2%ns		+7%ns	85
15	4W	18N	FRD			−2%ns			0%ns		69
20	4W	38IGT	FRD		−5%				−9%***	−10%*	86
Cellulose											
15	10D	8I	MD	BR	−6%ns			0%			87

					Psyllium				
10.8	7D	9I	FRD	MM	+6%ns	0%			35
3.6	2M	20N	FRD	MM	−19%**		−5%*	−6%ns	88
7.2	2M	20N	FRD	MM	−18%**		−5%*	−11%ns	87
					Konjac Mannan				
3.6–7	30D	13N	MD		−29%+	Reduced	−11%		89
					Xanthan Gum				
12	6W	9N	FRD	MU	−38%*		−13%*	−25%ns	59

[a] Length: D = days; W = weeks; M = months. Subjects: N = noninsulin-dependent diabetes; I = insulin-dependent diabetes; IGT = impaired glucose tolerance.

[b] Diets: MD = metabolic diet; FRD = free-range diet. Form = type of fiber formulation; MM = "Metamucil"; BR = bread; MU = fiber in muffins.

[c] FBG = fasting blood glucose; HbA1c = glycoylated hemoglobin; UG = urinary glucose; Insulin = daily insulin dose; CHOL = serum cholesterol; TG = serum triglycerides. * = $p < 0.05$; + = $p < 0.025$; ** = $p < 0.01$; ++ = $p < 0.002$; *** = $p < 0.001$.

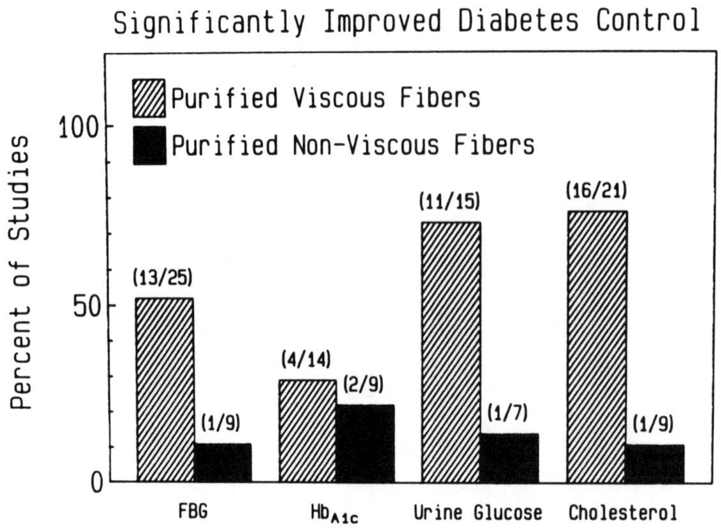

FIGURE 3. Effect of purified dietary fiber in the treatment of diabetes. Proportion of studies with statistically significant improvements in fasting blood glucose (FBG), glycosylated hemoglobin (HbA1c), urinary glucose excretion, and serum cholesterol concentration (data from Tables 7 and 8).

of total test meal calories) does it significantly reduce postprandial glucose and insulin responses (Table 11). In addition, fat taken at one meal may impair carbohydrate tolerance in the subsequent meal.[238] Large amounts of protein enhance insulin secretion (Table 11), but have little effect on the blood glucose response in the smaller amounts normally eaten, e.g., bread with cheese.[49,90,103]

Particle size is particularly important in determining the responses of starchy foods (Table 12). The glycemic response to wheat and barley breads increases linearly as the proportion of flour, as opposed to whole grains, in the bread increases;[135] finely ground flour produces higher glycemic responses than coarse flour;[136] and the whole grain rye breads popular in Northern Europe have relatively flat glycemic and insulinemic responses.[94] Increased particle size is probably related to the reduced glycemic effect after swallowing foods without adequate chewing.[239] In addition, cooking and processing of foods markedly affect their *in vitro* digestibility and these changes are reflected in similar alterations of metabolic responses *in vivo* (Table 13). Differences in food form may also be of great importance in determining the glycemic index of a food as exemplified by the similar composition but very different GI values of white bread and spaghetti (Table 9). Variables such as food variety (e.g., new vs. russet potato; Table 9), the degree of ripeness (e.g., banana; Tables 9, 10), and differences in cooking and processing (e.g., rice; Table 9) may therefore explain some of the differences in GI values obtained for the same food by different investigators.

Clinical Utility of the Glycemic Index

The GI of mixed meals can be estimated from the weighted mean of the GI values of the individual carbohydrate foods in the meal, with the weighting based on the proportion of the total carbohydrate contributed by each food (Table 14). In our hands, the GI value of mixed meals predicts almost exactly the relative differences between their mean glycemic responses (Figure 5). To be of predictive value, accurate GI values for the foods fed must be used, the calculation of meal GI must take into account all of the carbohydrate foods in the meal, and the method of calculation of area under the curve must be the same as that

TABLE 9
Glycemic Index Values of Foods Tested in Several Studies

Food	Individual GI values[a]	Studies[b]	Mean ± SD	CV[c]
Breads				
Rye (crispbread)	90, 100	C, A	95	
Rye (whole meal)	82, 89, 97, 105, 119	Ti, G, Tn, #, #	98 ± 14	15%
Rye (Whole grain-pumpernickel)	58, 78	C, G	68	
Wheat (white)	100 (Defined)	A–K, M	100	
Wheat (whole meal)	93, 95, 96, 96, 100, 104, 106, 106, 108	C, Tn, Ti, G, B, A, J, S, #	100 ± 6	6%
Pasta				
Spaghetti (white)	46, 59, 68, 72, 88	I, B, C, A, Z	67 ± 16	23%
Cereal Grains				
Barley (pearled)	31, 41	F, Xi	36	
Buckwheat	70, 74, 90	Xn, A, Xi	78 ± 11	14%
Rice (polished)	68, 70, 73, 77, 78, 83, 92, 104	M, L, C, Z, B, H, W, A	81 ± 12	15%
Rice (parboiled)	58, 66, 72, 78	D, H, E, P	69 ± 9	12%
Sweet corn	66, 67, 85, 86, 87, 90	E, L, P, A, J, D	80 ± 11	13%
Breakfast Cereals				
"All Bran"	71, 74, 76	B, A, N	74 ± 3	3%
Cornflakes	107, 116, 121, 139	L, A, B, W	121 ± 13	11%
Porridge oats	71, 88, 93, 96, 96	A, C, K, B, W	89 ± 10	12%
Cookies				
Digestive	77, 86	B, A	82	
Plain crackers (water biscuits)	91, 108	A, S	100	

TABLE 9 (continued)
Glycemic Index Values of Foods Tested in Several Studies

Food	Individual GI values[a]	Studies[b]	Mean ± SD	CV[c]
Root Vegetables				
Carrots	96, 131	¢, A	114	
Potato (instant mashed)	116, 119, 126	A, L, Y	120 ± 5	4%
Potato (mashed)	96, 100	Y, J	98	
Potato (new/white boiled)	67, 75, 77, 78, 101	C, B, Y, L, A	80 ± 13	16%
Potato (Russett, baked)	80, 112, 134, 137	Y, E, P, D	116 ± 26	23%
Legumes				
Baked beans (canned)	60, 69, 80	A, £, U	70 ± 10	14%
Bengal gram dal	7, 16	J, M	12	
Butter beans	39, 52	J, A	46	
Chick peas (dried)	44, 46, 52	U, B, A	47 ± 4	9%
Green peas (dried)	32, 68	C, A	50	
Green peas (frozen)	55, 74	C, A	65	
White beans (dried)	18, 27, 43, 44, 45, 46, 56, 84	@n, @h, U, O, A, £, Pn, Pi	45 ± 20	43%
Kidney beans (dried)	27, 31, 32, 42, 60, 65	M, W, Z, A, U, B	43 ± 16	38%
Lentils (green, dried)	31, 41	U, Z	36	
Lentils (red, dried)	25, 30, 42, 43, 45, 45	R, Xn, A, B, β, Xi, W	39 ± 8	21%
Pinto beans (dried)	55, 65	U, B	60	
Peanuts	10, 19	J, A	15	
Fruit				
Apple	48, 52, 57	C, V, A	52 ± 5	9%
Banana	66, 75, 81, 90, 99	C, $, B, A, J	82 ± 13	16%
Orange	46, 58, 73	J, A, C	59 ± 14	23%
Orange juice	56, 67, 90	V, A, V	71 ± 17	24%

Sugars

Food	Studies	Value	CV
Fructose	9, 29, 30, 35	26 ± 11	45%
Glucose	122, 131, 132, 137, 137, 140, 141, 145, 158	138 ± 10	7%
	V, A, C, K		
	E, K, Q, C, D, W, J, A, M		
Lactose	45, 69	57	
	V, K		
Sucrose	61, 85, 86, 87, 91, 92, 100	86 ± 12	14%
	V, C, A, @h, K, J, @n		

Dairy Products

Food	Studies	Value	CV
Ice cream	52, 54, 84, 86	69 ± 19	27%
	A, @h, @n, S		
Whole milk	26, 29, 39, 49	36 ± 10	29%
	@h, @n, S, A		

Snack Foods

Food	Studies	Value	CV
Potato chips	74, 79	77	
	A, L		

[a] Individual mean values from groups of subjects. Values have been adjusted proportionately so that the glycemic index (GI) of white bread = 100. Values have also been adjusted proportionately (studies C, peas; T, breads; Z, instant potatoes) for unequal amounts of carbohydrate. Where glucose, but not white bread, was given, the GI values were multiplied by 1.38 (the GI of glucose/100).

[b] The studies are listed in the same order as the values: A(49), B(90), C(46), D(91), E(92), F(93), G(94), H(95), I(96), J(97), K(98), L(99), M(100), N(101), O(102), P(103), Q(104), R(105), S(106), T(107), U(108), V(109), W(110), X(111), Y(112), Z(113), β(114), $(115), £(116), ¢(117), #(118), @(119), &(120): h = healthy subjects; i = IDDM; n = NIDDM.

[c] CV = coefficient of variation (100 × SD/Mean).

TABLE 10
Glycemic Index (GI) of Foods Tested Only Once

Food	GI	Ref[a]
Breads		
Wheat (French baguette)	131	Z
Wheat (puffed crispbread)	112	S
Pasta		
Fettuccine (nondurum)	44	#
Ravioli (durum)	54	#
Macaroni (white, boiled 5')	64	I
Spaghetti (brown, boiled 15')	61	I
Spaghetti (white, boiled 5')	45	I
Spaghetti (protein enriched)	38	I
Spirali (durum)	59	#
Star pasta (white, boiled 5')	54	I
Vermicelli (nondurum)	48	#
Cereal Grains		
Bulgur (cracked wheat)	65	G
Millet	103	A
Rice (instant, boiled 1')	65	H
Rice (instant, boiled 6')	121	L
Rice (polished, boiled 5')	58	H
Rice (parboiled, boiled 5')	54	H
Rye kernels	47	6
Unrefined maize meal porridge	71	J
Refined maize meal porridge	74	J
Wheat kernels	63	G
Wheat kernels (quick cooking)	75	S
Breakfast Cereals		
Muesli	96	A
Puffed rice	132	L
Puffed wheat	110	S
Shredded wheat	97	A
"Weetabix"	109	A
Cookies		
Oatmeal	78	A
"Rich Tea"	80	A
Shortbread	88	S
Miscellaneous		
Mars bar	99	A
Corn chips	99	L
Tomato soup	55	A

TABLE 10 (continued)
Glycemic Index (GI) of Foods Tested Only Once

Food	GI	Ref[a]
Root Vegetables		
Beetroot	93	A
Cassava (flakes)	113	&
Cassava (Eba)	99	&
Cassava (Lafun)	73	&
M'fino	68	J
Sweet potato	70	A
Yam	74	A
Pumpkin	75	J
Legumes		
Chick peas (canned)	60	U
Kidney beans (canned)	74	U
Lentils (green, canned)	74	U
Pinto beans (canned)	64	U
Black-eyed peas	48	A
Brown beans	24	J
Soybeans (canned)	20	A
Soybeans (dried)	22	A
Fruit		
Apple juice	45	V
Banana (slightly underripe)	59	$
Banana (slight overripe)	90	$
Cherries (raw)	32	C
Grapefruit	36	C
Grapes	62	C
Peaches	40	C
Pears	47	C
Plums	34	C
Raisins	93	A
Sugars		
Honey	126	A
Maltose	152	A
Dairy Products		
Custard	59	S
Skim milk	46	A
Yogurt	52	A

[a] See legend of Table 9 for identification of references.

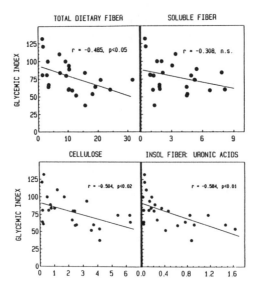

FIGURE 4. Relationship between the glycemic index value of 25 foods and their content of total dietary fiber, and selected fiber fractions (grams/50 g available carbohydrate portion; data from Reference 235).

used for the GI.[160,240] In a meta-analysis of data from the literature (Table 14), the Stanford group has been unable to predict mixed meal glycemic responses using the GI of foods. However, data from 11 other groups worldwide (Lund, Melbourne, Morgantown, Minneapolis (2 different groups), Toronto, Naples, Aarhus, London (Canada), Bristol, Sydney) are grouped around the line of identity (Figure 6). For small numbers of subjects, the most appropriate use of the GI is to help in determining which of two meals is likely to produce the greater glycemic response. The chance of a correct prediction depends upon the day-to-day variability of glycemic responses in the subjects being tested, the expected difference in meal GI, and the number of subjects or repeat tests done.[161,228] For a subject with NIDDM, there is a 95% chance of a correct prediction for a GI difference of 34 (i.e., 34 is the predictive difference); in subjects with IDDM, who have greater variability of glycemic responses, the predictive difference is 50. As the number of tests done increases, the predictive difference is reduced by a factor of $1/\sqrt{n}$.[161]

Treatment of Diabetes with High Carbohydrate, High Fiber Diets

High carbohydrate diets, in the absence of increased fiber, are not consistently effective in reducing fasting blood glucose and serum cholesterol levels (mean reductions, 3.4 ± 2.0% and 3.4 ± 2.2%, respectively [ns], Table 15) and may increase postprandial blood glucose and insulin responses, increase fasting triglyceride levels, and reduce HDL cholesterol, at least in the short term (2 to 6 weeks; Table 15, Figure 7). For these reasons the safety of high carbohydrate diets in diabetes has been questioned.[241] However, the use of foods rich in dietary fiber may offset the deleterious effects of high carbohydrate diets on blood glucose, insulin, and triglycerides and enhance their cholesterol lowering effects.

The use of high fiber foods in the diet, where overall carbohydrate content is kept constant, improves diabetic blood glucose and lipid control, but only when the increase in fiber comes from low glycaemic index foods (Table 16, Figure 8). In the limited number of studies done in this situation, fiber appears to be more effective at higher rather than lower carbohydrate intakes (Table 16). When guar gum was added to the diets of diabetic patients for 5 days, a similar phenomenon was observed.[242] Those patients whose diets contained more than 40% carbohydrates had a larger reduction of their urinary glucose output

TABLE 11
Effect of Fat and Protein on Metabolic Responses to Foods

Effect of Adding Fat Alone

Test meal constituents	CHO (g)	Added (g) PRO	Added (g) FAT	Sub[a]	% Change[b] Glucose	% Change[b] Insulin	% Change[b] GIP	Ref.
Flummery ± fat	50	0	10	N	−49%*	−8%ns	+100%ns	121
Flummery ± fat	50	0	10	NID	0%ns	+5%ns	+400%**	121
Flummery ± fat	50	0	10	ID	0%ns		+700%*	121
Potatoes ± olive oil	50	0	18	N	+40%			122
Rice ± olive oil	50	0	18	N	+108%			122
Lentils ± olive oil	50	0	18	N	−27%			122
Bread ± butter	50	0	23	NID	−16%ns			103
Potato ± butter	75	0	38	N	−58%*	−9%ns	+640%**	123
Lentils ± butter	75	0	38	N	−52%*	−26%ns	+650%**	123
Potato ± corn oil	50	0	28	N	−85%**	−89%**		124
Glucose ± avocado oil	50	0	40	NID	−12%ns	+14%ns		125
Potato ± intralipid (ileum)[c]	50	0	41	N	−87%**	−79%***		125
Potato ± intralipid (duodenum)[c]	50	0	41	N	−85%	−63%		125
Potato ± butter	50	0	50	N	−52%++	−7%ns	+800%++	126

Effect of Adding Protein Alone

Test meal constituents	CHO (g)	Added (g) PRO	Added (g) FAT	Sub[a]	Glucose	Insulin	GIP	Ref.
Glucose ± lean hamburger	50	10	3	NID	+9%ns	+25%ns		127
Bread ± cottage cheese	50	12	2	NID	−2%ns			90
Bread ± skim milk cheese	50	12	2	NID	−21%ns			103
Potato ± tuna	25	25	1	NID	−8%*	+59%***		128
Spaghetti ± tuna	25	25	1	NID	+9%ns	+69%***		128
Glucose ± beef	50	25	8	NID	−10%ns	+230%*		129
Glucose ± turkey	50	25	3	NID	−20%*	+230%*		129
Glucose ± gelatin	50	25	0	NID	−33%*	+260%*		129
Glucose ± egg white	50	25	0	NID	0%ns	+190%*		129
Glucose ± cottage cheese	50	25	0	NID	−34%*	+360%*		129
Glucose ± fish	50	25	1	NID	−10%ns	+230%*		129
Glucose ± soy	50	25	0	NID	−33%ns	+220%*		129

TABLE 11 (continued)
Effect of Fat and Protein on Metabolic Responses to Foods

Effect of Adding Fat Alone

Test meal constituents	CHO (g)	Added (g) PRO	Added (g) FAT	Sub[a]	% Change[b] Glucose	% Change[b] Insulin	% Change[b] GIP	Ref.
Glucose ± casein	50	30	0	NID	−37%	+99%**		125
Potatoes ± veal	50	42	1	N	+29%			122
Rice ± veal	50	42	1	N	+52%			122
Lentils ± veal	50	42	1	N	+12%			122
Glucose ± lean hamburger	50	30	9	NID	−9%ns	+100%*		127
Glucose ± lean hamburger	50	50	15	NID	−35%***	+207%***		127
Sugars ± milk/soy protein	58	16	tr	N	−40%***	+102%***		130
Sugars ± milk/soy protein	58	25	tr	N	−51%***	+117%***		130
Sugars ± milk/soy protein	58	34	tr	N	−70%***	+115%***		130
Sugars ± milk/soy protein	58	50	tr	N	−78%***	+129%***		130

Effect of Adding Fat and Protein

Test meal constituents	CHO (g)	Added (g) PRO	Added (g) FAT	Sub[a]	% Change[b] Glucose	% Change[b] Insulin	% Change[b] GIP	Ref.
Bread, rice, spaghetti, or barley ± fat and protein cheddar cheese	50	8	11	NID	+3%ns			111
	50	8	11	ID	+25%*			111
Flummery ± fat and protein	50	21	10	N	−89%*	+70%*	+340%**	121
Flummery ± fat and protein	50	21	10	NID	0%ns	+185%**	+600%**	121
Flummery ± fat and protein	50	21	10	ID	+63%**	+1000%**		121
Bread, potato, rice, spaghetti, or beans ± cheese and butter	50	4–20	19	NID	−20%ns	+56%*		113
Bread ± skim cheese and butter	50	12	25	NID	−4%ns			103
Bread ± peanut butter	50	14	25	NID	−27%**			103
Bread ± peanut butter	50	14	25	ID	+2%ns			103
Potato ± tuna and margarine	25	25	26	NID	−27%***	+70%***		128
Spaghetti ± tuna and margarine	25	25	26	NID	−7%ns	+85%***		128
Glucose ± casein and avocado oil	50	30	40	NID	−60%***	+16%ns		125

[a] Sub = subjects: NID = noninsulin-dependent diabetes; ID = insulin-dependent diabetes; N = normal.
[b] Change in incremental area under curve or peak rise compared to low protein/fat: * = $p < 0.05$; + = $p < 0.025$; ** = $p < 0.01$; ++ = $p < 0.005$; *** = $p < 0.001$; ns = not significant.
[c] The fat was infused into the intestine and the potato taken by mouth.

TABLE 12
Effect of Grinding on Metabolic Responses

Carbohydrate (g) and source	Degree of grinding	Sub[a]	% Change[b] Glucose	Insulin	GIP	Ref.
75, White rice	Fine	N	+38%**	+138%++		131
75, Brown rice	Fine	N	+46%***	+95%***		128
75, Brown rice	Fine	D	+67%*	+46%*	+60%+	132
75, Brown rice	Fine	N	+48%*	+54%**	+54%*	132
50, Cooked lentils	Fine	N	+6%ns			133
50, Lentils	Fine	N	+80%+	−11%ns		134
50, Cracked wheat[c]	25% Flour	D	+5%ns			135
50, Cracked wheat	50% Flour	D	+26%*			135
50, Cracked wheat	100% Flour	D	+39%*			135
50, Barley[c]	25% Flour	D	0%ns			135
50, Barley	50% Flour	D	+59%*			135
50, Barley	100% Flour	D	+146%*			135
50, Wheat kernels	100% Flour	D	+52%*			94
50, Wheat kernels	Cracked(bulgur)	D	+3%ns			94
50, Rye kernels	100% Flour	D	+89%*			94
50, Rye kernels	Pumpernickel[d]	D	+66%			94
50, Wheat[e]	Cracked grains	N	+7%ns	+16%ns		136
50, Wheat	Coarse flour	N	+34%ns	+42%*		136
50, Wheat	Fine flour	N	+32%ns	+95%***		136
50, Corn[e]	Cracked grains	N	−21%ns	+18%ns		136
50, Corn	Flour	N	−3%ns	+89%**		136
50, Oats[e]	Rolled oats	N	+29%ns	+53%ns		136
50, Oats	Flour	N	+75%ns	+19%ns		136

[a] Sub = subjects: D = diabetic; N = normal.
[b] Change in incremental area under the curve or peak rise: * = $p < 0.05$; + = $p < 0.025$; ** = $p < 0.01$; ++ = $p < 0.005$; *** = $p < 0.001$; ns = not significant.
[c] Varied proportions of whole grain and flour in breads compared to whole grain alone. Wheat breads made with bulgur (cracked, parboiled wheat) plus various proportions of whole meal flour; barley bread vs. cooked pearled barley.
[d] Rye kernels vs. pumpernickel bread (bread containing whole kernels).
[e] Wheat: cracked, each kernel broken into 6 pieces; coarse, 17% retained on 2200-μm sieve, 52% retained on 710-μm sieve; fine, 0% retained on 710-μm sieve. Corn; cracked, each kernel broken into 23 pieces; flour, 0.2% retained on 710-μm sieve. Oats, flour, 0.2% retained on 710-μm sieve.

on guar than those patients whose diets contained less than 40% carbohydrates (64% compared with 33%, $p < 0.02$).

The combined use of high carbohydrate/high fiber diets has benefited both IDDM and NIDDM patients in terms of improved blood glucose control, reduced serum lipid levels, and lower insulin dosage, but only in those studies where the increase in carbohydrate and fiber was achieved with low GI foods such as legumes and pasta (Table 16, Figure 8). In studies where the carbohydrate and fiber intakes were increased using high GI, cereal products (e.g., whole meal bread), fasting blood glucose, and cholesterol levels were improved, but this was achieved often at the expense of increased postprandial blood glucose and serum triglyceride levels (Table 16, Figure 8).

A number of dietary trials have been undertaken where the GI of the diet has been reduced without changing its overall macronutrient or fiber content (Table 17, Figure 7). In these studies, blood glucose and lipid lowering effects similar to those produced by high carbohydrate/high fiber diets were seen with no changes in carbohydrate or fiber intake. This suggests that the long-term metabolic effects of high carbohydrate/high fiber diets depends, at least in part, upon the ability to reduce the rate of carbohydrate absorption and

TABLE 13
Effect of Cooking/Processing on Metabolic Responses

Carbohydrate (g) and source	Cooking/Processing procedures	Sub[a]	% Change[b] Glucose	Insulin	Ref.
50, Red lentils	Boiled: 1 h vs. 20 min	N	+24% ns		133
50, Red lentils	Boiled 20 min, ground and dried 12 h at 250°F vs. boiled 20 min and ground	N	+78% +		133
1g/kg, Corn starch	Heated in water at 68 to 70°C until gelled vs. raw	N	+160% **	+133% **	137
50, Yam[c]	Roasted vs. boiled	N	+15%ns		138
50, Plantain[c]	Roasted vs. boiled	N	−2% ns		138
50, Potatoes	Raw vs boiled 20 min	D	+196% ++		139
25, Carrots	Raw vs. boiled 20 min	D	+3% ns		139
50, Polished rice	Boiled 5 min vs. boiled 15 min	D	+43% **		95
50, Parboiled rice	Boiled 5 min vs. boiled 15 min	D	+24% ns		95
50, Parboiled rice	Boiled 5 min vs. boiled 25 min	D	+22% ns		95
50, Spaghetti	Boiled 5 min vs. boiled 15 min	D	+2% ns		96
50, Spaghetti	Boiled 11 min vs. boiled 16.5 min	N	+10% ns	+8% ns	140
50, Spaghetti	Boiled 11 min vs. boiled 22 min	N	−22% ns	0% ns	140
50, Baked beans	Home cooked vs. canned	N	+50% +	+100% **	116
50, White beans	Home cooked vs. canned	D	+86% *		108
50, Green lentils	Home cooked vs. canned	D	+139% **		108
50, Pinto beans	Home cooked vs. canned	D	+16% **		108
50, Chick peas	Home cooked vs. canned	D	+36% ns		108
50, Kidney beans	Home cooked vs. canned	D	+23% ns		108

[a] Sub = subjects: D = diabetic; N = normal.
[b] Change in incremental area under the curve or peak rise: * = $p < 0.05$; + = $p < 0.025$; ** = $p < 0.01$; ++ = $p < 0.005$; *** = $p < 0.001$; ns = not significant.
[c] Tested in different groups of nonstandardized subjects.

hence reduce the acute postprandial blood glucose response. The mechanism for the lipid-lowering effect of slow absorption may relate to reduced insulin secretion and hence reduced stimulus to lipid synthesis. Recent studies where the rate of absorption was reduced by nibbling small meals at regular intervals throughout the day instead of consuming exactly the same food in three large meals indicate that nibbling reduces mean day-long insulin levels by about 30%[243,244] and is associated with significant reductions in serum total and LDL cholesterol and apolipoprotein B levels.[244]

CONCLUSIONS

Long-term benefits have been demonstrated using high carbohydrate/high fiber diets in both insulin- and noninsulin-dependent diabetes. These are associated with, and may be due to, slowing the rate of carbohydrate absorption within the gastrointestinal tract. Slow-release carbohydrate may be obtained by the addition of viscous types of dietary fiber, the use of low glycemic index foods, increased meal frequency, or by pharmacologic intervention with amylase inhibitors such as Acarbose.[245,246] Fiber has been shown to alter gut morphology in experimental animals.[247-252] Increased starch consumption,[253,254] low glycemic index foods,[255-260] and dietary fiber[261-264] also increase the amount of fermentable carbohydrate which enters the colon. This will result in the formation and absorption of the short-chain fatty acids, acetic, propionic, and butyric acids,[265-268] which influence carbohydrate and lipid metabolism[269-271] and may be part of the mechanism of action of high carbohydrate/high fiber diets.[272-274] The long-term consequences of these morphologic and absorptive changes are likely to be important and remain to be explored.

TABLE 14
Utility of Glycemic Index of Foods in Predicting the Relative Blood Glucose Responses of Single Mixed Meals

Text meal	Meal GI	Percent difference[a]				Ref.
		GI	BG-NIDDM	BG-Normal	BG-IDDM	
1. White bread	89					141
2. Whole grain bread	56	−38%	−39%* (8)			
1. Flummery	96					142
2. Salad and apple	100	+4%	0%ns (12)	+5%ns (13)		
1. Potato and sucrose	110					143
2. Rice and corn	85	−22%	−28%+ (12)	−8%ns (22)		144
1. Formula	117					145
2. Brown rice and beans	74	−37%		−31%* (7)		
1. Low fiber	84					146
2. High fiber	85	+1%		0%ns (8)		
1. Cornflakes, banana	113					147
2. Cornflakes, juice	90	−21%	−31%* (8)			
3. Potato, bread, juice	88	−27%	−31%* (8)			
4. Griddle cakes, juice	99	−12%	−20%ns (8)			
1. Glucose, rice	111					148
2. Fructose, rice	53	−52%	−46%* (12)	−78%* (10)	−55%ns (10)	
3. Sucrose, rice	82	−26%	−23%ns (12)	−60%* (10)	−16%ns (10)	
4. Potato starch, rice	92	−17%	−7%ns (12)	−56%* (10)	−6%ns (10)	
5. Wheat starch, rice	94	−16%	0%ns (12)	−25%ns (10)	−8%ns (10)	
1. Potato meal	123					149
2. Rice meal	89	−28%	−23%** (8)			
3. Spaghetti meal	77	−37%	−31%** (8)			
4. Lentils meal	62	−50%	−43%** (8)			
1. Potato meal	97					150
2. Bread meal	86	−10%	−13%ns (6)			
3. Rice meal	76	−22%	−26%** (6)			
4. Spaghetti meal	65	−33%	−44%** (6)			
5. Barley, lentils meal	47	−52%	−56%** (6)			
1. Mashed potato, bread	92					151
2. Sweet potato, orange	66	−29%	−5%ns (12)	−11%ns (13)		
3. Beans, cherries	53	−42%	−9%ns (12)	−44%ns (13)		
1. Bread meal	75					152
2. Potato meal	67	−11%	−12%			
3. Spaghetti meal	60	−20%	−41%** (7)			
1. Potato meal	80					153
2. Spaghetti meal	66	−17%			−49%***(7)	
1. Rice meal	71					154
2. Spaghetti meal	48	−32%	−13%ns (9)	−6%ns (6)		
3. Lentils meal	34	−52%	−19%ns (9)	−6%ns (6)		

TABLE 14 (continued)
Utility of Glycemic Index of Foods in Predicting the Relative Blood Glucose Responses of Single Mixed Meals

	Meal	Percent difference[a]				
Text meal	GI	GI	BG-NIDDM	BG-Normal	BG-IDDM	Ref.
1. Mashed potato meal	105					155
2. Lentils, barley meal	41	−61%		−61%* (5)		
1. Cornflakes, juice	95					156
2. "All Bran", juice	68	−28%		−24%* (11)		
1. Candy bar, tea	110					157
2. Cola, potato chips	105	−4%		−7%ns (10)		
3. Raisins, peanuts	87	−21%		−2%ns (10)		
4. Banana, peanuts	75	−32%		−51%ns (10)		
1. Lebanese meal	69					158
2. Western meal	69	0%		−27% (8)		
3. Chinese meal	65	−6%		−15% (8)		
4. Indian meal	60	−13%		−30% (8)		
5. Italian meal	40	−42%		−40% (8)		
6. Greek meal	38	−45%		−53% (8)		

[a] Percent difference from meal 1 for each study for GI = glycemic index, BG = blood glucose response incremental area, NIDDM = noninsulin-dependent diabetic subjects, IDDM = insulin-dependent diabetic subjects. GI values have been adjusted for unequal carbohydrate in meals. Figures in brackets = number of subjects. Meal GI for references 141 through 149, 152, 153, 156, and 157 were not reported in the original references. The meal GI calculations for studies 141 through 146 are presented in (159), for studies 147 and 148 in (102), for study 149 (160), for studies 152 and 153 in (161), and for study 156 in (162). The GI values for the meals in study 157 have not been presented previously.

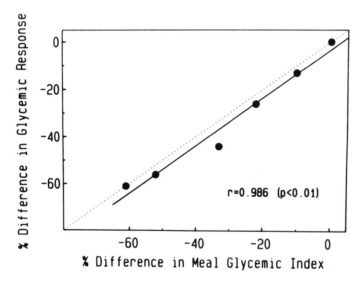

FIGURE 5. Prediction of mixed meal glycemic response using the glycemic index by Wolever et al.[150,155] Solid line = regression equation (% difference in glycemic response = 3.3 + 1.01 × % difference in GI); dotted line = line of identity.

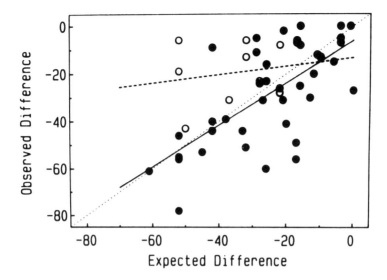

FIGURE 6. Prediction of mixed meal glycemic response using the glycemic index using the data from Table 14. Expected difference (ED) = percent difference of the glycemic index of each mixed meal from that of the meal with the highest glycemic index; observed difference (OD) = percent difference of glycemic response of each meal from that of the meal with the highest glycemic index. Dashed line, open circles = regression equation of data from the Stanford group (OD = −13 + 0.18 × ED, r = 0.168, n = 9,ns); solid line, closed circles = regression equation of data from 11 other groups worldwide (OD = −6 + 0.88 × Ed, r = 0.690, n = 41, $p < 0.001$); dotted line = line of identity.

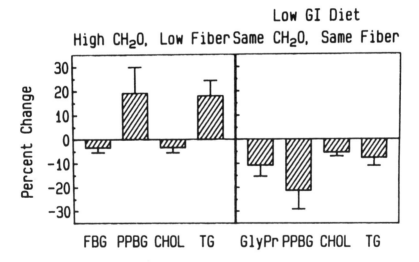

FIGURE 7. Left: effect of increasing dietary carbohydrate with no change in fiber on fasting (FBG) and postprandial (PPBG) blood glucose and serum cholesterol (CHOL) and triglyceride (TG) levels (mean ± SEM of data from Table 15). Right: effect of decreasing dietary glycemic index with no change in carbohydrate or fiber intake on glycosylated hemoglobin or albumin (GlyPr), postprandial blood glucose (PPBG) and serum cholesterol (CHOL) and triglyceride (TG) levels (mean ± SEM of data from Table 18).

TABLE 15
Metabolic Effects of High Carbohydrate, Low Fiber Diets

Diet composition[a]						% Change on high carbohydrate diet[b]			
CARB	FAT	Comment	LEN[c]	SUB[d]	FBG	GTT	CHOL	TG	Ref.
44 → 77%	36 → 16%	MD,NF	7D	IGt	−15%*	G −7%ns		+36%**	163
40 → 55%	45 → 30%	FD	10D	N	−2%ns	D 0%ns	0%ns	+42%***	164
40 → 60%	41 → 21%	HD,NF	10D	N	0%ns	D 0%ns	−2%ns	+49%***	165
45 → 85%	40 → 0%	FD	7–10D	UD	+7%ns				166
45 → 85%	40 → 0%	FD	7–10D	TD	−13%+				166
45 → 85%	40 → 0%	FD	10D	IGT	−10%***	G −8%*			167
42 → 53%	37 → 30%	MD,NF	10D	D	−2%ns	D +3%ns	+5%ns	ns	168
41 → 60%	41 → 20%	OPD	10D	ID	+6%ns	D +36%***	−2%ns	+19%ns	169
35 → 60%	47 → 22%	OPD	4W	NID	−10%*	D +11%+	0%ns	+11%ns	170
40 → 60%	40 → 20%	MD,NF	6W	NID	+2%ns	D +65%***	+2%ns	+25%***	171
42 → 55%	39 → 29%	OPD	6W	NID	−14%ns		−2%ns		172
41 → 56%	43 → 28%	OPD	40W	NID	0%ns		ns	ns	173
40 → 54%	40 → 26%	OPD	12M	NDN	+3%ns		−11%*	0%ns	174
53 → 58%	33 → 29%	OPD	12M	IDC	+1%ns[e]		−6%*	+33%*	175
41 → 64%	42 → 20%	OPD	13M	ID	0%ns		−21%***	−17%ns	176

[a] % of energy as carbohydrate (CARB) or fat on low → high carbohydrate diet. MD = metabolic diet, NF = normal foods, FD = formula diet, OPD = outpatient diets.

[b] % change of: FBG = fasting blood glucose; GTT = area under blood glucose curve after a standard oral glucose load (G) or while actually eating the diet (D); CHOL = serum cholesterol; TG = serum triglyceride. * = $p < 0.05$; + = $p < 0.025$; ** = $p < 0.01$; *** = $p < 0.001$.

[c] Study length: D = days; W = weeks; M = months.

[d] Subjects: N = normal; IGT = impaired glucose tolerance; UD = untreated diabetics; TD = treated diabetics; NID = noninsulin-dependent diabetics; NDN = newly diagnosed, noninsulin requiring diabetes; ID = insulin-dependent diabetes; D = combined ID and NID; IDC = insulin-dependent diabetic children.

[e] Change in HbA1c.

TABLE 16
Metabolic Effects of Increasing Fiber Intake from Whole Foods with no Change in Available Carbohydrate

Diet composition[a]				LEN[b]	SUB[c]	% Change on high fiber diet[d]					Ref.
CHO	PRO	FAT	FIBER			FBG	PPBG	UGO	CHOL	TG	

Fiber Increased with LOW Glycemic Index Foods

CHO	PRO	FAT	FIBER	LEN	SUB	FBG	PPBG	UGO	CHOL	TG	Ref.
53	17	30	16 → 54	10D	8D	−34%*	−37%**	−82%+	−14%*	−12%*	177
53	17	30	16 → 54	10D	14D	−6%ns	−24%++		−20%**	ns	168
39	20	40	2 → 20[e]	15D	8D	−24%++	−18%++				178
55	15	30	19 → 56	6W	10C	−38%**	−30%***	−76%**			179
35	17	47	18 → 33	6W	16D		−20%*	−19%ns	0%ns		180
40	13	46	18 → 36	6W	10CSII		+1%ns		−5%ns	−26%ns	181
53		30	14 → 23	6W	25NID	−9%ns	−5%[h]ns		−13%*		172

Fiber Increased with HIGH Glycemic Index Foods

CHO	PRO	FAT	FIBER	LEN	SUB	FBG	PPBG	UGO	CHOL	TG	Ref.
47	21	34	19 → 42	3W	14NID	−6%*	−13%**	−37%*	+2%ns	+11%ns	182
59	17	23	11 → 27[f]	4W	6NID	+10%ns	ns	−10%ns	+5%ns	+8%ns	183
44	19	37	+14−24 g[g]	4W	12ID	−14%	−15%				184
44	23	33	16 → 44	8W	14NID	−6%**	+6%ns		−4%+	+10%ns	185
53	16	28	30 → 41	8W	42NID	−7%[h]			−6%ns	−7%ns	186

[a] Percent of calories from carbohydrate (CHO), protein (PRO), and fat, and increase in dietary fiber (FIBER) from low → high fiber diet.
[b] Study length: D = days; W = weeks.
[c] Subjects: D = diabetic; NID = noninsulin-dependent diabetic; C = diabetic children; CSII-ID on continuous insulin infusion therapy.
[d] % change of: FBG = fasting blood glucose; PPBG = postprandial blood glucose levels; UGO = urinary glucose output; CHOL = serum cholesterol; TG = serum triglyceride. * = $p < 0.05$; + = $p < 0.025$; ** = $p < 0.01$; ++ = $p < 0.005$; *** = $p < 0.001$.
[e] Crude fiber.
[f] Grams dietary fiber per 1000 Kcal.
[g] Increase in fiber of 14 to 24 g/day.
[h] Change in HbA1c, ns.

TABLE 17
Metabolic Effects of High Carbohydrate, High Fiber Diets

Diet composition[a]						% Change on high carbohydrate diet[b]				
CARB	FAT	FIBER	LEN[c]	SUB[d]	FBG	HbA1c	UGO/ID/BG	CHOL	TG	Ref.

Fiber and Carbohydrate Increased with LOW Glycemic Index Foods

CARB	FAT	FIBER	LEN	SUB	FBG	HbA1c	UGO/ID/BG	CHOL	TG	Ref.
42 → 53%	37 → 37%	20 → 54 g	10D	D	−13%ns		U-56%ns	−19%***	+23%ns	177
42 → 53%	37 → 30%	20 → 54 g	10D	D	−7%ns		B-15%+	−16%***	ns	168
40 → 50%	51 → 38%	22 → 65 g	10D	D,R	0%ns		B-20%*	−18%*	−6%ns	187
43 → 75%	34 → 9%	5 → 14[e]	2W	NID	−26%++		I-56%+	−24%***	−15%ns	188
43 → 70%	37 → 9%	26 → 65 g	16D	NID	−7%ns		I-58%***	−29%***	−2%ns	189
43 → 68%	42 → 14%	17 → 78 g	3–4W	H	−5%*			−22%**	+21%ns	190
43 → 65%	42 → 21%	9 → 19[f]	5W	NID	+5%ns		U-11%ns	−10%ns	ns	191
40 → 61%	39 → 18%	18 → 97 g	6W	NID	−15%***	−10%+	U-94%*	−14%ns	−14%ns	192
40 → 61%	39 → 18%	18 → 97 g	6W	ID	−38%ns	−2%ns	U-80%*	−15%*	−18%ns	192
42 → 50%	39 → 32%	8 → 23 g	6W	NID	−23%*	−19%*		−15%*		172
40 → 58%	40 → 30%	30 → 70 g	2M	ID	−5%	−12%**	U-64%ns	−4%ns	+11%ns	193
43 → 55%	34 → 27%	26 → 40 g	15M	NID	−25%***		I-90%***	−5%ns	−43%++	194
? → 66%	? → 13%	? → 25 g	48M	NID	−18%*			−13%*	−15%*	195

Fiber and Carbohydrate Increased with HIGH Glycemic Index Foods

CARB	FAT	FIBER	LEN	SUB	FBG	HbA1c	UGO/ID/BG	CHOL	TG	Ref.
46 → 60%	35 → 23%	22 → 64 g	14D	ID	−11%ns		B-ns		+10%ns	196
28 → 60%	49 → 21%	21 → 57 g	3W	NID	−18%**		U-33%ns	−10%***	+20%**	197
45 → 65%	40 → 20%	28 → 50 g	4W	ID	−1%ns		U-14%ns	−22%**	−6%ns	198
34 → 61%	50 → 23%	36 → 78 g	6W	NID	−12%**	−11%**	R-+26%+	−14%***	−9%ns	199
34 → 61%	50 → 23%	36 → 78 g	6W	ID	−36%**	+1%ns	I-6%**	−10%***	+61%**	200
45 → 65%	40 → 20%	28 → 50 g	6W	ID	−1%ns	+2%ns	I-0%ns	−22%**	−17%*	201
47 → 53%	40 → 25%	20 → 42 g	12W	NH		−15%***		−2%ns		202
38 → 45%	43 → 34%	20 → 32 g	4M	ID		+19%**				203
40 → 65%	40 → 15%	20 → 65 g	4M	D,P		−30%	I-65%*			204
35 → 40%	45 → 41%	19 → 35 g	6M	PC	+17%**	+6%ns	B-+7%			205

a % of energy as carbohydrate (CARB), fat, and dietary fiber (FIBER) on low → high carbohydrate diet.
b + change of: FBG = fasting blood glucose; HbA1c = glycosylated haemoglobin; UGO = urinary glucose output (U); ID = insulin dose (I) or rate of glucose disposal during euglycemic insulin clamp (R); mean blood glucose on the diet (B); CHOL = serum cholesterol; TG = serum triglyceride. * = $p < 0.05$; + = $p < 0.025$; ** = $p < 0.01$; *** = $p < 0.001$.
c Study length: D = days; W = weeks; M = months.
d Subjects: D = diabetic, unspecified or mixed types; R = chronic renal failure; NID = noninsulin-dependent diabetes; ID = insulin-dependent diabetes; H = healthy; NH = hypertensive NID; P = pregnant; PC = NID in poor control.
e Grams of crude fiber.
f Grams dietary fiber per 1000 Kcal.

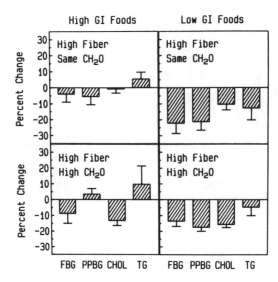

FIGURE 8. Effect of high carbohydrate, high fiber diets on fasting (FBG) and postprandial (PPBG) blood glucose and serum cholesterol (CHOL) and triglyceride (TG) levels. Left: increased fiber from foods with high glycemic index (GI). Right: increased fiber from foods with low GI. Top: effects of increasing fiber intake with no change in available carbohydrate intake (data from Table 16). Bottom: effect of increasing both fiber and available carbohydrate intakes (data from Table 17).

TABLE 18
Long-term Effects of Low Glycemic Index (GI) Diets

Diet composition[a]							Change on low GI diet[b]					
CHO	FAT	PRO	DF	LEN	SUBJ	Diet GI	PPBG	GlyPr	Ins/CP	CHOL	TG	Ref.
61%	20%	19%	29 g	2W	6N	−41(39%)	−37%**	F−2%ns	C−39%**	−11%*	−13%ns	206
50%	29%	21%	21 g	1M	12HT	−13(16%)				−9%**	−16%***	93
49%	29%	19%	22 g	1M	24HT	−11(13%)				−9%**	−19%**	207
49%	29%	19%	22 g	1M	6HC	−11(13%)				−3%ns	−1%ns	207
60%	20%			4W	24N + I	−7(12%)	−13%	H−0%ns				208
54%	25%	21%	31 g	2W	8NID	−23(26%)		H−3%ns	0%ns	−3%ns	0%ns	209
48%	35%	17%	32 g[c]	6W	7IDC	−12(15%)		F−27%*	I−14%ns	−9%**	−3%ns	210
46%	36%	17%	31 g[d]	3W	8IDA	−14(23%)		F−22%	I−9%*	0%ns	−16%*	211
45%	31%	21%	26 g	3M	16NID	−13(14%)	−14%*	H−11%*		0%ns	+6%ns	212

[a] These studies were designed to have equivalent dietary composition during the high and low GI periods, but in some cases there were small differences in macronutrients. CHO = carbohydrate as % of energy; FAT = fat as % of energy; PRO = protein as percent of energy; DF = dietary fiber in grams per day; LEN = study length (W = weeks; M = months); SUBJ = subjects (N = normal; HT = hypertriglyceridemic; HC = type 2a hypercholesterolemia; NID = noninsulin-dependent diabetes; IDC = insulin-dependent diabetes, children; IDA = insulin-dependent diabetes, adults; N + I = NID and IDA.

[b] PPBG = postprandial blood glucose high GI diet vs. low GI diet; GlyPr = glycosylated protein (F = fructosamine; H = hemoglobin); Ins/CP = Insulin dose (I) or urinary c-peptide output (C); CHOL = serum cholesterol; TG = serum triglycerides.

[c] Significant increase in dietary fiber on low GI diet (39 vs. 24 g/d).

[d] Significant decrease in dietary fiber on low GI diet (28 vs. 34 g/d).

REFERENCES

1. **Edwards, C. A., Blackburn, N. A., Craigen, L., Davison, P., Tomlin, J., Sugden, K., Johnson, I. T., and Read, N. W.**, Viscosity of food gums determined in vitro related to their hypoglycemic actions, *Am. J. Clin. Nutr.*, 46, 72, 1987.
2. **Jaris, H. A., Blackburn, N. A., Redfern, J. S., and Read, N. W.**, The effect of ispaghula (Fybogel and Metamucil) and guar gum on glucose tolerance in man, *Brit. J. Nutr.*, 51, 371, 1984.
3. **O'Connor, N., Tredger, J., and Morgan, L.**, Viscosity differences between various guar gums, *Diabetologia*, 20, 612, 1981.
4. **Morgan, L. M., Tredger, J. A., Madden, A., Kwasowski, P., and Marks, V.**, The effect of guar gum on carbohydrate-, fat- and protein-stimulated gut hormone secretion: modification of postprandial gastric inhibitory polypeptide and gastrin responses, *Brit. J. Nutr.*, 53, 467, 1985.
5. **Wolever, T. M. S., Jenkins, D. J. A., Nineham, R., and Alberti, K. G. M. M.**, Guar gum and reduction of post-prandial glycaemia: effect of incorporation into solid food, liquid food and both, *Brit. J. Nutr.*, 41, 505, 1979.
6. **Williams, D. R. R., James, W. P. T., and Evans, I. E.**, Dietary fibre supplementation of a normal breakfast administered to diabetics, *Diabetologia*, 18, 379, 1980.
7. **Smith, C. J., Roseman, M. S., Levitt, N. S., and Jackson, W. P. U.**, Guar biscuits in the diabetic diet, *S. Afr. Med. J.*, 61, 196, 1982.
8. **Gabbe, S. G., Cohen, A. W., Refhman, O. G., and Schwartz, S.**, Effect of dietary fiber on the oral glucose tolerance test in pregnancy, *Am. J. Obstet. Gynecol.*, 143, 514, 1982.
9. **Jenkins, D. J. A., Wolever, T. M. S., Taylor, R. H., Barker, H. M., Fielden, H., and Jenkins, A. L.**, Effect of guar crispbread with cereal products and leguminous seeds on blood glucose concentrations of diabetics, *Brit. Med. J.*, 281, 1248, 1980.
10. **Morgan, L. M., Gondler, T. J., Tsiolakis, D., Marks, V., and Alberti, K. G. M. M.**, The effects of unabsorbable carbohydrate on gut hormones: modification of postprandial GIP secretion by guar, *Diabetologia*, 17, 85, 1979.
11. **Fuessl, S., Adrian, T. E., Bacarese-Hamilton, A. J., and Bloom, S. R.**, Guar in NIDD: effect of different modes of administration on plasma glucose and insulin responses to a starch meal, *Practical Diabetes*, 3(5), 258, 1986.
12. **Gatti, E., Catenazzo, G., Camisasca, E., Torri, A., Denegri, E., and Sirtori, D. R.**, Effects of guar-enriched pasta in the treatment of diabetes and hyperlipidemia, *Annu. Nutr. Metab.*, 28, 1, 1984.
13. **Nestler, J. E., Bariascini, C. O., Clore, J. N., and Blackard, W. G.**, Absorption characteristic of breakfast determines insulin sensitivity and carbohydrate tolerance for lunch, *Diabetes Care*, 11, 755, 1988.
14. **Blackburn, N. A., Redfern, J. S., Jarjis, H., Holgate, A. M., Hanning, I., Scarpello, J. H. B., Johnson, I. T., and Read, N. W.**, The mechanism of action of guar gum in improving glucose tolerance in man, *Clin. Sci.*, 66, 329, 1984.
15. **Jenkins, D. J. A., Nineham, R., Craddock, C., Craig-McFeely, P., Donaldson, K., Leigh, T., and Snook, J.**, Fibre and diabetes, *Lancet*, 1, 434, 1979.
16. **Jenkins, D. J. A., Wolever, T. M. S., Leeds, A. R., Gassull, M. A., Dilawari, J. B., Goff, D. V., Metz, G. L., and Alberti, K. G. M. M.**, Dietary fibres, fibre analogues and glucose tolerance: importance of viscosity, *Brit. Med. J.*, 1, 1392, 1978.
17. **Walquist, M. L., Morris, M. J., Littlejohn, G. O., Bond, A., and Jackson, R. V. J.**, The effect of dietary fiber on glucose tolerance in healthy males, *Aust. N.Z. J. Med.*, 9, 154, 1979.
18. **Leatherdale, B. A., Green, D. J., Harding, L. K., Griffin, D., and Bailey, C. J.**, Guar and gastric emptying in non-insulin dependent diabetes, *Acta Diabetol. Lat.*, 19, 339, 1982.
19. **Levitt, N. S., Vinik, A. I., Sive, A. A., Child, P. T., and Jackson, W. P. U.**, The effect of dietary fiber on glucose and hormone responses to a mixed meal in normal subjects and in diabetic subjects with and without autonomic neuropathy, *Diabetes Care*, 3, 515, 1980.
20. **Kanter, Y., Eitan, N., Brook, G., and Barzilae, D.**, Improved glucose tolerance and insulin response in obese and diabetic patients on fiber-enriched diet, *Ist. J. Med. Sci.*, 16, 1, 1980.
21. **Jenkins, D. J. A., Leeds, A. R., Gassull, M. A., Wolever, T. M. S., Goff, D. V., Alberti, K. G. M. M., and Hockaday, T. D. R.**, Unabsorbable carbohydrates and diabetes: decreased postprandial hyperglycaemia, *Lancet*, 2, 172, 1976.
22. **Monnier, L. H., Colette, C., Aguirre, L., Orsetti, A., and Combeaux, D.**, Restored synergistic entro-hormonal response after addition of dietary fiber to patients with impaired glucose tolerance and reactive hypoglycemia, *Diabete Metab.*, 8, 217, 1982.
23. **Gold, L. A., McCourt, J. P., and Merimee, T. J.**, Pectin: an examination in normal subjects, *Diabetes Care*, 3, 50, 1980.
24. **Poynard, T., Slama, G., and Tchobroutsky, G.**, Reduction of post-prandial insulin needs by pectin as assessed by the artificial pancreas in insulin-dependent diabetics, *Diabete Metab.*, 8, 187, 1982.

25. **Vaaler, S., Hanssen, K. F., and Aagenase, O.,** Effect of different kinds of fibre on postprandial blood glucose in insulin-dependent diabetics, *Acta Med. Scand.*, 208, 389, 1980.
26. **Leeds, A. R., Ralphs, D. N. L., Ebied, F., Metz, G. L., and Dilawari, J.,** Pectin in the dumping syndrome: reduction of symptoms and plasma volume changes, *Lancet*, 1, 1075, 1981.
27. **Monnier, L., Pham, T. C., Aguirre, L., Orsetti, A., and Mirouze, J.,** Influence of indigestible fibers on glucose tolerance, *Diabetes Care*, 1, 83, 1978.
28. **Jenkins, D. J. A., Gassull, M. A., Leeds, A. R., Metz, G., Dilawari, J. B., Slavin, B., and Blendis, L. M.,** Effect of dietary fiber on complications of gastric surgery: prevention of postprandial hypoglycemia by pectin, *Gastroenterology*, 72, 215, 1977.
29. **Jenkins, D. J. A., Leeds, A. R., Bloom, S. R., Sarson, D. L., Albuquerque, R. H., Metz, G. L., and Alberti, K. G. M. M.,** Pectin and post-gastric surgery complications: normalisation of postprandial glucose and insulin responses, *Gut*, 21, 574, 1980.
30. **Holt, S., Heading, R. C., Carter, D. C., Prescott, L. F., and Tothill, P.,** Effect of gel fibre on gastric emptying and absorption of glucose and paracetomol, *Lancet*, 1, 636, 1979.
31. **Jefferys, D. B.,** The effect of dietary fibre on the response to orally administered glucose, *Proc. Nutr. Soc.*, 33, 11A, 1974.
32. **McMurry, J. F. and Baumgardner, B.,** A high-wheat bran diet in insulin-treated diabetes mellitus: assessment with the artificial pancreas, *Diabetes Care*, 7, 211, 1984.
33. **Hamberg, O., Rumessen, J. J., and Gudmand-Høyer, E.,** Blood glucose response to pea fiber: comparisons with sugar beet fiber and wheat bran, *Am. J. Clin. Nutr.*, 50, 324, 1989.
34. **Hall, S. E. H., Bolton, T. M., and Hetenyi, G.,** The effect of bran on glucose kinetics and plasma insulin in noninsulin-dependent diabetes mellitus, *Diabetes Care*, 3, 520, 1980.
35. **Ebihara, K., Masuhara, R., and Kiriyama, S.,** Effect of Konjac mannan, a water-soluble dietary fiber on plasma glucose and insulin responses in young men undergone (sic) glucose tolerance test, *Nutr. Rep. Int.*, 23, 577, 1981.
36. **Florholmen, J., Ardvidssonlenner, R., Jorde, R., and Burhol, P. G.,** The effect of Metamucil on postprandial blood glucose and plasma gastric inhibitory peptide in insulin-dependent diabetics, *Acta Med. Scand.*, 212, 237, 1982.
37. **Sartor, G., Carlstrom, S., and Schersten, B.,** Dietary supplementation of fiber (lunelax) as a means to reduce postprandial glucose in diabetics, *Acta Med. Scand.*, 656(Suppl.), 51, 1981.
38. **Wolever, T. M. S., Vuksan, V., Eshuis, H., Spadafora, P., Peterson, R. D., Chao, E. S. M., Storey, M. L., and Jenkins, D. J. A.,** Effect of method of administration of psyllium on the glycemic response and carbohydrate digestibility, *J. Am. Col. Nutr.*, in press.
39. **Tredger, J., Sheard, C., and Marks, V.,** Blood glucose and insulin levels in normal subjects following a meal with and without added sugar beet pulp, *Diabete Metab.*, 7, 169, 1981.
40. **Tsai, A. C., Vinik, A. I., Lasichak, A., and Lo, G. S.,** Effects of soy polysaccharide on postprandial plasma glucose, insulin, glucagon, pancreatic polypeptide, somatostatin, and triglyceride in obese diabetic patients, *Am. J. Clin. Nutr.*, 45, 596, 1987.
41. **Thomas, B. L., Laine, D. C., and Goetz, F. C.,** Glucose and insulin response in diabetic subjects: acute effect of carbohydrate level and the addition of soy polysaccharide in defined formula diets, *Am. J. Clin. Nutr.*, 48, 1048, 1988.
42. **Jenkins, D. J. A., Wolever, T. M. S., Taylor, R. H., Barker,, H. M., Fielden, H., and Gassull, M. A.,** Lack of effect of refining on the glycemic response to cereals, *Diabetes Care*, 4, 509, 1981.
43. **Jenkins, D. J. A., Wolever, T. M. S., Jenkins, A. L., Lee, R., Wong, G. S., and Josse, R. G.,** Glycemic response to wheat products: reduced response to pasta but no effect of fiber, *Diabetes Care*, 6, 155, 1983.
44. **Vaaler, S., Hanssen, K. F., and Aagenaes, O.,** Plasma glucose and insulin responses to orally administered carbohydrate-rich foodstuffs, *Nutr. Metab.*, 24, 168, 1980.
45. **Brodribb, A. J. M. and Humphreys, D. M.,** Diverticular disease: three studies. Part III. Metabolic effect of bran in patients with diverticular disease, *Brit. Med. J.*, 1, 428, 1976.
46. **Otto, H. and Niklas, L.,** Differences d'action sur la glycemie d'aliments contenant des hydrates de carbone. Consequences pour le traitment dietetique du diabete sucre, *Med. Hyg.*, 38, 3424, 1980.
47. **O'Dea, K., Nestel, P. J., and Antonoff, L.,** Physical factors influencing postprandial glucose and insulin responses to starch, *Am. J. Clin. Nutr.*, 33, 760, 1980.
48. **Walker, A. R. P. and Walker, B. R.,** Glycaemic index of South African foods determined in rural blacks — a population at low risk to diabetes, *Hum. Nutr. Clin. Nutr.*, 36C, 215, 1984.
49. **Jenkins, D. J. A., Wolever, T. M. S., Taylor, R. H., Barker, H. M., Fielden, H., Baldwin, J. M., Bowling, A. C., Newman, H. C., Jenkins, A. L., and Goff, D. V.,** Glycemic index of foods: a physiological basis for carbohydrate exchange, *Am. J. Clin. Nutr.*, 34, 362, 1981.
50. **Bolton, R. P., Heaton, K. W., and Burroughs, L. F.,** The role of dietary fiber in satiety, glucose, and insulin: studies with fruit and fruit juice, *Am. J. Clin. Nutr.*, 34, 211, 1981.
51. **Kay, R. M.,** Food form, post-prandial glycemia, and satiety, *Am. J. Clin. Nutr.*, 31, 738, 1978.

52. **Haber, G. B., Heaton, K. W., Murphy, D., and Burroughs, L. F.,** Depletion and disruption of dietary fibre: effects on satiety, plasma-glucose, and insulin, *Lancet,* 2, 679, 1977.
53. **McLean Ross, A. H., Eastwood, M. A., Brydon, W. G., Anderson, J. R., and Anderson, D. M. W.,** A study of the effects of dietary gum arabic in humans, *Am. J. Clin. Nutr.,* 37, 368, 1983.
54. **Jenkins, D. J. A., Leeds, A. R., Houston, H., Hinks, L., Alberti, K. G. M. M., and Cummings, J. H.,** Carbohydrate tolerance in man after six weeks of pectin administration, *Proc. Nutr.Soc.,* 36, 60A, 1977.
55. **Kestin, M., Moss, R., Clifton, P. M., and Nestel, P. J.,** Comparative effects of three cereal brans on plasma lipids, blood pressure, and glucose metabolism in mildly hypercholesterolemic men, *Am. J. Clin. Nutr.,* 52, 661, 1990.
56. **Villaume, C., Beck, B., Gariot, P., Desalme, A., and Debry, G.,** Long-term evolution of the effect of bran ingestion on meal-induced glucose and insulin response in healthy man, *Am. J. Clin. Nutr.,* 40, 1023, 1984.
57. **Munoz, J. A., Sandstead, H. H., Jacob, L. K., Johnson, L., and Mako, M. E.,** Effects of dietary fiber on glucose tolerance of normal men, *Diabetes,* 28, 496, 1979.
58. **Schweizer, T. F., Bekhechi, A. R., Koellreutter, B., Reimann, S., Pometta, D., and Bron, B. A.,** Metabolic effects of dietary fiber from dehulled soybeans in humans, *Am. J. Clin. Nutr.,* 38, 1–11, 1983.
59. **Osilesi, O., Trout, D. L., Glover, E. E., Harper, S. M., Koh, E. T., Behall, K. M., O'Dorisio, T. M., and Tartt, J.,** Use of xanthan gum in dietary management of diabetes mellitus, *Am. J. Clin. Nutr.,* 42, 597, 1985.
60. **Groop, P. H., Groop, L., Totterman, K. J., and Fyhrquist, F.,** Relationship between changes in GIP concentrations and changes in insulin and c-peptide concentrations after guar gum therapy, *Scand. J. Clin. Lab. Invest.,* 46, 505, 1986.
61. **Jenkins, D. J. A., Wolever, T. M. S., Hockaday, T. D. R., Leeds, A. R., Haworth, R., Bacon, S., Apling, E. C., and Dilawari, J.,** Treatment of diabetes with guar gum, *Lancet,* 2, 779, 1977.
62. **Jenkins, D. J. A., Wolever, T. M. S., Nineham, R., Taylor, R. H., Metz, G. L., Bacon, S., and Hockaday, T. D. R.,** Guar crispbread in the diabetic diet, *Brit. Med. J.,* 2, 1744, 1978.
63. **Kuhl, C., Molsted-Pedersen, L., and Hornnes, P. J.,** Guar gum and glycemic control of pregnant insulin-dependent diabetic patients, *Diabetes Care,* 6, 152, 1983.
64. **Smith, U. and Holm, G.,** Effect of a modified guar gum preparation on glucose and lipid levels in diabetics and healthy volunteers, *Atherosclerosis,* 45, 1, 1982.
65. **Johansen, K.,** Decreased urinary glucose excretion and plasma cholesterol level in non-insulin-dependent diabetic patients with guar, *Diabete Metab.,* 7, 87, 1981.
66. **Koepp, P. and Hegewisch, S.,** Effects of guar on plasma viscosity and related parameters in diabetic children, *Eur. J. Pediatr.,* 137, 31, 1981.
67. **Carroll, D. G., Dykes, V., and Hodgson, W.,** Guar gum is not a panacea in diabetes management, *NZ Med. J.,* 93, 292, 1981.
68. **Najemnik, C., Kritz, H., Irsigler, K., Laube, H., Knick, B., Klimm, H. D., Wahl, P., Vollmar, J., and Brauning, C.,** Guar and its effects on metabolic control in type II diabetic subjects, *Diabetes Care,* 7, 215, 1984.
69. **Fuessl, H. S., Williams, G., Adrian, T. E., and Bloom, S. R.,** Guar sprinkled on food: effect on glycaemic control, plasma lipids and gut hormones in non-insulin dependent diabetic patients, *Diabetic Med.,* 4, 463, 1987.
70. **Eberling, P., Yki-Jarvinen, H., Aro, A., Helve, E., Sinisalo, M., and Kiovisto, V.,** Glucose and lipid metabolism and insulin sensitivity in type 1 diabetes: the effect of guar gum, *Am. J. Clin. Nutr.,* 48, 98, 1988.
71. **Atkins, T. W., Al-Hussary, N. A. J., and Taylor, K. G.,** The treatment of poorly controlled non-insulin-dependent diabetic subjects with granulated guar gum, *Diabetes Res. Clin. Practice,* 3, 153, 1987.
72. **Sels, J. P., Flendrig, J. A., and Postmes, T. H. J.,** The influence of guar-gum brerad on the regulation of diabetes mellitus type II in elderly patients, *Brit. J. Nutr.,* 57, 177, 1987.
73. **Paganus, A., Maenpaa, J., Akerblom, H. K., Stenman, U. H., Knip, M., and Simell, O.,** Beneficial effects of palatable guar and guar plus fructose diets in diabetic children, *Acta Paediatr. Scand.,* 76, 76, 1987.
74. **Jones, D. B., Slaughter, P., Lousley, S., Carter, R. D., Jelfs, R., and Mann, J. I.,** Low-dose guar improves diabetic control, *J. Roy. Soc. Med.,* 78, 546, 1985.
75. **Beattie, V. A., Edwards, C. A., Hosker, J. P., Cullen, D. R., Ward, J. D., and Read, N. W.,** Does adding fibre to a low energy, high carbohydrate, low fat diet confer any benefit to the management of newly diagnosed overweight type II diabetics?, *Brit. Med. J.,* 296, 1147, 1988.
76. **Holman, R. R., Steemson, J., Darling, P., and Turner, R. C.,** No glycemic benefit from guar administration in NIDDM, *Diabetes Care,* 10, 68, 1987.

77. **Ray, T. K., Mansell, K. M., Knight, L. C., Malmud, L. S., Owen, O. E., and Boden, G.**, Long-term effects of dietary fiber on glucose tolerance and gastric emptying in noninsulin-dependent diabetic patients, *Am. J. Clin. Nutr.*, 37, 376, 1983.
78. **Aro, A., Uusitupa, M., Vontilainen, E., Hersio, K., Korhonen, T., and Siitonen, O.**, Improved diabetic control and hypocholesterolemic effect induced by long-term dietary supplementation with guar gum in type 2 (insulin-independent) diabetes, *Diabetologia*, 21, 29, 1981.
79. **Botha, A. P. J., Steyn, A. F., Esterhuysen, A. J., and Slabbert, M.**, Glycosylated haemoglobin, blood glucose and serum cholesterol levels in diabetics treated with guar gum, *S. Afr. Med. J.*, 59, 333, 1981.
80. **Cohen, M., Leong, V. W., Salmon, E., and Martin, F. I. R.**, The role of guar and dietary fibre in the management of diabetes mellitus, *Med. J. Aust.*, 1, 59, 1980.
81. **Uusitupa, M., Siitonen, O., Savolainen, K., Silvasti, M., Penttila, I., and Parviainen, M.**, Metabolic and nutritional effects of long-term use of guar gum in treatment of noninsulin-dependent diabetes of poor metabolic control, *Am. J. Clin. Nutr.*, 49, 345, 1989.
82. **Jenkins, D. J. A., Wolever, T. M. S., Taylor, R. H., Reynolds, D., Nineham, R., and Hockaday, T. D. R.**, Diabetic glucose control, lipids, and trace elements on long term guar, *Brit. Med. J.*, 1, 1353, 1980.
83. **Mahalko, J. R., Sandstead, H. H., Johnson, L. K., Inman, L. F., Milne, D. B., Warner, R. C., and Haunz, E. A.**, Effect of consuming fiber from corn bran, soy hulls, or apple powder on glucose tolerance and plasma lipids in type II diabetes, *Am. J. Clin. Nutr.*, 39, 25, 1984.
84. **Mayne, P. D., McGill, A. R., Gormley, T. R., Tomplin, G. H., Julian, T. R., and O'Moore, R. R.**, The effect of apple fibre on diabetic control and plasma lipids, *Ir. J. Med. Sci.*, 151, 36, 1982.
85. **Monnier, L. H., Blotman, M. J., Colette, C., Monnier, M. P., and Mirouze, J.**, Effects of dietary fibre supplementation in stable and labile insulin-independent diabetics, *Diabetologia*, 20, 12, 1981.
86. **Bosello, O., Ostuzzi, R., Armellini, F., Micciolo, R. M., and Ludovico, A. S.**, Glucose tolerance and blood lipids in bran fed patients with impaired glucose tolerance, *Diabetes Care*, 3, 46, 1980.
87. **Miranda, P. M. and Horwitz, D. L.**, High fiber diets in the treatment of diabetes mellitus, *Ann. Intern. Med.*, 88, 482, 1978.
88. **Fagerberg, S. E.**, The effects of a bulk laxative (metamucil) on fasting blood glucose, serum lipids, and other variables in constipated patients with noninsulin-dependent diabetes, *Current Therapeutic Res.*, 31, 166, 1982.
89. **Doi, K., Matsuura, M., Kawara, A., and Baba, S.**, Treatment of diabetes with glucomannan (Konjac mannan), *Lancet*, 1, 987, 1979.
90. **Jenkins, D. J. A., Wolever, T. M. S., Jenkins, A. L., Thorne, M. J., Lee, R., Kalmusky, J., Reichert, R., and Wong, G. S.**, The glycaemic index of foods tested in diabetic patients: a new basis for carbohydrate exchange favouring the use of legumes, *Diabetologia*, 24, 257, 1983.
91. **Crapo, P. A., Reaven, G., and Olevsky, J.**, Post-prandial plasma-glucose and -insulin responses to different complex carbohydrates, *Diabetes*, 26, 1178, 1977.
92. **Crapo, P. A., Insel, J., Sperling, M., and Kolterman, O. G.**, Comparison of serum glucose, insulin and glucagon responses to different types of complex carbohydrate in noninsulin-dependent diabetic patients, *Am. J. Clin. Nutr.*, 34, 184, 1981.
93. **Jenkins, D. J. A., Wolever, T. M. S., Kalmusky, J., Giudici, S., Giordano, C., Wong, G. S., Bird, J. H., Patten, R., Hall, M., Buckley, G. C., and Little, J. A.**, Low glycemic index food in the management of hyperlipidemia, *Am. J. Clin. Nutr.*, 42, 604, 1985.
94. **Jenkins, D. J. A., Wolever, T. M. S., Jenkins, A. L., Giordano, C., Giudici, S., Thompson, L. U., Kalmusky, J., Josse, R. G., and Wong, G. S.**, Low glycemic response to traditionally processed wheat and rye products: bulgur and pumpernickel bread, *Am. J. Clin. Nutr.*, 43, 516, 1986.
95. **Wolever, T. M. S., Jenkins, D. J. A., Kalmusky, J., Jenkins, A. L., Giordano, C., Giudici, S., Josse, R. G., and Wong, G. S.**, Comparison of regular and parboiled rices: explanation of discrepancies between reported glycemic responses to rice, *Nutr. Res.*, 6, 349, 1986.
96. **Wolever, T. M. S., Jenkins, D. J. A., Kalmusky, J., Giordano, C., Giudici, S., Jenkins, A. L., Josse, R. G., and Wong, G. S.**, Glycemic response to pasta: effect of food form, cooking and protein enrichment, *Diabetes Care*, 9, 401, 1986.
97. **Walker, A. R. P. and Walker, B. R.**, Glycaemic index of South African foods determined in rural blacks — a population at low risk to diabetes, *Hum. Nutr. Clin. Nutr.*, 36C, 215, 1984.
98. **Wolever, T. M. S., Wong, G. S., Kenshole, A., Josse, R. G., Thompson, L. U., Lam, K. Y., and Jenkins, D. J. A.**, Lactose in the diabetic diet: a comparison with other carbohydrates, *Nutr. Res.*, 5, 1335, 1985.
99. **Brand, J. C., Nicholson, P. L., Thorburn, A. W., and Truswell, A. S.**, Food processing and the glycemic index, *Am. J. Clin. Nutr.*, 42, 1192, 1985.
100. **Dilawari, J. B., Kamath, P. S., Batta, R. P., Mukewar, S., and Raghavan, S.**, Reduction of postprandial plasma glucose by bengal gram dal (*Cicer arietnum*) and rajmah (*Phaseolus vulgaris*), *Am. J. Clin. Nutr.*, 34, 2450, 1981.

101. **Potter, J. G., Coffman, K. P., Reid, R. L., Krall, J. M., and Albrink, M. J.,** Effect of test meals of varying dietary fiber content on plasma insulin and glucose response, *Am. J. Clin. Nutr.,* 34, 328, 1981.
102. **Wolever, T. M. S., Nuttall, F. Q., Lee, R., Wong, G. S., Josse, R. G., Csima, A., and Jenkins, D. J. A.,** Prediction of the relative blood glucose response of mixed meals using the white bread glycemic index, *Diabetes Care,* 8, 418, 1985.
103. **Jenkins, D. J. A., Wolever, T. M. S., Wong, G. S., Kenshole, A., Josse, R. G., Thompson, L. U., and Lam, K. Y.,** Glycemic responses to foods: possible differences between insulin-dependent and non-insulin-dependent diabetics, *Am. J. Clin. Nutr.,* 40, 971, 1984.
104. **Crapo, P. A., Kolterman, O. G., Waldeck, N., Reaven, G. M., and Olefsky, J. M.,** Postprandial hormonal responses to different types of complex carbohydrate in individuals with impaired glucose tolerance, *Am. J. Clin. Nutr.,* 33, 1723, 1980.
105. **Yoon, J. H., Thompson, L. U., and Jenkins, D. J. A.,** The effect of phytic acid on in vitro rate of starch digestibility and blood glucose response, *Am. J. Clin. Nutr.,* 38, 835, 1983.
106. **Ross, S. W., Brand, J. C., Thorburn, A. W., and Truswell, A. S.,** Glycemic index of processed wheat products, *Am. J. Clin. Nutr.,* 46, 631, 1987.
107. **Heinonen, L., Korpela, R., and Mantere, S.,** The effect of different types of Finnish bread on postprandial glucose responses in diabetic patients, *Hum. Nutr. Appl. Nutr.,* 39A, 108, 1985.
108. **Wolever, T. M. S., Jenkins, D. J. A., Thompson, L. U., Wong, G. S., and Josse, R. G.,** Effect of canning on the blood glucose response to beans in patients with type 2 diabetes, *Hum. Nutr. Clin. Nutr.,* 41C, 135, 1987.
109. **Gannon, M. C.,Nuttall, F. Q., Krezowski, P. A., Billington, C. J., and Parker, S.,** The serum insulin and plasma glucose responses to milk and fruit products in Type 2 (non-insulin-dependent) diabetic patients, *Diabetologia,* 29, 784, 1986.
110. **Krezowski, P. A., Nuttall, F. Q., Gannon, M. C., Billington, C. J., and Parker, S.,** Insulin and glucose responses to various starch-containing foods in type II diabetic subjects, *Diabetes Care,* 10, 205, 1987.
111. **Wolever, T. M. S., Jenkins, D. J. A., Josse, R. G., Wong, G. S., and Lee, R.,** The glycemic index: similarity of values derived in insulin-dependent and non-insulin-dependent diabetic patients, *J. Am. Col. Nutr.,* 6, 295, 1987.
112. **Wolever, T. M. S., Kalmusky, J., Giudici, S., Giordano, C., and Jenkins, D. J. A.,** Effect of processing/preparation on the blood glucose response to potatoes, *Can. Inst. Food. Sci. Technol. J.,* 18, xxxv, 1985.
113. **Bornet, F. R. J., Costagliola, D., Blayo, A., Fontvielle, A., Haardt, M. J., Letanoux, M., Tchobroutsky, G., and Slama, G.,** Insulinogenic and glycemic indexes of six starch-rich foods taken alone and in a mixed meal by type 2 diabetics, *Am. J. Clin. Nutr.,* 45, 588, 1987.
114. **Wolever, T. M. S., Jenkins, D. J. A., Collier, G. R., Ehrlich, R. M., Josse, R. G., Wong, G. S., and Lee, R.,** The glycaemic index: effect of age in insulin dependent diabetes mellitus, *Diabetes Res.,* 7, 71, 1988.
115. **Wolever, T. M. S., Jenkins, D. J. A., Vuksan, V., Wong, G. S., and Josse, R. G.,** Effect of ripeness on the glycaemic response to banana, *J. Clin. Nutr. Gastroenterol.,* 3, 85, 1988.
116. **Traianedes, K. and O'Dea, K.,** Commercial canning increases the digestibility of beans in vitro and postprandial metabolic responses to them in vivo, *Am. J. Clin. Nutr.,* 44, 390, 1986.
117. **Philippides, P., Katsilambros, N., Galanopoulos, A., Peppas, T., Kofotzouli, L., Frangaki, D., Siskoudis, P., and Sfikakis, P.,** Glycaemic response to carrot in Type II diabetic patients, *Diab. Nutr. Metab.,* 1, 363, 1988.
118. **Brand, J. C., Foster, K. A. F., Crossman, S., and Truswell, A. S.,** The glycaemic and insulin indices of realistic meals and rye breads tested in healthy subjects, *Diab. Nutr. Metab.,* 3, 137, 1990.
119. **Bucalossi, A., Conti, A., Lombardo, S., Marsilii, A., Petruzzi, E., Piazza, E., and Pulini, M.,** Glycaemic and insulinaemic responses to different carbohydrates in Type II (NIDD) diabetic patients, *Diab. Nutr. Metab.,* 3, 143, 1990.
120. **Akanji, A. O., Adeyefa, I., Charles-Davies, M., and Osotimehin, B. O.,** Plasma glucose and thiocyanate responses to different mixed cassava meals in non-diabetic Nigerians, *Eur. J. Clin. Nutr.,* 44, 71, 1990.
121. **Simpson, R. W., McDonald, J., Walqvist, M. L., Atley, L., and Outch, K.,** Macronutrients have different metabolic effects in nondiabetics and diabetics, *Am. J. Clin. Nutr.,* 42, 449, 1985.
122. **Calle-Pascual, A. L., Bordiu, E., Romeo, S., Romero, C., Martin-Alvarez, P. J., and Maranés, J. P.,** Food glycaemic index or meal glycaemic response?, *Hum. Nutr. Appl. Nutr.,* 40A, 282 1986 and 41A, 435(letter), 1987.
123. **Collier, G., McLean, A., and O'Dea, K.,** Effect of co-ingestion of fat on the metabolic responses to slowly and rapidly absorbed carbohydrates, *Diabetologia,* 26, 50, 1984.
124. **Welch, I., Bruce, C., Hill, S. E., and Read, N. W.,** Duodenal and ileal lipid suppresses postprandial blood glucose and insulin responses in man: possible implications for the dietary management of diabetes mellitus, *Clin. Sci.,* 72, 209, 1987.
125. **Estrich, D., Ravnick, A., Schlierf, G., Fukayama, G., and Kinsell, L.,** Effects of co-ingestion of fat and protein upon carbohydrate-induced hyperglycemia, *Diabetes,* 16, 232, 1967.

126. **Collier, G. and O'Dea, K.,** The effect of coingestion of fat on the glucose, insulin and gastric inhibitory polypeptide responses to carbohydrate and protein, *Am. J. Clin. Nutr.,* 37, 941, 1983.
127. **Nuttall, F. Q., Mooradian, A. D., Gannon, M. C., Billington, C., and Krezowski, P.,** Effect of protein ingestion on the glucose and insulin response to a standardized oral glucose load, *Diabetes Care,* 7, 465, 1984.
128. **Guilliford, M. C., Bicknell, E. J., and Scarpello, J. H.,** Differential effect of protein and fat ingestion on blood glucose responses to high- and low-glycemic-index carbohydrates in noninsulin-dependent diabetic subjects, *Am. J. Clin. Nutr.,* 50, 773, 1989.
129. **Gannon, M. C., Nuttall, F. Q., Neil, B. J., and Westphal, S. A.,** The insulin and glucose responses to meals of glucose plus various proteins in type II diabetic subjects, *Metabolism,* 37, 1081, 1988.
130. **Spiller, G. A., Jensen, C. D., Pattison, T. S., Chuck, C. S., Whittam, J. H., and Scala, J.,** Effect of protein dose on serum glucose and insulin response to sugars, *Am. J. Clin. Nutr.,* 46, 474, 1987.
131. **O'Dea, K., Nestel, P. J., and Antonoff, L.,** Physical factors influencing postprandial glucose and insulin responses to starch, *Am. J. Clin. Nutr.,* 33, 760, 1980.
132. **Collier, G. and O'Dea, K.,** Effect of physical form of carbohydrate on the post-prandial glucose, insulin and gastric inhibitory polypeptide responses in type 2 diabetes, *Am. J. Clin. Nutr.,* 36, 10, 1982.
133. **Jenkins, D. J. A., Thorne, M. J., Camelon, K., Jenkins, A. L., Rao, A. V., Taylor, R. H., Thompson, L. U., Kalmusky, J., Reichert, R., and Francis, T.,** Effect of processing on digestibility and the blood glucose response: a study of lentils, *Am. J. Clin. Nutr.,* 36, 1093, 1982.
134. **O'Dea, K. and Wong, S.,** The rate of starch hydrolysis in vitro does not predict the metabolic responses to legumes in vivo, *Am. J. Clin. Nutr.,* 38, 382, 1983.
135. **Jenkins, D. J. A., Wesson, V., Wolever, T. M. S., Jenkins, A. L., Kalmusky, J., Giudici, S., Csima, A., Josse, R. G., and Wong, G. S.,** Wholemeal versus wholegrain breads: proportion of whole or cracked grain and the glycaemic response, *Brit. Med. J.,* 297, 958, 1988.
136. **Heaton, K. W., Marcus, S. N., Emmett, P. M., and Bolton, C. H.,** Particle size of wheat, maize, and oat test meals: effects on plasma glucose and insulin responses and on the rate of starch digestion in vitro, *Am. J. Clin. Nutr.,* 47, 675, 1988.
137. **Collings, P., Williams, C., and MacDonald, I.,** Effect of cooking on serum glucose and insulin responses to starch, *Br. Med. J.,* 282, 1032, 1981.
138. **Oli, J. M., Ikeakor, I. P., and Onwuameze, I. C.,** Blood glucose responses to common Nigerian foods, *Trop. Geog. Med.,* 34, 317, 1982.
139. **Vaaler, S., Hanssen, K. F. and Aagenaes, O.,** The effect of cooking upon the blood glucose response to ingested carrots and potatoes, *Diabetes Care,* 7, 221, 1984.
140. **Bornet, F. R. J., Cloarec, D., Barry, J., Colonna, P., Gouilloud, S., Laval, J. D., and Calmiche, J.,** Pasta cooking time: influence on starch digestion and plasma glucose and insulin responses in healthy subjects, *Am. J. Clin. Nutr.,* 51, 421, 1990.
141. **Asp, N-G., Agardh, C-D., Ahren, B., Dencker, I., Johansson, C-G., and Lundquist, I., Nyman, M., Sartor, G., and Schersten, B.,** Dietary fiber in type II diabetes, *Acta Med. Scand.,* 656(Suppl.), 47, 1981.
142. **Simpson, R. W., McDonald, J., Wahlqvist, M., Balaza, N., and Dunlop, M.,** Effect of naturally occurring dietary fibre in Western foods on blood glucose, *Aust. NZ J. Med.,* 11, 484, 1981.
143. **Coulston, A. M., Greenfield, M. S., Enger, F., Tokay, T., and Reaven, G. M.,** Effect of source of dietary carbohydrate on plasma glucose and insulin responses to test meals in normal subjects, *Am. J. Clin. Nutr.,* 33, 1279, 1980.
144. **Coulston, A. M., Greenfield, M. S., Kraemer, F. B., Tobey, R. A., and Reaven, G. M.,** Effect of differences in source of dietary carbohydrate on plasma glucose and insulin responses to meals in patients with impaired carbohydrate tolerance, *Am. J. Clin. Nutr.,* 34, 2716, 1981.
145. **Albrink, M. J., Newman, T., and Davidson, P. C.,** Effect of high- and low-fiber diets on plasma lipids and insulin, *Am. J. Clin. Nutr.,* 32, 1486, 1979.
146. **Ullrich, I. H. and Albrink, M. J.,** Lack of effect of dietary fiber on serum lipids, glucose, and insulin in healthy young men fed high starch diets, *Am. J. Clin. Nutr.,* 36, 1, 1982.
147. **Nuttall, F. Q., Mooradian, A. D., DeMarais, R., and Parker, S.,** The glycemic effect of different meals approximately isocaloric and similar in protein, carbohydrate, and fat content as calculated using the ADA exchange lists, *Diabetes Care,* 6, 432, 1983.
148. **Bantle, J. P., Laine, D. C., Castle, G. W., Thomas, J. W., Hoogwerf, B. J., and Goetz, F. C.,** Postprandial glucose and insulin responses to meals containing different carbohydrates in normal and diabetic subjects, *New Engl. J. Med.,* 309, 7, 1983.
149. **Coulston, A. M., Hollenbeck, C. B., Liu, G. C., Williams, R. A., Starich, G. H., Mazzaferri, E. L., and Reaven, G. M.,** Effect of source of dietary carbohydrate on plasma glucose, insulin, and gastric inhibitory polypeptide responses to test meals in subjects with noninsulin-dependent diabetes mellitus, *Am. J. Clin. Nutr.,* 40, 965, 1984.

150. **Collier, G. R., Wolever, T. M. S., Wong, G. S., and Josse, R. G.,** Prediction of glycemic response to mixed meals in non-insulin dependent diabetic subjects, *Am. J. Clin. Nutr.,* 44, 349, 1986.
151. **Laine, D. C., Thomas, W., Levitt, M. D., and Bantle, J. P.,** Comparison of predictive capabilities of diabetic exchange lists and glycemic index of foods, *Diabetes Care,* 10, 387, 1987.
152. **Parillo, M., Giacco, R., Riccardi, G., Pacioni, D., and Rivellese, A.,** Different glycaemic responses to pasta, bread, and potatoes in diabetic patients, *Diabetic Med.,* 2, 374, 1985.
153. **Hermansen, K., Rasmussen, O., Arnfred, J., Winther, E., and Schmitz, O.,** Glycemic effects of spaghetti and potato consumed as part of mixed meal on IDDM patients, *Diabetes Care,* 10, 401, 1987.
154. **Coulston, A. M., Hollenbeck, C. B., Swislocki, A. L. M., and Reaven, G. M.,** Effect of source of dietary carbohydrate on plasma glucose and insulin responses to mixed meals in subjects with NIDDM, *Diabetes Care,* 10, 395, 1987.
155. **Wolever, T. M. S., Jenkins, D. J. A., Ocana, A. M., Rao, A. V., and Collier, G. R.,** Second-meal effect: low-glycemic-index foods eaten at dinner improve subsequent breakfast glycemic response, *Am. J. Clin. Nutr.,* 48, 1041, 1988.
156. **Behme, M. T. and Dupre, J.,** All bran vs. corn flakes: plasma glucose and insulin responses in young females, *Am. J. Clin. Nutr.,* 50, 1240, 1989.
157. **Oettle, G. J., Emmett, P. M., and Heaton, K. W.,** Glucose and insulin responses to manufactured and whole-food snacks, *Am. J. Clin. Nutr.,* 45, 86, 1987.
158. **Chew, I., Brand, J. C., Thorburn, A. W., and Truswell, A. S.,** Application of glycemic index to mixed meals, *Am. J. Clin. Nutr.,* 47, 53, 1988.
159. **Wolever, T. M. S. and Jenkins, D. J. A.,** Effect of dietary fiber and foods on carbohydrate metabolism, in *CRC Handbook of Dietary Fiber in Human Nutrition,* Spiller, G. A., Ed., CRC Press, Boca Raton, FL, 1986, 87.
160. **Wolever, T. M. S. and Jenkins, D. J. A.,** Use of the glycemic index in predicting the blood glucose response to mixed meals, *Am. J. Clin. Nutr.,* 43, 167, 1986.
161. **Wolever, T. M. S., Csima, A., Jenkins, D. J. A., Wong, G. S., and Josse, R. G.,** The glycemic index: variation between subjects and predictive difference, *J. Am. Col. Nutr.,* 8, 235, 1989.
162. **Wolever, T. M. S.,** Glycemic index and mixed meals, *Am. J. Clin. Nutr.,* 51, 1113, 1990.
163. **Anderson, J. W.,** Effect of carbohydrate restriction and high carbohydrate diets in men with chemical diabetes, *Am. J. Clin. Nutr.,* 30, 402, 1977.
164. **Ginsberg, H., Olefsky, J. M., Kimmerling, G., Crapo, P. A., and Reaven, G. M.,** Induction of hypertriglyceridemia by a low fat diet, *J. Clin. Endocrinol. Metab.,* 42, 729, 1976.
165. **Coulston, A. M., Liu, G. C., and Reaven, G. M.,** Plasma glucose, insulin and lipid responses to high carbohydrate low fat diets in normal humans, *Metabolism,* 32, 52, 1983.
166. **Brunzell, J. D., Lerner, R. L., Porte, D., and Bierman, E. L.,** Effect of a fat free, high carbohydrate diet on diabetic subjects with fasting hyperglycemia, *Diabetes,* 23, 138, 1974.
167. **Brunzell, J. D., Lerner, R. L., Hazard, W. R., Porte, D., and Bierman, E. L.,** Improved glucose tolerance with high carbohydrate feeding in mild diabetes, *New Engl. J. Med.,* 284, 521, 1971.
168. **Riccardi, G., Rivellese, A., Pacioni, D., Genovese, S., Mastranzo, P., and Mancini, M.,** Separate influence of dietary carbohydrate and fibre on the metabolic control in diabetes, *Diabetologia,* 26, 116, 1984.
169. **Perrotti, N., Santoro, D., Genovese, S., Giacco, A., Rivellese, A., and Riccardi, G.,** Effect of digestible carbohydrates on glucose control in insulin-dependent diabetic patients, *Diabetes Care,* 7, 354, 1984.
170. **Simpson, H. C. R., Carter, R. D., Lousley, S., and Mann, J. I.,** Digestible carbohydrate — an independent effect on diabetic control in type II (non-insulin-dependent) diabetic patients?, *Diabetologia,* 23, 235, 1982.
171. **Coulston, A. M., Hollenbeck, C. B., Swislocki, A. L. M., and Reaven, G. M.,** Persistence of hypertriglyceridemic effect of low-fat high-carbohydrate diets in NIDDM patients, *Diabetes Care,* 12, 94, 1989.
172. **Stevens, J., Burgess, M. B., Kaiser, D. L., and Sheppa, C. M.,** Outpatient management of diabetes mellitus with patient education to increase dietary carbohydrate and fiber, *Diabetes Care,* 8, 359, 1985.
173. **Weinsier, R. L., Seeman, A., Henera, M. G., Assal, J. P., Soeldner, J. S., and Gleason, R. E.,** High and low carbohydrate diets in diabetes mellitus. Study of effects on diabetic control, insulin secretion and blood lipids, *Ann. Intern. Med.,* 80, 332, 1974.
174. **Hockaday, T. D. R., Hockaday, J. M., Mann, J. I., and Turner, R. C.,** Prospective comparison of modified-fat-high-carbohydrate with standard low-carbohydrate dietary advice in the treatment of diabetes: one year follow-up study, *Brit. J. Nutr.,* 39, 357, 1978.
175. **Chiarelli, F., Verrotti, A., Tumini, S., and Morgese, G.,** Effects of normal carbohydrate/low fat diet on lipid metabolism in insulin-dependent diabetes mellitus in childhood, *Diab. Nutr. Metab.,* 2, 285, 1989.
176. **Stone, D. B. and Connor, W. E.,** Prolonged effects of a low cholesterol, high carbohydrate diet upon the serum lipids in diabetic patients, *Diabetes,* 12, 127, 1965.

177. **Rivellese, A., Riccardi, G., Giacco, A., Pancioni, D., Genovese, S., Mattioli, P. L., and Mancini, M.**, Effect of dietary fibre on glucose control and serum lipoproteins in diabetic patients, *Lancet,* 2, 447, 1980.
178. **Garcia, R., Garza, S., De La Garza, S., Espinosa-Campos, J., and Ovalle-Berumen, F.**, Dieta alta in fibras preparada con alimentos regionales como complemento in il control de la diabetes, *Rev. Invest. Clin. (Mex.),* 34, 105, 1982.
179. **Kinmonth, A-L., Angus, R. M., Jenkins, P. A., Smith, M. A., and Baum, D.**, Whole foods and increased dietary fibre improve blood glucose control in diabetic children, *Arch. Dis. Child.,* 57, 187, 1982.
180. **Manhire, A., Henry, C. L., Hartog, M., and Heaton, K. W.**, Unrefined carbohydrate and dietary fibre in treatment of diabetes mellitus, *J. Hum. Nutr.,* 35, 99, 1981.
181. **Venhous, A. and Chantelau, E.**, Self-selected unrefined and refined carbohydrate diets do not affect metabolic control in pump-treated diabetic patients, *Diabetologia,* 31, 153, 1988.
182. **Karlström, B., Vessby, B., Asp, N. G., Boberg, M., Gustafsson, I. B., Lithell, H., and Werner, I.**, Effects of an increased content of cereal fibre in the diet of Type 2 (non-insulin-dependent) diabetic patients, *Diabetologia,* 26, 272, 1984.
183. **Hollenbeck, C. B., Coulston, A. M., and Reaven, G. M.**, To what extent does increased dietary fiber improve glucose and lipid metabolism in patients with non-insulin-dependent diabetes mellitus (NIDDM)?, *Am. J. Clin. Nutr.,* 43, 16, 1986.
184. **Nygren, C., Hallmans, G., and Lithner, F.**, Effects of high-bran bread on blood glucose control in insulin-dependent diabetic patients, *Diabete Metab. (Paris),* 10, 39, 1984.
185. **Hagander, B., Asp, N. G., Efendic, Nilsson-Ehle, P., and Schersten, B.**, Dietary fiber decreases fasting blood glucose levels and plasma LDL concentration in noninsulin-dependent diabetes mellitus patients, *Am. J. Clin. Nutr.,* 47, 852, 1988.
186. **Silvis, N., Vorster, H. H., Mollentzer, W. F., de Jager, J., and Huisman, H. W.**, Metabolic and haemostatic consequences of dietary fibre and n-3 fatty acids in black type 2 (NIDDM) diabetic subjects: a placebo controlled study, *Int. Clin. Nutr. Rev.,* 10, 362, 1990.
187. **Parillo, M., Riccardi, G., Pacioni, D., Iovine, C., Contaldo, F., Isernia, C., DeMarco, F., Perrotti, N., and Rivellese, A.**, Metabolic consequences of feeding a high-carbohydrate, high-fiber diet to diabetic patients with chronic kidney failure, *Am. J. Clin. Nutr.,* 48, 255, 1988.
188. **Kiehm, T. G., Anderson, J. W., and Ward, K.**, Beneficial effects of a high carbohydrate high fiber diet in hyperglycemic men, *Am. J. Clin. Nutr.,* 29, 895, 1976.
189. **Anderson, J. W. and Ward, K.**, High carbohydrate, high fiber diets for insulin treated men with diabetes mellitus, *Am. J. Clin. Nutr.,* 32, 2312, 1979.
190. **Fukagawa, N. K., Anderson, J. W., Hageman, G., Young, V. R., and Minaker, K. L.**, High-carbohydrate, high-fiber diets increase peripheral insulin sensitivity in healthy young and old adults, *Am. J. Clin. Nutr.,* 52, 524, 1990.
191. **Abbott, W. G. H., Boyce, V. L., Grundy, S. M., and Howard, B. V.**, Effects of replacing saturated fat with complex carbohydrate in diets of subjects with NIDDM, *Diabetes Care,* 12, 102, 1989.
192. **Simpson, H. R. C., Simpson, R. W., Lousley, S., Carter, R. D., Geekie, M., Hockaday, T. D. R., and Mann, J. I.**, A high carbohydrate leguminous fibre diet improves all aspects of diabetic control, *Lancet,* 1, 1, 1981.
193. **Bruttomesso, D., Briani, G., Bilardo, G., Vitale, E., Lavagnini, T., Marescotti, C., Duner, E., Giorato, C., and Tiengo, A.**, The medium-term effect of natural or extractive dietary fibers on plasma amino acids and lipids in type 1 diabetes, *Diab. Res. Clin. Prac.,* 6, 149, 1989.
194. **Anderson, J. W. and Ward, K.**, Long-term effects of high carbohydrate, high fiber diets on glucose and lipid metabolism: a preliminary report in patients with diabetes, *Diabetes Care,* 1, 77, 1978.
195. **Barnard, R. J., Massey, M. R., Cherny, S., O'Brien, L. T., and Pritikin, N.**, Long-term use of a high-complex-carbohydrate, high-fiber, low-fat diet and exercise in the gratement of NIDDM patients, *Diabetes Care,* 6, 268, 1983.
196. **Lindsay, A. N., Hardy, S., Jarrett, L., and Rallinson, M. L.**, High-carbohydrate, high-fiber diet in children with type I diabetes mellitus, *Diabetes Care,* 7, 63, 1984.
197. **Simpson, R. W., McDonald, J., Wahlqvist, M. L., Balasz, N., Sissons, M., and Atley, L.**, Temporal study of metabolic change when poorly controlled noninsulin-dependent diabetics change from low to high carbohydrate and fiber diet, *Am. J. Clin. Nutr.,* 48, 104, 1988.
198. **Hollenbeck, C. B., Connor, W. E., Riddle, M. C., Alaupovic, P., and Leklem, J. E.**, The effects of a high-carbohydrate low-fat cholesterol-restricted diet on plasma lipid, lipoprotein, and apoprotein concentrations in insulin-dependent (Type I) diabetes mellitus, *Metabolism,* 34, 559, 1985.
199. **Simpson, R. W., Mann, J. I., Eaton, J., Moore, R. A., Carter, R., and Hockaday, T. D. R.**, Improved glucose control in maturity onset diabetes treated with high carbohydrate-modified fat diet, *Brit. Med. J.,* 1, 1752, 1979.

200. **Simpson, R. W., Mann, J. I., Eaton, J., Carter, R. D., and Hockaday, T. D. R.**, High carbohydrate diets in insulin-dependent diabetes, *Brit. Med. J.*, 2, 523, 1979.
201. **Hollenbeck, C. B., Riddle, M. C., Connor, W. E., and Leklem, J. E.**, The effects of subject-selected high carbohydrate, low fat diets on glycemic control in insulin dependent diabetes mellitus, *Am. J. Clin. Nutr.*, 41, 293, 1985.
202. **Dodson, P. M., Pacy, P. J., Bal, P., Kubicki, A. J., Fletcher, R. F., and Taylor, K. G.**, A controlled trial of a high fibre, low fat and low sodium diet for mild hypertension in Type 2 (non-insulin-dependent) diabetic patients, *Diabetologia*, 27, 522, 1984.
203. **McCulloch, D. K., Mitchell, R. D., Ambler, J., and Tattersall, R. B.**, A prospective comparison of 'conventional' and high carbohydrate/high fiber/low fat diets in adults with established Type 1 (insulin dependent) diabetes, *Diabetologia*, 28, 208, 1985.
204. **Ney, D., Hollingsworth, D. R., and Cousins, L.**, Decreased insulin requirement and improved control of diabetes in pregnant women given a high-carbohydrate, high-fiber, low-fat diet, *Diabetes Care*, 5, 529, 1982.
205. **Scott, A. R., Attenborough, Y., Peacock, I., Fletcher, E., Jeffcoate, W. J., and Tattersall, R. B.**, Comparison of high fibre diets, basal insulin supplements, and flexible insulin treatment for non-insulin dependent (type II) diabetics poorly controlled with sulphonylureas, *Brit. Med. J.*, 297, 707, 1988.
206. **Jenkins, D. J. A., Wolever, T. M. S., Collier, G. R., Ocana, A., Rao, A. V., Buckley, G., Lam, K. Y., Meyer, A., and Thompson, L. U.**, The metabolic effects of a low glycemic index diet, *Am. J. Clin. Nutr.*, 46, 968, 1987.
207. **Jenkins, D. J. A., Wolever, T. M. S., Kalmusky, J., Giudici, S., Giordano, C., Patten, R., Wong, G. S., Bird, J. N., Hall, M., Buckley, G., Csima, A., and Little, J. A.**, Low-glycemic index diet in hyperlipidemia: use of traditional starchy foods, *Am. J. Clin. Nutr.*, 46, 66, 1987.
208. **Calle-Pascual, A. L., Gomez, V., Leon, E., and Bordiu, E.**, Foods with a low glycemic index do not improve glycemic control of both type 1 and type 2 diabetic patients after one month of therapy, *Diabete Metab. (Paris)*, 14, 629, 1988.
209. **Jenkins, D. J. A., Wolever, T. M. S., Buckley, G., Lam, K. Y., Giudici, S., Kalmusky, J., Jenkins, A. L., Patten, R. L., Bird, J., Wong, G. S., and Josse, R. G.**, Low glycemic-index starchy food in the diabetic diet, *Am. J. Clin. Nutr.*, 48, 248, 1988.
210. **Collier, G. R., Giudici, S., Kalmusky, J., Wolever, T. M. S., Helman, G., Wesson, V., Ehrlich, R. M., and Jenkins, D. J. A.**, Low glycaemic index starchy foods improve glucose control and lower serum cholesterol in diabetic children, *Diab. Nutr. Metab.*, 1, 11, 1988.
211. **Fontvieille, A. M., Acosta, M., Rizkalla, S. W., Bornet, F., David, P., Letanoux, M., Tchobroutsky, G., and Slama, G.**, A moderate switch from high to low glycaemic-index foods for 3 weeks improves metabolic control of Type I (IDDM) diabetic subjects, *Diab. Nutr. Metab.*, 1, 139, 1988.
212. **Brand, J. C., Colagiuri, S., Crossman, S., Allen, A., Roberts, D. C. K., and Truswell, A. S.**, Low glycemic index foods improve long term glycemic control in non-insulin-dependent diabetes mellitus, *Diabetes Care*, 14, 95, 1991.
213. **Elsenhaus, B., Sufke, U., Blume, R., and Caspary, W. F.**, The influence of carbohydrate gelling agents on rat intestinal transport of monosaccharides and neutral amino acids in vitro, *Clin. Sci.*, 59, 373, 1980.
214. **Rainbird, A. L., Low, A. G., and Zebrowska, T.**, Effect of guar gum on glucose absorption from isolated loops of jejunum in conscious growing pigs, *Proc. Nutr. Soc.*, 39, 48A, 1982.
215. **Isaksson, G., Lundquist, I., and Ihse, I.**, Effect of dietary fiber on pancreatic enzyme activity in vitro: the importance of viscosity, pH, ionic strength, adsorption, and time of incubation, *Gastroenterology*, 82, 918, 1982.
216. **Leatherdale, B. A., Green, D. J., Harding, L. K., Griffin, D., and Bailey, C. J.**, Guar and gastric emptying in non-insulin dependent diabetes, *Acta Diabet. Lat.*, 19, 339, 1982.
217. **Thompson, L. U., Button, C. L., and Jenkins, D. J. A.**, Phytic acid and calcium affect the in vitro rate of navy bean starch digestion and blood glucose response in humans, *Am. J. Clin. Nutr.*, 46, 467, 1987.
218. **Rea, R. L., Thompson, L. U., and Jenkins, D. J. A.**, Lectins in foods and their relation to starch digestibility, *Nutr. Res.*, 5, 919, 1985.
219. **Thompson, L. U., Yoon, J. H., Jenkins, D. J. A., Wolever, T. M. S., and Jenkins, A. L.**, Relationship between polyphenol intake and blood glucose response of normal and diabetic individuals, *Am. J. Clin. Nutr.*, 39, 745, 1984.
220. **Marshall, J. J. and Lauda, C. M.**, Purification and properties of phaseolamin, an inhibitor of alpha-amylase from the kidney bean *phaseolus vuloaris*, *J. Biol. Chem.*, 250, 8030, 1975.
221. **Wolever, T. M. S., Chan, C., Law, C., Bird, L., Ramdath, D., Moran, J. J., and Jenkins, D. J. A.**, The in vitro and in vivo anti-amylase activity of starch blockers, *J. Plant Foods*, 5, 23, 1983.
222. **Jenkins, D. J. A., Thorne, M. J., Wolever, T. M. S., Jenkins, A. L., Rao, A. V., and Thompson, L. U.**, The effect of starch-protein interaction in wheat on the glycemic response and rate of in vitro digestion, *Am. J. Clin. Nutr.*, 45, 946, 1987.

223. Holm, J., Bjork, I., Ostrowska, S., Eliasson, A. C., Asp, N. G., Larsson, K., and Lundquist, I., Digestibility of amylose-lipid complexes in-vitro and in-vivo, *Starch/starke,* 35, 294, 1983.
224. Behall, K. M., Scholfield, D. J., and Canary, J., Effect of starch structure on glucose and insulin responses in adults, *Am. J. Clin. Nutr.,* 47, 428, 1988.
225. Goddard, M. S., Young, G., and Marcus, R., The effect of amylose content on insulin and glucose responses to ingested rice, *Am. J. Clin. Nutr.,* 39, 388, 1984.
226. Mourot, J., Thouvenot, P., Couet, C., Antoine, J. M., Krobicka, A., and Debry, G., Relationship between the rate of gastric emptying and glucose and insulin responses to starchy foods in young healthy adults, *Am. J. Clin. Nutr.,* 48, 1035, 1988.
227. Gannon, M. C. and Nuttall, F. Q., Factors affecting interpretation of postprandial glucose and insulin areas, *Diabetes Care,* 10, 759, 1987.
228. Wolever, T. M. S., Jenkins, D. J. A., Vuksan, V., Josse, R. G., Wong, G. S., and Jenkins, A. L., Glycemic index in individual subjects, *Diabetes Care,* 13, 126, 1990.
229. Jenkins, D. J. A., Wolever, T. M. S., Taylor, R. H., Ghafari, H., Jenkins, A. L., Barker, H., and Jenkins, M. J. A., Rate of digestion of foods and postprandial glycaemia in normal and diabetic subjects, *Brit. Med. J.,* 2, 14, 1980.
230. Jenkins, D. J. A., Ghafari, H., Wolever, T. M. S., Taylor, R. H., Barker, H. M., Fielden, H., Jenkins, A. L., and Bowling, A. C., Relationship between the rate of digestion of foods and postprandial glycaemia, *Diabetologia,* 22, 450, 1982.
231. O'Dea, K., Snow, P., and Nestel, P., Rate of starch hydrolysis in vitro as a predictor of metabolic responses to complex carbohydrate in vivo, *Am. J. Clin. Nutr.,* 34, 1991, 1981.
232. Jenkins, D. J. A., Wolever, T. M. S., Thorne, M. J., Jenkins, A. L., Wong, G. S., Josse, R. G., and Csima, A., The relationship between glycemic response, digestibility, and factors influencing the dietary habits of diabetics, *Am. J. Clin. Nutr.,* 40, 1175, 1984.
233. Thorburn, A. W., Brand, J. C., and Truswell, A. S., Slowly digested and absorbed carbohydrate in traditional bushfoods: a protective factor against diabetes?, *Am. J. Clin. Nutr.,* 45, 98, 1987.
234. Bornet, F. R. J., Fontvieille, A. M., Rizkalla, S., Colonna, P., Blayo, A., Mercier, C., and Slama, G., Insulin and glycemic responses in healthy humans to native starches processed in different ways: correlation with in vitro alpha-amylase hydrolysis, *Am. J. Clin. Nutr.,* 50, 315, 1989.
235. Wolever, T. M. S., Relationship between dietary fiber content and composition in foods and the glycemic index, *Am. J. Clin. Nutr.,* 51, 72, 1990.
236. Del Toma, E., Clementi, A., Marcelli, M., Cappelloni, M., and Lintas, C., Food fiber choices for diabetic diets, *Am. J. Clin. Nutr.,* 37, 667, 1988.
237. Thomas, E. J., Mechanics and regulation of gastric emptying, *Physiol. Rev.,* 37, 453, 1957.
238. Collier, G. R., Wolever, T. M. S., and Jenkins, D. J. A., Concurrent ingestion of fat and reduction in starch content impairs carbohydrate tolerance to subsequent meals, *Am. J. Clin. Nutr.,* 45, 963, 1987.
239. Read, N. W., Welch, I. M. L., Austen, C. J., et al., Swallowing food without chewing; a simple way to reduce postpranidal glycaemia, *Brit. J. Nutr.,* 55, 43, 1986.
240. Jenkins, D. J. A., Wolever, T. M. S., and Jenkins, A. L., Starchy foods and the glycemic index, *Diabetes Care,* 11, 149, 1988.
241. Reaven, G. M., Dietary therapy for non-insulin-dependent diabetes mellitus, *New Engl. J. Med.,* 319, 862, 1980.
242. Jenkins, D. J. A., Wolever, T. M. S., Bacon, S., Nineham, R., Lees, R., Rowden, R., Love, M., and Hockaday, T. D. R., Diabetic diets: high carbohydrate combined with high fiber, *Am. J. Clin. Nutr.,* 33, 1729, 1980.
243. Wolever, T. M. S., Metabolic effects of continuous feeding, *Metabolism,* 39, 947, 1990.
244. Jenkins, D. J. A., Wolever, T. M. S., Vuksan, V., Brighenti, F., Cunnane, S. C., Rao, A. V., Jenkins, A., Buckley, G., Patten, R., Singer, W., Corey, P., and Josse, R. G., "Nibbling versus gorging": Metabolic advantages of increased meal frequency, *New Engl. J. Med.,* 321, 929, 1989.
245. Creutzfeldt, W., Ed., Proceedings of first international symposium on acarbose, Montreux, Oct. 1981, *Excerpta Med.,* Amsterdam, 1982.
246. Hanefeld, M., Fischer, S., Schulze, J., Lüthke, C., and Spengler, M., Potential use of acarbose as first line drug in non-insulin dependent diabetes mellitus insufficiently treated with diet alone, *Diab. Nutr. Metab.,* 3(Suppl. 1), 51, 1990.
247. Tasman-Jones, C., Effects of dietary fiber on the structure and function of the small intestine, in *Medical Aspects of Dietary Fiber,* Spiller, G. A. and Kay, R. M., Eds., Plenum Medical Books, New York, 1980, 67.
248. Cassidy, M. M., Lightfoot, F. G., Gray, L. E., Story, J. A., Kritchevsky, D., and Vahouny, G. V., Effect of chronic intake of dietary fibers on the ultrastructural topography of rat jejunum and colon: a scanning electron microscopy study, *Am. J. Clin. Nutr.,* 34, 218, 1981.
249. Tasman-Jones, C., Owen, R. L., and Jones, A. L., Semipurified dietary fiber and small bowel morphology in rats, *Dig. Dis. Sci.,* 27, 519, 1982.

250. **Jacobs, L. R. and Schneeman, B. O.,** Effects of dietary wheat bran on rat colonic structure and mucosal cell growth, *J. Nutr.,* 111, 798, 1981.
251. **Jacobs, L. R. and White, F. A.,** Modulation of mucosal cell proliferation in the intestine of rats fed a wheat bran diet, *Am. J. Clin. Nutr.,* 37, 945, 1983.
252. **Jacobs, L. R.,** Effects of dietary fiber on mucosal growth and cell proliferation in the small intestine of the rat: a comparison of oat bran, pectin, and guar with total fiber derpivation, *Am. J. Clin. Nutr.,* 37, 954, 1983.
253. **Shetty, P. S. and Kurpad, A. V.,** Increased starch intake in the human diet increases fecal bulking, *Am. J. Clin. Nutr.,* 43, 210, 1986.
254. **Flourié, B., Leblond, A., Florent, Ch., Rautureau, M., Bisalli, A., and Rambaud, J-C.,** Starch malabsorption and breath gas excretion in healthy humans consuming low- and high-starch diets, *Gastroenterology,* 95, 356, 1988.
255. **Stephen, A. M., Haddad, A. C., and Phillips, S. F.,** Passage of carbohydrate into the colon: direct measurements in humans, *Gastroenterology,* 85, 589, 1983.
256. **Wolever, T. M. S., Cohen, Z., Thompson, L. U., Thorne, M. J., Jenkins, M. J. A., Prokipchuk, E. J., and Jenkins, D. J. A.,** Ileal loss of available carbohydrate in man: comparison of a breath hydrogen method with direct measurement using a human ileostomy model, *Am. J. Gastroenterol.,* 81, 115, 1986.
257. **Jenkins, D. J. A., Cuff, D., Wolever, T. M. S., Knowland, D., Thompson, L. U., Cohen, Z., and Prokipchuk, E.,** Digestibility of carbohydrate foods in an ileostomate: relationship to dietary fiber, in vitro digestibility, and glycemic response, *Am. J. Gastroenterol.,* 82, 709, 1987.
258. **Levitt, M. D., Hirsh, P., Fetzer, C. A., Sheahan, M., and Levine, A. S.,** H2 excretion after ingestion of complex carbohydrates, *Gastroenterology,* 92, 383, 1987.
259. **McBurney, M. I., Thompson, L. U., Cuff, D. J., and Jenkins, D. J. A.,** Comparison of ileal effluents, dietary fibers, and whole foods in predicting the physiological importance of colonic fermentation, *Am. J. Gastroenterol.,* 83, 536, 1988.
260. **McBurney, M. I., Thompson, L. U., and Jenkins, D. J. A.,** Colonic fermentation of some breads and its implication for energy availability in man, *Nutr. Res.,* 7, 1229, 1987.
261. **Cummings, J. H., Southgate, D. A. T., Branch, W. J., Wiggins, H. S., Houston, H., Jenkins, D. J. A., Jivraj, T., and Hill, M. J.,** The digestion of pectin in the human gut and its effect on calcium absorption and large bowel function, *Brit. J. Nutr.,* 41, 477, 1979.
262. **Holloway, W. D., Tasman-Jones, C., and Lee, S. P.,** Digestion of certain fractions of dietary fiber in humans, *Am. J. Clin. Nutr.,* 31, 927, 1978.
263. **Holloway, W. D., Tasman-Jones, C., and Maher, K.,** Pectin digestion in humans, *Am. J. Clin. Nutr.,* 37, 253, 1983.
264. **McBurney, M. I. and Thompson, L. U.,** In vitro fermentabilities of purified fiber supplements, *J. Food Sci.,* 54, 347, 1989.
265. **Bond, J. H. and Levitt, M. D.,** Fate of soluble carbohydrate in the colon of rats and man, *J. Clin. Invest.,* 57, 1158, 1976.
266. **Bond, J. A., Currier, B. E., Buchwald, H., and Levitt, M. D.,** Colonic conservation of malabsorbed carbohydrate, *Gastroenterology,* 78, 444, 1980.
267. **Cummings, J. H.,** Short chain fatty acids in the human colon, *Gut,* 22, 763, 1981.
268. **Cummings, J. H., Pomare, E. W., Branch, W. J., Naylor, C. P. E., and MacFarlane, G. T.,** Short chain fatty acids in human large intestine, portal, hepatic and venous blood, *Gut,* 28, 1221, 1987.
269. **Wolever, T. M. S., Brighenti, F., Royall, D., Jenkins, A. L., and Jenkins, D. J. A.,** Effect of rectal infusion of short chain fatty acids in human subjects, *Am. J. Gastroenterol.,* 84, 1027, 1989.
270. **Royall, D., Wolever, T. M. S., and Jeejeebhoy, K. N.,** Clinical significance of colonic fermentation, *Am. J. Gastroenterol.,* 85, 1307, 1990.
271. **Wolever, T. M. S., Spadafora, P., and Eshuis, H.,** Interaction between colonic acetate and propionate in man, *Am. J. Clin. Nutr.,* 53, 681, 1991.
272. **Chen, W-J. L., Anderson, J. W., and Jennings, D.,** Propionate may mediate the hypocholesterolemic effects of certain soluble plant fibers in cholesterol fed rats, *Proc. Soc. Exp. Biol. Med.,* 175, 215, 1984.
273. **Illman, R. J., Topping, D. L., McIntosh, G. H., Trimble, R. P., Storer, G. B., Taylor, M. N., and Cheng, B. Q.,** Hypocholesterolaemic effects of dietary propionate: studies in whole animals and perfused rat liver, *Ann. Nutr. Metab.,* 32, 97, 1988.
274. **Thacker, P. A., Salomons, M. O., Aherne, F. X., Milligan, L. P., and Bowland, J. P.,** Influence of propionic acid on the cholesterol metabolism of pigs fed hypercholesterolemic diets, *Can. J. Anim. Sci.,* 61, 969, 1981.

Chapter 4.2

EFFECTS OF DIETARY FIBER ON INTESTINAL ABSORPTION OF LIPIDS

Marie M. Cassidy and Richard J. Calvert

The increased intake of dietary fiber in humans is generally associated with increases in fecal volume and increases in the lipid contents of feces.[1-5] These increases are observed either when the diet has been modified to increase fiber intake or when the diet is supplemented with isolated polysaccharides (Table 1). The source of the increased fecal fat is uncertain. It could be derived either from poorly digestible lipids in the fiber source itself or from other dietary or endogenous lipids. In this connection, Southgate and co-workers[7] were unable to detect changes in fecal lipids, which were a reflection of the decreased digestibility in the lipids of ingested bran. The data from these human studies, although indirect, suggest that dietary fiber, and particularly polysaccharides which form viscous solutions (Table 2), may interfere with specific aspects of the emulsification and lipolysis of dietary fat, most likely at the level of micellar solubilization and absorption of fat digestion products and cholesterol.[8]

The emulsification of dietary fat, which is required for efficient lipolysis and for the solubilization of lipolytic products and cholesterol, is dependent on the concentration and composition of the biliary bile acid pool. This pool is derived from enterohepatic recirculation of luminal bile acids and by synthesis of bile acids from precursor cholesterol. A prolonged increase in fecal excretion of bile acids (acidic steroids) is taken to represent a potential reduction in the enterohepatic bile acid pool and to predict a reduction in the bioavailability of dietary and endogenous lipids particularly cholesterol. Furthermore, the increased excretion of neutral sterols (cholesterol and bacterial metabolites) represents an indirect assessment of reduced cholesterol absorption or of increased biliary output of cholesterol (Table 3).

Thus, the measurement of fecal acidic and neutral sterol output indicates that increased intake of dietary fiber, and particularly of supplements containing gelling or mucilaginous fibers, may interfere with the enterohepatic circulation of bile acids (Table 2). The fibers studied include oat bran, psyllium fiber, pectin, and guar, but may also include other natural food sources of fiber and fiber supplements. As shown in Table 2, increased intakes of dietary fibers or fiber supplements generally do not significantly alter the output of fecal neutral sterols in humans. In addition, the effect of increasing dietary fiber intakes on the plasma cholesterol level of normocholesterolemic subjects is generally modest. Nor are changes in plasma cholesterol consistently correlated with changes in fecal bile acid and neutral sterol output (Table 2).

The direct effects of dietary fiber supplements on certain aspects of fat digestion and on the absorption of fatty acids and cholesterol have been assessed in animal models. Early studies, which employed either balance techniques[34] or the use of isotopic tracers, suggested that pectin could cause increased output of fecal acidic steroids and reduced absorption of cholesterol (Table 3). In an acute study on the absorption of [^{14}C] cholesterol into thoracic duct lymph,[36] pectin given in two doses of 125 mg, 1 h apart, caused a 19% reduction in recovery of lymph cholesterol. The bile acid sequestrant cholestyramine, in contrast, resulted in 27% inhibition of cholesterol absorption, when given at a 50-mg dose, and 71% inhibition when included at a dose of 238 mg.

These and other early studies[7,32] have suggested that the hypocholesteremic effects of pectins and certain other viscous fiber derivatives appear to be most pronounced when

TABLE 1
Dietary Fiber and Fat Excretion in Human[6]

Change in dietary fiber intake (g/d)	Change in fecal fat (g/d)	(%)	Change in apparent digestibility (%)	Ref.
9.8 (diet)	+0.68	22.6	−0.4	1
11.8 (diet)	+2.27	55.0	−2.8	1
25.7 (diet)	+3.23	107.3	−3.6	1
16.0 (cellulose)	+0.60	21.4	−0.9	5
20.0 (ispaghula)	+2.85	40.1	−1.9	4
36.0 (pectin)	+1.18	80.3	—	3

TABLE 2
Effect of Dietary Fiber on Fecal Steroid Excretion in Humans[a]

Fiber source	Amount (g/d)	Plasma cholesterol (% change)	Fecal bile acids (% change)	Fecal neutral sterols (% change)	Ref.
Mixed	33	−7	0	+40	9
	60	0	+111	—	10
	93	0	0	0	11
	26.2	−4.5	+13	0	12
Legumes	—	−22	+55	0	13
	15	—	+25	—	14
	100	−25	+45	—	15
Soy fiber	25	0	0	0	16
Wheat grain	16	0	0	0	17
	35	—	0	0	18
	36	0	0	0	19
	39	0	0	0	20
	54	0	0	0	21
	60	—	+90	—	22
	70	0	−49	0	23
	13.2	—	0	0	24
	39.6	—	+65	0	24
	66.0	—	+60	0	24
	60	0	+16	+8	25
Psyllium	10	−10	+302	0	26
	15	0	+70	—	14
	21	−16	0	0	27
Pectin	15	−13	+33	+17	28
	36	−15	+34	—	29
	45	−13	+75	0	30
Guar gum	36	−16	+84	—	29
Oat bran	40	0	+111	—	11
	100	−13	+51	0	31

[a] Modified from Kay, R. M., *J. Lipid Res.*, 23, 221, 1982.

TABLE 3
Effect of Fiber Supplements on Fecal Bile Acids and Cholesterol Absorption in the Rat

Fiber supplement	Response	Ref.
Commercial rat chow (alfalfa)	Increased fecal bile acid	33
Alfalfa	Increased fecal neutral sterols	34
	Decreased cholesterol absorption	
Pectin (500 mg/day)	Increased fecal acidic and neutral steroids	35
	Decreased cholesterol absorption by balance techniques	
Pectin (5%)	Increased fecal acidic steroids	36
	Decreased cholesterol absorption by fecal isotope recovery	
Pectin (250 mg)	Decreased lymphatic absorption of cholesterol	37
Pectin (5%)	Decreased cholesterol absorption	38
Gum arabic (5%)	Decreased cholesterol absorption	38
Agar (5%)	Decreased cholesterol absorption	38

included in diets containing cholesterol. Thus, fiber-induced modifications of bile salt availability for micellar solubilization of luminal cholesterol have been considered as direct mechanisms by which dietary fiber influences cholesterol absorption.[7,32]

The sequestration ability of commercial bile acid-binding resins and certain types of fiber derivatives is not merely confined to bile acids. The ability of cholestyramine, cereal fibers, and alfalfa to adsorb cholesterol from bile acid micelles has been reported,[7,39,40] and this binding approximates that for bile acids. Other studies (Table 4) suggest that all components of micelles, typical of those in the intestinal lumen, may be adsorbed by resins and dietary fibers in approximately equal proportions.[7] These *in vitro* data, however, demonstrate binding capability but do not necessarily reflect the actual effect of these materials *in vivo*.

The effects of dietary fiber supplements on the absorption of cholesterol and triglycerides may involve mechanisms other than the bile acid- and micellar lipid-sequestering effects noted for these fibers *in vitro*. Wheat germ and wheat bran demonstrate a significant inhibitory effect on the hydrolytic capability of pancreatic lipase *in vitro*. When these same wheat fractions were fed to rats for 4 weeks, mucosal uptake of [^{14}C]lipids and [^{3}H]cholesterol from a test meal was significantly reduced and dietary lipids accumulated in the cecum.[42] These authors believe that the mechanism underlying the hypocholesteremic effect is one of impaired fat lipolysis. This hypothesis is attractive since it offers an explanation for the many observations that these wheat fractions have a much larger impact on cholesterol and triglyceride levels in rats when fed with a high fat diet, and little or no effect in conjunction with a low fat diet.

It has been reported that in the presence of viscous fiber derivatives (e.g., guar gum and pectins) the *in vitro* transport rate of water-soluble molecules is inhibited.[43,44] The effect

TABLE 4
Binding of Micellar Components by Ion-Exchange Resin and Dietary Fiber Derivatives[8]

Test material	Percentage bound				
	Bile salt[a]	Lecithin	Cholesterol	Monoolein	Fatty acids[b]
Cholestyramine	82	99	95	96	96
DEAE-Sephadex	49	99	100	99	98
Guar gum	36	22	23	23	33
Lignin	20	9	5	13	13
Alfalfa	7	4	1	19	18
Wheat bran	4	6	0	11	12
Cellulose	1.5	0.5	8	4	4

[a] Sodium taurocholate.
[b] Equimolar mixture of palmitic, oleic, and linoleic acids.

is reversible by washing the intestinal tissue prior to transport studies,[43] and it has been suggested that the gelling fibers may modify the resistance of the surface-associated, unstirred water layer,[43-45] which can influence nutrient flux and absorption in the intestine. Similar studies on intestinal cholesterol transport have been reported either with intestinal segments incubated with micellar cholesterol and guar gum or with intestinal loops *in vivo*.[46] The presence of the gelling fiber reduced cholesterol transport by both preparations. When intestinal segments were preincubated with guar gum prior to transport studies, cholesterol uptake was also reduced, but to a lesser extent when gum was present in the lumen. These and other studies[47] suggest that viscous fibers like guar gum can interfere with bulk-phase diffusion of lipids and may also have a residual effect in limiting transmural transport of lipids. Studies conducted *in vivo*,[46] however, suggested that prolonged feeding of diets containing guar gum did not lead to adaptive reduction of either cholesterol or glucose disappearance from intestinal loops in subsequently fasted animals.[46] These latter data are, however, inconsistent with other reports demonstrating dramatic modifications of both structural and functional aspects of the intestine in response to prolonged intake of various fiber supplements.[7,48,49]

Recent studies on the effects of fiber feeding on gastrointestinal mucin (probably the major constituent of the unstirred water layer) have suggested that long-term adaptive changes in mucin quantity may be at least partly responsible for fiber's effects on lipid absorption. Feeding rats either wheat bran[50] or citrus fiber[51] produced significant increases in small intestinal mucin quantity as determined by a sensitive enzyme-linked immunosorbent assay (ELISA) method. Consistent with these findings, human[25] and animal[52] studies have documented reduced cholesterol absorption following chronic wheat bran consumption.

Measurement of the disappearance of radioactivity from the small intestine of rats fed fiber-containing test meals incorporating [^{3}H]cholesterol and [^{14}C]triolein was recently used to assess the initial *in vivo* effects of dietary fiber on lipid absorption. The effects of guar gum, konjac mannan (a viscous fiber), and chitosan (an aminopolysaccharide derived from the chitin potion of arthropod exoskeletons) were examined.[53] Rats were killed 2 h after consuming test meals containing one of these three fibers or cellulose (control). Guar gum and konjac mannan significantly delayed the disappearance of ^{14}C and ^{3}H radioactivity from the small intestinal lumen, in addition to reducing the amount found in the small intestinal wall. These results suggest interference by these gelling fibers with the diffusion of lipid-containing micelles within the small intestine. Although chitosan bound micellar components as documented by decreased amounts of bile acids and phospholipids found in the aqueous

TABLE 5
Influence of Feeding Fiber Supplements in Defined Diets on the Lymphatic Absorption of Cholesterol in Fasted Rats[50,53]

Dietary supplement (%)	Cholesterol absorption (percent of fiber-free control)	
	0–12 h	0–24 h
Wheat bran (15)	67	79
Cellulose (15)	14	24
Alfalfa (15)	42	51
Pectin (15)	60	70
Cholestyramine (2) (5)	28	38(32)
Chitosan (5)	—	(41)

portion of the small intestinal contents, it did not retard the disappearance of ^{3}H or ^{14}C from the lumen. This contrasts with the results of lymph cannulation studies,[54] which have shown chitosan to delay lymphatic recovery of cholesterol and fatty acids. The much shorter time course (2 h vs. 24 h) of the radioactive tracer studies may partly explain this difference in findings.

Lipid recoveries in thoracic duct or mesenteric lymph have been examined in animal models as a direct measure of dietary fiber influences on lipid digestion and absorption.[47,52] In one study,[47] the output of mesenteric lymph triglycerides (in chylomicrons) was followed at hourly intervals after the last meal. Lymph triglyceride concentrations already peaked within the first hour in animals fed fiber-free diets and decreased rapidly thereafter. In cellulose-fed rats, lymph triglycerides peaked at 2 h after the first meal and decreased slowly thereafter. In guar-fed rats, lymph triglycerides reach a lower plateau, but only 6 to 10 h after the last meal. The lymph triglyceride changes were paralleled by changes in the lymph levels of apoprotein A1. In another study,[54] fiber sources were infused as a part of lipid test emulsions containing unlabeled triglyceride and radiolabeled cholesterol. Thoracic duct recovery of fatty acids (minus endogenous lymphatic fatty acids from lymph collected in the fasted state) and radiolabeled cholesterol were measured. Compared to cellulose (which served as the control), the aminopolysaccharide chitosan significantly slowed the rate of cholesterol and fatty acid recovery, while guar gum had no effect on cholesterol absorption and produced only a statistically insignificant reduction in the rate of fatty acid recovery in lymph. A zero fiber treatment for comparison was not included in this study. Considered together, these studies suggest that the lymphatic absorption of both cholesterol and fatty acids is slowed by the presence of either soluble or insoluble fiber in test meals.

Indirect or adaptive changes in lipid absorption as a result of prolonged intake of fiber supplements have also been demonstrated by direct measurement of lipid recoveries in lymph.[52] In these studies, rats were fed for 4 weeks on defined diets containing various dietary fiber supplements. Lymphatic drainage catheters were surgically introduced and animals were fasted for 18 to 24 h before study. Cholesterol and triglyceride fatty acid absorption into lymph was assessed after a single intragastric dose of a lipid emulsion containing cholesterol and triolein. Since all animals were fasted, differences in absorption were taken to represent prolonged effects on gastric emptying, effects of residual fiber associated with the intestinal lumen or absorptive surface, or modified cellular transport of lipids. The first possibility may be unlikely since the lipid dose was a dilute aqueous emulsion. The data shown in Table 5 suggest that residual or adaptive responses to fiber supplements

TABLE 6
Effect of 4-Week Intakes of Fiber Supplements on Cholesterol Absorption in Fasted Rats[56]

Dietary supplement (%)	Cholesterol absorption (percent of fiber-free control)	
	0–4 h	0–24 h
Cellulose (10)	55[a]	75
Alfalfa (10)	44[a]	77
Bran-pectin (3:1) (10)	34[a]	38[a]
Pectin (5)	33[a]	37[a]
Guar gum (5)	41[a]	58[a]
Metamucil (5)	22[a]	25[a]
Cholestyramine (2)	21[a]	45[a]

[a] $p < 0.5$ from fiber-free control.

TABLE 7
Effect of 4-Week Intakes of Fiber Supplement on Oleic Acid Absorption in Fasted Rats[56]

Dietary supplement	Oleic acid absorption (percent of fiber-free control)	
	0–4 h	0–24 h
Cellulose	80	92
Alfalfa	71	81
Bran-pectin	51[a]	60
Pectin	55[a]	79
Guar gum	69[a]	71
Metamucil	41[a]	33[a]
Cholestyramine	46[a]	76

[a] $p < 0.05$ from fiber-free control.

such as bran, cellulose, alfalfa, and pectin, as well as to the bile acid sequestrant cholestyramine, can result in impaired lymphatic absorption (or recovery) of luminal cholesterol. Furthermore, the same effects are observed for the digestion and/or absorption of emulsified triglyceride with a correlation coefficient for absorption of cholesterol and triglyceride fatty acids of 0.962. These observations have been extended to include the partially acetylated derivative of polyglucosamine, chitosan.[55]

This approach has been extended[56] to eliminate the possible adaptive responses on gastric emptying and to circumvent possible effects of lipolysis of triolein. Animals were fed for 4 weeks on defined diets, provided a thoracic duct drainage catheter, and fasted 18 to 24 h. In these studies, animals were given the aqueous lipid emulsion intraduodenally rather than intragastrically, and the emulsion contained cholesterol and unesterfied oleic acid. The effects on cholesterol absorption under these conditions (Table 6) suggest that all fiber supplements modified intestinal absorption of cholesterol during the initial 4 h of lymph collection, but this effect was persistent only in animals fed viscous fiber preparations or the bile acid-binding resin. As shown in Table 7, studies on free fatty acid absorption suggest

TABLE 8
Lipoprotein Distribution of Absorbed Cholesterol and Oleic Acid in the Thoracic Duct Lymph of Rats Fed Dietary Fiber Supplements[56]

Dietary supplement	Percent distribution of absorbed cholesterol			Percent distribution of absorbed oleic acid		
	Chylomicrons + VLDL[a]	LDL	HDL	Chylomicrons + VLDL	LDL	HDL
None	88.1	7.2	4.7	96.2	2.6	1.1
Cellulose	90.1	6.2	3.7	91.3	7.6	1.1
Alfalfa	86.1	6.0	7.9	95.6	2.2	2.2
Bran-pectin	91.8	5.6	2.6	96.5	2.5	0.9
Pectin	89.3	5.6	5.0	89.1	7.8	3.1
Guar gum	92.7	4.8	2.5	97.4	1.4	0.9
Metamucil	81.2	14.4[a,b]	4.4	95.3	3.1	1.2
Cholestyramine	90.0	8.7	1.2	95.5	3.9	0.7

[a] Abbreviations: VLDL = very low density lipoprotein; LDL = low density lipoprotein; HDL = high density lipoprotein.
[b] $p < 0.05$ from fiber-free control.

TABLE 9
Lipid Distribution of Absorbed Oleic Acid in Thoracic Duct Lymph of Rats Fed Dietary Fiber Supplements[56]

Dietary supplement	Percent distribution of oleic acid				
	TG[a]	MG-DG	FA	PL	CE
None	85	4	7	3	1
Cellulose	87	2	7	3	2
Alfalfa	84	3	9	3	1
Bran-pectin	84	4	5	4	3
Pectin	89	3	3	2	3
Guar gum	87	2	5	4	2
Metamucil	88	2	4	4	2
Cholestyramine	83	3	7	6	2

[a] Abbreviations: TG, triglycerides; MG-DG, mono- and diglycerides; FA, unesterified fatty acids; PL, phospholipids; CE, cholesterol esters.

that only the viscous fiber preparations reduced the initial absorption of the lipid, but that, except for animals fed Metamucil, the overall 24-h absorption of fatty acid was statistically the same as for animals fed fiber-free diets. Data on the lipoprotein distributions of the absorbed lipids and on distribution of absorbed oleic acid among the major lymph lipids are summarized in Tables 8 and 9. Except for Metamucil, none of these distributions are significantly different from those in the rats fed fiber-free, defined diets. Furthermore, there were no differences in chylomicron sizes in any of the groups as assessed by scanning electron microscopy.

Finally, the effects of fiber on lipid absorption have been examined in a few human studies using radioisotopic methods to assess cholesterol absorption. An isotope ratio method[57] was used in two studies to estimate cholesterol absorption by comparing the ratio of ^{3}H/^{14}C in serum of patients given simultaneous doses of intravenous [^{3}H]cholesterol and oral [^{14}C]cholesterol. Wheat bran (60 g/d for 4 weeks) produced a 16% mean decrease in cholesterol absorption (from 50% absorption pre-bran to 42% after 4 weeks of bran consumption) in 12 human subjects.[25] Consumption of guar gum (15 to 30 g/d) by a single subject over a 10-month period reduced cholesterol absorption by 25% to a mean level of 47% (average of 7 time points) from a pretreatment level of 63%.[57] In contrast to these two studies demonstrating significant effects of fiber, a trial of a high fiber diet utilizing a mixture of soluble and insoluble fiber derived from both foods and purified supplements showed no difference in cholesterol absorption between high and low fiber periods in 34 male subjects.[12] This study utilized a fecal [^{14}C]cholesterol/[^{3}H]sitosterol method to assess cholesterol absorption after oral administration of [^{14}C]cholesterol and the nonabsorbable [^{3}H]sitosterol. Thus, while human studies suggest that some types of fiber diminish lipid absorption, these studies are few in number and not entirely consistent in their findings. Additional studies in humans, possibly using stable isotopes rather than ratio isotopes, would be useful to explore further the effect of fiber on lipid absorption in humans.

The available evidence to date suggests that:

1. Dietary fibers supplements, including particulate fibers such as cellulose,[47] and chitosan[54] and particularly the viscous fibers,[43,44,46,47,53] when present in the intestine, can modify the rates of absorption of fatty acids and cholesterol. This effect may be related to disruption of micellar solubility of lipids due to bile acid sequestration[7,40] or to interference with bulk phase diffusion of lipids.[45,46,50,51]
2. Prolonged intake of fiber supplements may modify the nutriture of the upper intestine and result in morphological[47,48] and functional[7,47,58] changes in the intestine with respect to lipid absorption.
3. Direct studies on lymphatic absorption of lipids suggest that either direct or adaptive responses to fiber intake may interfere with triglyceride digestion[7,47,54] and delay absorption of unesterified fatty acids.[47,56] Under these same conditions, cholesterol absorption is reduced.[7,56]
4. Human studies using noninvasive techniques to assess cholesterol absorption also show that fiber consumption may reduce cholesterol absorption, although these studies are not consistent.[12,25,57]

REFERENCES

1. **Southgate, D. A. T. and Durnin, J. V. G. A.**, Calorie conversion factors: an experimental re-assessment of the factors used in the calculation of energy value of human diets, *Br. J. Nutr.*, 24, 517, 1970.
2. **Losowsky, M. S.**, Effects of dietary fibre on intestinal absorption, in *Dietary Fibre: Current Development of Importance to Health*, Heaton, K. W., Ed., John Libbey, London, 1978, 129.
3. **Cummings, J. H., Southgate, D. A. T., Branch, W., Wiggens, H. S., Houston, H., Jenkins, D. J. A., Jibraj, T., and Hill, M. W.**, The digestion of dietary pectin in the human gut, and its effect on calcium absorption and large bowel function, *Br. J. Nutr.*, 41, 477, 1979.
4. **Prynne, C. J. and Southgate, D. A. T.**, The effects of a supplement of dietary fibre on fecal excretion by human subjects, *Br. J. Nutr.*, 41, 495, 1979.
5. **Slavin, J. L. and Marlett, J. A.**, Effect of refined cellulose on apparent energy, fat, and nitrogen digestibilities, *J. Nutr.*, 100, 2020, 1980.
6. **Southgate, D. A. T.**, *Dietary Fiber in Health and Disease*, Vahouny, G. V. and Kritchevsky, D., Eds., Plenum Press, New York, 1982, 45.

7. **Southgate, D. A. T., Branch, W. J., Hill, M. J., Draser, B. S., Walter, R. L., Davies, P. S., and McLean Baird, I.,** Metabolic responses to dietary supplements of bran, *Metabolism,* 25, 1129, 1976.
8. **Vahouny, G. V.,** Dietary fibers and the intestinal absorption of lipids, in *Dietary Fiber in Health and Disease,* Vahouny, G. V. and Kritchevsky, D., Eds., Plenum Press, New York, 1982, 203.
9. **Stasse-Wolthuis, J. G., Hautvast, R. J., Hermus, M. B., Katan, J. E., Bausch, J. G., Rietberg-Brussar, J. H., Velema, J. P., Zondervan, J. H., Eastwood, M. A., and Brydon, W. G.,** The effect of a natural high-fiber diet on serum lipids, fecal lipids and colonic function, *Am. J. Clin. Nutr.,* 32, 1881, 1979.
10. **Raymond, T. L., Connor, W. E., Lin, D. S., Warner, S., Fry, M. M., and Connor, S. L.,** The interaction of dietary fibers and cholesterol upon the plasma lipids and lipoproteins, sterol balance and bowel function in human subjects, *J. Clin. Invest.,* 60, 1429, 1977.
11. **Kretsch, M. J., Crawford, L. K., and Calloway, D. H.,** Some aspects of bile acid and urobilinogen excretion and fecal elimination in men given a rural Guatemalan diet and egg formulas with and without added oat bran, *Am. J. Clin. Nutr.,* 32, 1492, 1979.
12. **Kesaneimi, Y. A., Tarpila, S., and Miettinen, T. A.,** Low vs. high dietary fiber and serum, biliary, and fecal lipids in middle-aged men, *Am. J. Clin. Nutr.,* 51, 1007, 1990.
13. **Mathur, K. S., Khan, M. A., and Sharma, R. D.,** Hypocholesterolemic effect of bengal gram: a long-term study in man, *Br. Med. J.,* 1, 30, 1968.
14. **Stanley, M. M., Paul, S., Gacke, D., and Murphy, J.,** Effect of cholestyramine, metamucil and cellulose on fecal bile acid excretion in man, *Gastroenterology,* 565, 889, 1973.
15. **Shurpalekar, K. S., Doraiswany, T. R., Sundaravalli, O. E., and Reo, M. N.,** Effect of inclusion of cellulose in an "atherogenic" diet on the blood lipids of children, *Nature (London),* 232, 554, 1971.
16. **Tsai, A. C., Mott, E. L., Owen, G. M., Bennick, M. R., Lo, G. S., and Steinke, F. H.,** Effects of soy polysaccharide on gastrointestinal functions, nutrient balance, steroid excretion, glucose tolerance, serum lipids, and other parameters in humans, *Am. J. Clin. Nutr.,* 38, 504, 1983.
17. **Eastwood, M. A., Kirkpatrick, J. R., Mitchell, W. D., Bone, A., and Hamilton, T.,** Effects of dietary supplements of wheat bran on feces and bowel function, *Br. Med. J.,* 4, 392, 1973.
18. **Van Berge Henegouwen, G. P., Huibregts, A. W., Hectors, M., Schaik van, A., and Werf de van, S.,** Bran feeding and vegetarian diet do not alter biliary lipids and bile acid kinetics in young males, *Gut,* 20, A930, 1979.
19. **Jenkins, D. J. A., Hill, M. J., and Cummings, J. H.,** Effect of wheat fiber on blood lipids, fecal steroid excretion and serum iron, *Am. J. Clin. Nutr.,* 28, 1408, 1975.
20. **Walters, R. L., McLean-Baird, Davies, P. S., Hill, M. J. K., Drasar, B. S., Southgate, D. A. T., and Morgan, R.,** Effects of two types of dietary fibre on fecal steroid and lipid excretion, *Br. Med. J.,* 2, 536, 1975.
21. **Kay, R. M. and Truswell, A. S.,** Effect of wheat fibre on gastrointestinal function, plasma lipids and steroids excretion in man, *Br. J. Nutr.,* 37, 227, 1977.
22. **Cummings, J. H., Hill, M. J., Jenkins, D. J. A., Pearson, J. R., and Wiggins, H. S.,** Changes in fecal composition and colonic function due to cereal fibre, *Am. J. Clin. Nutr.,* 29, 1468, 1976.
23. **Tarpila, S., Miettinin, T. A., and Metasaranta, L.,** Effects of bran on serum cholesterol, faecal mass, fat, bile acids and neutral steroids and biliary lipids in patients with diverticular disease of colon, *Gut,* 19, 137, 1978.
24. **Spiller, G. A., Story, J. A., Wong, L. G., Nunes, J. D., Alton, M., Petro, M. S., Furumoto, E. J., Whittam, J. H., and Scala, J.,** Effect of increasing levels of hard wheat fiber on fecal weight, minerals and steroids and gastrointestinal transit time in healthy young women, *J. Nutr.,* 116, 778, 1986.
25. **Salvioli, G., Lugli, R., and Pradelli, J. M.,** Cholesterol absorption and sterol balance in normal subjects receiving dietary fiber or urosodeoxycholic acid, *Dig. Dis. Sci.,* 30, 301, 1985.
26. **Forman, D. T., Garvin, J. E., Forestner, J. E., and Taylor, C. B.,** Increased excretion of bile acids by an oral hydrophilic colloid, *Proc. Soc. Exp. Biol. Med.,* 126, 1060, 1968.
27. **Abraham, Z. D. and Mehta, T.,** Three-week psyllium-husk supplementation: effect of plasma cholesterol concentrations, fecal steroid excretion, and carbohydrate absorption in men, *Am. J. Clin. Nutr.,* 47, 67, 1988.
28. **Kay, R. M. and Truswell, A. S.,** Effect of citrus pectin on blood lipids and fecal steroid excretion in man, *Am. J. Clin. Nutr.,* 30, 171, 1977.
29. **Jenkins, D. J. A., Leeds, A. R., Gassull, M. A., Houston, H., Goff, D. V., and Hill, M. J.,** The cholesterol-lowering properties of guar and pectin, *Clin. Sci. Mol. Med.,* 51, 8, 1976.
30. **Miettinen, T. A. and Tarpila, S.,** Effects of pectin on serum cholesterol, fecal bile acids and biliary lipids in normolipidemic and hyperlipidemic individuals, *Clin. Chim. Acta,* 79, 471, 1977.
31. **Kirby, R. W., Anderson, J. W., Sieling, B., Rees, E. D., Chen, W. J. L., Miller, R. E., and Kay, R. M.,** Oat bran intake selectively lowers serum low density lipoprotein concentrations: studies of hypercholesterolemic men, *Am. J. Clin. Nutr.,* 34, 824, 1981.

32. **Kay, R. M.**, Dietary fiber, *J. Lipid Res.*, 23, 221, 1982.
33. **Portman, O. W. and Murphy, O.**, Excretion of bile acids and β-hydroxy sterols by rats, *Arch. Biochem. Biophys.*, 76, 367, 1958.
34. **Kritchevsky, D., Tepper, S. A., and Story, J. A.**, Isocaloric, isogravic diets in rats. III. Effects of nonnutritive fiber (alfalfa or cellulose) on cholesterol metabolism, *Nutr. Rep. Int.*, 9, 301, 1974.
35. **Lin, T. M., Kim, K. S., Karvinen, E., and Ivy, A. C.**, Effect of dietary pectin, "protopectin" and gum arabic on cholesterol excretion in rats, *Am. J. Physiol.*, 188, 66, 1957.
36. **Leveille, G. A. and Sauberlich, H. E.**, Mechanism of the cholesterol-depressing effect of pectin in the cholesterol fed rat, *J. Nutr.*, 88, 209, 1966.
37. **Hyun, S. A., Vahouny, G. V., and Treadwell, C. R.**, Effect of hypocholesterolemic agents on intestinal cholesterol absorption, *Proc. Soc. Exp. Biol. Med.*, 112, 496, 1963.
38. **Kelly, J. J. and Tsai, A. C.**, Effect of pectin, gum arabic and agar on cholesterol absorption, synthesis and turnover in rats, *J. Nutr.*, 108, 630, 1978.
39. **Balmer, J. and Zilversmit, D. B.**, Effects of dietary roughage on cholesterol absorption, *J. Nutr.*, 104, 1319, 1974.
40. **Eastwood, M. and Mowbray, L.**, The binding of components of mixed micelles to dietary fiber, *Am. J. Clin. Nutr.*, 29, 1461, 1976.
41. **Lairon, D., Lafont, H., Vigne, J. L., Nalbone, G., Leonardi, J., and Hauton, J. C.**, Effects of dietary fibers and cholestyramine on the activity of pancreatic lipase in vitro, *Am. J. Clin. Nutr.*, 42, 629, 1985.
42. **Borel, P., Lairon, D. M., Senft, M., Chauban, M., and Lafont, H.**, Wheat bran and wheat germ: effect on digestion and intestinal absorption of dietary lipids in the rat, *Am. J. Clin. Nutr.*, 49, 1192, 1989.
43. **Elsenhans, B., Sufke, U., Blume, R., and Caspary, W. F.**, The influence of carbohydrate gelling agents on rat intestinal transport of monosaccharides and neutral amino acids in vitro, *Clin. Sci.*, 59, 373, 1980.
44. **Johnson, I. T., and Gee, J. M.**, Effect of gel-forming gums on the intestinal unstirred layer and sugar transport in vitro, *Gut*, 22, 398, 1981.
45. **Gerencser, G. A., Cerda, J., Burgin, C., Barg, M. M., and Guild, R.**, Unstirred water layers in rabbit intestine: effects of pectin, *Proc. Soc. Exp. Biol. Med.*, 176, 183, 1984.
46. **Gee, J. M., Blackburn, N. A., and Johnson, I. T.**, The influence of guar gum on intestinal cholesterol transport in the rat, *Br. J. Nutr.*, 50, 215, 1983.
47. **Imaizumi, K., Tominaga, A., Maivatari, K., and Sugano, M.**, Effect of cellulose and guar gum on the secretion of mesenteric lymph chylomicrons in meal-fed rats, *Nutr. Rep. Int.*, 26, 263, 1982.
48. **Cassidy, M. M., Lightfoot, F. G., and Vahouny, G. V.**, Morphological aspects of dietary fiber in the intestine, *Adv. Lipid Res.*, 19, 203, 1982.
49. **Leeds, A. R.**, Modification of intestinal absorption by dietary fiber and components, in *Dietary Fiber in Health and Disease*, Vahouny, G. V. and Kritchevsky, D., Eds., Plenum Press, New York, 1982, 53.
50. **Satchithanandam, S., Jahangeer, S., Cassidy, M. M., Floor, M. K., Calvert, R. J., Leeds, A. R., and Alabaster, O.**, Quantitative effects of wheat bran feeding on rat small intestinal mucin, *FASEB J.*, 3, A1066, 1989.
51. **Satchithandam, S., Vargyofcak-Apker, M., Calvert, R. J., Leeds, A. R., and Cassidy, M. M.**, Alteration of gastrointestinal mucin by fiber feeding in rats, *J. Nutr.*, 120, 1179, 1990.
52. **Vahouny, G. V., Roy, T., Gallo, L. L., Story, J. A., Kritchevsky, D., and Cassidy, M. M.**, Dietary Fibers. III. Effects of chronic intake on cholesterol absorption and metabolism in the rat, *Am. J. Clin. Nutr.*, 33, 2182, 1980.
53. **Ebihara, K. and Schneeman, B. O.**, Interaction of bile acids, phospholipids, cholesterol and triglyceride with dietary fibers in the small intestine of rats, *J. Nutr.*, 119, 1100, 1989.
54. **Ikeda, I., Tomari, Y., and Sugano, M.**, Interrelated effect of dietary fiber and fat on lymphatic cholesterol and triglyceride absorption in rats, *J. Nutr.*, 199, 1383, 1989.
55. **Vahouny, G. V., Satchithanandam, S., Cassidy, M. M., Lightfoot, F. G., and Furda, I.**, Comparative effects of chitosan and cholestyramine on lymphatic absorption of lipids in rat, *Am. J. Clin. Nutr.*, 38, 278, 1983.
56. **Vahouny, G. V., Satchithanandam, S., Chen, I., Tepper, S. A., Kritchevsky, D., Lightfoot, F. G., and Cassidy, M. M.**, Dietary fiber and intestinal adaptation: effects on lipid absorption and lymphatic transport in the rat, *Am. J. Clin. Nutr.*, 47, 201, 1988.
57. **Samuel, P., McNamara, D. J., Ahrens, E. H., Crouse, J. R., and Parker, T.**, Further validation of the plasma isotope ratio method for measurement of cholesterol absorption in man, *J. Lipid Res.*, 23, 480, 1982.
58. **Schwartz, S. E., Starr, C., Bachman, S., and Holtzapple, P. G.**, Dietary fiber decreases cholesterol and phospholipid synthesis in rat intestine, *J. Lipid Res.*, 24, 746, 1983.

Chapter 4.3

INFLUENCE OF DIETARY FIBER ON CHOLESTEROL METABOLISM IN EXPERIMENTAL ANIMALS

David Kritchevsky and Jon A. Story

INTRODUCTION

What may be referred to as the modern "fiber era" has precipitated a number of lay and professional suggestions concerning the amount and type of fiber which will yield results beneficial to health. Many of the suggestions have related to effects on plasma or serum cholesterol levels and most of these have, in turn, been based on data derived from animal experiments. Several suggested mechanism(s) by which fiber may affect cholesterol levels involve aspects of bile acid metabolism, including inhibition of absorption of cholesterol due to binding of bile acids or increased cholesterol turnover because of fiber-enhanced excretion of bile acids. The following chapter will be devoted mainly to tabulation of effects of dietary fiber on plasma or serum and liver cholesterol levels.

INFLUENCE OF DIETARY FIBER ON BLOOD AND LIVER LIPIDS

Table 1 is devoted to a summary of experimental results obtained in rats. This species has been studied more widely than any other. Because of the rat's ability to regulate its own cholesterol level, many of the studies have entailed addition of cholesterol to the diet; in some instances, the sterol has been fed together with bile acids or bile salts. Table 1 is a selection of papers which illustrate the different effects of various types of fiber. The data summarized in Table 1 show clearly that different types of fiber exert different effects. Pectin and other gelling fibers such as guar gum or mannan can reduce serum cholesterol levels in rats regardless of whether the diet contains cholesterol or not. Cellulose, gum arabic, and agar are not hypocholesterolemic. The effects on liver cholesterol levels are more marked than those seen in serum or plasma, but here too not all fibers act similarly. The effect of fiber can be mediated by the type of carbohydrate present in the diet[7] or the amount and type of fat.[9,10] It is also interesting to note that dietary fiber is a more effective hypolipidemic agent in germ-free rats than in conventional rats.[20,21]

Table 2 presents a summary of the effects of fiber in rabbits. Cellulose and cellophane offer little protection against cholesterolemia. The type of fat[23] and protein[27] present in the diet modulates the effects of fiber. These findings underscore the observation that all facets of the diet influence lipidemia and atherosclerosis.[28]

Data available from experiments in which fiber was fed to chickens are presented in Table 3. The experiments in which fiber was used in monkey diets are described in Table 4 and those in which pigs were the test animal are summarized in Table 5. Twelve baboons (*Papio ursinus*) were fed a "Western diet" or the same diet augmented with 5% Konjac mannan for 9 weeks. In animals fed Konjac mannan, serum cholesterol was decreased by 17%, percentage of HDL-cholesterol was increased by 10%, and liver cholesterol was decreased by 31%.[68] The data in Table 5 suggest that the level of dietary fat may enhance action[38] and hints at the possibility of a male-female difference.[40] Two experiments carried out in guinea pigs are described in Table 6. Wells and Ershoff[1] also fed hamsters a semi-purified diet containing 1% cholesterol or the same diet with 5% fiber. After 6 weeks, animals fed pectin exhibited 7% lower plasma cholesterol and 8% higher liver cholesterol.

TABLE 1
Effect of Dietary Fiber on Blood and Liver Cholesterol in Rats

Fiber Source	%	Rat* strain	Duration (weeks)	Comparison diet	Dietary cholesterol	ΔCholesterol (%) Plasma or serum	Liver	Ref.
Pectin	5	H	6	SF	1%	−29	−30	1
Pectin	5	H	4	SF	1%	−12	−65	2
Pectin	10					−9	−75	
Guar gum	10					−12	−62	
Locust bean gum	10					−2	−53	
Carrageenan	10					−16	−66	
Pectin	5	H	4	SF	1%	−9	−27	3
Pectin	5	CFE	4	SF	1%	0	−32	4
Pectin	10					−10	−41	
Guar gum	5					−8	−35	
Guar gum	10					−21	−71	
Pectin	5	CFE	4	L	1%	+4	−20	4
Pectin	10					−6	−26	
Guar gum	5					−3	−46	
Guar gum	10					−16	−20	
Citrus pectin	5	N	4	SF	1%	−13	−26	5
Tomato pectin	5					−17	−53	
Carboxymethyl cellulose	5	W	2	SF	1%[a]	−9	−25	6
Pectin	5					−19	−34	
Alginic acid	5					−1	+21	
Cellulose	5					+12	+44	
Cellulose	14[b]	W		L	0	+9	−7	7
Alfalfa	30[b]					0	+7	
Cellulose	14[c]					+21	−30	
Alfalfa	30[c]					+23	−37	
Lignin	3	SD	3	SC	0.5%	−15	—	8
Pectin	7[d]	SD	6	SF		−21	−64	9
Carrageenan	7[d]					−22	+9	
Agar	7[d]					−8	+105	
Cellulose	7[d]					−1	+32	

Fiber	Level	Animal	n	Diet	Chol	Δ Chol	Δ Athero	Ref
Pectin	7[e]	SD	5	SF	0.5%	+13	−31	9
Carragenan	7[e]					+4	+29	
Gum arabic	7[e]					+16	+65	
Cellulose	7[e]					+13	0	
Wheat bran	7					+9	−14	
Agar	7	SD	5	SF	0	−12	−5	9
Gum arabic	2.5[f]	W	2	SC	0.5%	−8	−21	10
Pectin	2.5[g]					−15	−59	
						−10	−27	
Carob pod	5	SD	9	SF	1%	+2	0	11
	10					−7	−55	
Pectin, citrus	5	W	1	SF	1%[h]	−12	+21	12
Pectic acid	5					−12	+17	
Pectin, orange	5					−43	−39	
Pectin, persimmon	5					−37	−33	
Pectin, radish	5					−39	−22	
Pectin, carrot	5					−28	−11	
Pectin, peach	5					−17	−6	
Pectin	10	SD	3	SC	1%[i]	−37[j]	−74	13
Guar gum	10					−21	−55	
Oat bran	10					−15	−47	
Cellulose	10	Z	12	SF	0.1%	+6	−4	14
Bran	12.5					+2	−19	
Pectin	5	SD	6	SC	0	−32[k]		15
Guar gum	5					−36		
Pectin	5		15			−36[l]		
Guar gum	5					−43		
Pectin	10	SD	3	SC	1%[j]	−27[m]	−46	16
Oat bran	10					−41	−74	
Oat gum	10					−44	−86	
Alfalfa	5	W	4	SF	1%	+32	−3	17
Cellulose	5					+11	+15	
Lignin	5					+6	−19	
Pectin	5	W	4	SF	0.5%	+3	−75	17
Cellulose	5					0	−30	
Lignin	5					−4	−66	
Alginic acid	10[n]	W	3	SF	0	+3	0	18
Cellulose	10					+11	+9	

TABLE 1 (continued)
Effect of Dietary Fiber on Blood and Liver Cholesterol in Rats

Fiber Source	%	Rat* strain	Duration (weeks)	Comparison diet	Dietary cholesterol	ΔCholesterol (%) Plasma or serum	Liver	Ref.
Guar gum	10					+11	−22	
Mannan	10					+4	−25	
Pectin	10					+11	−22	
Cellulose	15[a]	W	3	SF	0	+4	+38	19
Hemicellulose	15					+20	−27	
Pectin	15					+10	−9	
Lignin	15					+4	−19	
Bagasse alkaline extract	1	W	8	SP	0.5°	−11	−6	60
Bagasse (alk ext) (B)	3.0	W	2	SP	0.5°	−35	−29	61
αAmylase hydrolysate(H)						−40	−27	
(H) Long chain	2.7					+15	−7	
(H) Short chain	2.3							
Pectin	3	SD	2	SP	0.5[p]	−7	−32	62
Gum arabic	3					+4	+4	
Wheat bran + Fish oil (12%)	7[a]	W	1.4	WB/RB	0	−37	+6	63
Rice bran + Fish oil (12%)	7					−28	+23	
Oat bran	5[s]	SD	3	SP	1[s]	−10	−19	64
	10					−25	−39	
Cellulose	8	SD	8–10	SP	0	−25	+2	65
Pectin	8					−2	−12	
Oat bran	8[a]					−6	−15	
Wheat bran	8[a]					+30	−18	
Celery	6[a]	SD	3	SP	0	−5		66
Parsnip	6					−7		
Rutabaga	6					−1		
Wheat bran	6					+11		
Oat bran	6					+1		
Cellulose	6	W	3	SP	0.5	+15[u]	+11	67
Oat bran	6[a]					+12	−12	
Barley	4					−3	−39	
Barley	6					−8	−48	

Note: The single asterisk indicates the rat strain: H, Holtzman; CFE, Carworth Farms; N, not given; W, Wistar; SD, Sprague-Dawley; Z, Zucker. The double asterisk indicates the comparison diet: SC, semipurified containing cellulose: SF, semipurified fiber free; L, laboratory ration.

a Plus 0.25% bile salts.
b Dextrose.
c Sucrose.
d 10% soybean oil.
e 15% soybean oil.
f 5% Fat (2% corn oil; 3% tallow).
g 20% Fat (2% corn oil, 18% tallow).
h Plus 0.3% cholic acid.
i Plus 0.2% cholic acid.
j HDL-cholesterol/total cholesterol: pectin +122%; guar gum +114%; oat bran +62%.
k HDL-cholesterol/total cholesterol: pectin −14%; guar gum +7%.
l HDL-cholesterol/total cholesterol: pectin +4%; guar gum −0.2%.
m HDL-cholesterol/total cholesterol: oat bran +112%; oat gum +197%; pectin +19%.
n Meal-fed.
o 0.15% Na cholate.
p 0.25% Na cholate.
q Effective fiber content.
r Effective fiber 5 or 10%. Publication describes effects of 0–10% fiber in 1% increments.
s 0.1% cholic acid.
t % HDL-cholesterol: celery +4%; parsnip +7%; rutabaga −5%; wheat bran −1%; oat bran −3%.
u % HDL-cholesterol: cellulose −17%; oat bran +1%; barley (≡4% fiber) −5%; barley (≡6% fiber) +29%.

TABLE 2
Effect of Dietary Fiber on Blood and Liver Cholesterol in Rabbits

Fiber Source	%	Duration (weeks)	Comparison diet	Dietary cholesterol	Cholesterol (%) Plasma or serum	Liver	Ref.
Pectin	15	6	SC	1%	+15	−12	1
Alfalfa	90	10	M	0.6%	−97		22
Wheat straw	19[a]	40	SC	0	−14[b]		23
Cellophane	19				+62		
Cellophane: peat	14.5				+6		
Wheat straw	19[c]	40	SC	0	−62[d]		23
Cellophane	19				+16		
Pectin	5	2	L	1%	−33[e]		24
Cellulose	15	24	L	0	+131[f]	+56	25
Alfalfa	36.3	4	SF	0	−70		26
Wheat	62.1				−33		
Oats	62.5				−38		
Oat groats	59.9				−20		
Wheat straw	42.8				−3		
Oat hulls	59.3				−28		
Sawdust	16				−8		
Cellulose	4				+78		
Cellulose	20				+40		
Wheat straw	15[g]	40	SC	0	−17[h]	−4	27
Alfalfa	15[g]				−52	−10	
Wheat straw	15[i]	40	SC	0	+2[j]	−9	27
Alfalfa	15[i]				−36	−17	

Note: SC, Semipurified diet containing cellulose; M, calf meal; L, laboratory ration; SF, semipurified fiber-free diet.

[a] 20% Butter oil.
[b] Compared to cellulose, average atherosclerosis:wheat straw −39%; cellophane +80%; cellophane-peat 14:5 −49%.
[c] Corn oil.
[d] Compared to cellulose:wheat straw −46%; cellophane +285%.
[e] HDL-cholesterol/total cholesterol: −41%.
[f] Atherosclerosis in test group, none in group fed commercial ration.
[g] Contained casein.
[h] Average atherosclerosis:wheat straw −31%; alfalfa −58%.
[i] Contained soy protein.
[j] Average atherosclerosis:wheat straw −27%; alfalfa −42%.

Hamsters were fed a very low fat (0.2 to 1.2%) diet including 10% brewer's spent grain or 10% crushed barley for 6 weeks. Serum cholesterol rose by 6% in hamsters fed the spent grain and was reduced by 6% in hamsters fed barley.

DIETARY FIBER-BILE SALT INTERACTIONS

Interactions between bile salts and dietary fiber have been suggested as a possible mechanism for the observed effects of dietary fiber on serum cholesterol. Eastwood and Boyd[42] found that a significant portion of bile salts is associated with the insoluble contents of the intestine. This led to the further observation of Eastwood and Hamilton[43] that dry grain preparations (high in unavailable carbohydrate) absorbed bile salts *in vitro*. A series of experiments were designed to quantitate the level of adsorption for various food sources

TABLE 3
Effect of Dietary Fiber on Blood and Liver Cholesterol in Chickens

Fiber Source	%	Duration (weeks)	Comparison diet	Dietary cholesterol	Cholesterol (%) Plasma or serum	Liver	Ref.
Guar gum	0.5	4	SF	3%	−18		29
Guar gum	2				−18		
Guar gum	3				−27		
Pectin	3				+6		
Carrageenan	3				−42		
Pectin	3	24	SC	0.65%	−23[a]	−16	30
Pectin	3	3	G	0.65%	−24		31
Oat hulls	15				−30	−47	
Cellulose	15	29	M	0	+8		32
Cellulose	15			1%	−12		
Sunflower meal	4.41[b]	20	SF	0	+4	+6	33
	6.68				+17	+21	
	8.79				+13	+34	
Cellulose	4	2	SF	0	−1	−43	34
Rice hull	15				+11	−15	
Rice hull NDF	15				+7	−32	
Alfalfa meal	15				+3	−27	
Peanut meal NDF	15				+18	+10	

Note: SF, Semipurified fiber-free diet; SC, semipurified diet containing cellulose; G, grains; M, mash.

[a] Atherosclerosis, −20%.
[b] Comparison diet contained 2.05% fiber.

TABLE 4
Effect of Dietary Fiber on Blood and Liver Cholesterol in Monkeys

Fiber Source	%	Duration (weeks)	Comparison diet	Dietary cholesterol	Cholesterol (%) Plasma or serum	Liver	Ref.
Alfalfa Pellets	51	72	a	0.1%	−41 −54		35[b]
Wheat bran	48.6	36	SF	0.07%	+46		36[b]
Rice bran	50.0			0.09%	+159		
Soy bean	46.4			0.07%	+26		
Alfalfa	15	23	SF	0	−12[a,c]	−12	37[d]
Wheat straw	15				−4	−15	

[a] Monkeys placed on low cholesterol diets following hypercholesterolemic regimen.
[b] Cynomolgus monkeys (*Macaca fasicularis*).
[c] HDL-cholesterol/total cholesterol:alfalfa +29%; wheat straw +23%.
[d] Vervet monkeys (*Cercopithecus aethiops*).

of dietary fiber (Table 7). These data suggest that most food sources of dietary fiber adsorb bile acids but that there is considerable variation among various foods. No food fibers were as effective as bile acid sequestrants (e.g., cholestyramine), but the similarity of properties led to the hypothesis that bile acid adsorption resulted in increased steroid excretion and negative steroid balance.[46]

Differences in the bile salt or bile acid employed, pH, and incubation conditions affected the amount of adsorption. In addition, the question of bile acids absorbed with solvent held

TABLE 5
Effect of Dietary Fiber on Blood and Liver Cholesterol in Pigs

| Fiber | | Duration | Comparison | Dietary | Cholesterol (%) | | Ref. |
Source	%	(weeks)	diet	cholesterol	Plasma or serum	Liver	
All bran	36.4[a]	2	M	1%	+27		38
All bran	36.4[b]				+60		
All bran	36.4[c]				+93		
Cellulose	12.8				+153		
All bran	36.4[a]	2	M	1%	+5		38
Wheat Chex	66.1[a]				+5		
Pectin	5	12	L	—	+18		39
Wheat middlings	10	1	M	—	−20		40[d]
Wheat middlings	20				−6		
Wheat middlings	30				−5		
Wheat middlings	10	1	M	—	−2		40[e]
Wheat middlings	20				−2		
Wheat middlings	30				+2		

Note: M, Mash; L, laboratory ration.

[a] 10% Fat.
[b] 20% Fat.
[c] 30% Fat.
[d] Boars.
[e] Sows.

TABLE 6
Effect of Dietary Fiber on Blood and Liver Cholesterol in Guinea Pigs

| Fiber | | Duration | Comparison | Dietary | Cholesterol (%) | | Ref. |
Source	%	(weeks)	diet	cholesterol	Plasma or serum	Liver	
Pectin	5	4	SCA	1%	−18	−6	1
Cellulose	15	3	SF	0	+10	+12	41
Hydrolyzed cellulose	15				+61	+19	
Alfalfa	15				+30	−2	

Note: SCA, semipurified diet containing cellulose (10%) and agar (5%).

by the dietary fiber was not adequately answered by the early experiments. Eastwood et al.[47] devised a method which, after an initial incubation, employed several washings with buffer to remove unbound bile acids or salts and leave only those which were more tightly adsorbed (Table 8). His results indicated that levels of bile acid binding measured by other techniques include both adsorption of the bile acids or salts to the dietary fiber and absorption of solvent with dissolved bile acids or salts. The possible physiological significance of these two "pools" has not been determined.

Using this method, Story et al.[48] attempted to better understand the nature of the plant component responsible for the adsorption of bile acids by wheat brain and alfalfa. These two dietary fiber sources were subjected to a sequential extraction of various components and the adsorption of cholic and deoxycholic acids was measured at each step (Table 9). Removal of lignin reduced adsorption dramatically in all cases, but a significant level of adsorption still remained, associated with the holocellulose (cellulose and hemicellulose). Since the cellulose has not been shown to adsorb bile salts, hemicellulose may be responsible

TABLE 7
Bile Acid Adsorption to Dietary Fiber Sources

Binding substance	Bile acid or salt (% adsorbed)			
	Taurocholate	Glycocholate	Cholate	Deoxycholate
Experiment 1[a]				
Alfalfa	16.9 ± 0.7	16.7 ± 1.0	—	—
Cellulose	0.5 ± 0.5	0.4 ± 1.4	—	—
Wheat bran	0.7 ± 0.7	2.4 ± 0.4	—	—
Oat hulls	0.4 ± 0.6	—	—	—
Cholestyramine	81.5 ± 0.2	62.8 ± 0.4	—	—
Experiment 2[b]				
Alfalfa	6.9 ± 1.0	11.5 ± 0.5	19.9 ± 0.7	10.4 ± 1.3
Cellulose	1.0 ± 0.4	1.2 ± 0.6	3.0 ± 0.9	0.2 ± 0.2
Wheat bran	1.4 ± 0.7	3.8 ± 1.0	10.2 ± 0.7	5.4 ± 0.9
Cholestyramine	80.7 ± 0.3	63.1 ± 0.5	60.7 ± 0.7	92.4 ± 0.2

[a] 40 mg of each material were incubated with 5 ml of a 20-m M bile salt solution in 0.15 M NaCl (Reference 44).
[b] 50 mg of each material were incubated with 5 ml of 10-m M bile acid solution in phosphate buffer (pH 7.0) (Reference 45).

TABLE 8
Alteration by Water Holding Capacity of Bile Acid Adsorption by Sources of Dietary Fiber

Fiber source[a]	Wash[b]	Adsorptions[c]			
		Deoxycholic		Glycocholic	
		2.5 mM	5.0 mM	2.5 mM	5.0 mM
		(%)	(%)	(%)	(%)
Carrot	0	79	79	71	75
	I	64	64	56	54
	II	42	42	34	30
Pea	0	72	67	61	54
	I	50	51	42	37
	II	35	44	36	29
Wheat bran	0	51	41	35	32
	I	31	23	19	16
	II	28	20	15	12
Celery	0	62	61	58	37
	I	31	32	25	8
	II	16	14	9	7

[a] Dietary fiber sources were washed with deionized water and freeze-dried.[47]
[b] After initial adsorption (zero wash) the dietary fiber source with adsorbed bile salt was washed for 16 h with a volume of phosphate buffer (pH 8.0) equal to initial volume removed.
[c] 1 g dietary fiber source incubated with 35 ml (pea and wheat bran) or 60 ml (carrot and celery) bile salt solution in phosphate buffer (pH 8.0) for 16 h.

TABLE 9
Adsorption of Cholic and Deoxycholic Acids by Components of Alfalfa and Wheat Bran

Extraction process	Substance removed	Alfalfa[a]		Wheat bran[a]	
		No wash (%)	One wash (%)	No wash (%)	One wash (%)
None	None	38	27	29	19
Petroleum ether-acetone	Fats, hydrocarbons, terpenes, etc.	39	26	35	21
95% ethanol, 50% ethanol	Saponins, glycosides, alkaloids, etc.	44	31	49	31
Hot water	Pectins, starches, gums, mucilages, etc.	39	25	38	23
Sodium chlorite	Lignin	13	9	11	8

[a] Adsorption of deoxycholic (5.0 mM) from phosphate buffer (pH 8.0) (5 ml) using 50 mg of dried material. Wash as described in Table 2.[46]

for this adsorption. The amount of bile salts which could be removed by washing remained fairly constant until lignin was removed. At this point, the structure of the dietary fiber was completely changed and the ability to hold water was lost. This change is probably responsible for the change in bile acid removed by washing. It should also be noted that the removal of lignin and the ensuing structural changes may increase the adsorption capacity of the remaining holocellulose beyond its original level.

A method has recently been developed for measuring adsorption of bile acids by water-soluble components of dietary fiber. This method employs a membrane filter which retains the bile acid-polysaccharide complex (Table 10). Hemicellulose does indeed adsorb bile acids as predicted from earlier fractionation studies. However, pectin and gums also adsorb a significant quantity of bile acid which might not have been predicted from the earlier work. The membrane filter method provides a valuable tool for assessing the adsorption of water-soluble materials, but still does not provide a foolproof assessment of adsorption *in vivo*.

ALTERATION OF FECAL STEROID EXCRETION BY DIETARY FIBER

If the hypothesis concerning the effect of dietary fiber on bile acid excretion and, in turn, on cholesterol balance is valid, one should expect to see an increase in fecal steroid excretion in response to ingestion of sources of dietary fiber which adsorb bile acids *in vitro*. As can be seen in Table 11, dietary fiber alters both the concentration of bile acids in feces and the total daily excretion. The concentration of bile acids excreted is highest in animals fed fiber-free diets, indicating the importance of fiber in diluting intestinal contents. Feeding of wheat bran generally results in lower fecal bile acid concentrations and feeding of pectin or oats in higher concentrations. This correlates to some extent with their interaction with bile acids *in vitro*. Daily fecal excretion of bile acids is generally high when wheat bran is fed, despite the low concentration and an apparent inability of bran to alter cholesterol balance. Water-soluble polysaccharides have been shown to lead to high levels of daily excretion in some experiments.

Recently, several sources of dietary fiber and isolated polysaccharides were fed to rats at appropriate levels (Table 12). Neutral and acidic steroid concentrations in feces were

TABLE 10
Adsorption of Bile Acids by Various Isolated Polysaccharides

Polysaccharide	Adsorption[a]	
	Cholic (%)	Deoxycholic (%)
Cellulose[b]	4.9	1.5
Hemicellulose A[c]	8.1	20.8
Hemicellulose B[c]	9.8	23.8
Pectin[b]	1.4	11.2
Carrageenan[b]	5.8	19.5
Guaran[b]	11.7	31.0
Locust bean bum[b]	13.9	20.0

[a] 50 mg of polysaccharide were incubated with 5 ml of a 5 mM bile acid solution in phosphate buffer (pH 8.0)
[b] Commercial preparation.
[c] Isolated from corn bran.

TABLE 11
Steroid Excretion in Experimental Animals in Response to Various Sources of Dietary Fiber

Fiber source (% in diet)	Neutral steroids		Bile acids		Ref.
	mg/g	mg/day	mg/g	mg/day	
Cellulose (15)	—	—	2.5	22.5	49
Alfalfa (15)	—	—	3.8	15.8	
Oats (whole) (15)	—	—	6.2	8.7	
Low fiber (2.5)	—	—	13.1	16.8	50
Wheat bran (20)	—	—	3.6	5.5	
Cellulose (15)	5.9	20.4[a]	4.9	16.7[a]	51
Wheat bran (15)	3.8	18.6	2.9	14.1	
Pectin (15)	10.1	44.7	9.6	43.7	
Alfalfa (15)	2.8	18.6	4.0	26.7	
Carrageenan (15)	2.9	30.7	5.7	58.4	
Control (0)	—	—	17.5	10.7	52
Wheat bran (21)	—	—	7.7	27.0	
Agar (7.4)	—	—	5.9	18.6	
Carrageenan (7.4)	—	—	3.1	12.8	

[a] Reported as milligram per kilogram body weight per day.

increased by all added dietary fiber sources in comparison to cellulose, as might be predicted from the adsorption data. However, due to the differences in changes in fecal weight, daily excretion did not parallel changes in bile acid concentration. Only Metamucil and the wheat bran-pectin mixture caused increased excretion of bile acids and then by only 10 to 20%. (A summary of changes in fecal steroid excretion in humans in response to dietary fiber has been given elsewhere.)

A second possible effect of dietary fiber on bile acid metabolism could be alteration of the spectrum of bile acids present in bile and feces. Changes in the relative amounts of bile acids, especially increases in chenodeoxycholic acid (CDC) derivatives, can alter bile sat-

TABLE 12
Steroid Excretion in Response to Various Sources of Dietary Fiber

Fiber source/ level in diet	Neutral steroids		Bile acids	
	mg/g	mg/d	mg/g	mg/d
Control/0	239	66	194	55
Cellulose/10%	100[a]	100[a]	100[a]	100[a]
Wheat bran/10%	164	102	108	67
Alfalfa/10%	137	96	125	84
Metamucil/5%	189	121	175	110
Wheat bran-pectin (3–1)/5%	153	113	148	109
Pectin/5%	226	46	150	35
Guar gum/5%	189	107	108	61

[a] Cellulose adjusted to 100 for comparison purposes.

TABLE 13
Changes in Fecal Bile Acid Spectrum in Rats in Response to Dietary Fiber

Fiber source (% in diet)	Primary bile acids (%)	CDC[a] derivatives (%)	Ref.
Cellulose (15)	32	49	49
Alfalfa (15)	42	61	
Oats (whole) (15)	47	60	
Low fiber (2.5)	21	80	50
Wheat bran (20)	27	80	
No fiber	21	60	[b]
Cellulose (10)	30	66	
Alfalfa (10)	30	66	
Wheat bran (10)	28	63	
Wheat bran, pectin (3:1) (5)	29	56	
Pectin (5)	23	59	
Guar gum (5)	24	61	
Metamucil (5)	30	71	
Cellulose (5)	24	68	51
Wheat bran (15)	28	69	
Pectin (15)	15	69	
Alfalfa (15)	28	67	
Carageenan (15)	9	45	

[a] Chenodeoxycholate.
[b] Unpublished data.

uration, cholesterol absorption, and reabsorption of bile acids from the small intestine.[53] In animal studies (Table 13), an increase in CDC derivatives in response to feeding of alfalfa and oats might be in part responsible for changes in bile acid excretion and cholesterol levels observed earlier.[49] Similar changes have not been observed consistently in subsequent studies. Some sources of dietary fiber (alfalfa and oat products) seem to cause a consistent increase in CDC, whereas other sources do not. In general, most sources of dietary fiber cause an increase in primary bile acid excretion, possibly as a result of changes in the environment of the large intestine.

TABLE 14
Modification of Human Fecal Bile Acid Spectrum by Dietary Fiber

Treatment	Fecal bile acids (mg/day)	Percent CDC[a] derivatives	Ref.
16 g wheat bran per day; 3 weeks	−4 −11	−3 −6	54
15 g pectin per day; 3 weeks	+106	−2	55
40–50 g pectin per day; 2 weeks	+196	−3	56
Hard red spring wheat bran; 2 weeks			57
5.7 g/day	+38	−4	
17.1 g/day	+65	+9	
28.5 g/day	+60	+13	
100 g oat bran;			58
10 days	+54	+2	
21 days	+65	−21	
100 g beans			59
21 days	−30	+24	

[a] Chenodeoxycholate.

Changes in the amount of CDC derivatives excreted by humans in response to dietary fiber have also been inconsistent (Table 14). Only hard red spring wheat bran has been shown to cause increased excretion of CDC derivatives in response to increasing levels of fiber in the diet. Interestingly, including 100 g of beans in the diet causes a significant increase in CDC derivatives, but reduces bile acid excretion.

Dietary fiber effects on bile acid metabolism appear at best to comprise only part of the overall mechanism(s) related to fiber influences on serum or plasma and liver cholesterol levels.

REFERENCES

1. **Wells, A. F. and Ershoff, B. H.,** Comparative effects of pectin N.F. administration on the cholesterol-fed rabbit, guinea pig, hamster and rat, *Proc. Soc. Exp. Biol. Med.,* 111, 147, 1962.
2. **Ershoff, B. H. and Wells, A. F.,** Effects of guar gum, locust bean gum and carrageenan on liver cholesterol of cholesterol-fed rats, *Proc. Soc. Exp. Biol. Med.,* 110, 580, 1962.
3. **Leveille, G. A. and Sauberlich, A. E.,** Mechanism of the cholesterol-depressing effect of pectin in the cholesterol-fed rat, *J. Nutr.,* 88, 209, 1966.
4. **Riccardi, B. A. and Fahrenbach, M. J.,** Effect of guar gum and pectin N.F. on serum and liver lipids of cholesterol-fed rats, *Proc. Soc. Exp. Biol. Med.,* 124, 749, 1967.
5. **Anderson, T. A. and Bowman, R. D.,** Comparative cholesterol lowering activity of citrus and tomato pectin, *Proc. Soc. Exp. Biol. Med.,* 130, 665, 1969.
6. **Kiriyama, S., Okazaki, Y., and Yoshida, A.,** Hypocholesterolemic effect of polysaccharides and polysaccharide-rich foodstuffs in cholesterol-fed rats, *J. Nutr.,* 97, 382, 1969.
7. **Kritchevsky, D., Tepper, S. A., and Story, J. A.,** Isocaloric, isogravic diets in rats. III. Effect of non-nutritive fiber (alfalfa or cellulose) on cholesterol metabolism, *Nutr. Rep. Int.,* 9, 301, 1974.

8. **Judd, P. A., Kay, R. M., and Truswell, A. S.,** Cholesterol lowering effect of lignin in rats, *Proc. Nutr. Soc.*, 35, 71A, 1976.
9. **Tsai, A. C., Elias, J., Keeley, J. J., Lin, R-S. C., and Robson, J. R. K.,** Influence of certain dietary fibers on serum and tissue cholesterol levels in rats, *J. Nutr.*, 106, 118, 1976.
10. **Chang, M. L. W. and Johnson, M. A.,** Influence of fat level and type of carbohydrate on the capacity of pectin in lowering serum and liver lipids of young rats, *J. Nutr.*, 106, 1562, 1978.
11. **Wursch, P.,** Influence of tannin-rich carob pod fiber on the cholesterol metabolism in the rat, *J. Nutr.*, 109, 685, 1979.
12. **Ebihara, K., Kiriyama, S., and Manabe, M.,** Cholesterol-lowering activity of various natural pectins and synthetic pectin derivatives with different physico-chemical properties, *Nutr. Rep. Int.*, 20, 519, 1979.
13. **Chen, W. J. L. and Anderson, J. W.,** Effects of plant fiber in decreasing plasma total cholesterol and increasing high density lipoprotein cholesterol, *Proc. Sco. Exp. Biol. Med.*, 162, 310, 1979.
14. **Van Beresteyn, E. C. H., Van Schaik, M., and Mogot, M. F. K.,** Effect of bran and cellulose on lipid metabolism in obese female Zucker rats, *J. Nutr.*, 109, 2085, 1979.
15. **Koo, S. I. and Stanton, P.,** Effects of cellulose, pectin and guar gum on the distribution of serum cholesterol among lipoprotein fraction, *Nutr. Rep. Int.*, 24, 395, 1981.
16. **Chen, W. J. L., Anderson, J., and Gould, M. R.,** Effects of oat bran, oat gum and pectin on lipid metabolism of cholesterol-fed rats, *Nutr. Rep. Int.*, 24, 1093, 1981.
17. **Story, J. A., Baldino, A., Czarnecki, S. K., and Kritchevsky, D.,** Modification of liver cholesterol accumulation by dietary fiber in rats, *Nutr. Rep. Int.*, 24, 1213, 1981.
18. **Kritchevsky, D., Ryder, E., Fishman, A., Kaplan, M., and DeHoff, J. L.,** Influence of dietary fiber on food intake, feed efficiency and lipids in rats, *Nutr. Rep. Int.*, 25, 783, 1982.
19. **Mueller, M. A., Cleary, M. P., and Kritchevsky, D.,** Influence of dietary fiber on lipid metabolism in meal fed rats, *J. Nutr.*, 113, 2229, 1983.
20. **Sacquet, E., Leprince, C., and Riottot, M.,** Dietary fiber and cholesterol and bile acid metabolism in anexic (germfree) and halonexic (conventional) rats. I. Effect of wheat bran, *Reprod. Nutr. Dev.*, 22, 291, 1982.
21. **Sacquet, E., Leprince, C., and Riottot, M.,** Dietary fiber and cholesterol and bile acid metabolisms in anexic (germfree) and halonexic (conventional) rats. II. Effect of pectin, *Reprod. Nutr. Dev.*, 22, 575, 1982.
22. **Cookson, F. B., Altschul, R., and Federoff, S.,** The effects of alfalfa on serum cholesterol and in modifying or preventing cholesterol-induced atherosclerosis in rabbits, *J. Atheroscler. Res.*, 7, 69, 1967.
23. **Moore, J. H.,** The effect of the type of roughage in the diet on plasma cholesterol levels and aortic atherosis in rabbits, *Br. J. Nutr.*, 21, 207, 1967.
24. **Berenson, L. M., Bhandaru, R. R., Radhakrishnamurty, B., Srinivasan, S. R., and Berenson, G. S.,** The effect of dietary pectin on serum lipoprotein cholesterol in rabbits, *Life Sci.*, 16, 1533, 1975.
25. **Kritchevsky, D., Tepper, S. A., Kim, H. K., Moses, D. E., and Story, J. A.,** Experimental atherosclerosis in rabbits fed cholesterol-free diets. IV. Investigations into the source of cholesterolemia, *Exp. Mol. Pathol.*, 22, 11, 1975.
26. **Hamilton, R. M. G. and Carroll, K. K.,** Plasma cholesterol levels in rabbits fed low fat, low cholesterol diets: effects of dietary proteins, carbohydrates and fiber from different sources, *Atherosclerosis*, 24, 47, 1976.
27. **Kritchevsky, D., Tepper, S. A., Williams, D. E., and Story, J. A.,** Experimental atherosclerosis in rabbits fed cholesterol-free diets. VII. Interaction of animal and vegetable protein with fiber, *Atherosclerosis*, 26, 397, 1977.
28. **Kritchevsky, D.,** Diet and atherosclerosis, *Am. J. Pathol.*, 84, 615, 1976.
29. **Fahrenbach, M. J., Riccardi, B. A., and Grant, W. C.,** Hypocholesterolemic activity of mucilaginous polysaccharides in white leghorn cockerels, *Proc. Soc. Exp. Biol. Med.*, 123, 321, 1966.
30. **Fisher, H., Soller, W. G., and Griminger, P.,** The retardation by pectin of cholesterol-induced atherosclerosis in the fowl, *J. Atheroscler. Res.*, 6, 292, 1966.
31. **Fisher, H. and Griminger, P.,** Cholesterol-lowering effects of certain grains and of oat fraction in the chick, *Proc. Soc. Exp. Biol. Med.*, 126, 108, 1967.
32. **Menge, H., Littlefield, L. H., Frobish, L. T., and Weinland, B. T.,** Effect of cellulose and cholesterol on blood and yolk lipids and reproductive efficiency of the hen, *J. Nutr.*, 104, 1554, 1974.
33. **McNaughton, J. L.,** Effect of dietary fiber on egg yolk, liver and plasma cholesterol concentrations of the laying hen, *J. Nutr.*, 10, 1842, 1978.
34. **Okita, Y. and Matsumato, T.,** Effects of several types of dietary fibers on lipid content in liver and plasma nutrient retentions and plasma transaminase activities in force-fed growing chicks, *J. Nutr.*, 110, 1112, 1980.
35. **Malinow, M. R.,** Hypotholesterolemic effect of alfalfa meal in monkeys is not due to thyroid stimulation, *Proc. Soc. Exp. Biol. Med.*, 169, 110, 1982.

36. **Malinow, M. R., McLaughlin, P., Papworth, L., Naito, H. K., and Lewis, L. A.,** Effect of bran and cholestyramine on plasma lipids in monkeys, *Am. J. Clin. Nutr.,* 29, 905, 1976.
37. **Kritchevsky, D., Davidson, L. M., Krendel, D. A., Van der Watt, J. J., Russell, D., Friedland, S., and Mendelsohn, D.,** Influence of dietary fiber on aortic sudanophilia in vervet monkeys, *Ann. Nutr. Metab.,* 25, 125, 1981.
38. **Kim, D. N., Lee, K. T., Reiner, J. M., and Thomas, W. A.,** Lack of beneficial effects of wheat bran cereals in cholesterol balance in swine, *Exp. Mol. Pathol.,* 35, 301, 1981.
39. **Fausch, H. D. and Anderson, T. A.,** Influence of citrus pectin feeding on lipid metabolism and body composition of swine, *J. Nutr.,* 85, 145, 1965.
40. **Collings, G. F., Erickson, J. P., Yokayama, M. T., and Miller, E. R.,** Effect of wheat middlings on fiber digestibility, serum cholesterol and glucose and fecal bile acids in pigs, *J. Anim. Sci.,* 19, 528, 1979.
41. **Fahey, G. C., Jr., Miller, B. L., and Hadfield, H. W.,** Metabolic parameters affected by feeding various types of fiber to guinea pigs, *J. Nutr.,* 109, 77, 1979.
42. **Eastwood, M. A. and Boyd, G. S.,** The distribution of bile salts along the small intestine of rats, *Biochim. Biophys. Acta,* 137, 393, 1967.
43. **Eastwood, M. A. and Hamilton, D.,** Studies on the adsorption of bile salts to nonabsorbed components of diet, *Biochim. Biophys. Acta,* 152, 165, 1968.
44. **Kritchevsky, D. and Story, J. A.,** Binding of bile salts *in vitro* by non-nutritive fiber, *J. Nutr.,* 104, 458, 1974.
45. **Story, J. A. and Kritchevsky, D.,** Comparison of the binding of various bile acids and bile salts *in vitro* by several types of fiber, *J. Nutr.,* 106, 1292, 1976.
46. **Story, J. A. and Kritchevsky, D.,** Dietary fiber and lipid metabolism, in *Fiber in Human Nutrition,* Spiller, G. A. and Amen, R. J., Eds., Plenum Press, New York, 1976, 171.
47. **Eastwood, M. A., Anderson, R., Mitchell, W. D., Robertson, J., and Pocock, S.,** A method to measure the adsorption of bile salts to vegetable fiber of differing water holding capacity, *J. Nutr.,* 106, 1429, 1976.
48. **Story, J. A., White, A., and West, L. G.,** Adsorption of bile acids by components of alfalfa and wheat bran *in vitro, J. Food Sci.,* 47, 1276, 1982.
49. **Kelley, M. J., Thomas, J. N., and Story, J. A.,** Modification of spectrum of fecal bile acids in rats by dietary fiber, *Fed. Proc. Fed. Am. Soc. Exp. Biol.,* 40, 845, 1981.
50. **Brydon, W. G., Tadesse, K., Eastwood, M. A., and Lawson, M. E.,** The effect of dietary fibre on bile acid metabolism in rats, *Br. J. Nutr.,* 43, 101, 1980.
51. **Reddy, B. S., Watanabe, K., and Sheinfil, A.,** Effect of dietary wheat bran, alfalfa, pectin and carrageenan on plasma cholesterol and fecal bile acid and neutral sterol excretion in rats, *J. Nutr.,* 110, 1247, 1980.
52. **Glauert, H. P. and Bennink, M. R.,** Influence of diet and intrarectal bile acid injections on colon epithelial cell proliferation in rats previously injected with 1,2-dimethylhydrazine, *J. Nutr.,* 113, 475, 1983.
53. **Story, J. A. and Thomas, J. N.,** Modification of bile acid spectrum by dietary fiber, in *Dietary Fiber in Health and Disease,* Vahouny, G. V. and Kritchevsky, D., Eds., Plenum Press, New York, 1982, 192.
54. **Eastwood, M. A., Kirkpatrick, J. R., Mitchell, W. D., Bone, A., and Hamilton, T.,** Effects of dietary supplements of wheat bran and cellulose on faeces and bowel function, *Br. Med. J.,* 4, 392, 1973.
55. **Kay, R. M. and Truswell, A. S.,** Effect of citrus pectin on blood lipids and fecal steroid excretion in man, *Am. J. Clin. Nutr.,* 30, 171, 1977.
56. **Miettinen, T. A. and Tarpila, S.,** Effect of pectin on serum cholesterol, fecal bile acids and biliary lipids in normolipidemic and hyperlipidemic individuals, *Clin. Chim. Acta,* 79, 471, 1977.
57. **Spiller, G. A., Wong, L. G., Nunes, J. D., Story, J. A., Petro, M. S., Furumoto, E. J., Alton-Spiller, M., Whittam, J. H., and Scala, J.,** Effect of four levels of hard wheat bran on fecal composition and transit time in healthy young women, *Fed. Proc. Fed. Am. Soc. Exp. Biol.,* 43, 392, 1984.
58. **Kirby, R. W., Anderson, J. W., Sieling, B., Rees, E. D., Chen, W-J. L., Miller, R. E., and Kay, R. M.,** Oat bran intake selectively lowers serum low density lipoprotein cholesterol concentrations of hypercholesterolemic men, *Am. J. Clin. Nutr.,* 34, 824, 1981.
59. **Anderson, J. W., Story, L., Sieling, B., Chen, W-J. L., Petro, M. S., and Story, J. A.,** Hypocholesterolemic effects of oat bran and bean intake for hypercholesterolemic mean, *Am. J. Clin. Nutr.,* 40, 1156, 1984.
60. **Fukuda, N., Machida, M., Oku, H., and Chinen, I.,** Hypocholesterolemic activity of bagasse alkaline extract in rats fed a high cholesterol diet, *Agric. Biol. Chem.,* 53, 3097, 1989.
61. **Oku, H., Kayano, K., Miyagi, M., and Chinen, I.,** Hypocholesterolemic activity of α-amylase hydrolysate of bagasse alkaline extract in rats fed atherogenic diet, *J. Nutr. Sci. Vitaminol.,* 35, 481, 1989.
62. **Koseki, M., Tsuji, K., Nakagawa, Y., Kawamura, M., Ichikawa, T., Kazama, M., Kitabatake, M., and Doi, E.,** *Agric. Biol. Chem.,* 53, 3127, 1989.
63. **Topping, D. L., Illman, R. J., Roach, P. D., Trimble, R. P., Kambouris, A., and Nestel, P. J.,** Modulation of the hypolipidemic effect of fish oils by dietary fiber in rats: studies with rice and wheat bran, *J. Nutr.,* 120, 325, 1990.

64. **Shinnick, F. L., Ink, S. L., and Marlett, J. A.**, Dose response to a dietary oat bran fraction in cholesterol-fed rats, *J. Nutr.*, 120, 561, 1990.
65. **Nishina, P. M. and Freedland, R. A.**, The effects of dietary fiber feeding on cholesterol metabolism in rats, *J. Nutr.*, 120, 800, 1990.
66. **Mongeau, R., Siddiqui, I. R., Emery, J., and Brassard, R.**, Effect of dietary fiber concentrated from celery, parsnip and rutabaga on intestinal function, serum cholesterol and blood glucose response in rats, *J. Agric. Food. Chem.*, 38, 195, 1990.
67. **Kritchevsky, D., Tepper, S. A., Davidson, L. M., and Klurfeld, D. M.**, Effect of barley fiber on serum and liver cholesterol in rats, *FASEB J.*, 4, A782, 1990.
68. **Venter, C. S., Vorster, H. H., and Van der Nest, D. G.**, Comparison between physiological effects of Konjac-Glucomannan and propionate in baboons fed "Western" diets, *J. Nutr.*, 120, 1046, 1990.
69. **Zhang, J-X, Bergman, F., Hallmans, G., Johansson, G., Lundin, E., Stenling, R., Theander, O., and Westerlund, E.**, The influence of barley fibre on bile composition, gallstone formation, serum cholesterol and intestinal morphology in hamsters, *APMIS*, 98, 568, 1990.

Chapter 4.4

EFFECT OF DIETARY FIBER ON PROTEIN DIGESTIBILITY AND UTILIZATION

Daniel D. Gallaher and Barbara O. Schneeman

Determination and prediction of the quality of dietary protein has been a research interest almost since the beginning of nutrition as a science. For many years attention focused primarily on the evaluation of particular protein sources, either by chemical analysis or by biological assay using standardized diets. However, there is considerable interest in the influence of dietary components other than protein on protein quality. For example, the influence of digestible carbohydrates, particularly starch, has been studied extensively.[9] Dietary fiber, an indigestible carbohydrate, has recently received considerable attention with regard to its effect on protein digestibility and utilization. This chapter is a collation of data from these studies.

Three pairs of tables have been presented. For each pair the first table contains information from studies using purified dietary fibers, with the second describing studies where fiber-rich sources were utilized. In all tables information on diet composition, species studied, time period evaluated, and the method of fiber incorporation has been included to assist in evaluating the results of each study. The method of incorporation of the fiber or fiber source into the diet is of particular interest since it influences the protein to calorie ratio of the diet. One or two methods are usually employed. The more common method employed is incorporation by substitution, in which the fiber is added to the diet at the expense of the digestible carbohydrate source. With the second method, called the dilution (or addition) method, the fiber is added to the basal or control diet, thus causing a dilution of all components of the diet. With the substitution method, the protein content remains unchanged on a weight basis, but the protein:calorie ratio is increased. In contrast, with a fiber-diluted diet the protein:calorie ratio remains unchanged. As animals will normally consume diets to meet their energy needs,[31,32,37] incorporation of moderate amounts of fiber usually causes an increased food intake. Hence with incorporation of fiber by substitution, animals will be consuming a greater proportion of their diet as protein than will the animals being fed a fiber-free or low fiber diet. Animals fed a fiber diluted diet, however, are likely to consume an equivalent amount of protein compared to control animals. In some studies in which very high levels of fiber have been fed and/or weanling animals used, the animals have not been able to increase food intake sufficiently to meet their energy needs. This problem is a complicating factor whether fiber is incorporated by substitution or dilution. The difference in the incorporation method becomes potentially significant when one considers that utilization of a protein varies with the amount of protein consumed.[26] This problem has been examined experimentally by Delorme et al.[7] The results of their study showed that when rats were fed cellulose in the diet by the substitution method, the protein efficiency ratio (PER) decreased with increasing cellulose. However, when the diet was diluted with cellulose the PER did not change, except at the very highest level of cellulose where a slight decrease was noted. Thus, for experiments investigating the effect of dietary fiber on measures of protein utilization, it would appear the diet dilution is the better method of fiber incorporation.

The effect of purified dietary fibers on protein digestibility in animals and humans is presented in Table 1. In most cases, only apparent digestibility was determined. However, in those instances where both apparent and true digestibility were reported, the trend was similar for both. In most instances, these fibers reduced digestibility significantly in animals. This is consistent with several reports of increased protein in the small intestinal contents when cellulose or wheat bran is fed.[34,35] The two human studies reported, however, showed no effect of fiber on digestibility. Protein digestibility during consumption of fiber-rich

TABLE 1
Effect of Purified Dietary Fibers on Protein Digestibility

Fiber	Method of incorporation[a]	Species studied	Time on diet[b] adaptation → balance (days)	Concentration in diet Fiber (%)	Concentration in diet Protein[c] (%)	Protein digestibility Apparent (%)	Protein digestibility True (%)	Ref.
Cellulose	Substitution	Rats, weanling ♂ and ♀	10	2.0 7.0 12.0	(10.0)	92.5 NR[d] 92.0 90.0		46
Cellulose	Substitution	Rats, weanling ♂	5 → 4	0.0 10.0 20.0	(12.0)	89.0 ± 4.7[e]NR 86.0 ± 5.5 85.3 ± 6.9		28
Cellulose	Substitution	Rats, weanling ♂	25 → 3	0.0 2.5 5.0 10.0 20.0	(8.5)	93.0 ± 1.0 92.0 ± 0.7 90.4 ± 0.6 89.8 ± 1.1 81.6 ± 2.3 r = 0.85[f]		19
Cellulose	Substitution	Rats, weanling ♂	25 → 3	0.0 2.5 5.0 10.0 20.0	(22.0)	94.9 ± 0.6 96.1 ± 0.6 95.5 ± 0.8 92.6 ± 0.7 91.6 ± 0.5 r = −0.80[f]		19
Cellulose	Dilution	Rats, weanling ♂	21	0.0 5.0 10.0 20.0	(10.0) (9.5) (9.0) (8.0)	92.3 ± 0.5 88.7 ± 0.6* 86.4 ± 0.9* 81.9 ± 0.6*	92.9 ± 0.5 90.8 ± 0.8 89.2 ± 0.9* 86.2 ± 0.6*	36
Cellulose	Substitution	Rats, weanling ♂	21 → 7	0.2 5.9 11.4 21.0 34.9	12.4 11.6 11.9 12.1 11.8	93.0 NR 91.9 91.4 90.9 87.0		7

Fiber	Method	Subject	Days	Fiber added	Dietary fiber	Digestibility		N
Cellulose	Dilution	Rats, weanling ♂	21 → 7	0.1	10.4	89.3 NR		7
				4.9	9.9	90.3		
				8.9	10.0	85.9		
				16.2	8.6	85.8		
				27.5	8.3	74.7		
Cellulose	Substitution	Rats, ♂	4 → 5	5.2	9.3		100.0	2
				15.2			99.4	
Cellulose	Substitution	Mice, weanling ♂	28	5.0	(10.0)	86.7 ± 0.7		21
				10.0		82.2 ± 2.5		
				20.0		77.5 ± 3.9*		
Cellulose	Dilution	Dogs, ♀	14 → 5	0.0		37.8	90.8 ± 0.9	3
				2.9		29.5	88.8 ± 0.5	
				5.6		30.2	87.7 ± 1.0	
				8.3		28.5	87.0 ± 1.4	
							r = −0.59^f	
Cellulose	Substitution	Rats, weanling ♂	35	0.0	10.0	92.8		12
				10.0	9.0	85.4*		
Cellulose	Dilution	Human, adult, ♀	20 → 30	9.5	23.0	93.2 ± 0.8		38
				g/d NDF^g 23.5		92.9 ± 0.5		
Hemicellulose	Substitution	Mice, weanling ♂	28	g/d NDF 5.0	(10.0)	74.4 ± 2.6		21
				10.0		67.0 ± 3.7*		
				20.0		62.0 ± 6.1*		
Xylan	Substitution	Rats, weanling ♂	35	0.0	10.0	92.8		12
				10.0	9.8	80.8		
Raffinose	Substitution	Rats, weanling ♂	35	0.0	10.0	92.8		12
				1.0	8.8	90.9		
Lignin	Substitution	Mice, weanling ♂	28	5.0	(10.0)	74.4 ± 2.6		21
				10.0		67.0 ± 3.7*		
				20.0		62.0 ± 6.1*		
Lignin	Dilution	Rats, weanling ♂	21	0.0	(10.0)	92.3 ± 0.5	92.9 ± 0.5	36
				3.0	(9.7)	89.5 ± 0.7*	90.6 ± 0.8*	
				6.0	(9.4)	84.8 ± 0.4*	87.4 ± 0.5*	
Acid detergent fiber	Substitution	Rats, ♂ and ♀	7 → 10	0.0	16.0	90.9 ± 0.8		14
				5.0		87.8 ± 1.6*		
				10.0		83.6 ± 2.1*		
				15.0		82.6 ± 1.3*		

TABLE 1 (continued)
Effect of Purified Dietary Fibers on Protein Digestibility

Fiber	Method of incorporation[a]	Species studied	Time on diet[b] adaptation → balance (days)	Concentration in diet Fiber (%)	Concentration in diet Protein[c] (%)	Protein digestibility Apparent (%)	Protein digestibility True (%)	Ref.
Pectin	Substitution	Rats, weanling ♂ and ♀	10	0.0	(10.0)	92.5 NR		17
				5.0[h]		85.5		
				10.0[h]		79.5		
				10.0[i]		79.0		
Pectin	Substitution	Rats, weanling ♂	25 → 3	0.0	(8.5)	93.3 ± 0.5		19
				2.5		88.3 ± 1.4		
				5.0		88.7 ± 0.6		
				7.5		86.0 ± 0.8		
				10.0		85.1 ± 21.		
						r = −0.78[f]		
Pectin	Substitution	Rats, weanling ♂	25 → 3	0.0	(22.0)	95.4 ± 0.1		19
				2.5		94.8 ± 0.5		
				5.0		94.6 ± 0.8		
				7.5		92.3 ± 1.5		
				10.0		91.5 ± 0.8		
						r = −0.68[f]		
Pectin	Dilution	Rats, weanling ♂	21	0.0	(10.0)	92.3 ± 0.5	92.9 ± 0.5	36
				5.0	(9.5)	86.3 ± 0.2*	88.9 ± 0.3*	
				10.0	(9.0)	83.4 ± 0.4*	88.4 ± 0.5*	
				20.0	(8.0)	79.1 ± 1.0*	86.9 ± 0.9*	
Pectin	Substitution	Rats, weanling ♂	3 → 7	0.0	(10.0)	92.0 ± 0.3		1
				10.0	(HMW,HDE)[j]	79.4 ± 2.2*		
				10.0	(HMW,LDE)	87.4 ± 0.06*		
				10.0	(LMW,HDE)	81.6 ± 1.0*		
				10.0	(LMW,LDE)	87.4 ± 0.6*		
Pectin	Substitution	Rats, ♂	4 → 5	0.0	(10.0)	92.8 ± 1.2	101.8 ± 1.2	30
				9.3	(HDE)	77.7 ± 1.0*	86.9 ± 1.0*	
				9.4	(LDE)	81.9 ± 1.0*	91.1 ± 1.0*	
Pectin	Substitution	Rats, weanling ♂	35	0.0	10.0	92.8		12
				10.0		78.2*		

Fiber	Method	Subject	Duration	Level (%)	Control	Treatment	Ref
Guar gum	Dilution	Rats, weanling ♂	21	0.0	92.3 ± 0.5	92.9 ± 0.5	36
				5.0	81.4 ± 0.8*	83.9 ± 0.8*	
				10.0	79.9 ± 0.9*	84.5 ± 1.1*	
				20.0	63.3 ± 1.3*	70.8 ± 1.3*	
Guar gum	Substitution	Rats, ♂	4 → 5	0.0	92.8 ± 1.2	101.8 ± 1.2	30
				10.0	78.3 ± 2.3*	87.2 ± 5.1*	
Guar gum	Substitution	Rats, weanling ♂	3 → 8	0.0	87.8 ± 0.5		16
				10.0	78.0 ± 0.4*		
Guar gum	Dilution	Rats, weanling ♂	21	0.0	89.4 ± 0.4		15
				4.8	82.3 ± 0.3*		
				0.0	80.0 ± 1.3		
				4.8	70.4 ± 1.4*		
Agar	Substitution	Rats, weanling ♂	3 → 8	0.0	87.8 ± 0.5		16
				10.0	79.5 ± 0.2*		
Alginate, Na	Substitution	Rats, weanling ♂	3 → 8	0.0	87.7 ± 0.5		16
				10.0	81.0 ± 0.2*		
Alginate, Na	Substitution	Rats, weanling ♂ and ♀	10	0.0	92.5 NR		46
				(10.0)	88.5		
Carrageenan	Substitution	Rats, weanling ♂	3 → 8	0.0	87.8 ± 0.5		16
				10.0	82.6 ± 0.6*		
Carob bean gum	Substitution	Rats, weanling ♂	3 → 8	0.0	87.8 ± 0.5		16
				10.0	75.0 ± 0.8*		
Ispaghula husk (Isogel)	Dilution	Humans, adult ♂ and ♀	14 → 5	0 g	88.5 NR		33
				(19.7 g)ᵏ			
				25 g	87.3		
				(43.5 g)			
Mixed (cellulose, pectin, xylan, 3.33%, raffinose, 0.25%)	Substitution	Rats, weanling ♂	35	0.0	92.8		12
				10.2	82.2*		

TABLE 1 (continued)
Effect of Purified Dietary Fibers on Protein Digestibility

Note: An asterisk indicates that the value is significantly different from fiber-free or low fiber control group ($p < 0.05$).

a   Indicates method by which fiber or fiber source was incorporated into the diet. Substitution signifies addition to the diet at the expense of the digestible carbohydrate source. Dilution signifies addition to the diet, resulting in a whole diet dilution. In the case of dilution, the fiber or fiber source concentration in the diet indicates the actual concentration of fiber in the diet, not the percent of fiber added to the diet. See text for further explanation.
b   Indicates time of the experimental diet. Where two values appear separated by an arrow, the first value is the time allowed for adaptation to the experimental diet. The value after the arrow, or where only one value is present, incidates the length of time for which sample collections were made.
c   Values in parentheses indicate concentration of protein sources (usually casein) in diet, as the actual crude protein concentration was not reported, otherwise reported as grams per day or grams nitrogen (N) per day.
d   NR, no statistics reported.
e   Mean ± SEM.
f   Correlation between the percent fiber in the diet and the apparent protein digestibility. The correlation is statistically significant.
g   NDF, neutral detergent fiber.
h   Slow setting, 55% esterified.
i   Fast setting, 65% esterified.
j   MW, molecular weight; DE, degree of esterification; H, high; L, low.
k   Total dietary fiber.

sources is shown in Table 2. As with the purified fibers, the presence of fiber-rich sources in the diet led to significant decreases in both apparent and true digestibility in animals for all fibers for which statistics were reported. In contrast to the diets containing purified fibers, protein digestibility was lower in humans consuming the fiber-rich sources.

Fiber-rich sources usually contain significant quantities of protein which can influence the digestibility data since part of this protein is indigestible.[13] This points out a potential difference in the source of fecal nitrogen between the purified fibers and the fiber-rich sources. For the purified fibers containing no protein (guar gum, usually considered a purified fiber, often contains a small amount of protein), the source of fecal protein must be from incomplete digestion of the dietary protein, the secreted digestive enzymes, sloughed mucosal cells, and microbial protein. In the case of fiber-rich sources, the protein associated with the fiber source will contribute to the fecal nitrogen. Thus, a low protein digestibility may be due in part to the presence of indigestible protein within the fiber source. This possibility was examined in cirrhotic subjects fed an animal or vegetable diet by Weber et al.[48] They found that little fecal nitrogen was associated with the fecal fiber fraction regardless of the diet. Large increases in fecal nitrogen with the vegetable diet were due to increases in the bacterial fraction and to a lesser extent the soluble fraction. Thus, at least for vegetable sources of fiber, fiber-associated protein appears to contribute little to fecal nitrogen.

Tables 3 and 4 show the effect of fibers on nitrogen excretion and on nitrogen balance for the purified and fiber-rich sources. It is apparent from the data that fiber consumption causes a shift in the pattern of nitrogen excretion. Fecal nitrogen increases are often accompanied by a decrease in urinary nitrogen. This occurred with all types of fibers and fiber sources. However, in most instances the decrease in urinary nitrogen did not fully compensate for the increase in fecal nitrogen, such that nitrogen balance was often significantly reduced, although in all cases it remained positive.

The effect of dietary fibers on several measures of protein utilization are found in the last two tables (Tables 5 and 6). The most common measure of protein utilization is the protein efficiency ratio, undoubtedly due to its ease of determination. It should be understood, however, that this is not the same PER as described by the AOAC since the cellulose concentrations differed from 1% and the protein concentrations were not always in the 9.5 to 10.5% range. However, the term is retained since the PER is calculated in the same way (body weight gain/protein consumed). Given the decrease in protein digestibility and the consequent increase in fecal nitrogen, one might expect a decrease in protein utilization parameters that have a digestibility component, such as PER and net protein utilization, (NPU) and an increase in parameters measuring the utilization of absorbed protein, such as biological value (BV). However, the results from protein utilization studies are quite variable. For example, in rats the PER of diets containing 10 to 12% cellulose are either significantly higher,[12] lower,[7] or unchanged[38,47] than in fiber-free controls. The fiber with the most consistent effect on PER is pectin. A level of 10% or greater in the diet almost invariably led to a significant reduction in this measure of protein utilization. Interestingly, two other soluble fibers showed divergent effects on the PER. Guar gum at 10% of the diet led to a significant reduction in PER,[36] whereas alginate did not.[46] Few studies have investigated the effect of fibers on NPU and, consequently, no trends can be discerned regarding the effect of fibers on NPU. Although a large number of studies have reported the BV of fiber-containing diets, the results are too inconsistent to make any meaningful statements about the effect of fibers as a whole. Unfortunately, because of differences in the protein and/or fiber concentrations of the diets, as well as the method of fiber incorporation into the diet, comparisons between studies using the same fiber type are often not possible. As work continues in this area perhaps some methodological standardization will evolve that will allow such comparisons to be made. Until that time, it seems unlikely that a clear pattern will then emerge concerning the effects of dietary fibers on protein utilization.

This review covers the published literature through July 1991.

TABLE 2
Effect of Fiber-Rich Sources on Protein Digestibility

Fiber	Method of incorporation[a]	Species studied	Time on diet[b] adaptation → balance (days)	Concentration in diet Fiber (%)	Concentration in diet Protein[c] (%)	Protein digestibility Apparent (%)	Protein digestibility True (%)	Ref.
Wheat bran	Substitution	Rats, ♂	4 → 5	0.0	(10.0)	92.8 ± 1.2[d]	101.8 ± 1.2	30
				10.0		87.4 ± 1.2*	96.2 ± 1.3*	
Wheat bran	Dilution	Rats, weanling ♂	21	0.0	(10.0)	92.3 ± 0.5	92.9 ± 0.5	36
				5.0	(9.5)	89.0 ± 0.4*	89.9 ± 0.5	
				10.0	(9.0)	86.3 ± 0.4*	87.9 ± 0.4*	
				20.0	(8.0)	77.0 ± 1.0*	77.7 ± 0.8*	
Wheat bran	Substitution	Rats, weanling ♂	35	0.0	10.0	92.8		12
				16.8	12.5	83.0*		
Wheat bran	Dilution	Humans, adult ♂	18 → 4	0 (33.0 g/d)[e]	15.4 g N/d	89.7 ± 0.6		11
				12 g (53.5 g/d)	16.4 g N/d	87.6 ± 0.5*		
Wheat bran	Substitution	Rats, ♂	9 → 5	0(4.3)[h]	9.8		97.9	8
				5.2[i]			97.2	
				6.1			96.3	
				7.9			95.2*	
				11.6			92.6*	
Wheat bran	Dilution	Pigs, ♂	20 → 10	0.0	16.9	97.0[j]		42
				6.9[e]	16.3	93.4		
				12.8	16.3	91.8		
				18.0	15.6	88.5		
				22.4	15.6	78.9		
Corn bran	Substitution	Rats, weanling ♂	35	0.0	10.0	92.8		12
				16.8	12.5	83.0*		
Oat bran	Dilution	Humans, adult ♂	14	0 (3.8 g/d)[e]	10.7 g N/d	91 ± 3 NR[f]		4
				45 g (12.0 g/d)	10.5 g N/d	85 ± 4		
Sorghum meal	Substitution	Humans, adult	5 → 6	3.3[e]	10.6 g N/d	65.4 ± 1.8		5
				4.8		60.5 ± 2.1*		
				5.4		56.9 ± 2.3*		
Barley hulls	Substitution	Rats, ♂	4 → 5	0.0	9.3	100.0		2
				10.0		97.3*		

Source	Method	Animal	n	Dose	Value	Digestibility	Ref
Barley husk	Substitution	Rats, ♂	4 → 5	0.0	9.7	87.8	10
				7.7e	12.8	86.9*	
Barley husk	Substitution	Rats, ♂	9 → 5	0(4.3)h	9.8	97.9	8
				5.1i	9.7	98.4	
				6.0	9.7	96.7	
				7.9		96.1*	
				11.7		94.9*	
Maize hulls	Dilution	Pigs, ♂	20 → 10	0.0	16.9	97.0i	42
				7.4e	15.6	94.7	
				14.7	14.4	91.3	
				21.7	13.8	88.0	
				23.6	12.5	83.7	
Oat hulls	Dilution	Pigs, ♂	20 → 10	0.0	16.9	97.0i	42
				7.4e	15.6	95.5	
				14.7	14.4	94.1	
				21.8	13.1	92.6	
				28.7	11.9	90.7	
Soybean hulls	Dilution	Pigs, ♂	20 → 10	0.0	16.9	97.0i	42
				7.3e	14.4	93.0	
				14.1	15.6	88.6	
				20.6	15.0	82.9	
				26.6	14.4	80.3	
Soybean hulls	Substitution	Rats, ♂	16	0	13	98	47
				12	14	92*	
Lupin hulls	Dilution	Pigs, ♂	20 → 10	0.0	16.9	97.0i	42
				7.4e	15.6	91.9	
				14.5	14.4	90.7	
				21.6	13.1	86.0	
				28.5	12.5	81.4	
Pea hulls	Dilution	Pigs, ♂	20 → 10	0.0	16.9	97.0i	42
				7.2e	15.6	89.6	
				13.8	14.4	81.7	
				19.8	13.1	74.8	
				25.4	12.5	65.3	
Canola hulls	Substitution	Rats, ♂	16	0	13	98	47
				12	15	87*	
Bean cell wall	Substitution	Rats, weanling ♂	35	0.0	10.0	92.8	12
				10.0	11.8	85.8*	

TABLE 2 (continued)
Effect of Fiber-Rich Sources on Protein Digestibility

Fiber	Method of incorporation[a]	Species studied	Time on diet[b] adaptation → balance (days)	Concentration in diet Fiber (%)	Concentration in diet Protein[c] (%)	Protein digestibility Apparent (%)	Protein digestibility True (%)	Ref.
Soybean cell wall	Substitution	Rats, ♂	16	0.0	13	98		47
				12	14	90*		
Soy polysaccharide	Formulated[h]	Humans, ♂ and ♀	3 → 4–5	0.0 g/d	13.1 g/d	92.2 ± 2.9		18
				8.8 g/d	14.3 g/d	90.0 ± 1.6		
Canola cell wall	Substitution	Rats, ♂	16	0.0	13	98		47
				12	13	90*		
Sugar beet fiber	Substitution	Rats, ♂	4 → 5	0.0	(10.0)	92.8 ± 1.2	101.8 ± 2.6	30
				10.0		84.6 ± 0.8*	92.5 ± 0.8*	
				10.0[g]		83.0 ± 1.5*	92.0 ± 1.5*	
Brown rice	Substitution	Humans, adult ♂	1 → 14	5.7 g/d[e]	4.74 g N/d	68.0 ± 3.5	83.2 ± 3.5	27
				13.9 g/d[e]	4.65 g N/d	48.4 ± 3.8*	63.8 ± 36.	
Fruits, vegetables, and wholemeal bran	Unclear	Human, ♂	2 → 7	6.2 g/d	13.1 g N/d	92.1 ± 0.6NR		40
				16.2 g/d	13.9 g N/d	90.8 ± 0.5		
				31.9 g/d	14.7 g N/d	85.2 ± 0.5		
Fruits and vegetables	Unclear	Humans, adult ♂	19 → 7	3.6 g/d[e]	93.0 g/d	90.4 ± 0.9		22
				20.0 g/d	96.0 g/d	81.1 ± 1.1*		
Fruits and vegetables	Unclear	Humans, adult ♂	14 → 7	1.9 g/d[e]	13.6 N/d	89.9 ± 0.5		23
				10.0 g/d	14.1 g N/d	86.9 ± 0.7*		
				19.4 g/d	13.8 g N/d	83.5 ± 0.8*		
				25.6 g/d	13.9 g N/d	81.2 ± 1.1*		
Fruits and vegetables	Substitution	Humans, adult ♂	21 → 7	17.8 g/d	15.8 g N/d	90 ± 2		25
				41.0 g/d	16.5 g N/d	84 ± 4*		
Konjac and seaweed	Substitution	Humans, adult ♂	5	0.0	26 g/d	81.2		20
				18 g/d[e]	27 g/d	55.5*		
"Guatemalan" diet	Dilution	Humans, adult ♂	14	3.8 g/d	10.7 g N/d	91 ± 3 NR		4
				93.0 g/d	10.8 g N/d	69 ± 2		

Note: An asterisk indicates that the value is significantly different from fiber-free or low fiber control group ($p < 0.05$).

a See footnote a of Table 1.
b See footnote b of Table 1.
c See footnote c of Table 1.
d Mean ± SEM.
e Neutral detergent fiber.
f NR, no statistics reported.
g Treated with hot water to increase the solubility of pectin.
h Enteral formulas.
i Total dietary fiber.

TABLE 3
Effect of Purified Dietary Fibers on Nitrogen Excretion and Balance

Fiber	Method of incorporation[a]	Species studied	Time on diet[b] adaptation → balance (days)	Fiber in diet	Nitrogen intake (g/day)	Nitrogen excretion Fecal (mg/day)	Urinary (mg/day)	Nitrogen balance (mg/day)	Ref.
Cellulose	Substitution	Rats, weanling ♂	5 → 4	0.0	0.121	22.9 ± 3.2[c]NR[d]	10.4 ± 1.4 NR	40.0 ± 4.6 NR	18
				10.0	0.132	20.2 ± 2.9	11.1 ± 1.5	45.1 ± 5.6	
				20.0	0.132	19.8 ± 3.1	12.7 ± 1.6	51.3 ± 6.8	
Cellulose	Dilution	Rats, weanling ♂	21	0.0	0.289	22.0(6)[e]			36
				5.0	0.276	31.0*(10*)			
				10.0	0.266	36.0*(12*)			
				20.0	0.264	47.0*(16*)			
Cellulose[f]	Dilution	Rats, ♂	35 → 7	0.0	0.188	16.0 ± 2.4 NR	163.4 ± 8.3 NR	8.2 NR	44
				2.0 g/d		25.5 ± 5.0	249.4 ± 4.3	12.7	
Cellulose[g]	Substitution	Rats, ♂	21 → 7	0.0	0.289	18.0	9.60	181.0	29
				2.1	0.287	17.0	106.0	165.0	
Cellulose[h]	Substitution	Rats, ♂	21 → 7	0.0	0.319	20.0	139.0	154.0	29
				2.1	0.316	21.0	114.0*	186.0*	
Cellulose	Substitution	Mice, weanling, ♂	28	5.0	0.080	10.0 ± 1	10.0 ± 3	50.0 ± 7	21
				10.0	0.070	10.0 ± 1	10.0 ± 2	50.0 ± 9	
				20.0	0.070	20.0 ± 2	10.0 ± 3	50.0 ± 10	
Cellulose	Substitution	Rats, growing ♂ and ♀	30 → 1	0.0	0.256	133.0 ± 30			17
				15.0		131.0 ± 12			
Cellulose	Dilution	Monkeys, ♂	7 → 7	1.0 g/d		250			41
				7.0 g/d		200			
				16.0 g/d		225			
				20.0 g/d		275			
Cellulose	Dilution	Humans, adult, ♀	3 → 4	0	7.910	970	5840	1100	24
				(6.8 g/d)[i]					
				14.2 g/d		1140*	5950	820*	
				(21.0 g/d)[i]					
Cellulose	Dilution	Humans, adult, ♂ and ♀	3 → 7	0	7.880	910	5750	1220	24
				(6.8 g/d)[i]					
				14.2 g/d		1170*	5740	970*	
				(21.0 g/d)[i]					

Fiber	Method	Subjects	Duration	Dose					Ref
Cellulose	Dilution	Humans, adolescent, ♂	3 → 4	0 (6.8 g/d)ⁱ 14.2 g/d (21.0 g/d)	7.850	860 920	5080 5570	1910 1360*	24
Hemicellulose	Substitution	Mice, weanling, ♂	28	5.0 10.0 20.0	0.060 0.070 0.060	20.0 ± 4 20.0 ± 4* 20.0 ± 5*	10.0 ± 4 10.0 ± 4 10.0 ± 5	30.0 ± 4 40.0 ± 6 30.0 ± 6	21
Hemicellulose	Dilution	Human, adult, ♀	3 → 4	0 (6.8 g/d)ⁱ 14.2 g/d (21 g/d)	7.910	970 1180*	5840 5990	1100 740*	24
Hemicellulose	Dilution	Humans, adult, ♂ and ♀	3 → 7	0 (6.8 g/d)ⁱ 14.2 g/d (21 g/d)	7.880	910 1290*	5750 5730	1220 860*	24
Hemicellulose	Dilution	Humans, adolescent, ♂	3 → 4	0 (6.8 g/d)ⁱ 14.2 g/d (21 g/d)	7.850	860 1110*	5080 5730	1910 1380*	24
Lignin	Dilution	Rats, weanling, ♂	21	0.0 3.0 6.0	0.289 0.275 0.264	22.0(6)ᶜ 29.0(10*) 40.0*(14*)			36
Lignin	Substitution	Mice, weanling, ♂	28	5.0 10.0 20.0	0.070 0.070 0.050	10.0 ± 3 10.0 ± 2 10.0 ± 4	10.0 ± 5 20.0 ± 6 20.0 ± 7	40.0 ± 15 40.0 ± 9 20.0 ± 8*	21
Neutral detergent fiber (wheat bran)ᵍ	Substitution	Rats, ♂	21 → 7	0.0 2.1	0.289 0.297	18.0 26.0*	96.0 80.0	181.0 187.0	29
Neutral detergent fiber (wheat bran)ʰ	Substitution	Rats, ♂	21 → 7	0.0 2.1	0.319 0.332	20.0 34.0*	139.0 118.0*	154.0 172.0	29
Acid detergent fiber (wheat bran)ʰ	Substitution	Rats, ♂	21 → 7	0.0 2.1	0.289 0.289	18.0 22.0*	96.0 90.0	181.0 182.0	29

TABLE 3 (continued)
Effect of Purified Dietary Fibers on Nitrogen Excretion and Balance

Fiber	Method of incorporation[a]	Species studied	Time on diet[b] adaptation → balance (days)	Fiber in diet	Nitrogen intake (g/day)	Nitrogen excretion Fecal (mg/day)	Urinary (mg/day)	Nitrogen balance (mg/day)	Ref.
Acid detergent fiber (wheat bran)	Substitution	Rats, ♂	21 → 7	0.0	0.319	20.0	13.9	154.0	29
				2.1	0.321	25.0	122.0*	174.0*	
Pectin	Substitution	Rats, ♂	4 → 5	0.0		10.5			30
				9.3 (LDE)[j]		23.7*			
				9.4 (HDE)		30.0*			
Pectin[g]	Substitution	Rats, ♂	21 → 7	0.0	0.289	18.0	96.0	181.0	29
				2.1	0.288	24.0*	97.0	182.0	
Pectin[h]	Substitution	Rats, ♂	21 → 7	0.0	0.319	20.0	139.0	154.0	29
				2.1	0.316	25.0	132.0	159.0	
Pectin[h]	Substitution	Rats, ♂	21 → 7	0.0	0.319	20.0	139.0	154.0	29
				2.1	0.316	25.0	132.0	159.0	
Pectin	Dilution	Humans, adult, ♂ and ♀	3 → 4	0	7.910	970.0	5840.0	1100.0	24
				(6.8 g/d)[j]					
				14.2 g/d					
				(21.0 g/d)		1060.0	5510.0	1090.0	
Pectin	Dilution	Humans, adult, ♂ and ♀	3 → 7	0	7.880	910	5750	1220	24
				(6.8 g/d)[j]					
				14.2 g/d					
				(21.0 g/d)		1060	5510	1310	
Pectin	Dilution	Humans, adolescent, ♂	3 → 4	0	7.850	860	5080	1910	24
				(6.8 g/d)[j]					
				14.2 g/d					
				(21.0 g/d)		1010	5010*	1830	
Pectin	Dilution	Monkeys, ♂	7 → 7	1.0 g/d		190			41
				7.0 g/d		250			
				13.0 g/d		210			
				20.0 g/d		230			

Fiber	Type	Subject	n	Level	Col 1	Col 2	Col 3	Col 4	Ref
Pectin	Dilution	Rats, weanling, ♂	21	0.0	0.289	22.0(6)e			36
				5.0	0.241*	33.0*(11*)			
				10.0	0.191*	31.0*(15*)			
				20.0	0.146*	30.0*(19*)			
Guar gum	Substitution	Rats, weanling, ♂	3 → 8	0.0	0.142	17.3 ± 0.6	58.9 ± 1.6	66.0k	16
				10.0	0.152	33.5 ± 1.0*	43.8 ± 1.3*	75.0	
Guar gum[l]	Dilution	Rats, ♂		0.0	0.335	6.0	92.0	234.0	45
				5.0	0.311	18.0*	56.0	228.0	
Guar gum	Dilution	Rats, weanling, ♂	8	Casein					15
				0.0	0.234	24.5	152.3	57.2k	
				5.0	0.237	42.0	129.5*	65.6	
				Egg albumin					
				0.0	0.109	21.8	69.4	17.7	
				5.0	0.114	33.8*	57.6*	22.5	
Guar gum	Substitution	Rats, ♂	4 → 5	0.0		10.5			30
				5.0		26.8*			
Guar gum	Dilution	Rats, weanling, ♂	21	0.0	0.289	22.0(6)e			36
				5.0	0.259	48.0*(12*)			
				10.0	0.217	44.0*(17*)			
				20.0	0.168	61.0*(20*)			
Carrageenan	Substitution	Rats, ♂ and ♀	148	0.0			55.0 ± 4.8m		17
				2.0			49.0 ± 3.0%		
				5.0			53.0 ± 2.9%		
				10.0			52.0 ± 3.0%		
				15.0			44.0 ± 3.0%		
				20.0			43.0 ± 4.2%		
Carrageenan	Substitution	Rats, weanling, ♂	3 → 8	0.0	0.142	17.3 ± 0.6	58.9 ± 1.6	66.0*	16
				10.0	0.138	24.8 ± 0.5*	61.9 ± 0.6*	51.0	
Carob bean gum	Substitution	Rats, weanling, ♂	3 → 8	0.0	0.142	17.3 ± 0.6	58.9 ± 1.6	66.0k	16
				10.0	0.154	38.4 ± 1.4*	49.5 ± 1.3*	66.0	
Na-alginate	Substitution	Rats, weanling, ♂	3 → 8	0.0	0.142	17.3 ± 0.6	58.9 ± 1.6	66.0k	16
				10.0	0.149	28.2 ± 1.0*	51.4 ± 1.9*	70.0	
Agar	Substitution	Rats, weanling, ♂	3 → 8	0.0	0.142	17.3 ± 0.6	58.9 ± 1.6	66.0	16
				10.0	0.134	27.5 ± 1.6*	61.2 ± 1.8	45.0	
Vegetable	Substitution	Humans, adult	3 → 6	0.15 g/kg	118.2 mg/kg	11.7 ± 1.7 mg/kg	106.0 ± 6.5 mg/kg	−3.4 ± 4.1 mg/kg	48
				0.67 g/kg	124.8 mg/kg	27.6 ± 4.7 mg/kg	85.3 ± 4.1* mg/kg	6.4 ± 6.5 mg/kg	

TABLE 3 (continued)
Effect of Purified Dietary Fibers on Nitrogen Excretion and Balance

Note: An asterisk indicates that these values are significantly different from the fiber-free of low fiber control group ($p < 0.05$).

a   See footnote a in Table 1.
b   See footnote b in Table 1.
c   Mean ± SEM.
d   NR, no statistics reported.
e   Endogenous fecal nitrogen, uncorrected for nitrogen content of nonprotein diet.
f   Rats were made obese, then fed an energy-restricted regime with or without cellulose.
g   Metabolizable energy of diet was 57 kcal/day.
h   Metabolizable energy of diet was 67 kcal/day.
i   Total dietary fiber intake.
j   DE, degree of esterification; L, low; H, high.
k   Calculated from intake and excretion means.
l   Data chosen from 1.2% dietary arginine groups. Nitrogen intake and balance calculated from data presented in article.
m   Values are mean ± SEM for nitrogen excreted per day as a percent of ingested nitrogen.

TABLE 4
Effect of Fiber-Rich Sources on Nitrogen Excretion and Balance

Fiber	Method of incorporation[a]	Species studied	Time on diet[b] adaptation → balance (days)	Fiber in diet	Nitrogen intake (g/day)	Fecal (mg/day)	Urinary (mg/day)	Nitrogen balance (mg/day)	Ref.
Wheat bran	Substitution	Rats, ♂	4 → 5	0.0%		10.5			30
				10.0%		19.7			
Wheat bran	Substitution	Rats, ♂	28 → 7	0.0%	0.289	18.0	96.0	181.0	29
				2.0%	0.287	26.0*	80.0	185.0	
Wheat bran	Dilution	Rats, ♂	3 → 15	0.0%	0.335	6.0	92.0	237.0[c]	45
				5.0%	0.322	12.0*	87.0*	223.0	
Wheat bran (largely)	Dilution	Humans, adult	18 → 4	0.0%			6300		11
				12.0%					
Wheat bran	Substitution	Humans, adult, ♂ and ♀	4–5 → 7	0.0	18.2 ± 0.8[d]	1150 ± 210 NR[e]	8200*		39
				5.0 g	19.1 ± 0.9	1650 ± 220			
Wheat bran	Not stated	Humans	14 → 7	0.0		1400 NR			43
				18.0g		2000			
Wheat fiber[f]	Substitution	Humans, ♂	21	0	21.9	1400 ± 300			6
				(21.8 g/d)[g]					
				31 g/d	26.9	2490 ± 100*			
				(53.2 g/d)					
Sorghum fiber	Substitution	Humans	5 → 6	3.3%[h]	10.6	4020 ± 270	5500 ± 360	2020 ± 230	5
				4.8%	10.6	4139 ± 240	4830 ± 200	1470 ± 310*	
				5.4%	10.6	4730 ± 390	4960 ± 270	1110 ± 310*	
Oat bran[i]	Substitution	Human, ♂	14	3.8 g/d[j]	10.7 ± 0.9	1000 ± 320 NR	8390 ± 420 NR	800 ± 440[k] NR	4
				12.0 g/d	10.5 ± 0.8	1610 ± 560	8160 ± 280	260 ± 320	
Sugar beet fiber	Substitution	Rats, ♂	4 → 5	0.0%	10.5				30
				10.0%	26.2*				
Locust bean gum	Dilution	Monkeys, ♂	7 → 7	1.0 g/d	260				41
				15.0 g/d[l]	280				
Slippery elm	Dilution	Monkeys, ♂	7 → 7	1.0 g/d	190				41
				20.0 g/d[l]	390				
Rice hulls	Dilution	Monkeys, ♂	7 → 7	1.0 g/d		200			41
				16.0 g/d[l]		335			

TABLE 4 (continued)
Effect of Fiber-Rich Sources on Nitrogen Excretion and Balance

Fiber	Method of incorporation[a]	Species studied	Time on diet[b] adaptation → balance (days)	Fiber in diet	Nitrogen intake (g/day)	Nitrogen excretion Fecal (mg/day)	Urinary (mg/day)	Nitrogen balance (mg/day)	Ref.
Oat straw	Dilution	Monkeys, ♂	7 → 7	1.0 g/d		200			41
				15.0 g/d[l]		385			
Soy husks	Dilution	Monkeys, ♂	7 → 7	1.0 g/d		205			41
				20.0 g/d[l]		470			
Psyllium seed	Dilution	Monkeys, ♂	7 → 7	1.0 g/d		335			41
				18.0 g/d[l]		320			
Fruits and vegetables	Substitution (?)	Humans, ♂	19 → 7	3.6 g/d[j]	14.9	1350	11450	1090	22
				20.0 g/d	15.4	2480	10810	740	
Fruits and vegetables	Substitution	Humans, ♂	14 → 7	1.9 g/d[j]	13.6			1380 ± 80	23
				10.1 g/d	14.1			1840 ± 120*	
				19.4 g/d	13.8			2280 ± 140*	
				25.6 g/d*	13.9			2600 ± 180*	
Cabbage	Not stated	Humans	4 → 7	0.0 g/d		1400			43
				18.3 g/d		2100			
Vegetables	Substitution	Humans, adult (cirrhotic)	3 → 6	12.5 g/d	9.8	955	8798	−282	48
				55.6 g/d	10.4	2291*	7080*	531	
Brown rice	Substitution	Humans, adult ♂	1 → 15	5.7 g/d[j]	4.74 ± 0.65	1500 ± 140	3950 ± 390	−710 ± 290	27
				13.9 g/d	4.65 ± 0.64	2410 ± 430	3330 ± 510	−1090 ± 330	

Note: A single asterisk indicates that the value is significantly different from the fiber-free or low fiber control group (p < 0.05).

[a] See footnote a in Table 1.
[b] See footnote b in Table 2.
[c] Calculated from intake and excretion means.
[d] Mean ± SEM.
[e] NR, no statistics reported.
[f] High protein diets.
[g] Total dietary fiber.
[h] Crude fiber.
[i] Date from untoasted oat bran group only.
[j] Neutral detergent fiber.
[k] Corrected balance, with one subject omitted.
[l] Highest level fed.

TABLE 5
Effect of Purified Dietary Fibers on Measures of Protein Utilization

Fiber	Method of incorporation[a]	Species studied	Concentration in diet		Measures of protein utilization[c]			Ref.
			Fiber (%)	Protein[b](%)	PER	NPU	BV	
Cellulose	Substitution	Rats	0.0	7.6			76.0	19
			2.5	(8.5)			78.0	
			5.0				76.0	
			10.0				79.0	
			20.0				76.0	
			0.0	19.7			64.0	
			2.5	(22.0)			72.0	
			5.0				61.0	
			10.0				65.0	
			20.0				69.0	
Cellulose	Substitution	Rats	0.0	9.98	2.89(2.50)[d]			12
			10.0	8.98	3.94*(3.41)			
Cellulose	Substitution	Rats	0.0	10.0		79.1 ± 4.6[e]NR[f]	60.4 ± 3.6 NR	28
			10.0	(12.0)		80.2 ± 5.3	57.8 ± 3.1	
			20.0			78.1 ± 4.2	63.4 ± 3.8	
			0.0	9.5%		83.7 ± 6.1	64.7 ± 5.0	
			10.0	of calories		84.9 ± 5.7	58.9 ± 4.3	
			20.0	(12.0)		80.7 ± 5.6	59.3 ± 4.0	
Cellulose	Substitution	Rats	0.0	12.38	2.24 ± 0.21			7
			5.0	11.61	2.29 ± 0.10			
			10.0	11.89	2.06 ± 0.05*			
			20.0	12.05	2.06 ± 0.12*			
			40.0	11.82	1.98 ± 0.06*			
	Dilution		0.0	10.38	2.70 ± 0.24			
			5.0	9.94	2.72 ± 0.12			
			10.0	9.95	2.57 ± 0.11			
			20.0	8.58	2.82 ± 0.22			
			40.0	8.25	2.36 ± 0.19*			
Cellulose	Substitution	Rats	0.0	(10.0)	3.2 ± 0.2			46
			5.0		3.3 ± 0.1			
			10.0		2.8 ± 0.7			

TABLE 5 (continued)
Effect of Purified Dietary Fibers on Measures of Protein Utilization

Fiber	Method of incorporation[a]	Species studied	Concentration in diet Fiber (%)	Protein[b] (%)	Measures of protein utilization[c] PER	NPU	BV	Ref.
Cellulose	Substitution	Mice	5.0	10.0	1.7 ± 0.2			21
			10.0	(10.0)	1.7 ± 0.5			
			20.0		1.4 ± 0.3			
Cellulose	Dilution	Rats	0.0	10.0	3.98 ± 0.14^g(87)^h		4.31 ± 0.15^i	36
							(4.28 ± 0.14)^j	
			5.0		3.90 ± 0.21 (85)		4.40 ± 0.29	
							(4.30 ± 0.28)	
			10.0		3.71 ± 0.37 (81)		4.30 ± 0.50	
							(4.16 ± 0.47)	
			20.0		3.79 ± 0.20 (83)		4.63 ± 0.19*	
							(4.40 ± 0.19)	
Cellulose	Substitution	Rats	0.0^k	12.78	2.89		75.4	29
			2.1	(2.044% N)	2.95		70.2	
			0.0^l		1.86		63.9	
			2.1		1.98*		74.4*	
Cellulose	Substitution	Rats	5.2	9.38		87.4	95.7	2
			15.2	(1.5% N)		87.7	93.3*	
Cellulose	Substitution	Rats, ♂	0.0	13	3.00			47
			12	13	2.99			
Xylan	Substitution	Rats	0.0	9.98	2.89 (2.50)^c			12
			10.0	9.75	3.79* (3.28)			
Hemicellulose	Substitution	Mice	5.0	10.0	1.1 ± 0.3			17
			10.0	(10.0)	2.3 ± 0.5*			
			20.0		1.9 ± 0.7			
Lignin	Substitution	Mice	5.0	10.0	1.2 ± 0.6			21
			10.0	(10.0)	2.3 ± 0.4			
			20.0		1.0 ± 0.9			
Lignin	Dilution	Rats	0.0	10.0	3.98 ± 0.14^g(87)^h		4.31 ± 0.15^i	36
							(4.28 ± 0.14)^j	
			3.0		3.48 ± 0.22 (76)		3.89 ± 0.20	
							(3.83 ± 0.20)	

Fiber	Type	Animal	Dose			Ref
			6.0		3.05 ± 0.20 (67)	3.60 ± 0.24 (3.49 ± 0.23)
Neutral detergent fiber (wheat bran)	Substitution	Rats	0.0[k] 2.1 0.0[k] 2.1		2.89 2.91 1.86 1.96*	75.4 78.0 63.9 71.3*	29
Acid detergent fiber (wheat bran)	Substitution	Rats	0.0[k] 2.1 0.0[j] 2.1		2.89 2.91 1.86 1.99*	75.4 77.7 63.9 70.7*	29
Pectin	Substitution	Rats	0.0 2.5 5.0 10.0 20.0 0.0 2.5 5.0 10.0 20.0	7.6 (8.5) 19.7 (22.0)		75.0 83.0 78.0 76.0 72.0 66.0 66.0 63.0 64.0 63.0	19
Pectin	Substitution	Rats	0.0 5.0[i] 10.0[i] 10.0[j]	10.0	3.2 ± 0.2 3.6 ± 0.5 2.8 ± 0.3 2.3 ± 0.3*		46
Pectin	Substitution	Rats	0.0 10.0	9.98 9.95	2.89 (2.50)[d] 2.21* (1.91)		12
Pectin	Substitution	Rats	0.0 10.0 (HDE, HMW)[m] 10.0 (LDE, HMW) 10.0 (HDE, LMW) 10.0 (LDE, LMW)	(10.0)		64.3 ± 8.0 60.0 ± 11.5 71.3 ± 5.2* 67.4 ± 5.3 74.5 ± 6.4*	67.9 ± 8.9 76.4 ± 18.1 81.6 ± 5.5* 82.7 ± 7.0* 85.4 ± 8.0*	1
Pectin	Substitution	Rats	0.0 2.1 0.0 2.1	12.78 (2.044% N)	2.89 2.96 1.86 2.11*	75.4 78.2 63.9 66.4	29
Pectin	Dilution	Rats	0.0	(10.0)	3.98 ± 0.14[g](87)[h]	4.31 ± 0.15[i] (4.28 ± 0.14)[j]	36

TABLE 5 (continued)
Effect of Purified Dietary Fibers on Measures of Protein Utilization

Fiber	Method of incorporation[a]	Species studied	Concentration in diet		Measures of protein utilization[c]			Ref.
			Fiber (%)	Protein[b](%)	PER	NPU	BV	
Pectin			5.0		3.05 ± 0.33*(66)		3.54 ± 0.04*	
							(3.44 ± 0.38)*	
			10.0		3.00 ± 0.42*(65)		3.59 ± 0.47*	
							(3.39 ± 0.47)*	
			20.0		1.83 ± 0.31*(40)		2.32 ± 0.40*	
							(2.11 ± 0.37)*	
Pectin	Substitution	Rats	0.0	(10.0)			82.9 ± 4.4	30
			9.3 (HDE)[m]				81.6 ± 3.1	
			9.4 (LDE)				79.9 ± 5.0	
Guar gum	Substitution	Rats	0.0	(10.0)			82.9 ± 4.4	30
							84.3 ± 3.1	
Guar gum	Dilution	Rats	0.0	(10.0)	3.98 ± 0.14g(87)[h]		4.31 ± 0.15[i]	36
							(4.28 ± 0.14)[j]	
							4.48 ± 0.35	
			5.0		3.65 ± 0.38(79)		4.35 ± 0.32)	
			10.0		3.45 ± 0.18*(76)		4.33 ± 0.30	
							(4.00 ± 0.30)	
			20.0		2.24 ± 0.32*(47)		3.57 ± 0.64*	
							(3.19 ± 0.56)*	
Algin	Substitution	Rats	0.0	(10.0)	3.2 ± 0.2			46
			10.0		2.9 ± 0.4			

Note: An asterisk indicates that the value is significantly different from the fiber-free or low fiber control group ($P < 0.05$).

[a] See footnote a of Table 1.
[b] Values in parentheses are the concentrations of the protein source (usually casein) or the percent nitrogen (where so indicated) in the diet.
[c] PER, protein efficiency ratio; NPU, net protein utilization; BV, biological value.
[d] PER, corrected for fiber-free group = 2.50.
[e] Mean ± SD.
[f] NR, no statistics reported.
[g] Net protein ratio (NPR).
[h] Relative net protein ration (RNPR).
[i] NPR ÷ apparent digestibility (NPR/AD).
[j] NPR ÷ true digestibility (NPR/TD).
[k] Metabolizable energy of diet was 57 kcal/day.
[l] Metabolizable energy of diet was 67 kcal/day.
[m] DE, degree of esterification; MW, molecular weight; L, low; H, high.

TABLE 6
Effect of Fiber-Rich Sources on Measures of Protein Utilization

Fiber	Method of incorporation[a]	Species studied	Concentration in diet Fiber (%)	Protein[b] (%)	Measures of protein utilization[c] PER	NPU	BV	Ref.
Wheat bran	Substitution	Rats	0.0	9.98%	2.87 (2.50)[d]			12
			10.0	12.50%	3.02 (2.61)			
Wheat bran	Substitution	Rats	0.0	(10.0)			82.9 ± 4.4	24
			10.0	(10.0)			77.1 ± 5.1	
Wheat bran	Dilution	Rats	0.0	(10.0)	2.98 ± 0.14[e,f](87)[g]		4.31 ± 0.15[h] (4.28 ± 0.14)[i]	36
			5.0		3.22 ± 0.22*(70)		3.61 ± 0.26* (3.57 ± 0.26*)	
			10.0		2.92 ± 0.18*(64)		3.38 ± 0.22* (3.33 ± 0.22*)	
			20.0		2.52 ± 0.12*(55)		3.28 ± 0.17* (3.16 ± 0.16*)	
Wheat bran	Substitution	Rats	0.0[j]	12.78 (2.044% N)	2.89		75.4	29
			5.0		3.03*		80.1	
			0.0[k]		1.86		63.9	
			5.0		2.07*		69.5*	
Wheat bran	Substitution	Rats, ♂	0(4.3)[n]	9.8		82.6	84.3	8
			5.2[l]	9.8		83.3	85.8	
			6.1[l]	9.8		83.3	86.5	
			7.9[l]	9.8		83.4	88.3*	
			11.6[l]	10.0		83.3	90.1	
Corn bran	Substitution	Rats	0.0	9.98	2.89 (2.50)[d]			12
			10.0	10.59	3.26 (2.82)			
Barley hulls	Substitution	Rats	0.0	9.38 (1.5% N)		87.4	95.7	2
			10.0			87.5	94.2*	
Barley husk	Substitution	Rats, ♂	0(4.3)[n]	9.8		82.6	84.3	8
			5.1[l]	9.7		80.7	83.5	
			6.0[l]	9.7		80.7*	83.5	
			7.9[l]	9.8		80.1*	83.4	
			11.7[l]	9.8		79.5*	83.7	
Barley husk	Substitution	Rats, ♂	0.0	9.7		68.0	77.4	10
			7.7[o]	12.8		67.9	78.1	

Sugar beet fiber	Substitution	Rats	0.0 10.0(7.67)^l 10.0^m(7.43)	(10.0)		92.9 ± 4.4 75.2 ± 3.3* 74.4 ± 4.3*	24
Bran cell wall fiber	Substitution	Rats	0.0 10.0	9.98 11.78	2.89 (2.50)^d 2.97 (2.57)		10

Note: An asterisk indicates that the value is significantly different from the fiber-free or low fiber control group ($p < 0.05$).

a   See footnote a in Table 1.
b   See footnote b in Table 5.
c   See footnote c in Table 5.
d   PER, corrected for fiber-free group = 2.50.
e   Mean ± SD.
f   Net protein ratio (NPR).
g   Relative net protein ratio (RNPR).
h   NPR ÷ apparent digestibility (NPR/AD).
i   NPR ÷ true digestibility (NPR/TD).
j   Metabolizable energy of diet was 57 kcal/day.
k   Metabolizable energy of diet was 67 kcal/day.
l   Total dietary fiber.
m   Treated with hot water to increase the solubility of pectin.
n   Cellulose content of 0% fiber diet.
o   Neutral detergent fiber.

REFERENCES

1. **Atallah, M. T. and Melnik, T. A.**, Effect of pectin structure on protein utilization by growing rats, *J. Nutr.*, 112, 2027, 1982.
2. **Beames, R. M. and Eggum, B. O.**, The effect of type of and level of protein fiber and starch on nitrogen excretion patterns in rats, *Br. J. Nutr.*, 46, 301, 1981.
3. **Burrows, C. F., Kronfeld, D. S., Banta, C. A., and Merritt, A. M.**, Effects of fiber on digestibility and transit time in dogs, *J. Nutr.*, 112, 1726, 1982.
4. **Calloway, D. H. and Kretsch, M. J.**, Protein and energy utilization in men given a rural Guatamalan diet and egg formulas with and without added oat bran, *Am. J. Clin. Nutr.*, 31, 1118, 1978.
5. **Cornu, A. and Delpeuch, F.**, Effect of fiber in sorghum on nitrogen digestibility, *Am. J. Clin. Nutr.*, 34, 2454, 1981.
6. **Cummings, J. H., Hill, M. I., Bone, E. S., Branch, W. J., and Jenkins, D. J. A.**, The effect of meat protein and dietary fiber on colonic function and metabolism. II. Bacterial metabolites in feces and urine, *Am. J. Clin. Nutr.*, 32, 2094, 1979.
7. **Delorme, C. B., Wojcik, J., and Gordon, C.**, Method of addition of cellulose to experimental diets and its effect on rat growth and protein utilization, *J. Nutr.*, 111, 1522, 1981.
8. **Donangelo, C. M. and Eggum, B. O.**, Comparative effects of wheat bran and barley husk on nutrient utilization in rats, *Br. J. Nutr.*, 54, 741, 1985.
9. **Dreher, M. L., Dreher, C. J., and Berry, J. W.**, Starch digestibility of foods: a nutritional perspective, in *CRC Crit. Rev. Food Sci. Nutr.*, 20, 47, 1984.
10. **Eggum, B. O., Beames, R. M., Wolstrup, J., and Bach Knudsen, K. E.**, The effect of protein quality and fibre level in the diet and microbial activity in the digestive tract on protein utilization and energy digestibility in rats, *Br. J. Nutr.*, 51, 305, 1984.
11. **Farrell, D. J., Girle, L., and Arthur, J.**, Effects of dietary fiber on the apparent digestibility of major food components and on blood lipids in men, *Aust. J. Exp. Biol. Med. Sci.*, 56, 469, 1978.
12. **Fleming, S. E. and Lee, B.**, Growth performance and intestinal transit time of rats fed purified and natural dietary fibers, *J. Nutr.*, 113, 592, 1983.
13. Food and Agriculture Organization, Amino Acid Content of Foods and Biological Data on Protein, Nutritional Studies No. 24, FAO, Rome, 1970.
14. **Garrison, M. V., Rein, R. L., Fawley, P., and Breidenstein, C. P.**, Comparative digestibility of acid detergent fiber by laboratory albino and wild Polynesian rats, *J. Nutr.*, 108, 191, 1978.
15. **Harmuth-Hoene, A. E., Jakubick, V., and Schelenz, R.**, Der einfluss von guarmehl in der nahrung auf die stickstoffbilanz, den proteinstoff-wechsel und die transitzeit der nahrung in ratten, *Nutr. Metab.*, 22, 32, 1978.
16. **Harmuth-Hoene, A. E. and Schwerdtfeger, E.**, Effect of indigestible polysaccharides on protein digestibility and nitrogen retention in growing rates, *Nutr. Metab.*, 23, 399, 1979.
17. **Hawkins, W. W. and Yaphe, W.**, Carrageenan as a dietary constituent for the rat: faecal excretion, nitrogen absorption and growth, *Can. J. Biochem.*, 43, 479, 1965.
18. **Heymsfield, S. B., Roongspisuthipong, C., Evert, M., Casper, K., Heller, P., and Akrabawi, S. S.**, Fiber supplementation of enteral formulas: effects on the bioavailability of major nutrients and gastrointestinal tolerance, *J. Parenter. Enteral. Nutr.*, 12, 265, 1988.
19. **Hove, E. L. and King, S.**, Effects of pectin and cellulose on growth, feed efficiency and protein utilization, and their contribution to energy requirement and cecal VFA in rats, *J. Nutr.*, 109, 1274, 1979.
20. **Kaneko, K., Nishida, K., Yatsuda, J., Osa, S., and Koike, G.**, Effect of fiber on protein, fat and calcium digestibilities and fecal cholesterol excretion, *J. Nutr. Vitaminol.*, 32, 317, 1986.
21. **Keim, K. and Kies, C.**, Effects of dietary fiber on nutritional status of weanling mice, *Cereal Chem.*, 56, 73, 1979.
22. **Kelsay, J. L., Behail, K. M., and Prather, E. S.**, Effect of fiber from fruits and vegetables on metabolic responses of human subjects. I. Bowel transit time, number of defecations, fecal weight, urinary excretions of energy and nitrogen and apparent digestibilities of energy, nitrogen and fat, *Am. J. Clin. Nutr.*, 31, 1149, 1978.
23. **Kelsay, J. L., Clark, W. M., Herbst, B. J., and Prather, E. S.**, Nutrient utilization by human subjects consuming fruits and vegetables as sources of fiber, *J. Agric. Food Chem.*, 29, 461, 1981.
24. **Kies, C. and Fox, H. M.**, Fiber and protein nutritional status, *Cereal Foods World*, 23, 249, 1978.
25. **Miles, C. W., Kelsay, J. L., and Wong, N. P.**, Effect of dietary fiber on the metabolizable energy of human diets, *J. Nutr.*, 118, 1075, 1988.
26. **Miller, D. S. and Payne, P. R.**, Problems in the prediction of protein values of diets. The influence of protein concentration, *Br. J. Nutr.*, 15, 11, 1961.

27. **Miyoshi, H., Okuda, T., Okuda, K., and Koishi, K.,** Effects of brown rice on apparent digestibility and balance of nutrients in young mean on low protein diets, *J. Nutr. Sci. Vitaminol.,* 33, 207, 1987.
28. **Narayana Rao, M. and Sunderavalli, O. E.,** Extraneous cellulose: effect on protein utilization, *J. Am. Dietet. Assoc.,* 57, 517, 1970.
29. **Nomani, M. Z., Fashandi, E. F., Davis, G. K., and Bradac, C. J.,** Influence of dietary fiber on the growth and protein metabolism of the rat, *J. Food Sci.,* 44, 745, 1979.
30. **Nyman, M. and Asp, N-G.,** Fermentation of dietary fiber components in the rat intestinal tract, *Br. J. Nutr.,* 47, 357, 1982.
31. **Peterson, A. D. and Baumgardt, B. R.,** Food and energy intake of rats fed diets varying in energy concentration and density, *J. Nutr.,* 101, 1059, 1971.
32. **Peterson, A. D. and Baumgardt, B. R.,** Influence of level of energy demand on the ability of rats to compensate for diet dilution, *J. Nutr.,* 101, 1069, 1971.
33. **Prynne, C. J. and Southgate, D. A. T.,** The effects of a supplement of dietary fiber on fecal excretion by human subjects, *Br. J. Nutr.,* 41, 495, 1979.
34. **Schneeman, B. O. and Gallaher, D.,** Changes in small intestinal digestive enzyme activity and bile acids with dietary cellulose in rats, *J. Nutr.,* 110, 584, 1980.
35. **Schneeman, B. O., Richter, B. D., and Jacobs, L. R.,** Response to dietary wheat bran in the exocrine pancreas and intestine of rats, *J. Nutr.,* 112, 283, 1982.
36. **Shah, N., Attallah, M. T., Mahoney, R. R., and Pellett, P. L.,** Effect of dietary fiber components on fecal nitrogen excretion and protein utilization in growing rats, *J. Nutr.,* 112, 658, 1982.
37. **Sibbald, I. R., Berg, R. T., and Bowland, J. P.,** Digestible energy in relation to food intake and nitrogen retention in the weanling rat, *J. Nutr.,* 59, 385, 1956.
38. **Slavin, J. E. and Marlett, J. A.,** Effect of refined cellulose on apparent energy, fat and nitrogen digestibilities, *J. Nutr.,* 110, 2020, 1980.
39. **Southgate, D. A. T., Branch, W. J., Hill, M. J., Draser, B. S., Walters, R. L., Davies, P. S., and Baird, I. M.,** Metabolic responses to dietary supplements of bran, *Metabolism,* 25, 1129, 1976.
40. **Southgate, D. A. T. and Durnin, J. V.,** Calorie conversion factors. An experimental reassessment of the factors used in the calculation of the energy value of human diets, *Br. J. Nutr.,* 24, 517, 1970.
41. **Spiller, G. A.,** Effect of graded dietary levels of plant fibers on fecal output in pig-tailed monkeys, *Nutr. Rep. Int.,* 23, 313, 1981.
42. **Stanogias, G. and Pearce, G. R.,** The digestion of fibre by pigs. I. The effects of amount and type of fibre on apparent digestibility, nitrogen balance and rate of passage, *Br. J. Nutr.,* 53, 513, 1985.
43. **Stephan, A. M. and Cummings, J. H.,** The influence of dietary fiber on fecal nitrogen excretion in man, *Proc. Nutr. Soc.,* 38, 141A, 1979.
44. **Sundaravalli, O. E., Shurpalekar, K. S., and Narayana Rao, M.,** Inclusion of cellulose in calorie-restricted diets, *J. Am. Dietet. Assoc.,* 62, 41, 1973.
45. **Ulnan, E. A. and Fisher, H.,** Arginine utilization of young rats fed diets with simple versus complex carbohydrates, *J. Nutr.,* 113, 131, 1983.
46. **Viola, S., Zimmerman, G., and Mokady, S.,** Effect of pectin and algin upon protein utilization, digestibility of nutrients and energy in young rats, *Nutr. Rep. Int.,* 1, 367, 1970.
47. **Ward, A. T. and Reichert, R. D.,** Comparison of the effect of cell wall and hull fiber from canola and soybean on the bioavailability for rats of minerals, protein and lipid, *J. Nutr.,* 116, 233, 1986.
48. **Weber, F. L., Minco, D., Fresard, K. M., and Banwell, J. G.,** Effects of vegetable diets on nitrogen metabolism in cirrhotic subjects, *Gastroenterology,* 89, 538, 1985.

Section 5: Effect of Dietary Fiber on Vitamin and Mineral Metabolism

Chapter 5.1

BIOAVAILABILITY OF MINERALS FROM CEREALS

Wenche Frølich

INTRODUCTION

Whole grain cereals and cereal products are some of the best sources not only for dietary fiber, but also for minerals and trace elements in our diet. An increased consumption of flours with high extraction rates of these compounds is therefore a nutritional aim in many countries. Most minerals and trace elements in the cereals are closely related to the outer layers, especially the aleurone cells, where also dietary fiber and phytic acid are recovered. All these components have therefore, to a certain extent, been defined as a part of the dietary fiber complex.

The complexity of interactions that may take place between minerals and different components in the dietary fiber complex makes it very difficult to predict the bioavailability of minerals in whole grain cereals by chemical determinations of minerals and trace elements present in the cereal products. Due to the chelating properties of the dietary fiber components and the phytic acid, there has been a lot of concern about the effect of an unrefined high fiber diet with respect to mineral bioavailability. An increasing knowledge of the complexity of nutrient interactions and the number of dietary components that can influence bioavailability makes this field very complicated. This includes both the difficulties in the analysis of dietary fiber and the various physical and chemical conditions which may alter the interactions between the nutrients.

MINERALS STUDIED

Bioavailability problems of practical significance are known for some minerals of long established nutritional importance such as calcium, zinc, and iron, but there seem to be similar problems for other minerals and trace elements such as selenium, chromium, copper, and nickel. New knowledge of bioavailability is constantly being discovered, and it seems that currently only a small fraction of these problems are recognized and corrected for.

MINERALS AND UNREFINED CEREAL PRODUCTS

It has been claimed that the bioavailability of minerals and trace elements in diets rich in whole grain products can be reduced in comparison with diets rich in refined cereal products. Great controversies, in the terms of mineral interactions, have been connected with the chelating properties of dietary fiber vs. phytic acid. In earlier studies it was claimed that the phytic acid present in the whole grain cereal products was the component chiefly responsible for the chelating of divalent minerals. More recently it has been suggested that phytic acid is not the component which is solely responsible for the decreased mineral availability. Fiber itself or other polysaccharides seem to a great extent to complex with minerals. However, the results in the literature are conflicting, and it is still debatable whether it is the fiber components, the phytic acid, or both that are responsible for the decreased absorption of minerals from whole grain cereal products.

Dietary fiber is often divided into a soluble and an insoluble fraction due to relative solubilities and other chemical properties. The solubilities of the minerals may be decreased as a result of chelation to fiber components. Dietary fibers could increase the viscosity and reduce the rate of migration of minerals, which, in addition to reduced transit time, could result in changes in the bioavailability of minerals.

The binding behavior of different minerals to cereal fibers seems to be extremely variable, probably due to the various chelating properties of the different fiber components. The various cereals also have quite different dietary fiber compositions with different chemical structure and binding capacities, making the chelating properties of the same mineral special for each cereal. As dietary fiber and phytic acid most often occur together in the cereal foods, it is difficult to distinguish between the effect of the different dietary fiber components and the phytic acid.

In many studies isolated fiber components and phytic acid have been added to the diet to study the effects of the individual components on the mineral bioavailability. It is important to realize that addition of isolated components to the diet only indicates the effect of the same amount of native dietary fiber or phytate present in the original food item.

Generalization about the bioavailability of minerals can be misleading because the chelating properties are not the same in different cereals due to different amounts of fiber, different fiber composition, and different amounts of phytate present in the different cereals.

It is also important to stress that the refining of cereals leads to a marked fall in the mineral content. Therefore an inhibition of the percent uptake of minerals and trace elements from the whole grain cereal products does not necessarily mean a decreased absolute intake due to the considerably higher amount of minerals present in the whole grain.

BINDING BEHAVIOR OF MINERALS

The binding behavior of different minerals to cereal fibers seems to be quite variable, probably due to various chelating properties of the minerals. Little information on minerals other than Ca, Zn, Fe, Cu, and P is available and no agreement exists for the different minerals studied. Much of the older work is still relevant today and has been taken into consideration when conclusions have been drawn.

ENRICHMENT STUDIES

When a single mineral is added to the food, as has been done in various enrichment studies, the balance between this mineral and the rest of the minerals and trace elements present is changed. This type of enrichment study has given quite different results than studies with the corresponding amount of the mineral naturally occurring in the food, even if the same amounts of dietary fiber and phytic acid were present in the studies.

In many studies, both human and animal studies, dosages of dietary fiber and phytic acid which are not physiological have been used. The interpretation of these studies is difficult and extrapolation to normal diets often impossible.

HUMAN STUDIES/ANIMAL STUDIES

Much less is known about the mineral requirement and bioavailability in humans than in animals. Only limited studies on minerals connected with deficiency states can be carried out in humans. It is also difficult to carry out long-term studies, and studies which might cause risks to humans cannot be performed from an ethical point of view, e.g., studies on children and pregnant women. Evidence suggests, however, that many observations carried out in animals do have relevance to man. On the other hand, direct extrapolations from animals to humans do not give correct answers in all cases, and before any definite conclusions can be drawn human studies are needed.

IN VITRO/IN VIVO STUDIES

The mechanisms by which dietary fiber chelates to the minerals are largely unknown. Several *in vitro* studies have been published concerning dietary fiber components that are responsible for the mineral association. The different isolated fiber components have been shown to have different cation exchange potentials, and several factors must be taken into consideration when interpreting the results: (1) presence of different chelators such as phytic acid, oxalic acid, tannins, citrate, and amino acids, (2) pH in the solution, (3) concentration of minerals, (4) heat treatment that may affect the binding, (5) presence of type and amount of various dietary fiber components, and (6) concentration of minerals. It is important to realize that great care is needed when extrapolating results from *in vitro* studies to *in vivo* conditions. The ability of minerals to bind or chelate to the different cereal components or isolated fiber fractions seems to be different in an *in vitro* system than when ingested alone or together with a composite diet.

INFLUENCE OF PROCESSING

The heat treatment during processing of cereal foods, both during the milling procedure and baking of bread, also influences the bioavailability of the minerals present in the final product. This is mainly due to the breakdown of phytic acid, but also reorganization of dietary fiber components, changing the chelating properties of these components. This is important to bear in mind when conclusions concerning the final cereal products (e.g., bread) are to be drawn on the basis of the cereal ingredients like flour and bran. Fermentation and leavening seem to improve the utilization of the minerals.

OTHER FACTORS INFLUENCING BIOAVAILABILITY

The bioavailability, which is a measure of the degree of both absorption and utilization, is shown to be affected by both intrinsic and extrinsic factors. The individual need for the mineral due to nutritional and health status, sex, and age are intrinsic factors. Components in the diet are the extrinsic factors and could have both promoting and inhibitory effects. It is of importance to bear in mind that when studying mineral bioavailability, the composite diet should be taken into consideration and not only a single food component or fraction of the food. Studies on a single food item, on the other hand, can be used to identify the dietary components that are responsible for the changes in the mineral absorption.

The studies made with respect to the influence of other food items on mineral absorption from cereals are mainly done with respect to iron, with only a few studies on zinc. Ascorbic acid seems to be the most potent enhancer of iron absorption, while animal protein improves both zinc and iron absorption. Tea, on the other hand, seems to depress iron absorption.

LONG-TERM STUDIES NEEDED

Adaptation to a diminished availability of minerals is probably of importance after continuous addition of fiber from unrefined cereals. In experiments with a duration longer than 3 to 4 weeks, no change in mineral availability from whole grain cereals is observed. Most of the studies published are, however, short-term experiments, and it is therefore difficult to draw any definite conclusions about the inhibitory/promoting factors until more long-term studies have been performed.

CONCLUSIONS

There seems to be an inhibitory effect on the bioavailability of some minerals due to some of the components in the dietary fiber complex in cereals. Different cereals have different chelating properties due to different fiber components present in the various cereals. In the numerous human, animal, and *in vitro* studies on the effect of dietary fiber on mineral bioavailability, more controversy than consensus is found. There is a general agreement in the literature that further research is needed to clarify a number of questions still not solved.

In countries where the intake of minerals is limited and whole grain cereals account for the main part of energy, the somewhat decreased absorption could be of importance. In diets with extremely high dietary fiber and phytic acid content, deficiencies in both zinc and iron are likely to occur. There is, however, no evidence that the dietary fiber intake from a fiber-rich Western diet will interfere sufficiently with mineral absorption to cause deficiency in a healthy population. Such a diet is usually well balanced with a good quality standard, and animal products are a natural part of the diet. It is important to stress that a natural high fiber diet contains more minerals and trace elements than a low fiber diet, as fiber and minerals are located together in the cereals. On the other hand, if the increase in the dietary fiber content is due to increased intake of isolated fiber components, there is no additional intake of minerals. The chelating properties of these isolated dietary fiber components could have an influence on the utilization of minerals and trace elements. However, much work is still needed in this field. The studies so far completed only give us an idea of the complexity of the mineral bioavailability from cereals.

TABLE 1
References to Minerals Studied with Respect to Bioavailability from Cereals

Mineral	Increased absorption, ref. no.	Decreased or low absorption, ref. no.	No change in availability, ref. no.
Ca	16, 106, 130	6, 13, 16, 17, 18, 19, 33, 48, 58, 59, 61, 66, 74, 83, 87, 88, 89, 106, 108, 114, 121, 159, 163, 177, 184	4, 5, 11, 43, 44, 64, 75, 82, 84, 91, 94, 96, 99, 106, 109, 113, 115, 152, 153, 158, 169, 175, 176, 182, 183, 186
P	151	87, 157, 167, 168	4, 82, 96, 106, 114, 115, 158, 175, 182
Zn	52, 72, 97, 98, 111, 276	12, 20, 34, 42, 47, 48, 65, 69, 70, 71, 73, 84, 85, 87, 88, 89, 90, 96, 114, 115, 121, 125, 136, 138, 140, 149, 154, 158, 159, 173, 178	4, 5, 11, 14, 31, 38, 45, 81, 82, 89, 97, 99, 103, 113, 123, 152, 156, 177, 182, 183, 184
Mn			64, 158, 159, 160
Cu		21, 65, 115	69, 97, 152, 159, 177, 182
Mg	16, 77, 106, 113	12, 16, 48, 66, 93, 106, 115, 159	5, 19, 64, 79, 82, 96, 99, 110, 115, 152, 160, 175, 177, 184, 186
Se			182
Fe	83, 87, 88, 89, 3, 15, 39, 40, 53, 63, 95, 101, 116, 120, 130, 158, 178, 186, 187	1, 2, 7, 8, 10, 12, 13, 22, 23, 24, 28, 32, 37, 46, 47, 49, 51, 54, 55, 56, 75, 78, 80, 81, 86, 88, 100, 104, 105, 107, 117, 119, 131, 132, 133, 137, 171, 172, 179	4, 9, 16, 27, 30, 35, 36, 43, 57, 68, 82, 89, 96, 97, 99, 101, 106, 112, 113, 115, 122, 123, 124, 134, 135, 145, 156, 159, 160, 177, 182, 183, 184

TABLE 2
Description of Mineral Bioavailability Studies from Cereals

Mineral	Subject	Exp. design	Time	Diet	Fiber source	Result	Ref.
Fe	Human, 8 persons	Balance	49–91 days	Controlled 40–50% of energy from white flour	Whole wheat meal (extraction rate 92%) replace white bread	Decreased iron absorption by brown bread, but mean balance positive	107
Fe	Rat	Hgb-relation			Whole wheat bread	Lowered availability; iron from bread less available than inorganic iron	80
Fe	Human, 154 persons	Radioisotope technique	2-week period		Rice	Increased absorption with fortification with $FeSO_4$	39
Fe	Human	Hgb, serum iron, IBC radioassay, ^{59}Fe, ^{56}Fe	15 days	Controlled meal	Corn	Decreased Fe absorption	55
Fe, Ca, Mg	Human, 3 persons	Balance	7-day period, 3–5 weeks		Brown bread (1 lb)	Fe, P, not affected; Mg, Ca, absorption negative after 4 weeks; Mg, Ca absorption positive after 8 weeks	106
Fe	Human, 66 persons	Radioassay, food intrinsically labeled with ^{55}Fe		Controlled, 1 meal	Rice	Low availability	100
Fe	Human, 116 persons	Radio-Fe erythrocyte utilization method	14 days	Controlled, 1 meal	Maize meal porridge	Very low absorption (3.8%)	22
Fe	Human, 66 persons	Radio-Fe, erythrocyte utilization method		Controlled, 1 meal	Maize, wheat	Low absorption	101
Fe	Human, 42 children	^{59}Fe-labeled maize, whole body counter		Controlled, 1 meal	Maize	Low absorption (4.3%)	2
Fe, Mg, Ca	Human, 12 persons	Balance	3 weeks		Unpolished rice (27 oz)	Ca, Mg absorption lowered on unpolished rice for 3 weeks; long term (18	16

Mineral	Subject	Method	Duration	Diet control	Diet	Result	Ref
Fe, Zn, Cu	Human, 5 persons	Balance	28–30 days		26 g corn bran, 26 g wheat bran	weeks): Ca, Mg, retention improved, Fe not affected No significant effect of bran; Cu absorption better because of higher intake	97
Fe	Human	Hgb-measurements; balance			Wheat bread	Not affected	43
Fe	Human				Different cereals	Affected by phytic acid	1
Fe	Human	Serum iron measurements			Whole wheat bread	Affected, possible binder phytic acid	24
Fe	Human, 21 persons	Radioisotope technique; blood samples	17 days		Chapathi from whole meal wheat flour or white flour	Affected, but not significantly. Absorption higher from white flour than whole grain (3.2% contra 1.7%), possible binder phytate	27
Fe	Human, 6 persons, 28 persons	Radioisotope	10 days	Self-selected	1. Rolls containing 10 or 40% bran 2. Rolls containing 0.3 to 10% bran	Decreased Fe absorption	7
Fe	Human, 6 persons	Metabolic balance, serum Fe measurement	3 weeks	Metabolically controlled	36 g bran of wheat	Serum Fe level fell, hemoglobin decreased	49
Fe	Rat	Hgb-repletion test	3 weeks repletion		Whole grain wheat bread	Fe utilization negatively affected, unrelated to phytic acid or fiber	78
Fe, Ca	Human, 14 persons	Serum measurements	6 weeks	Self-controlled	20 g wheat bran	Serum iron fell, Ca unaltered	75
Fe, Zn, Ca, Mg	Human, 10 persons	Blood samples, serum mineral levels	6–12 weeks	Self-controlled	20 g wheat bran 1. Low phytate 2. Normal phytate level	Not affected by wheat bran, phytic acid no influence	99

TABLE 2 (continued)
Description of Mineral Bioavailability Studies from Cereals

Mineral	Subject	Exp. design	Time	Diet	Fiber source	Result	Ref.
Fe	Human, 9 persons	Radioassay			Bread, enriched with ferrum reductum or ferric ammonium citrate	Decreased absorption with bread	10
Fe	Rat	1. Chemical balance measurement 2. Radioassay	14 days	Semisynthetic 310 g bread/kg diet	Bread/white, 60.5 g fiber/kg; brown, 130.2 g fiber/kg; whole meal, 221.2 g fiber/kg	No differences in Fe absorption	30
Fe	Human, 2 persons	Balance experiment, serum iron		Bread 60% of energy	Wheat bread; White bread, 2 g fiber; brown bread, 15 g fiber; whole grain, 22 g fiber	Serum Fe decreased, decreased Fe balance	32
Fe					Oatmeal	Low availability, no correlation with phytate, possible binder phosphor	104
Fe	Human, 4 persons	Radioactivity measurements	10–15 days	Self-selected, 28 g bread	White bread, exchanged for whole meal bread	Lowered Fe absorption in wheat Fe from bran	28
Fe	Rat	Repletion experiment	24 days		Bread, wheat	Fe better absorption from $FeSO_4$ than bread	63
Fe	Human, 11 persons	Radioiron absorption		200 g rice (2 mg iron)	Rice	Low Fe absorption	54
Fe	Human, 42 persons	Radioiron absorption		Controlled, pancakes	Whole meal from wheat	Geometric mean wheat Fe absorption 5.1%; 1/4 of that of $FeSO_4$	46
Fe	Human, 4 persons			Self-selected, meal + bread	Bran	Fe absorption 6.4; in one iron-deficient 19%	9

Mineral	Subject	Method	Duration	Diet	Source	Result	Ref
Fe	Rat	Hemoglobin, regeneration technique			Monoferric phytate from bran	Relative biological value of Fe the same from bran and ferrous ammonium sulfate	68
Fe	Human, 60 persons	Double isotope technique		Controlled	Whole wheat bran, 12 g bran	Decreased Fe absorption 51 to 74%; not phytic acid, but the soluble fraction more than insoluble	105
Fe	Human	Isotope technique			Unmilled rice	Fe four times better absorption from milled than unmilled rice	8
Fe	Dog	Double radio isotope method, total body counting			Monoferric phytate	Absorption not influenced by phytic acid	57
Fe	Human	Radioisotope technique		Controlled meal; 100 g bread	Whole meal bread	Significantly lower Fe absorption from whole meal bread	51
Fe	Rat	Hemoglobin repletion			Corn, NFD up to 15%	Fe 50% less available than ferrous sulfate	37
Fe, Zn	Rat	Isotope dilution technique, fecal and urinary Zn		Semisynthetic diet; 180 g bran/kg diet	Bran	No differences in Fe absorption due to particle size; small effect on Zn-retention due to particle size	14
Fe	Pig	Hemoglobin repletion	7–9 weeks	Controlled, Fe intake constant	Wheat bran 20% of diet	No differences in Fe absorption	35
Mg		Phytate			Bread	May be affected, caused by phytate	93
Zn, Ca, Mg, P	Rat	Balance experiment	41 days, 2-week adaptation period	Controlled	Wheat bran, 10% and 15%	No adverse effect on mineral absorption; favored P retention, adaptation	5
Zn, Cu	Human, 7 persons	Balance	32 days	Controlled	Rice, corn, wheat	Cu absorption not affected; Zn negatively affected by fiber and phytate	69

TABLE 2 (continued)
Description of Mineral Bioavailability Studies from Cereals

Mineral	Subject	Exp. design	Time	Diet	Fiber source	Result	Ref.
Zn	Rat	Growth response, absorption in femur and serum	4 weeks	Controlled	Wheat bread	Not affected probably due to completely hydrolyzed phytate during breadmaking	81
Zn, Ca, P	Human, 3 persons	Balance	28–32 days	Bread, 350 g	Whole meal bread	Negative effect on Zn	90
Zn, Ca, P	Human	Balance, urine, feces	6 days	Controlled bread, 40% of energy; phytate content 680 and 1040 mg/day	Whole meal bread, unleavened	Negative effect on Ca, Zn, P	87
Zn	Swine	Growth measurements				Depressed growth due to phytic acid	70
Zn, Ca	Human	Balance, feces, plasma	20 days	Controlled, 500 g bread (60% of energy)	Whole meal bread (25 g fiber)	Negative Zn balance, negative Ca balance but not significant, binder is cellulose	84
Zn	Human, 4 persons	Balance	4 weeks	Self-selected + bran	Wheat bran, 14 g	Not significantly affected by bran	38
Zn, Mg	Human, 7 persons	Balance	7 days	Controlled	Wheat bran (10–20 g), cellulose, hemicellulose	Tendency to increase fecal Zn loss	72
Zn	Human, 28 persons	Balance, plasma	15 weeks	Controlled Zn intake constant	Wheatflakes, wheat bran	Negatively affected	42
Ca, Zn	Human, 2 persons	Balance	20 days	Controlled metabolic ward 50% of energy from bread	Whole wheat bread	Negative balance of Ca, Mg, Zn, P	85
Zn	Human, 66 persons	Radioisotope technique; whole-body counter		Controlled	Whole grain bread	Decreased percent absorption but increased total absorption; possible binder: phytic acid	98

Zn	Chicken	Growth response	4 weeks	Controlled	Corn	Decreased absorption; only 60% Zn utilized; possible binder phytic acid	71
Zn	Rat	Femur Zn measurement		Controlled	Rice, barley	Barley poorer source than mixed infant cereal (wheat, corn, oat); rice poorer than standard; no correlation between Zn availability and fiber/phytate	103
Zn	Rat	Repletion experiment and growth response	28 days		Wheat bran 50 g fiber/kg	Reduced growth; decreased zinc absorption (phytate possible binder)	20
Zn	Rat	Weight gain, femur Zn content			Iranian flat bread, bread and dough	Bread better Zn source than unfermented dough; no differences on dough with different fermenting time; no correlation between Zn and fiber/phytate	31
Zn	Rat	Growth response			Selected cereals	Phytic acid inversely related to Zn availability; ratio of Zn to phytate important; Zn availability; more inhibition of phytic acid in cereals than legumes	34
Zn	Rat				Grain	Availability of Zn in grain better than in legumes; phytic acid not the only factor responsible for decreased availability	52

TABLE 2 (continued)
Description of Mineral Bioavailability Studies from Cereals

Mineral	Subject	Exp. design	Time	Diet	Fiber source	Result	Ref.
Zn	Rat	Balance experiment and ^{65}Zn kinetic			Cereal	Phytic acid naturally occurring in food; affects Zn metabolism to the same extent as Na phytate	45
Zn	Rat	Balance; growth response		Controlled	Breakfast cereals: rice, corn	If molar ratio >15, depressed growth; biological response not directly correlated to dietary fiber in cereals; phytate to Zn ratio major factor affecting Zn availability	67
Zn, Ca	Rat	Metabolic balance			Wheat bran 0.5% 10% 15%	No significant changes	4
Zn	Rat	Balance studies			Rye	Apparent Zn absorption and retention in absolute values, higher from flour with high extraction rate	73
Ca, Mg, Na, Cl, K	Human, 6 persons	Balance experiment	3 weeks	Controlled	Different cereals, fiber intake increased from 17 to 45 g/day (bran, whole meal)	Decreased Ca absorption. K, Na, Cl small changes, fecal Mg increased, but probably due to higher Mg intake	19

Mineral	Subject	Study type	Duration	Diet control	Food	Result	Ref
Ca	Human	Balance studies	4–9 weeks		Whole meal bread	No change or adaptation	106
Zn, Ca, Mg	Human, 2 persons	Balance	5–6 weeks		Whole meal bread	Negatively affected Ca absorption, Ca, Zn adaptation	11
Ca	Human, 19 persons	Serum measurements	19 weeks	Controlled, 230 g bread	Whole meal bread	Not affected	43
Ca	Human, 27 persons	Balance	6 weeks		Bran (10–20 g)	Lowered Ca in serum	74
Ca	Human	Balance			Wheat whole meal bread, unleavened	Decreased Ca absorption, possible binder: phytic acid	6
Ca	Human	Balance	7 weeks		Whole meal bread chapathi	Decreased Ca absorption	83
Ca	Human	Balance	3 weeks		Whole meal bread	Decreased Ca absorption	33
Ca	Human	Balance			Whole meal bread, bran (22 g → 53 g fiber)	Negative Ca balance even if increased Ca intake	18
Ca	Human				Whole grain	Decreased Ca absorption	108
Ca	Human, 9 persons	Balance	9 month periods: 2–3 weeks	Flour, 40–50% of energy	Whole grain flour (extraction rate 92%)	Negative Ca balance; possible binder phytate; dephytinization gives better absorption	59
Zn, Ca, P	Human, 3 persons	Balance	28 + 32 days	Controlled	Whole grain bread, unleavened or leavened	Unleavened bread: negative Ca and Zn balance; high phytate intake can cause negative disturbance in Zn and Ca adaptation for serum Fe and serum Zn	89

TABLE 2 (continued)
Description of Mineral Bioavailability Studies from Cereals

Mineral	Subject	Exp. design	Time	Diet	Fiber source	Result	Ref.
Ca	Human, 4 persons	Balance	3 weeks		Wheat fiber, 31 g fiber	Negative Ca balance	17
Ca	Human, 6 persons	Balance	11 days	Controlled	Whole meal wheat bread fiber, 123 g (standard 106 g)	Negative Ca balance	58
Ca	Human, 14 persons	Balance (serum)	4–9 weeks	Controlled	Wheat bran, 38 g bran per day	No changes in plasma Ca	44
Ca	Human, 25 persons	Balance (serum)	5 weeks	Controlled	Wheat bran, 24 g bran per day	No changes in serum Ca	109
Ca	Survey, children	Balance	1940–1948	Self-selected	Whole meal bread	Ca adaptation	94
Ca, Mg, Zn, P	Human, 2 persons	Balance		Controlled, 60% of energy from bread	Whole meal bread; fiber, 12.6 g/day	Negative Zn balance, negative Ca balance, negative Mg balance	48
Zn, Cu, Fe, Mg	Rat	Balance			Phytic acid	Decreased absorption	21
Mg	Rat	Balance		Wheat flour, 55% Mg; the rest of Mg from magnesium carbonate	Whole grain wheat bread	Mg available	110
Mg	Rat	Balance	3 weeks		Whole grain wheat bread	Mg available	79
Mg	Rat	Balance	4 weeks		Whole grain wheat flour	Mg available; higher absorption from flour than from the same amount of added salt	77

Ca, P, Zn, Mg	Human, 68 persons	13 months	Self-selected	3 tsp. bran per day	No influence on mineral balance; bran does not cause deficiency	82
P, Ca, Zn, Mg, Fe	Human, 8 persons (ileostomy)	Metabolic balance technique	2–3 weeks	Controlled	Wheat bran, 16 g/day	No effect on mineral absorption except Zn	96

TABLE 2a
Description of Mineral Bioavailability Studies from Cereals (references after 1984)

Mineral	Subject	Exp. design	Time	Diet	Fiber source	Result	Ref.
Fe	Rat	Hgb regeneration assay in weanling anemic rats		Controlled, ± juice	Baked/unbaked wheat bran muffins	Baking + organic acids increased bioavailability	116
Fe	Rat	Whole body counter			Extruded maize	Extrusion no effect on Fe absorption	124
Fe	Rat	Hgb regeneration			Bran cereal, corn meal	Cereals significant contribution to available Fe in diet	187
Fe	Rat	Hgb repletion		Corn tortillas and cooked beans	Maize, beans	Fe availability reduced with 15% NDF; correlation between soluble Fe and repletion. Fe from corn tortillas, being 50% less available than $FeSO_4$	132
Fe, Mn, Cu, Zn, Mg, Ca	Human	Balance study	45 days	Controlled	Three levels of phytate	No effect on absorption of Fe, Mn, Cu; decreased absorption for Zn, Mg, Ca	159
Fe	Human	Isotope study, absorption test			Muffins baked with wheat bran	Fiber not the major determinant of food Fe availability, but Fe absorption lowered in bran muffins; fruit enhanced	119
Fe, Zn, Ca	Human	Metabolic balance	26 days	Controlled	Wheat bran, corn bran, soybean husk	Increased Fe excretion	120
Fe, Zn, Ca	Chicks	Metabolic balance and tissue conc	18 days	Controlled	Wheat bran	Minerals not effected	183
Fe	Rats	Balance	10 days	Controlled	Whole wheat, wheat bran	Digestibility lowest with wheat bran; no significant relation	112

Minerals	Species	Method	Duration	Diet	Food/Source	Result	Ref
Fe	Rat	Hgb regeneration		Controlled	Wheat bran	between Fe and phytate absorption / No change	134
Fe	Rat	Balance technique		Controlled	White bread 6% DF, brown bread 13% DF, whole meal bread 22% DF	Fe absorption higher in control, but no difference within the breads; fiber itself no effect	122
Fe, Zn	Human	Balance study	12 weeks		Cereals, fruit, vegetables increased from 20–30 g	No change in Fe or Zn absorption	156
Fe	Rat	Whole body radioassay procedure		Controlled	Different wheat varieties	Selection of wheat for high protein content, no effect on Fe bioavailability	145
Fe	Rat	Retention study on rat intestine			Maize and wheat fiber	Retention lowered by presence of fiber, polymerization	171
Fe	Human	Erythrocytes utilization of radioactive Fe			Sorghum	Polyphenol and phytate decreased Fe absorption; hemicellulose and lignin possible inhibitors of Fe absorption	133
Zn, Fe	Human	Isotopic retention from fecal extraction	4–7 days	40 g extruded/not extruded cereal + milk	Wheat bran and flour	Extrusion cooking, no effect on absorption	123
Zn	Rat	Balance	4 weeks	Dosa + milk	Dosa (rice and dal)	Zn absorption higher in plain dosa diet than in raw dosa mixture	111
Zn, Fe, Ca, Mg, P	Human	Whole body counter			Extruded high fiber cereals	The total effects of extrusion on bioavailability are small but observable; negative effect on Zn, Ca, Mg; no effect on Fe	150

TABLE 2a (continued)
Description of Mineral Bioavailability Studies from Cereals (references after 1984)

Mineral	Subject	Exp. design	Time	Diet	Fiber source	Result	Ref.
Zn	Human, 33 subjects	Whole body counter		Controlled	20 or 30% wheat bran	Zn absorption improved when extrusion was performed after phytate reduction	149
Zn	Rat	Growth response Zn retention Zn concentration in serum and bone	25 weeks	ad lib.	Endosperm, whole grain, bran enriched crisp bread	DF and phytate from bran; limit availability of Zn to minor degree when Zn is needed	138
Zn	Rat	Growth response Bone-Zn deposition	3 weeks	Controlled	Whole meal, wheat bread, and crisp bread	Lowered Zn absorption when high phytic acid/Zn ratio; improvement by enrichment of Zn	140
Zn	Human	Whole body counter		Meals based on 60 g cereals + milk	Rye, barley, oat meal, triticale, whole wheat	Food preparation that decreases the phytic acid improves Zn absorption	173
Zn, P	Rat	Balance study Femur consistence of Zn, Ca, P	9–12 days		Wheat bran, barley husk	Both sources had more negative effect on Zn than Ca absorption; phytate did not appear as a major factor affecting mineral absorption in barley husk	121
Zn	Human	Radio isotope technique			Browned and unbrowned corn products	Reduced Zn absorption in browned products, probably due to Maillard products	154
Zn, Se	Rat	Whole body isotope study		Controlled	Wheat grain	Se and Zn have antagonistic effects on each other	146

Minerals	Subject	Method	Duration	Diet type	Food	Result	Ref
Zn	Human	Rise in plasma zinc	6 hours		Wheat bran, phytate-reduced bran rice (low phytate, low fiber)	Decreased Zn rise, mainly due to phytate	136
Zn, Cu, Ca, Mg	Human	Metabolic balance	4 weeks	Controlled	Wheat bran (0.4 g/kg/day)	No change in mineral balance	152
Zn	Human	Zinc tolerance test, whole body monitor			Wheat bran	Wheat bran leads to significant reduction in Zn absorption	125
Zn, Fe	Rat	Whole body retention using radio isotopes	19 days	Controlled	Sorghum products	Fe highly available; Zn more available from fermented products with lower phytic acid	178
Ca	Rat	Balance study; bioavailability measured by TIBIA, Ca content reflecting retention	27 days	Controlled ad lib.	Whole wheat bread (enriched with Ca)	Ca bioavailability 95% from bread, same as milk diet	169
Ca, P, Mg	Rat	Balance study, urine, feces, tissue	7 months	ad lib.	Cellulose, wheat bran, oat bran, corn bran at 4 of 14% TDF	Diets did not appreciably affect mineral levels	175
Ca	Human	Balance		Controlled	Oat bran	No impact on Ca intake	176
Ca, Fe, Zn, Na, Mg	Human	Metabolic balance	72 days	Controlled	Wheat bran	Fecal excretion for minerals not changed, except Mg which increased	113
Ca, P, Mg, Fe, Zn, Cu, Se	Human	Balance serum, urine	3 months	Controlled	Wheat bran bread, guar gum bread	No change in serum or urinary concentration of any of the minerals	182
Ca, P, Mg, Na, K, Zn, Fe	Pig	Balance study	26 days	Controlled + 15% fiber	Oat husk, soybean husk	No effect on mineral utilization; Zn balance lower with oat husk; Fe balance higher with soya husk	158
Ca	Rat	Balance	6 weeks	Controlled	5, 10, 15% processed oat husk	No effect on Ca absorption	153

TABLE 2a (continued)
Description of Mineral Bioavailability Studies from Cereals (references after 1984)

Mineral	Subject	Exp. design	Time	Diet	Fiber source	Result	Ref.
Ca, Zn, Cu, Fe, Mg	Human	Balance study		Controlled	Hard red wheat bran baked in yeast leavened bread, 20—45 g DF/day	Increased loss of Ca, but not of Zn, Cu, Fe, or Mg for the increased DF	177
Ca	Human	Urinary Ca excretion	1–36 months		Rice bran	Phytic acid in rice bran decreased Ca absorption	163
Ca, Mg, Zn, Fe	Human	Balance	21 days	Controlled	Fiber 50 g/day; bread w/barley fiber; bread w/whole wheat bran; fruit, vegetables	No effects on mineral balance; improved absorption of Fe, Zn	186
Ca, Mg, Fe, Cu, Zn, Mn, Se	Pig	Balance study, urine, feces	2 weeks	Controlled cereals/ milk	Wheat, oat, barley	In comparison with mixed cereal diet: *barley* — decreased loss due to lower content of minerals; *wheat* — increased loss of minerals, no change of intake; *oat* — higher absorption, especially Fe, Ca	130
P, Ca, Zn	Pig	Balance study		Marginal Ca and P (0.5 and 0.35%) addition of Zn (20 vs. 100 mg/kg)	Barley, wheat, corn	Absorption of P higher in wheat; Zn supplement affected phytase activity in small intestine; Ca absorption influence negative by Zn supplement; mineral absorption different in different cereals	151

Minerals	Subject	Method	Duration	Diet	Source	Results	Ref.
P	Pig	Balance study	6 weeks	Controlled wheat diets	Corn triticale wheat	The higher the phytase activity of the diet, the greater the phytate P availability and the lower the bone mineral disorder; triticale and wheat higher in phytase than corn	167
P, Ca, Mg, Zn	Pig	Balance study	3 weeks	Controlled	Wheat bran, 20% DF	Wheat bran, a source of available P and Mg, but might have an unfavorable effect on the utilization of Ca and Zn; Low methoxylated pectin has deleterious effect on mineral balances	114
P	Pig	Balance	6 weeks	Controlled	Wheat or corn + 0.3% P	P utilization 1.7 times higher in wheat than corn due to phytase activity	168
P, Ca, Mg, Zn, Cu	Rat	Balance		Controlled corn, soybean meal + fiber	Wheat bran, rice, rice bran cellulose	Phytate more reduced in wheat bran diet than rice; cellulose no effect on serum or tissue mineral concentration; rice bran no effect on serum levels of Ca, P, Mg; lower concentration of Zn, Mg, Cu	115
Mg, Cu, Ca, Fe, Zn	Human	Metabolic balance	22 days	Controlled	Coarse bran bread (35 g NDF, 22 g NDF)	Balance value for Mg, Fe, Zn, and Cu did not differ by type of bread; Ca balance was negative; excretion significance greater when consum-	184

TABLE 2a (continued)
Description of Mineral Bioavailability Studies from Cereals (references after 1984)

Mineral	Subject	Exp. design	Time	Diet	Fiber source	Result	Ref.
Na, K, P	Human	Balance	14 days	Controlled	Brown rice	ing coarse than fine bran bread P balance lower in brown rice, other minerals not affected	157
Various minerals	Human (10 men)	Balance study	15 days		Whole or dephytinized wheat bran	No effect on mineral bioavailability	160

Note: OH = oat husk; NDF = neutral detergent fiber.

TABLE 3
in vitro Binding Studies

Mineral	Fiber source	Result	Ref.
Ca, Mg, Zn, Fe	Wheat bran and fractions of dietary fiber	Lignin, pectin; high metal binding capacity; metal binding: pH dependent	13
Fe, Cu, Zn	Rice bran	All three metals bound, probably to hemicellulose sequence of binding; Cu > Zn > Fe. Metals released with enzyme incubation; Zn affected dietary Cu binding	65
Zn, Fe	Whole meal wheat bread	Bran high binding capacity for Zn and Fe. Zn binding pH dependent; lignin and two fractions of hemicellulose high capacity for Zn; complexes with wheat fiber; can to some extent explain decreased availability of Fe and Zn	47
Fe	Wheat, rice	Ionizable iron nearly twice as high when compared with that from chapathi (wheat); percentage ionizable iron was lower in the parboiled rice than in raw rice, but actual amount the same; cereal, twofold increase of ionizable iron when germinating; cooking of rice/wheat did not influence ionizable iron	76
Fe	Wheat, maize	Neutral detergent fiber accounts for all binding capacity of iron. Binding pH-dependent; iron binding by fiber is strongly inhibited by ascorbic acid, citric acid, phytic acid, EDTA, cysteine, phosphate, and calcium; iron in wheat and maize strongly inhibited	86
Fe	Wheat bran	Ascorbic acid inhibits complete binding of ferrous iron; boiling for 1 h no effect on phytic acid; toasting for 1 h: 19% destruction of phytic acid boiling 1 h in 1 N HCL: 36% destruction of phytic acid	12
Zn	Rye bread and whole wheat bread	Higher availability with increased rising time	41
Zn	Whole wheat bread	Dephytinized fiber did bind Zn; adding of phytic acid lowered the ability to bind Zn	84
Zn	Bran, and components of bran	Soluble components responsible for 39% of total binding power of wheat bran; possible binder: phytate. Hemicellulose, cellulose, starch, pectin contribute only 10% of total binding capacity	32
Zn, Fe, Ca, Mg	Wheat bran	Zn, Fe, the only soluble metals of wheat bran associated with phytic acid; at least 70% of phytate does not exist as Ca_5Mg-phytate	26
Ca	Wheat bran	Only weakly binding; no important contribution to Ca binding; increased binding with lowered pH (pH under 5)	91
Ca, Mg	Cell wall fraction	Cellulose, hemicellulose: low availability	66

TABLE 3 (continued)
in vitro Binding Studies

Mineral	Fiber source	Result	Ref.
Mg, Mn, Ca	Rice bran	Minerals available for absorption; minerals released with incubation for 16 h	64
Fe	Phytate, oatmeal	No correlation with phytate and Fe absorption; oatmeal low availability, phosphate?	104
Ca, Zn, Fe	Bread	Cellulose important binder; fiber responsible more than phytic acid	88
Ca, Mg, Zn, Fe	Wheat bran	Binding to cellulose and lignin not affected by cooking; pH-dependent Ca binding diminished by boiling, not affected by toasting; Zn affected significantly by pH and type of cooking (toasting had no effect) boiling no effect at pH 6, decreasing binding by boiling pH 7	13
Zn, Cu, Fe	Corn	Cornflakes bound more Cu, and less Fe than corn grits at pH 5, 6, 7	50
Na, K, Ca, Mg, P	Wheat bran	Ash associated with soluble fiber, coprecipitation due to isolation procedure of fiber partly responsible; dependent on ionic strength and different buffers	102
Ash	Different cereals	Ash associated with soluble fiber components	36
Zn	Wheat bran	Soluble components responsible for 37% of total binding power of wheat bran; possible binder phytate; hemicellulose, cellulose, starch, pectin contribute only 10% of total binding capacity	92
Fe	Wheat bread	Insoluble iron generated due to baking process; the differences found between iron sources prior to baking vanished in final baked product	56

TABLE 3a
in vitro Binding Studies (references after 1984)

Mineral	Fiber source	Method	Result	Ref.
Fe	Breakfast cereals w/wheat bran and germ	*In vitro* procedure simulating gastro intestinal digestion	Wheat bran, germ reduced availability; processing affects availability	117
Fe	Sorghum	Solubility study	Germination, soak, fermentation increased soluble Fe	179
Fe	Maize	Solubility boiling	Availability of Fe same as for soluble Fe	135
Fe	Maize	Diffusing across a semipermeable membrane	Increased availability after extrusion cooking procedure, mainly due to refining of maize	142
Fe	Wheat roll	Digestion under similar physical conditions	Degradation of inositol hexa- and penta-phosphates significantly reduced inhibitory effect on Fe availability	172
Fe	Wheat flake cereal	Solubility during sequential pH treatment	Acid incubation to form an organic acid chelate with iron improved bioavailability with Fe fortification of cereals	161
Fe	Cereals with 0–973 mg tannins	Measurements of ionizable iron	Tannins as well as phytates may be responsible for low absorption of iron in Indian diets	131
Fe, Zn, Mg, Ca, P	Wheat bran and whole wheat flour	Isolation procedure	The different minerals chelated to different DF components; only 10% Fe associated with phytic acid; 60% Fe associated with insoluble fractions; 24% Zn, 60% Ca, 9% Mg associated with phytic acid	126
Zn	Polished rice	*In vitro* digestion; separation of gel; filtration of soluble Zn components	More than 30% of rice zinc solubilized; proteinaceous components increases soluble Zn	147
Zn, Cd, Cu	Wheat, barley, rye, oat	^{31}P-NMR spectroscopy; potentiometric methods; isolation procedures	Minerals associated with soluble fiber fractions; phytate potent inhibitor in wheat, but not in the other cereals studied	131
Ca, Mg, Zn, Cu	Different cereal products	Extraction precipitation	Organic ligand, EDTA, and citric acid prevented precipitation; naturally occurring soluble ligands important controlling factors for bioavailabilities	155

TABLE 3a (continued)
in vitro Binding Studies (references after 1984)

Mineral	Fiber source	Method	Result	Ref.
Ca, Cu, Fe, K, Mg, Mn, P, Zn	Whole oat grain	Isolation procedures	70% of minerals present in kernel associated with soluble fiber fractions, most probably phytic acid/glucans; Fe and Cu the only minerals that are associated with insoluble fraction	127
Ca, Zn	Ca fortified wheat flake	Solubility during sequential pH treatment (pH 2–7)	Citric acid increased solubility of Zn and Ca; his., cyst, alone and in combination enhanced Zn solubility, but not Ca; malate, citrate + malate, lactate + malate, citrate + lactate, glucan did not effect Zn and Ca solubility	118
Cu, Cd, Zn	Soluble fiber of wheat bran, whole wheat grain, inolaxol, cellulose	Potentiometric method	Phytic acid in wheat interacted strongly with minerals	165
Cu, Cd, Zn	Barley, rye, oat	Potentiometric method	Considerable association found between minerals and soluble fractions of all three cereals; the ability to bind was in order Cu (II) > Zn (II) > Cd (II) for cereals barley > oats = rye; between pH 3.5–5, phytic acid important chelator for oats; pure β-glucan from barley no complexing agent	166
	Wheat bran, oat	^{31}P-NMR	Phytase present in oats; breakdown of phytic acid in oats same as for wheat	129

TABLE 4
Effect of Addition of Other Foods on Bioavailability of Minerals

Mineral	Fiber source	Subject	Food addition	Result	Ref.
Fe	Rice	Human	Fish	Increased absorption	39
Fe	Corn maize, bread	Human	Vitamin C	Increased absorption	15
Fe	Rice	Human	Fruit, meat	Absorption increased 5 times	40
Fe	Maize	Human	50 g meat; 100 g fish; 150 g papaya (66 mg vitamin C)	Absorption increased 2 times with meat and fish, 5 times with papaya	53
Fe	Corn	Human	Fish or food of animal origin	Increased availability	55
Fe	Bread	Human	Tea	Decreased availability	23
Fe	Rice	Human	Ascorbic acid	Improved availability	100
Fe	Maize	Human	Tea, ascorbic acid	Tea reduced absorption from 3.8 to 2.1%; ascorbic acid increased absorption 10 times; inhibitory effect of tea overcome if ascorbic acid given	22
Fe	Maize, wheat	Human	Ascorbic acid	Enhanced absorption from maize, not from wheat	101
Fe	Cereals	Human	Ascorbic acid	Improved nonheme iron absorption	29
Zn	Whole grain bread	Human	Animal protein, milk (Ca)	Both improved absorption	71
Fe	Whole grain bread	Human	Tea, orange juice, egg yolk	Tea reduced to half; orange juice increased 2 times; egg yolk inhibitor	95
Fe	Whole meal bread	Human	Fruit juice, egg	Fruit juice enhanced absorption, egg no effect	28
Fe	Rice	Human	Fish	Absorption improved with fish	3
Fe	Wheat bread	Human	Orange juice	Improved absorption	10
Fe	Whole meal bread	Human	Ascorbic acid	Enhanced absorption	51
Zn	Flat bread	Rat	Protein (animal)	Could prevent complexation of Zn with phytic acid	31
Fe	Breakfast cereal foods	In vitro	Milk	Enhanced bioavailability	174

TABLE 4 (continued)
Effect of Addition of Other Foods on Bioavailability of Minerals

Mineral	Fiber source	Subject	Food addition	Result	Ref.
Fe	Whole wheat flour	*In vitro* (diffusion across a semipermeable membrane)	Various beverages and condiments	Choice of beverage and condiments influence Fe availability in either reducing or enhancing	144
Fe	Processed foods of white and whole meal bread, wheat bran, maize meal, corn flakes	*In vitro* (diffusion across a semipermeable membrane)	Fruit juices	Processing increased bioavailability compared to raw materials; Fe diffusibility was enhanced by fruit juices	143
Fe	Rice	Rats fed *ad libitum*	Various carbohydrates	Bioavailability higher in diets containing starch and lactose	150
Fe	Breakfast cereals	*In vitro*	Sugar, orange juice, citric acid	Sugar slight increase; orange juice dramatically enhanced; citric acid more potent enhancer than ascorbic acid	117
Fe	Cereal-based	1. *In vitro* solubilization 2. Isotope experiments on humans	Milk	1. Soluble Fe increased with milk 2. No change in Fe absorption	181
Fe	Wheat bran	Isotope experiments on humans	Ascorbic acid or meat	Iron absorption inhibited 50% by phytate; ascorbic acid/meat counteract the inhibition	137
Zn	Corn germ	Rat depletion experiments; growth development	Citric acid	Citric acid improved Zn availability	164
Zn	Corn germ (0.5% phytate)	Repletion experiment with rats	1% citric acid	Improved absorption with citric acid	164

REFERENCES

1. **Apte, S. V. and Venkatachalam, P. S.**, Iron absorption in human volunteers using high phytate cereal diet, *Ind. J. Med. Res.*, 50, 516, 1962.
2. **Ashworth, A., Milner, P. F., Waterlow, J. C., and Walker, R. B.**, Absorption of iron from maize (*Zea mays* L.) and soya beans (*Glycine hispida* Mx) in Jamaican infants, *Br. J. Nutr.*, 29, 269, 1973.
3. **Aung-Than-Batu, Thein-Than, and Thave-Toe**, Iron absorption from South East Asia rice based meals, *Am. J. Clin. Nutr.*, 29, 219, 1976.
4. **Bagheri, S. M. and Gueguen, L.**, Effects of wheat bran on the metabolism of ^{46}Ca and ^{65}Zn in rats, *J. Nutr.*, 112, 2047, 1982.
5. **Bagheri, S. M. and Gueguen, L.**, Influence of wheat bran diets containing unequal amounts of calcium, magnesium, phosphorus and zinc upon the absorption of these minerals in rats, *Nutr. Rep. Int.*, 24, 47, 1981.
6. **Berlyne, G. M., Ari, J. B., Nord, E., and Shainkin, R.**, Bedouin osteomalacia due to calcium deprivation caused by high phytic acid content of unleavened bread, *Am. J. Clin. Nutr.*, 26, 910, 1973.
7. **Björn-Rasmussen, E.**, Iron absorption from wheat bread. Influence of various amount of bran, *Nutr. Metab.*, 16, 101, 1974.
8. **Björn-Rasmussen, E., Hallberg, L., and Walker, R.**, Isotopic exchange of iron between labelled foods and between a food and iron salt, *Am. J. Clin. Nutr.*, 26, 1311, 1973.
9. **Callender, S. T. and Warner, G. T.**, Iron absorption from brown bread, *Lancet*, 1, 546, 1970.
10. **Callender, S. T. and Warner, G. T.**, Iron absorption from bread, *Am. J. Clin. Nutr.*, 21, 1170, 1968.
11. **Campell, G. J., Reinhold, J. G., Cannell, J. S., and Nourmana, I.**, The effect of prolonged consumption of whole meal bread upon metabolism of calcium, magnesium, zinc and phosphorus of two young American adults, *Pahlavi Med. J.*, 7, 1, 1976.
12. **Camire, A. L. and Clydesdale, F. M.**, Interactions of soluble iron with wheat bran, *J. Food Sci.*, 47, 1296, 1982.
13. **Camire, A. L. and Clydesdale, F. M.**, Effect of pH and heat treatment on the binding of calcium, magnesium zinc and iron to wheat bran and fraction of dietary fiber, *J. Food Sci.*, 46, 548, 1981.
14. **Caprez, A. and Fairweather-Tait, S. J.**, The effect of heat treatment and particle size of bran on mineral absorption in rats, *Br. J. Nutr.*, 48, 467, 1982.
15. **Cook, J. D. and Monsen, E. R.**, Vitamin C, the common cold and iron absorption, *Am. J. Clin. Nutr.*, 35, 235, 1977.
16. **Cullumbine, M., Basnayake, V., Le Motte, J., and Wickramanayaka, T. W.**, Mineral metabolism on rice diets, *Br. J. Nutr.*, 4, 101, 1950.
17. **Cummings, J. M., Hill, M. J., Jivraj, T., Houston, H., Branch, W. J., and Jenkins, D. J. A.**, The effect of meat protein and dietary fiber on colonic function and metabolism. I. Changes in bowel habit, bile acid excretion and calcium absorption, *Am. J. Clin. Nutr.*, 32, 2086, 1979.
18. **Cummings, J. M.**, Nutritional implications of dietary fiber, *Am. J. Clin. Nutr.*, 31, S21, 1978.
19. **Cummings, J. M., Hill, M. J., Jenkins, D. J. A., Pearson, J. R., and Wiggins, H. S.**, Changes in fecal composition and colonic function due to cereal fiber, *Am. J. Clin. Nutr.*, 29, 1468, 1976.
20. **Davis, N. T., Hristic, V., and Flett, A. A.**, Phytate rather than fibre in bran as the major determinant of zinc availability to rats, *Nutr. Rep. Inc.*, 15, 207, 1977.
21. **Davis, N. T. and Nightingale, R.**, The effects of phytate on intestinal absorption and secretion of zinc and whole body retention of zinc, copper, iron, manganese in rats, *Br. J. Nutr.*, 34, 243, 1975.
22. **Derman, D., Sayers, M., Lynch, S. R., Charlton, R. W., Bothwell, T. M., and Fatima Mayet**, Iron absorption from cereal based meal containing cane sugar fortified with ascorbic acid, *Br. J. Nutr.*, 38, 261, 1977.
23. **Disler, P. B., Lynch, S. R., Charlton, R. W., Torrance, J. D., Bothwell, T. M., Walker, R. B., and Fatima Mayet**, The effect of tea on iron absorption, *Gut*, 16, 193, 1975.
24. **Dobbs, R. J. and Baird, I. M.**, Effect of wholemeal and white bread on iron absorption, *Br. Med. J.*, 2, 1641, 1977.
25. **Drews, L. M., Kies, C., and Fox, H. M.**, Effect of dietary fiber on copper, zinc, magnesium utilization by adolescent boys, *Am. J. Clin. Nutr.*, 32, 1893, 1979.
26. **Ellis, R. and Morris, E. R.**, Relation between phytic acid and trace metals in wheat bran and soy bean, *Cereal Chem.*, 58, 367, 1981.
27. **Elwood, P. C., Benjamin, I. T., Fry, F.-A., Eakins, J. D., Brown, D. A., De Kock, P. C., and Shah, J. V.**, Absorption of iron from chapathi made from wheat flour, *Am. J. Clin. Nutr.*, 23, 1267, 1970.
28. **Elwood, P. C., Newton, D., Eakins, J. D., and Brown, D. A.**, Absorption of iron from bread, *Am. J. Clin. Nutr.*, 21, 1162, 1968.

29. **Erdman, J. W., Jr.,** Bioavailability of nutrients from food, *Contemp. Nutr.,* 3, 1, 1978.
30. **Fairweather-Tait, S. J.,** The effect of different levels of wheat bran on iron absorption in rats from bread containing similar amounts of phytate, *Br. J. Nutr.,* 47, 243, 1982.
31. **Faridi, H. A., Finney, P. L., and Rubenthaler, G. L.,** Iranian flat breads: relative bioavailability of zinc, *J. Food Sci.,* 48, 107, 1983.
32. **Faradji, B., Reinhold, J. G., and Abadi, P.,** Human studies of iron absorption from fiber-rich Iranian flatbreads, *Nutr. Rep. Int.,* 23, 267, 1981.
33. **Ford, J. A., Colhoun, E. M., McIntosh, W. B., and Dunningan, M. G.,** Biochemical response of late rickets and osteomalacia to a chapathi-free diet, *Br. Med. J.,* 3, 446, 1972.
34. **Franz, K. B., Kennedy, B. M., and Feller, F. A.,** Relative bioavailability of zinc from selected cereals and legumes using rat growth, *J. Nutr.,* 110, 2272, 1980.
35. **Frølich, W. and Lysø, A.,** Bioavailability of iron from wheat bran in pigs, *Am. J. Clin. Nutr.,* 37, 31, 1983.
36. **Frølich, W. and Asp, N. G.,** Dietary fiber content in cereals in Norway, *Cereals Chem.,* 58, 524, 1981.
37. **Garcia-Lopez, S. and Wyatt, C. J.,** Effect of fiber in corn tortillas and cooked beans on iron availability, *J. Agric. Food Chem.,* 30, 724, 1982.
38. **Guthrie, B. E. and Robinson, M. F.,** Zinc balance studies during wheat bran supplementation, *Fed. Proc. Fed. Am. Soc. Exp. Biol.,* 37, 254, 1978.
39. **Hallberg, L., Bjorn-Rasmussen, E., and Garby, L.,** Iron absorption from South-East Asian diets and the effect of iron fortification, *Am. J. Clin. Nutr.,* 31, 1403, 1978.
40. **Hallberg, L., Garby, L., Suwanik, R., and Bjorn-Rasmussen, E.,** Iron absorption from South-East Asian diets, *Am. J. Clin. Nutr.,* 27, 826, 1974.
41. **Harland, B. F. and Harland, J.,** Fermentative reduction of phytate in rye, white and whole wheat breads, *Cereal Chem.,* 57, 226, 1980.
42. **Harland, B. F., Stringfellow, D. E., Connor, D. H., Foster, W. D., and Heggie, C. M.,** Lower plasma zinc in humans ingesting wheat bran products, *Fed. Proc. Fed. Am. Soc. Exp. Biol.,* 38, 548, 1979.
43. **Heaton, K. W., Manning, A. P., and Hartog, M.,** Lack of effect on blood lipids and calcium concentrations of young mean on changing from white to wholemeal bread, *Br. J. Nutr.,* 35, 55, 1976.
44. **Heaton, K. W. and Pomare, E. W.,** Effect of bran of blood lipids and calcium, *Lancet,* 1, 49, 1974.
45. **House, W. E., Welch, R. M., and Van Campen, D. R.,** Effect of phytic acid on the absorption, distribution and endogenous excretion of zinc in rats, *J. Nutr.,* 112, 941, 1982.
46. **Hussain, R., Walker, R. B., Layrisse, M., Clark, P., and Finch, C. A.,** Nutritive value of food iron, *Am. J. Clin. Nutr.,* 16, 464, 1965.
47. **Ismail-Beigi, F., Faradji, B., and Reinhold, J. G.,** Binding of zinc and iron to wheat bread, wheat bran and their components, *Am. J. Clin. Nutr.,* 30, 1721, 1977.
48. **Ismail-Beigi, F., Reinhold, J. G., Faradji, B., and Abadi, P.,** Effect of cellulose added to diets of low and high fiber content upon the metabolism of calcium, magnesium, zinc and phosphorus by man, *J. Nutr.,* 107, 510, 1977.
49. **Jenkins, D. J. A., Hill, M. S., and Cummings, J. H.,** Effect of wheat fiber on blood lipids, fecal steroid excretion and serum iron, *Am. J. Clin. Nutr.,* 28, 1408, 1975.
50. **Johnson, P. E., Lykken, G., Mahalko, J., Milne, D., Inman, L., Sanstead, H. H., Garcia, W. J., and Inglett, G. E.,** The effect of browned and unbrowned corn products on absorption of zinc, iron and copper in humans, presented at ACS Meeting, Las Vegas, NV, 1982.
51. **Kobza, K. and Steenblock, V.,** Effect of wholemeal and white bread on iron absorption in normal people, *Br. Med. J.,* 1, 1641, 1977.
52. **Lantzsch, M. J., Schenkel, H., and Nickel, I.,** Zn availability in grains and legumes, in *Trace Element Metabolism in Man and Animals,* Vol. 3, Kirchgessner, M., Ed., Arbeitskries Teir ernährungsforschung Weihen stephan (ATW) Freising-Weihenstephan, West Germany, 1978, 460.
53. **Layrisse, M., Martinez-Torres, C., and Gonzales, M.,** Measurement of the total daily dietary iron absorption by intrinsic tag model, *Am. J. Nutr.,* 27, 152, 1974.
54. **Layrisse, M. and Martinez-Torres, C.,** Food iron absorption: iron supplementation of food, *Preg. Hematol.,* 7, 137, 1971.
55. **Layrisse, M., Martinez-Torres, C., and Roche, M.,** Effect of interaction of various foods on iron absorption, *Am. J. Clin. Nutr.,* 21, 1175, 1968.
56. **Lee, K. and Clydesdale, F. M.,** The effect of baking on the iron in iron enriched flour, *J. Food Sci.,* 45, 1500, 1980.
57. **Lipschitz, D. A., Simpson, K. M., Cook, J. D., and Morris, E. R.,** Absorption of monoferric phytate by dogs, *J. Nutr.,* 109, 1154, 1979.
58. **McCance, R. A. and Walsham, C. M.,** The digestibility and absorption of calories, proteins, purines, fat and calcium in wholemeal wheaten bread, *Br. J. Nutr.,* 2, 26, 1948.

59. **McCance, R. A. and Widdowson, E. M.**, Mineral metabolism of healthy adults on white and brown bread dietaries, *J. Physiol.*, 101, 44, 1942.
60. **McHale, A., Kies, C., and Fox, H. M.**, Calcium and magnesium nutritional status of adolescent humans fed cellulose and hemicellulose supplement, *J. Food Sci.*, 44, 1412, 1979.
61. **Mellanby, E.**, Anti-calcifying action of phytate, *J. Physiol.*, 109, 488, 1949.
62. **Miller, J.**, Effect of heat processing diet mixtures on bioavailability of iron, *Nutr. Res.*, 3, 351, 1983.
63. **Miller, J.**, Study of experimental conditions for most reliable estimates of relative biological value of iron in bread, *J. Agric. Food Chem.*, 25, 154, 1977.
64. **Mod, R. R., Ory, R. L., Morris, N. M., and Normand, F. L.**, In vitro interaction of rice hemicellulose with trace minerals and their release by digestive enzymes, *Cereal Chem.*, 59, 538, 1982.
65. **Mod, R. R., Ory, R. L., Morris, N. M., and Normand, F. L.**, Chemical properties and interactions of rice hemicellulose with trace minerals in vitro, *J. Agric. Food Chem.*, 29, 449, 1981.
66. **Molloy, L. F. and Richards, E. L.**, Complexing of calcium and magnesium by organic constituents of Yorkshire Fog (*Holcus lanatus*). II. Complexing of Ca^{2+} and Mg^{2+} by cell wall fraction and organic acid, *J. Food. Agric.*, 22, 397, 1971.
67. **Morris, E. R. and Ellis, R.**, Phytate-zinc molar ratio of breakfast cereals and bioavailability of zinc to rats, *Cereal Chem.*, 58, 363, 1981.
68. **Morris, E. R. and Ellis, R.**, Isolation of monoferric phytate from wheat bran and its biological value as an iron source to the rat, *J. Nutr.*, 106, 753, 1976.
69. **Obizoba, I. C.**, Zinc and copper metabolism of human adults fed combinations of corn, wheat, beans, rice and milk containing various levels of phytate, *Nutr. Rep. Int.*, 42, 203, 1981.
70. **Oberleas, D., Muhrer, M. E., and O'Dell, B. L.**, Some effects of phytic acid on zinc availability and physiology of swine, *J. Anim. Sci.*, 21, 57, 1962.
71. **O'Dell, B. L.**, Effect of dietary components upon zinc availability, *Am. J. Clin. Nutr.*, 22, 1315, 1969.
72. **Papakyrikos, H., Kies, C., and Fox, H. M.**, Zinc and magnesium utilization as affected by graded levels of hemicellulose, cellulose and wheat bran, *Fed. Proc. Fed. Am. Soc. Exp. Biol.*, 38, 549, 1979.
73. **Pedersen, B. and Eggum, B. O.**, The influence of milling on the nutritive value of flour cereal grains. I. Rye, *Qual. Plant Foods Hum. Nutr.*, 32, 185, 1983.
74. **Persson, I. K., Raby, P., Fønt-Beck, P., and Jensen, E.**, Effect of prolonged bran administration on serum levels of cholesterol, ionized calcium and iron in the elderly, *J. Am. Gerontol. Soc.*, 24, 334, 1976.
75. **Persson, I., Raby, K., Fonns-Beck, P., and Jensen, E.**, Bran and blood-lipids, *Lancet*, 2, 1208, 1975.
76. **Prabhavathi, T., and Narasinga Rao, B. S.**, Effect of domestic preparation of cereals and legumes on ionizable iron, *J. Sci. Food Agric.*, 30, 597, 1979.
77. **Ranhotra, G. S., Loewe, R. J., and Puyat, L. V.**, Bioavailability of magnesium from wheat flour and various organic and inorganic salts, *Cereal Chem.*, 53, 770, 1976.
78. **Ranhotra, G. S., Lee, C., and Gelroth, J. A.**, Bioavailability of iron in some commercial variety breads, *Nutr. Rep. Int.*, 19, 851, 1979.
79. **Ranhotra, G. S., Lee, C., and Gelroth, J. A.**, Expanded cereal fortification: bioavailability and functionality (flavor) of magnesium in bread, *J. Food Sci.*, 45, 915, 1980.
80. **Ranhotra, G. S., Lee, C., and Gelroth, J. A.**, Bioavailability of iron in high-cellulose bread, *Cereal Chem.*, 56, 156, 1979.
81. **Ranhotra, G. S., Lee, C., and Gelroth, J. A.**, Bioavailability of zinc in soy-fortified wheat bread, *Nutr. Rep. Int.*, 18, 487, 1978.
82. **Rattan, J., Levin, N., Graff, E., Weizer, N., and Gilat, T.**, A high fiber diet does not cause mineral and nutrient deficiences, *J. Clin. Gastroenterol.*, 3, 339, 1981.
83. **Reinhold, J. G.**, Rickets in Asian immigrants, *Lancet*, 2, 1132, 1976.
84. **Reinhold, J. G., Faradji, B., Abadi, P., and Ismail-Beigi, F.**, Binding of zinc to fiber and other solids of whole-meal bread, in *Trace Elements in Human Health and Disease*, Vol. 1., Prasad, A.-S. and Oberleas, D., Eds., Academic Press, New York, 1976, 163.
85. **Reinhold, J. G., Faradji, B., Abadi, P., and Ismail-Beigi, F.**, Decreased absorption of calcium, magnesium, zinc and phosphorus by humans due to increased fiber and phosphorus consumption as wheat bread, *J. Nutr.*, 106, 493, 1976.
86. **Reinhold, J. G., Garcia, J. S., and Garzon, P.**, Binding of iron by fiber of wheat and maize, *Am. J. Clin. Nutr.*, 34, 1384, 1981.
87. **Reinhold, J. G., Hedayati, H., Lahimgarzadeh, A., and Nasr, K.**, Zinc, calcium, phosphorus and nitrogen balances of Iranian villagers following a change from phytate-rich to phytate-poor diets, *Ecol. Food Nutr.*, 2, 157, 1973.
88. **Reinhold, J. G., Ismail-Beigi, F., and Faradji, B.**, Fiber vs phytate as determinant of the bioavailability of calcium, zinc and iron of bread stuff, *Nutr. Rep. Int.*, 12, 75, 1975.

89. **Reinhold, J. G., Lahimgarzadeh, A., Nasr, K., and Hedayati, M.,** Effects of purified phytate and phytate rich bread upon metabolism of zinc, calcium, phosphorus and nitrogen in man, *Lancet,* 1, 283, 1973.
90. **Reinhold, J. G., Nasr, K., Lahimgarzadeh, A., and Hedayati, M.,** Effect of purified phytate and phytate rich bread upon metabolism of zinc, calcium, phosphorus and nitrogen in man, *Lancet,* 1, 283, 1973.
91. **Rendelman, J. A.,** Cereal complexes: binding of calcium by bran and components of bran, *Cereal Chem.,* 59, 302, 1982.
92. **Rendelman, J. A. and Grobe, C. A.,** Cereal complexes: binding of zinc by bran and components of bran, *Cereal Chem.,* 59, 310, 1982.
93. **Roberts, A. H. and Yudkin, J.,** Dietary phytate as a possible cause of magnesium deficiency, *Nature (London),* 185, 823, 1960.
94. **Robertson, I., Ford, J. A., McIntosh, W. B., and Dunnigan, M. G.,** The role of cereals in the aetiology of nutritional rickets, the lesson of the Irish National Nutrition Survey 1943–1948, *Br. J. Nutr.,* 45, 17, 1981.
95. **Rossander, L., Hallberg, L., and Björn-Rasmussen, E.,** Absorption of iron from breakfast meals, *Am. J. Clin. Nutr.,* 32, 2484, 1979.
96. **Sandberg, A. S., Hasselblad, C., Hasselblad, K., and Hultén, L.,** The effect of wheat bran on the absorption of minerals in the small intestine, *Br. J. Nutr.,* 48, 185, 1982.
97. **Sandstead, M. M., Munoz, J. M., Jacob, R. A., Klevay, L. M., Reck, S. J., Logan, G. M., Dintzis, F. R., Inglett, G. E., and Shuey, W. C.,** Influence of dietary fiber on trace elements balance, *Am. J. Clin. Nutr.,* 31, S180, 1978.
98. **Sandström, B. M., Arvidsson, B., Cederblad, Å., and Björn-Rasmussen, E.,** Zinc absorption from composite meals. I. The significance of wheat extraction rate, zinc, calcium and protein content in meals based on bread, *Am. J. Clin. Nutr.,* 33, 739, 1980.
99. **Sandström, B. M., Andersson, H., Bosaeus, I., Falkheden, B. T., Göransson, H., and Melkersson, M.,** The effect of wheat bran on the intake of energy and nutrients and on serum mineral levels in constipated geriatric patients, *Hum. Nutr. Clin. Nutr.,* 37, 295, 1983.
100. **Sayers, M. H., Lynch, S. R., Charlton, R. W., Bothwell, T. M., and Fatima Mayet,** Iron absorption from rice meals cooked with fortified salt containing ferrous sulfate and ascorbic acid, *Br. J. Nutr.,* 31, 367, 1974.
101. **Sayers, M. H., Lynch, S. R., Jacob, P., Charlton, R. W., Bothwell, T. M., Walker, R. B., and Fatima Mayet,** The effects of ascorbic acid supplementation on the absorption of iron in maize, wheat, soya, *Br. J. Haematol.,* 24, 209, 1973.
102. **Schweizer, T. F., Frølich, W., Del Vedovo, S., and Besson, R.,** Minerals and phytic acid in the analysis of dietary fiber from cereals, *Cereal Chem.,* 61(2), 116, 1983.
103. **Shah, B. G., Giroux, A., and Belonje, B.,** Bioavailability of zinc in infant cereals, *Nutr. Metab.,* 23, 286, 1979.
104. **Sharpe, M., Peacock, W. C., Cooke, R., and Harris, R. S.,** The effect of phytate and other foods on iron absorption, *J. Nutr.,* 41, 435, 1950.
105. **Simpson, K. S., Morris, E. R., and Cook, J. D.,** The inhibitory effect of bran on iron absorption in man, *Am. J. Clin. Nutr.,* 34, 1469, 1981.
106. **Walker, A. R. P., Fox, F. W., and Irving, J. T.,** Studies in human mineral metabolism. I. The effect of bread rich in phytate phosphorus on the metabolism of certain mineral salts with special reference to calcium, *Biochem. J.,* 42, 452, 1948.
107. **Widdowson, E. M. and McCance, R. A.,** Iron exchanges of adults on white and brown bread diet, *Lancet,* 1, 588, 1942.
108. **Widdowson, E. M.,** Interactions of dietary calcium with phytates, phosphates and fats, *Nutr. Dieta,* 15, 38, 1970.
109. **Weinreich, J., Pedersen, O., and Dinesen, K.,** Role of bran in normals, *Acta Med. Scand.,* 202, 125, 1977.
110. **Winterringer, G. L. and Ranhotra, G. S.,** Relative bioavailability of magnesium from mineral and soy-fortified breads, *Cereal Chem.,* 60, 14, 1983.
111. **Ajit Kaur Labana and Kawatra, B. L.,** Studies on protein quality and availability of zinc from Dosa, *J. Food Sci. Technol.,* 23, 224, 1986.
112. **Akhtar, D., Begum, N., and Sattar, A.,** Effect of dietary phytate on bioavailability of iron, *Nutr. Res.,* 7, 833, 1987.
113. **Andersson, H., Navert, B., Bingham, S. A., Englyst, H. N., and Cummings, J. H.,** The effects of breads containing similar amounts of phytate, but different amounts of wheat bran on calcium, zinc and iron balance in man, *Br. J. Nutr.,* 50, 503, 1983.
114. **Bagheri, S. and Gueguen, L.,** Effect of wheat bran and pectin on the absorption and retention of phosphorus, calcium, magnesium and zinc by the growing pig, *Reprod. Nutr. Rev.,* 25, 705, 1985.

115. **Ballam, G. C., Nelson, T. S., and Kirby, L. K.**, The effect of phytate and fiber source on phytate hydrolysis and mineral availability in rats, *Nutr. Rep. Int.*, 30, 1089, 1984.
116. **Buchowski, M., Vanderstoep, J., and Kitts, D. D.**, Effects of heat treatment and organic acids on bioavailability of endogenous iron from wheat bran in rats, *Can. Inst. Food Sci. Technol. J.*, 21, 161, 1988.
117. **Carlson, B. L. and Miller, D. D.**, Effects of product formulation, processing and meal composition on *in vitro* estimated iron availability from cereal-containing breakfast cereals, *J. Food Sci.*, 48, 1211, 1983.
118. **Clydesdale, F. M.**, Effectiveness of organic chelators in solubilizing calcium and zinc in the fortified cereals under simulated gastrointestinal pH conditions, *J. Food Proc. Preserv.*, 13, 307, 1989.
119. **Cook, J. D., Noble, N. L., Morck, T. A., Lynch, S. R., and Petersburg, S. J.**, Effect of fiber on non-heme iron absorption, *Gastroenterology*, 85, 1354, 1983.
120. **Dintzis, F. R., Watson, P. R., and Sandstead, H. H.**, Mineral content of brans passed through the human G.I. tract, *Am. J. Clin. Nutr.*, 113, 653, 1983.
121. **Donangelo, C. M. and Eggum, B. O.**, Comparative effects of wheat bran and barley husk on nutrient utilization in rats. II. Zinc, calcium and phosphorus, *Br. J. Nutr.*, 56, 269, 1986.
122. **Fairweather-Tait, S. J.**, The effect of different levels of wheat bran on iron absorption in rats from bread containing similar amounts of phytate, *Brit. J. Nutr.*, 47, 243, 1982.
123. **Fairweather-Tait, S. J., Portwood, D. E., Symss, L. L., Eagles, J., and Minski, M. J.**, Iron and zinc absorption in human subjects from a mixed meal of extruded and non-extruded wheat bran and flour, *Am. J. Clin. Nutr.*, 49, 151, 1989.
124. **Fairweather-Tait, S. J., Symss, L. L., Smith, A. C., and Johnson, I. T.**, The effect of extrusion cooking on iron absorption from maize and potato, *J. Sci. Food Agric.*, 38, 73, 1987.
125. **Farah, D. A., Hall, M. J., Mills, P. R., and Russel, R. I.**, Effect of wheat bran on zinc absorption, *Hum. Nutr. Clin. Nutr.*, 38, 433, 1984.
126. **Frølich, W. and Asp, N.-G.**, Minerals and phytate in the analysis of dietary fiber from Cereals. III, *Cereal Chem.*, 62, 238, 1985.
127. **Frølich, W. and Nyman, M.**, Minerals, phytate and dietary fiber in different fractions of oat grain, *J. Cereal Sci.*, 7, 73, 1988.
128. **Frølich, W., Drakenberg, T., and Asp, N.-G.**, Enzymic degradation of phytate (myo-inositol hexaphosphate) in whole grain flour suspension and dough. A comparison between ^{31}P-NMR spectroscopy and a ferric ion method, *J. Cereal Sci.*, 4, 325, 1986.
129. **Frølich, W., Wahlgren, M., and Drakenberg, T.**, Studies on phytate in oats and wheat using ^{31}P-NMR spectroscopy, *J. Cereal Sci.*, 8, 47, 1988.
130. **Frølich, W. et al.**, Phytic acid, dietary fiber and minerals in wheat, oats and barley, Proc. 23rd Nordic Cereal Conf. 1987, 327, 1988.
131. **Frølich, W.**, Chelating properties of dietary fiber and phytate. The role for mineral availability, *Adv. Exp. Med. Biol.*, 270, 83, 1990.
132. **Garcia-Lopez, S. and Wyatt, C. J.**, Effect of fiber in corn-tortillas and cooked beans on iron availability, *J. Agric. Food Chem.*, 30, 724, 1982.
133. **Gillooly, M., Bothwell, T. H., Charlton, R. W., Torrance, J. D., Bezwoda, W. R., MacPhail, A. P., Derman, D. P., Novelli, L., Morrall, P., and Mayet, F.**, Factors affecting the absorption of iron from cereals, *Br. J. Nutr.*, 51, 37, 1984.
134. **Gordon, D. T. and Chao, L. S.**, Relationship of components in wheat bran and spinach to iron availability in the anemic rat, *J. Nutr.*, 114, 526, 1984.
135. **Gupta, H. O.**, Iron and its availability in maize (Zea mays L.), *J. Food Sci. Technol.*, 25, 179, 1988.
136. **Hall, M. J., Downs, L., Ene, M. D., and Farah, D.**, Effect of reduced phytate wheat bran on zinc absorption, *Eur. J. Clin. Nutr.*, 43, 4431, 1989.
137. **Hallberg, L.**, Wheat fiber, phytase and iron absorption, *Scand. J. Gastroenterol. Suppl.*, 129, 73, 1987.
138. **Hallmans, G., Sjöström, R., Wetter, L., and Wing, K. R.**, The availability of zinc in endosperm, whole grain and bran-enriched wheat crispbreads fed to rats on a zinc-deficient diet, *Br. J. Nutr.*, 62, 165, 1989.
139. **Harland, B. F. and Morris, E. R.**, Fiber and mineral absorption, in *Dietary Fibre Perspectives. Reviews and Bibliography*, Leeds, A. R., Ed., John Libbey, London, 1985, 72.
140. **Harmuth-Hoene, A. E. and Meuser, F.**, Improvement of the bioavailability of zinc in wholemeal bread and crispbread, *Z. Ernaehrungswiss.*, 27, 244, 1988.
141. **Harmuth-Hoene, A. E.**, Dietary fiber and bioavailability of essential trace elements, a controversial topic, in *Trace Element — Analytical Chemistry in Medicine and Biology*, Vol. 4, Walter de Gruyter, Berlin, 1987, 108.
142. **Hazell, T. and Johnson, I. T.**, Influence of food processing on iron availability *in vitro* from extruded maize-based snack foods, *J. Sci. Food Agric.*, 46, 365, 1989.
143. **Hazell, T. and Johnson, I. T.**, Effects of food processing and fruit juices on *in vitro* estimated iron availability from cereals, vegetables and fruit, *J. Sci. Food Agric.*, 38, 73, 1987.

144. **Hazell, T. and Johnson, I. T.,** The influence of beverages and condiments on *in vitro* estimate of iron availability from wheat flour and potato, *Food Chem.,* 27, 151, 1988.
145. **House, W. A. and Welch, R. M.,** Bioavailability to rats of iron in six varieties of wheat grain intrinsically labeled with radio iron, *J. Nutr.,* 117, 476, 1987.
146. **House, W. A. and Weelch, R.,** Bioavailability of and interactions between zinc and selenium in rats fed wheat grain intrinsically labelled with ^{65}Zn and ^{75}Se, *J. Nutr.,* 119, 916, 1989.
147. **Ikeda, S.,** Characterization of zinc components on *in vitro* enzymatic digestion of foods, *J. Food Sci.,* 49, 1297, 1984.
148. **Ink, S.,** Fiber. Mineral and fiber-vitamin interaction, in *Nutrient Interactions,* Bodwell, C. E. and Erdman, J. W., Eds., Marcel Dekker, New York, 1988, 253.
149. **Kivistö, B., Cederblad, A., Davidsson, L., Sandberg, A.-S., and Sandström, B. M.,** Effect of meal composition and phytate content on zinc absorption in humans from an extruded bran product, *J. Cereal Sci.,* 10, 189, 1989.
150. **Kivistö, B., Anderson, H., Cederblad, G., Sandberg, A. S., and Sandström, B. M.,** Extrusion cooking of a high-fiber cereal product. II. Effects on apparent absorption of zinc, iron, calcium, magnesium and phosphorus in humans, *Br. J. Nutr.,* 55, 255, 1986.
151. **Lantzsch, H.-J., Scheuermann, S. E., and Menke, K.-H.,** Influence of various sources on the phosphorus, calcium and zinc metabolism of young pigs at different dietary levels, *J. Anim. Physiol. Anim. Nutr.,* 60, 146, 1988.
152. **Liu, Z. Q., Chao, C. S., and Wu, H. W.,** Investigation of the effect of a diet with wheat bran on the metabolic balances of Zn, Cu, Ca and Mg in diabetics, *Chung Hua Nei Ko Tsa Chih,* 28, 741, 1989.
153. **Lopez-Guisa, J. M., Harned, M. C., Dubielzig, R., Rao, S. C., and Marlett, J. A.,** Processed oat hulls as potential dietary fiber sources in rats, *J. Nutr.,* 118, 953, 1988.
154. **Lykken, G. I., Mahalko, J., Johnson, P. E., Milne, D., Sandstead, H. H., Garcia, W. J., Dintzis, F. R., and Inglett, G. E.,** Effect of browned and unbrowned corn products intrinsically labeled with zinc-65 on absorption of zinc-65 in humans, *J. Nutr.,* 116, 7955, 1986.
155. **Lyon, D. B.,** Studies on the solubility of Ca, Mg, Zn and Cu in cereal products, *Am. J. Clin. Nutr.,* 39, 190, 1984.
156. **Mason, P. M., Judd, P. A., Fairweather-Tait, S. J., Eagles, J., and Miniski, M. J.,** The effect of moderately increased intakes of complex carbohydrates (cereals, vegetables and fruit) for 12 weeks on iron and zinc metabolism, *Br. J. Nutr.,* 63, 597, 1990.
157. **Miyoshi, H., Okuda, T., Okuda, K., and Koishi, H.,** Effects of brown rice apparent digestibility and balance of nutrients in young men on low protein diets, *J. Nutr. Sci. Vitaminol.* (Tokyo), 33, 207, 1987.
158. **Moore, R. J. and Kornegay, E. T.,** Effect of dietary fiber level and duration of feeding on fiber digestibility and mineral utilization by growing pigs fed high-fiber diets, *Animal Sci.,* Virginia Agric. Exp. Station, Virginia Polytech. Inst. and State Univ., 6, 96, 1986/1987.
159. **Morris, E. R., Ellis, R., Hill, A. D., Cottrell, S., Steele, P., Moy, T., and Moser, P. B.,** Trace elements nutriture of adult men consuming three levels of phytate, *Fed. Proc.,* 43, 846, 1984.
160. **Morris, E. R., Ellis, R., Steele, P., and Moser, P. B.,** Mineral balance of adult men consuming whole or dephytinized wheat bran, *Nutr. Res.,* 8, 445, 1988.
161. **Nadeau, D. B. and Clydesdale, F. M.,** Effect of acid pretreatment on the stability of citric and malic acid complexes with various iron sources in a wheat flake cereal, *J. Food Biochem.,* 10, 241, 1986.
162. **Narasinga Rao, B. S. and Prabhavathi, T.,** Tannin content of foods commonly consumed in India and its influence on ionizable iron, *J. Sci. Food Agric.,* 33, 889, 1982.
163. **Ohkawa, T., Ebisuno, S., Kitagawa, M., Morimoto, S., Miyazaki, Y., and Yasukawa, S.,** Rice bran treatment for patients with hypercalciuric stones: experimental and clinical studies, *J. Urol.,* 132, 1140, 1984.
164. **Pallauf, J., Kraemer, K., Markwitan, A., and Ebel, D.,** Effect of citric acid supplementation on the bioavailability of zinc from corn germs, *Z. Ernaehrungswiss.,* 29, 27, 1990.
165. **Persson, H., Nair, B. M., Frølich, W., Nyman, M., and Asp, N.-G.,** Binding of mineral elements by some dietary fibre components *in vitro*. II, *Food Chem.,* 26, 139, 1987.
166. **Persson, H., Nyman, M., Liljeberg, H., Önning, G., and Frølich, W.,** Binding of mineral elements by dietary fibre components in cereals — *in vitro*. III, *Food Chem.,* 40, 169, 1991.
167. **Pointillaert, A., Fourdin, A., and Fountaine, N.,** Importance of cereal phytase activity for phytate phosphorus utilization by growing pigs fed diets containing triticale or corn, *J. Nutr.,* 117, 907, 1987.
168. **Pointillart, A., Fontaine, N., and Thomasset, M.,** Phytate phosphorus utilization and intestinal phosphatases in pigs fed low phosphorus: wheat or corn diets, *Nutr. Rep. Inter.,* 29, 473, 1984.
169. **Poneros-Schneier, A. G. and Erdman, J. L.,** Bioavailability of calcium from sesame seeds, almond powder, whole wheat bread, spinach and non-fat dry milk in rats, *J. Food Sci.,* 54, 150, 1989.

170. **Reddy, N. S. and Reddy, P. R.**, Effect of different carbohydrates on the availability of iron from rice, *Nutr. Rep. Int.*, 31, 1117, 1985.
171. **Reinhold, J. G., Garcia Estrada, J., Garcia, P. M., and Garzon, P.**, Retention of iron by rat intestine *in vivo* as affected by dietary fiber, ascorbate and citrate, *J. Nutr.*, 116, 1007, 1986.
172. **Sandberg, A. S., Carlsson, N. G., and Svanberg, U.**, Effects of inositol tri-, tetra-, penta- and hexaphosphates on *in vitro* estimation of iron availability, *J. Food Sci.*, 54, 159, 1989.
173. **Sandström, B. M., Almgren, A., Kivistö, B., and Cederblad, A.**, Zinc absorption in humans from meals based on rye, barley, oatmeal, triticale and whole wheat, *J. Nutr.*, 117, 1898, 1987.
174. **Saxena, A. and Seshadri, S.**, The effect of whole milk, milk protein and some constituent amino acids on the *in vitro* availability of iron from cereal meals, *Nutr. Res.*, 8, 717, 1988.
175. **Shah, B. G., Malcolm, S., Belonje, B., Trick, K. D., Brassard, R., and Monge, A. R.**, Effect of dietary cereal brans on the metabolism of calcium, phosphorus and magnesium in a long term rat study, *Nutr. Res.*, 10, 1015, 1990.
176. **Spencer, H., Derler, J., and Osis, D.**, Calcium requirement, bioavailability and loss, *Fed. Proc.*, 46, 631, 1987.
177. **Spiller, G. A., Story, J. A., Wong, L. G., Nunes, J. D., Alton, M., Petro, M. S., Furumoto, E. J., Whittam, J. H., and Scala, J.**, Effect of increasing levels of hard wheat fiber on fecal weight, minerals and steroids and gastrointestinal transit time in healthy young women, *J. Nutr.*, 116, 778, 1986.
178. **Stuart, S. M. A., Johnson, P. E., Hamaker, B., and Kirleis, A.**, Absorption of zinc and iron by rats fed meals containing sorghum food products, *J. Cereal Sci.*, 6, 81, 1987.
179. **Svanberg, U. and Sandberg, A. S.**, Improved iron availability in weaning foods through the use of germination and fermentation, Household level food tech. Proceedings of a workshop held in Narirobi, Kenya, FSTA 22, 10G9, 1987.
180. **Toma, R. B. and Curtis, D. J.**, Effect on mineral bioavailability, *Food Technol.*, 111, 1986.
181. **Turnlund, J. R., Smith, R. G., Kretsch, M. J., Keyes, W. R., and Shah, A. G.**, Milks effect on the bioavailability of iron from cereal-based diets in young women by use of *in vitro* and *in vivo* methods, *Am. J. Clin. Nutr.*, 652, 373, 1990.
182. **Vaaler, S., Aaseth, J., Hanssen, K. F., Dahl-Jørgensen, K., Frølich, W., Ødegaard, B., and Agenæs, Ø.**, Trace elements in serum and urine of diabetes patients given bread enriched with wheat bran or guar gum, in Int. Symp. Trace Element Metabolism in Man and Animals, TEMA-5, 1985, 142.
183. **Van der Aar, P. J., Fahey, G. C., Bricke, S. C., Allen, S. E., and Berger, L. L.**, Effects of dietary fibers on mineral status of chicks, *J. Nutr.*, 113, 653, 1983.
184. **van Dokkum, W., Wesstra, A., and Schippers, F. A.**, Physiological effects of fibre-rich types of breads. I. The effect of dietary fibre from bread on mineral balance of young men, *Br. J. Nutr.*, 47, 451, 1982.
185. **Walker, A. R. P.**, Dietary fibre and mineral metabolism, *Molec. Aspects Med.*, 6, 69, 1987.
186. **Wisker, E., Schweizer, T. F., and Feldheim, W.**, Effects of dietary fiber on mineral balance in humans, in *Dietary Fibre, Chemical and Biological Aspects*, Southgate, D. A. T., Waldron, K., Johnson, I. T., and Fenwick, G. R., Eds., Royal Society of Chemistry, Norwich, Special Publication No. 83, 1990, 23.
187. **Zhang, D., Henricks, D. G., Mahoney, A. W., and Cornforth, D. P.**, Bioavailability of iron in green peas, spinach, bran cereal and corn meal fed to anemic rats, *J. Food Sci.*, 50, 426, 1985.

Chapter 5.2

OVERVIEW OF THE EFFECTS OF DIETARY FIBER ON THE UTILIZATION OF MINERALS AND TRACE ELEMENTS

Juan M. Munoz and Barbara F. Harland

The effects of dietary fiber on the function of the GI tract and the utilization of nutrients vary greatly with the amount and type of fiber consumed. Some sources of dietary fiber (water-insoluble) such as cellulose, lignin, and some hemicelluloses affect the motility of the GI tract and interfere with the absorption of nutrients.[1-3] Other sources (water-soluble) such as pectin, gums, and some hemicelluloses affect the metabolism of lipids and carbohydrates.[4]

The properties and metabolic effects of dietary fiber depend on the speces, age, and growth conditions of the source plant. No two sources of plant cell walls are identical. Because both chemical and physical properties influence physiologic attributes, dietary fibers from different plants may produce variations in experimental results, even when employed in the same experimental protocols. Disruption of the fiber by grinding and cooking may also affect the physiologic effects of dietary fiber. These factors must be considered in order to understand the conflicting results published in the literature, especially in reference to the effects of fiber on the utilization of minerals and trace elements.

The possibility that chelating effects of dietary fiber may produce deficiencies of minerals, vitamins, and trace elements has been extensively investigated in both animals and humans. Available studies permit no final conclusions. Most are short term and poorly controlled, and similar studies conducted by independent investigators often produce conflicting results.

The significance of cation binding by certain polysaccharides of dietary fibers (and the relative *roles* of phytates vs. fiber components in cation binding) is now better understood. McCance and Widdowson,[5] Walker et al.,[6] and others[7-10] have demonstrated that phytate-rich fiber in the diet causes deficiencies of zinc, calcium, and phosphorus. Others have established that effects of dietary fiber on mineral binding are primarily due to phytate alone. By calculating dietary phytate: mineral molar ratios, one may predict the extent to which mineral status may be compromised.

Increasing the intake of dietary fiber is usually associated with a dose-related increase in the fecal volume.[11] Associated with increased volume, the feces contain higher concentrations of fat, nitrogen, minerals, and race elements. This is in part due to the blocking effect that dietary fiber has on digestion and in part due to the fact that dietary fiber, in general, has higher concentrations of minerals and other nutrients.[12,13]

In general, it has been postulated that dietary fiber affects the utilization of nutrients by slowing the process of digestion (decreasing gastric emptying, increasing intestinal motility), by modifying intestinal morphology, and by altering the sites of nutrient transport.[14] Further studies, especially in humans, are needed to clarify the nutritional effects of dietary fiber.[71-73]

Several human and animal studies which look at the effect of dietary fiber on trace element and mineral metabolism are summarized in Figures 1 through 6.

Experimental Studies

Source of Fiber	Humans	Animals
Cellulose	↓ 8, 15, 16, 17, 19, 20, 21, 22, 23	↓ 29
	↔ 42	↔ 32
Wheat Bran	↔ 10, 37	↔ 9, 28, 32, 33
	↓ 14, 18, 24	↓ 30
Phytate	↓ 5, 6, 7, 34, 35, 83	↔ 62
		↓ 79
Pectin	↓ 27, 43	↔ 32
	↔ 42	
Guar	↔ 25, 26	↔ 31
Corn		↔ 32
Whole Meal Bread	↑ 74	

FIGURE 1. Influence of dietary fiber on the utilization of calcium.

Experimental Studies

Source of Fiber	Humans	Animals
Cellulose	↓ 8, 15, 17, 21, 23	
	↔ 42	
Wheat Bran	↔ 10	↓ 9
	↓ 18	↔ 28
Phytate	↓ 5, 7	↓ 45
Pectin	↔ 42	
	↓ 43	
Whole Meal Bread	↔ 74	

FIGURE 2. Influence of dietary fiber on the utilization of magnesium.

Experimental Studies

Source of Fiber	Humans	Animals
Cellulose	↓ 16	↔ 65, 68
Wheat Bran	↔ 10, 37	↓ 30, 65, 66
	↓ 18, 56, 59, 60, 76	↔ 49, 69
Phytate	↓ 52, 53, 70, 75, 77, 81	↓ 45, 48, 61, 82
		↔ 62
Pectin		↓ 68
Beans	↑ 43	↓ 67
	↓ 54	
Corn	↓ 54	↓ 63, 64, 67
Whole Meal Bread	↓ 51, 57, 58	
	↔ 55	
	↑ 74	

FIGURE 3. Influence of dietary fiber on the utilization of iron.

Experimental Studies

Source of Fiber	Humans	Animals
Cellulose	↓ 8, 22	↓ 50
	↔ 42	↔ 32, 47
Wheat Bran	↓ 10, 38, 44, 75	↓ 9, 32, 49
	↔ 37, 41	↔ 28, 33
Phytate	↓ 7, 34, 35, 39, 81, 83	↓ 45, 46, 48, 79, 82
	↔ 40	
Pectin	↓ 27	↔ 32
	↔ 41	
Beans	↓ 36	↓ 80
Guar	↔ 25	↔ 31
		↓ 31
Corn		↓ 32
Whole Meal Bread	↑ 74	

FIGURE 4. Influence of dietary fiber on the utilization of zinc.

Experimental Studies

Source of Fiber	Humans	Animals
Cellulose	↓ 22	↑ 47
Wheat Bran	↓ 18	
	↔ 37	
	↑ 38	
Phytate	↓ 81	↓ 45
Pectin	↓ 27	↑ 78
Guar		↓ 31

FIGURE 5. Influence of dietary fiber on the utilization of copper.

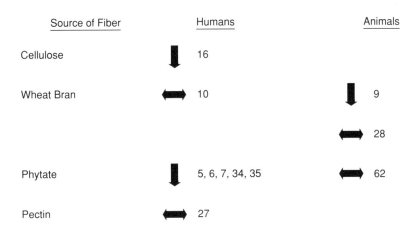

FIGURE 6. Influence of dietary fiber on the utilization of phosphorous.

REFERENCES

1. **Cummings, J. H.**, Consequences of the metabolism of fiber in the human large intestine, in *Dietary Fiber in Health and Disease*, Vahouny, G. V. and Kritchevsky, D., Eds., Plenum Press, New York, 1982, 9.
2. **Fernandez, R. and Phillips, S. F.**, Components of fiber bind iron in vitro, *Am. J. Clin. Nutr.*, 35, 100, 1982.
3. **Southgate, D. A. T.**, Digestion and absorption of nutrients, in *Dietary Fiber in Health and Disease*, Vahouny, G. V. and Kritchevsky, D., Eds., Plenum Press, New York, 1982, 45.
4. **Anderson, J. W. and Chen, W. L.**, Plant fiber: carbohydrate and lipid metabolism, *Am. J. Clin. Nutr.*, 32, 346, 1979.
5. **McCance, R. A. and Widdowson, E. M.**, Mineral metabolism of dephytinized bread, *J. Physiol.*, 101, 304, 1942.
6. **Walker, A. R. P., Fox, F. W., and Irving, J. R.**, The effect of bread rich in phytate phosphorus on the metabolism of certain mineral salts, with special reference to calcium, *Biochem. J.*, 42, 452, 1948.
7. **Reinhold, J. G., Faraji, B., Abadi, P., and Ismail-Beigi, F.**, Decreased absorption of calcium, magnesium, zinc and phosphorus by humans due to increased fiber and phosphorus consumption as wheat bread, *J. Nutr.*, 106, 493, 1976.
8. **Ismail-Beigi, F., Reinhold, J. G., Faraji, B., and Abadi, P.**, Effects of cellulose added to diets of low and high fiber content upon metabolism of calcium, magnesium, zinc and phosphorus, by man, *J. Nutr.*, 107, 510, 1977.
9. **Bagheri, S. M. and Guegeun, L.**, Bioavailability to rats of calcium, magnesium, phosphorus and zinc in wheat bran diets containing equal amounts of these minerals, *Nutr. Rep. Int.*, 25, 583, 1982.
10. **Sandberg, A.-S., Hasselbad, C., and Hasselbad, K.**, The effect of wheat bran on the absorption of minerals in the small intestine, *J. Nutr.*, 48, 185, 1982.
11. **Cummings, J. H., Southgate, D. A. T., Branch, W. J., Houston, H., Jenkins, D. J. A., and James, W. P. T.**, Colonic responses to dietary fiber from carrot, cabbage, apple, bran and guar gum, *Lancet*, 1, 5, 1978.
12. **Southgate, D. A. T. and Durnim, J. V. G. A.**, Colonic conversion factors: an experimental reassessment of the factors used in the calculation of the energy value of human diets, *Br. J. Nutr.*, 24, 517, 1970.
13. **Leeds, A. R.**, Modification of intestinal absorption by dietary fiber and fiber components, in *Dietary Fiber in Health and Disease*, Vahouny, G. V. and Kritchevsky, D., Eds., Plenum Press, New York, 1982, 53.
14. **Macleod, M. A. and Blacklock, N. J.**, The influence of glucose and crude fiber (wheat bran) on the rate of intestinal ^{47}Ca absorption. The influence of glucose and wheat bran on calcium absorption, *J. R. Nav. Med. Serv.*, 65, 143, 1979.

15. **Slavin, J. L., Marlett, M. S., and Marlett, J. A.**, Influence of refined cellulose on human bowel function and calcium and magnesium balances, *Am. J. Clin. Nutr.*, 33, 1932, 1980.
16. **Godara, R., Kaur, A. P., and Bhat, C. M.**, Effect of cellulose incorporation in a low fiber diet on fecal excretion and serum levels of calcium, phosphorus and iron in adolescent girls, *Am. J. Clin. Nutr.*, 34, 1083, 1981.
17. **McHale, M., Kies, C., and Fox, H. M.**, Calcium and magnesium nutritional status of adolescent humans fed cellulose or hemicellulose supplements, *J. Food Sci.*, 44, 1412, 1979.
18. **Van Dokku, W., Wesstra, A., and Schippers, F. A.**, Physiological effects of fiber-rich types of bread, *Br. J. Nutr.*, 47, 451, 1982.
19. **Berstad, A., Jorgensen, H., Frey, H., and Vogt, J. H.**, The acute effect of sodium cellulose phosphate on intestinal absorption and urinary excretion of calcium in man, *Acta Med. Scand.*, 197, 361, 1975.
20. **Pietrek, J. and Kokot, F.**, Treatment of patients with calcium containing renal stones with cellulose phosphate, *Br. J. Urol.*, 45, 136, 1973.
21. **Revusova, V. et al.**, Sodium cellulose phosphate-induced increment in urinary calcium/magnesium ratio, *Eur. Urol.*, 1, 294, 1975.
22. **Pak, C. Y. C.**, Sodium cellulose phosphate: mechanism of action and effect on mineral metabolism, *J. Clin. Pharmacol.*, 13, 15, 1973.
23. **Parfitt, A. M.**, Effect of cellulose phosphate on calcium and magnesium homeostasis: studies in normal subjects and patients with latent hypoparathyroidism, *Clin. Sci. Mol. Med.*, 49, 83, 1975.
24. **Cummings, J. H., Hill, M. J., Jivnay, J., Houston, H., Branch, W. J., and Jenkins, D. A. J.**, The effects of meat protein and dietary fiber on colonic function and metabolism. I. Changes in bowel habit, bile acid excretion and calcium absorption, *Am. J. Clin. Nutr.*, 32, 2086, 1979.
25. **Jenkins, D. J. A., Reynold, D., Wolever, T. H. S., Nineham, R., Taylor, R. H., and Hockaday, T. D. R.**, Diabetic glycose control, lipids and trace elements after six months on guar, *Clin. Sci.*, 58, 20P, 1980.
26. **Aro, A., Usiteyra, M., Korhonen, T., and Sitonen, O.**, Dietary fiber and calcium excretion in diabetes, *Br. Med. J.*, 281, 831, 1980.
27. **Kelsay, J. L., Jacob, R. A., and Prather, E. S.**, Effect of fiber from fruits and vegetables on metabolic responses of human subjects, *Am. J. Clin. Nutr.*, 32, 2307, 1979.
28. **Bagheri, S. M. and Gueguen, L.**, Influence of wheat bran diets containing unequal amounts of calcium, magnesium, phosphorus and zinc upon the absorption of these minerals in rats, *Nutr. Rep. Int.*, 24, 47, 1981.
29. **Momchiore, B. and Gruden, N.**, The effect of dietary fiber on ^{85}Sr and ^{47}Ca absorption in infant rats, *Experientia*, 37, 498, 1981.
30. **Thompson, A. S. and Weber, C. W.**, Effect of dietary fiber sources on tissue mineral levels in chicks, *Poultry Sci.*, 60, 840, 1981.
31. **Harmuth-Hoene, A. E. and Schalenz, R.**, Effect of dietary fiber on mineral absorption in growing rats, *J. Nutr.*, 110, 1774, 1980.
32. **Ari, V. D., Fahey, G. C., Ricke, S. C., Allen, S. C., and Beroper, L. L.**, Effects of dietary fibers on mineral status of chicks, *J. Nutr.*, 113, 653, 1983.
33. **Bagheri, S. M. and Guequen, L.**, Effects of wheat bran on the metabolism of calcium-45 and zinc-65 in rats, *J. Nutr.*, 112, 2047, 1982.
34. **Reinhold, J. G., Hedayati, H., Lahimgarzadeh, A., and Nasr, K.**, Zinc, calcium, phosphorus and nitrogen balance of Iranian villagers following a change from phytate-rich to phytate-poor diets, *Ecol. Food Nutr.*, 2, 157, 1973.
35. **Reinhold, J. G., Lahimgarzadeh, A., Nasr, K., and Hedayati, H.**, Effects of purified phytate and phytate-rich bread upon metabolism of zinc, calcium, phosphorus and nitrogen in man, *Lancet*, 1, 283, 1973.
36. **Solomons, N. W., Jacob, R. A., Pineda, O., and Viteri, F. E.**, Studies on the bioavailability of zinc in man. Effects of the Guatamalan rural diet and of the iron-fortifying agent NaFeEDTA, *J. Nutr.*, 10, 1519, 1979.
37. **Sandstead, H. H., Klevay, L. M., Jacob, R. A., Munoz, J. M., Logan, G. M., Jr., and Reck, S. J.**, Effects of dietary fiber and protein level on mineral element metabolism, in *Dietary Fibers: Chemistry and Nutrition*, Inglett, G. E. and Falkehag, S. I., Eds., Academic Press, New York, 1979, 147.
38. **Sandstead, H., Munoz, J. M., Jacob, R. A., Klevay, L. M., Reck, S. J., Logan, G. M., Jr., Dintzis, F. R., Inglett, G. E., and Shuey, W. C.**, Influence of dietary fiber on trace element balance, *Am. J. Clin. Nutr.*, 31, S180, 1978.
39. **Treuherz, J.**, Zinc and dietary fiber: observation on a group of vegetarian adolescents, *Nutr. Soc.*, 39, 10A, 1980.
40. **Ellis, R., Morris, E. R., Hill, A. D., and Smith, J. C., Jr.**, Phytate: zinc molar ratio, mineral and fiber content of three hospital diets, *J. Am. Dietet. Assoc.*, 81, 26, 1982.

41. **Guthrie, B. E. and Robinson, M.**, Zinc balance studies during wheat bran supplementations, *Fed. Proc. Fed. Am. Soc. Exp. Biol.,* 37, 256, 1978.
42. **Drews, L. M., Kies, C., and Fox, H. M.**, Effects of dietary fiber on copper, zinc and magnesium utilization in adolescent boys, *Am. J. Clin. Nutr.,* 32, 1893, 1979.
43. **Kelsay, J. L., Behall, K. M., and Prather, E. S.**, Effect of fiber from fruits and vegetables on metabolic responses of human subjects, *Am. J. Clin. Nutr.,* 32, 1876, 1979.
44. **Farah, D. A., Hall, M. H., Mills, P. R., and Russell, R. I.**, Effect of dietary fiber on zinc absorption, *Gut,* 23, A920, 1982.
45. **Davies, N. T. and Nightingale, R.**, The effects of phytate on intestinal absorption and secretion of zinc, and whole-body retention of zinc, copper, iron and manganese in rats, *Br. J. Nutr.,* 34, 243, 1975.
46. **Davies, N. T. and Olpin, S. E.**, Studies on the phytate: zinc molar contents in diets as a determinant of availability to young rats, *Br. J. Nutr.,* 41, 590, 1979.
47. **Tsai, R. C. Y. and Lei, K. Y.**, Dietary cellulose, zinc and copper: effects on tissue levels of trace minerals in the rat, *J. Nutr.,* 109, 1117, 1979.
48. **Morris, E. R. and Ellis, R.**, Bioavailability to rats of iron and zinc in wheat bran: response to a low-phytate bran and effect of the phytate/zinc molar ratio, *J. Nutr.,* 110, 2000, 1980.
49. **Caprez, A. and Fairweather-Tait, S. J.**, The effect of heat treatment and particle size of bran on mineral absorption in rats, *Br. J. Nutr.,* 48, 467, 1982.
50. **Tsai, C. Y. and Lei, K. Y.**, Dietary fiber zinc and copper: effects on tissue mineral levels in rats, *Fed. Proc. Fed. Am. Soc. Exp. Biol.,* 37, 562, 1978.
51. **Widdowson, E. M. and McCance, R. A.**, Iron exchanges of adults on white and brown bread diets, *Lancet,* 1, 588, 1942.
52. **McCance, R. A., Edgecombe, C. N., and Widdowson, E. M.**, Phytic acid and iron absorption, *Lancet,* 2, 126, 1943.
53. **Sharpe, L. M.**, The effect of phytate and other food factors on iron absorption, *J. Nutr.,* 41, 433, 1950.
54. **Layrisse, M., Martinez-Torres, C., and Roche, M.**, Effect of interaction of various foods on iron absorption, *Am. J. Clin. Nutr.,* 21, 1175, 1968.
55. **Callender, S. T. and Warner, G. T.**, Iron absorption from brown bread, *Lancet,* 1, 546, 1970.
56. **Jenkins, D. J. A., Hill, M. S., and Cummings, J. H.**, Effect of wheat fiber on blood lipids, fecal steroid excretion and serum iron, *Am. J. Clin. Nutr.,* 28, 1408, 1975.
57. **Kobza, K. and Steenblock, U.**, Effect of wholemeal and white bread on iron absorption in normal people, *Br. Med. J.,* 1, 1641, 1977.
58. **Bjorn-Rasmussen, E.**, Iron absorption from wheat bread: influence of various amounts of bran, *Nutr. Metab.,* 16, 101, 1974.
59. **Simpson, K. M., Morris, E. R., and Cook, J. D.**, The inhibitory effect of bran on iron absorption in man, *Am. J. Clin. Nutr.,* 34, 1469, 1981.
60. **McWhinnie, D. L. and Mack, A. J.**, The interaction of wheat bran and oral iron supplements in vivo, *Hum. Nutr. Clin. Nutr.,* 36C, 315, 1982.
61. **Cowan, J. W., Esfahani, M., Salji, J. P., and Azzam, S. A.**, Effect of phytate on iron absorption in the rat, *J. Nutr.,* 90, 423, 1966.
62. **Ranhotra, G. S., Loewe, R. J., and Puyat, L. V.**, Effect of dietary phytic acid on the availability of iron and phosphorus, *Cereal Chem.,* 51, 323, 1974.
63. **Miller, J.**, Uncooked grain corn as a source of iron for normal and anemic rats, *Cereal Chem.,* 53, 413, 1976.
64. **Miller, J.**, Iron utilization by rats fed high quality protein and iron at different temporal spacings, *Nutr. Rep. Int.,* 17, 645, 1978.
65. **Ranhotra, G. S., Lee, C., and Gelroth, J. A.**, Bioavailability of iron in some commercial variety breads, *Nutr. Rep. Int.,* 19, 851, 1979.
66. **Fairweather-Tait, S. J.**, The effect of different levels of wheat bran on iron absorption in rats from bread containing similar amounts of phytate, *Br. J. Nutr.,* 47, 243, 1982.
67. **Garcia-Lopez, S. and Wyatt, J. C.**, Effect of fiber in corn tortillas and cooked beans on iron availability, *J. Agric. Food Chem.,* 30, 725, 1982.
68. **Fernandez, R. and Phillips, S. F.**, Components of fiber impair iron absorption in the dog, *Am. J. Clin. Nutr.,* 35, 107, 1982.
69. **Frolich, W. and Lyso, A.**, Bioavailability of iron from wheat bran in pigs, *Am. J. Clin. Nutr.,* 37, 31, 1983.
70. **Faraji, S. F., Reinhold, J. G., and Abadi, P.**, Human studies of iron absorption from fiber-rich Iranian flat-breads, *Nutr. Rep. Int.,* 23, 267, 1981.
71. **Harland, B. F. and Morris, E. R.**, Fibre and mineral absorption, in *Fibre Perspectives,* Leeds, A. R., Ed., John Libbey and Son, London, 1985, 72.

72. **Harland, B. F. and Oberleas, D.,** Phytate in foods, in *World Review of Nutrition and Dietetics,* Bourne, G. H., Ed., 52, 235, 1987.
73. **Harland, B. F.,** Fibre and mineral bioavailability, *Nutr. Res. Rev.,* 2, 133, 1989.
74. **Wisker, E., Schweizer, T. F., and Feldheim, W.,** Effects of dietary fiber on mineral balances in humans, in *Dietary Fibre: Chemical and Biological Aspects,* Southgate, D. A. T., Waldron, K., Johnson, I. T., and Fenwick, G. R., Eds., Royal Society of Chemistry, Cambridge, England, 1990, 203.
75. **Brune, M., Rossander, L., and Hallberg, L.,** Iron absorption: no intestinal adaptation to a high phytate diet, *Am. J. Clin. Nutr.,* 49, 542, 1989.
76. **Fairweather-Tait, S. J., Portwood, D. E., Symss, L. L., Eagles, J., and Minski, M. J.,** Iron and zinc absorption in human subjects from a mixed meal of extruded and nonextruded wheat bran and flour, *Am. J. Clin. Nutr.,* 49, 151, 1989.
77. **Hallberg, L., Brune, M., and Rossander, L.,** Iron absorption in man: ascorbic acid and dose-dependent inhibition by phytate, *Am. J. Clin. Nutr.,* 49, 140, 1989.
78. **Lee, D.-Y., Schroeder, J., and Gordon, D. T.,** Enhancement of Cu bioavailability in the rat by phytic acid, *J. Nutr.,* 118, 712, 1988.
79. **Lonnerdal, B., Sandberg, A.-S., Sandstrom, B., and Kunz, C.,** Inhibitory effects of phytic acid and other inositol phosphates on zinc and calcium absorption in suckling rats, *J. Nutr.,* 119, 211, 1989.
80. **Moeljopawiro, S., Fields, M. L., and Gordon, D.,** Bioavailability of zinc in fermented soybeans, *J. Food Sci.,* 53, 460, 1988.
81. **Moser, P. B., Reynolds, R. D., Acharya, S., Howard, M. P., Andon, M. B., and Lewis, S. A.,** *Am. J. Clin. Nutr.,* 47, 729, 1988.
82. **Ali, H. L. and Harland, B. F.,** Effects of fiber and phytate in sorghum flour on iron and zinc in weanling rats: a pilot study, *Cereal Chem.,* 68, 234, 1991.
83. **Ferguson, E. R., Gibson, R. S., Thompson, L. U., and Ounpuy, S.,** Dietary calcium, phytate and zinc intakes and the calcium, phytate, and zinc molar ratios of the diets of a selected group of East African children, *Am. J. Clin. Nutr.,* 50, 1450, 1989.

Chapter 5.3

EFFECTS OF DIETARY FIBER ON VITAMIN METABOLISM

Heinrich Kasper

ABSORPTION OF VITAMINS

Fat Soluble Vitamins

Starting from the fact that fecal fat excretion is increased after a high fiber diet, the question arises whether dietary fiber substances (DF) affect ingested fat-soluble vitamins being utilized in the GI tract. The exact mechanism by which the intake of DF induces fecal fat excretion is not known. Interactions between DF and bile salts or the formation of micelles are discussed, as is the impaired activity of intestinal enzymes. DF binds components of mixed micelles, such as bile salts, fatty acids, monolene, phospholipids, etc. and may therefore impair fat absorption in the upper jejunum.[1] Reduced lymphatic absorption of both cholesterol and triglycerides in rats receiving pectin, alfalfa, and cellulose also supports this hypothesis.[2] Reports on the way different DF influence pancreatic enzyme activity, especially lipase activity, are contradictory.[3-6] Due to the close relationship between the absorption of triglycerides and fat-soluble vitamins, disorders of fat absorption are invariably always associated with a disorder of the absorption of fat-soluble vitamins. Esters of fat-soluble vitamins, dissolved in nutritional fat, are hydrolyzed in the intestinal lumen by pancreatic carboxylic ester hydrolases.[7,8] Hydrolysis takes place in the intestinal lumen during solubilization of the vitamin esters in the mixed micelles.[9] Across the unstirred water layer the fat-soluble nutrients have to be moved towards the cell membrane in the form of mixed micelles.

Vitamin A and Carotene
Experiments on Test Animals

Experiments on rats have shown that there is no decrease in vitamin A accumulation in the liver when vitamin A or carotene and 3% of pectin are added to the feed, whereas the same amount of pectin has a hypocholesterinemic effect when cholesterin is added to the diet.[10] Due to the different concentrations of vitamin A and cholesterin when pectin is administered, the authors believe that this DF substance does not affect the common steps of vitamin A and cholesterin absorption. Even the addition of 5 or 10% of microcrystalline cellulose had no effects on the postprandial serum vitamin A concentrations in rats when radioactively labeled vitamin A was administered orally.[11] Under these experimental conditions there were no indications of DF influencing vitamin A or carotene absorption. Polish investigators[12] have shown that DF, according to individual test conditions, can have a positive as well as a negative effect on vitamin A absorption. Increased vitamin A absorption in rats, indicated by accumulation in the liver and plasma concentration, was found when the daily vitamin A intake with feed was 30 or 90 IU and 10% methylcellulose, agar, pectin, or wheat bran was added to the feed. With the vitamin A dose increased to 300 IU/day, the same amount of DF had a negative effect on vitamin A absorption.

Experiments on Man

Among the fat-soluble vitamins, vitamin A has been the most extensively studied in man. Mahle and Patton[13] reported that subsequent to 8 g of a hydrophilic mucilloid laxative extracted from psyllium being administered daily neither the fecal excretion of vitamin A and carotene was increased nor were plasma vitamin A and carotene concentrations affected by long-term intake of hyrophilic mucilloid. In contrast to this, Kelsay et al.,[14] using other experimental conditions, reported that carotene excretion after a high fiber diet was approximately double that of a low fiber diet. In healthy subjects a mixed diet containing fiber from fruits and vegetables was compared with the same diet, in which fruit and vegetable juices replaced the fruits and vegetables. Carotene was added to the low fiber diet to make the two diets as equivalent as possible in all respects except fiber.

Wheat bran, pectin, carob seed flour, microcrystalline cellulose, and guar, administered together with a formula diet, had no negative effect on a vitamin A tolerance test in healthy subjects. Compared with the area under the postprandial serum concentration curve, there was an increase in vitamin A absorption subsequent to the above-mentioned DF being administered.[15] Barnard and Heaton[16] stress the point that in healthy subjects cholestyramine added to a test meal reduced vitamin A absorption, whereas lignin had no significant effect. In patients suffering from steatorrhea in the course of an excretory pancreatic insufficiency in chronic pancreatitis (mean daily fecal fat excretion 38 g), the additional ingestion of 10 g pectin together with a standard meal had no effect on the serum vitamin A concentrations when 300,000 IU vitamin A palmitate were added to the meal.[17]

Single tests are inappropriate to determine whether or not long-term administration of large amounts of DF leads to the concentration of an essential serum nutrient or impairment of the supply required. The three well-known long-term studies on man on serum vitamin A concentrations subsequent to increased ingestion of DF come to different conclusions. During an experiment on 68 patients receiving two tablespoons of bran per day over a period of at least 6 months, it was found that serum vitamin A concentrations were higher compared to the initial figures,[18] whereas in another experiment on 4 subjects after the daily intake of 15 g apple pectin or 30 g wheat bran over a period of 50 days, a decrease in vitamin A concentrations was found, while serum carotene concentrations remained unchanged.[16] Wahal and co-workers[19] tested the effect of wheat bran on serum vitamin A levels in healthy subjects during a 6-week trial. The addition of wheat bran to a standard diet with 20,000 units of vitamin A significantly lowered serum vitamin A levels within 1 week, and this trend continued over 3 weeks. They suggest that bran in the wheat flour which forms the staple diet in some parts of India may contribute towards the vitamin A deficiency state commonly observed in this country.

Vitamin D
Experiments on Test Animals

Investigations on chickens revealed that carboxymethylcellulose, pectin, and guar led to decreased fat and nitrogen utilization, and, if given with diets marginally deficient in vitamin D_3, led to the development of rickets. These findings indicate that the above-mentioned carbohydrates have a negative effect on vitamin D_3 absorption.[20]

Experiments on Man

Several findings indicate that a high intake of fiber from unleavened whole meal wheat flat bread is responsible for rickets occurring in population groups in Asia. The significance of the rich phytate concentration and the role of wheat fiber, especially its lignin component, is currently being discussed. Lignin combines with bile acids and increases their excretion. The authors postulate that vitamin D probably becomes attached to the fiber/bile-acid/ complex and is transported unabsorbed through the gut.[21] Serum or urinary calcium and phosphate concentrations and the serum alkaline phosphatase concentrations, obtained during investigations on children treated with bran for constipation, indicate that under this therapy vitamin D-deficiency rickets may develop.[22] Experimental high fiber diets have been reported to reduce plasma half-life of 25 (OH) D.[23] This finding in combination with a low vitamin D intake and bioavailability may explain the high incidence of rickets and low plasma 25 (OH) D concentrations in some population groups and in infants on macrobiotic diets.[24,25]

Vitamin E
Experiments on Test Animals

There have been several fiber and vitamin E studies conducted on rats. From these studies it appears that intakes of pectin decrease vitamin E bioavailability, but fiber-containing breads or cereals have only transient or no effects.[26-28]

Experiments in Man

The glucomannan konjac mannan has a lowering effect on vitamin E absorption in healthy volunteers and in diabetic patients. This could be demonstrated with the vitamin E tolerance test when the glucomannan was added to the test meal.[29]

Vitamin K

It is uncertain whether there are relations between vitamin K metabolism and ingestion of dietary fiber. Investigations on the influence of DF on vitamin K absorption and serum vitamin K concentration are not available. The prothrombin and thromboplastin times of diabetics who were treated with a high fiber diet (25 to 35 g dietary fiber per 1000 kcal) for an average of 21 months remained unchanged. This indicates that the high fiber diet does not impair vitamin K absorption.[30] From the fact that the concentration of coagulation factors is changed if the fat and dietary fiber content of the diet is altered, it must be inferred that coagulation factors are not sufficiently reliable parameters for judging vitamin K absorption.[31]

Water-Soluble Vitamins

The underlying mechanisms of water-soluble vitamins being absorbed are more complex and less uniform than those of the fat-soluble vitamins. Some of them, such as folic acid, must be transformed in the intestinal lumen prior to absorption.

Thiamin (Vitamin B_1), Pantothenic Acid, Biotin

No data published.

Riboflavin (Vitamin B_2)

The influence of high and low fiber diets on urinary riboflavin excretion was examined in healthy subjects. Compared to a control group receiving a low fiber diet, coarse and fine bran, cellulose, and cabbage increased urinary excretion for 8 h when 15 mg riboflavin-5'-phosphate were administered orally with breakfast. The authors concluded that dietary fiber accelerates GI riboflavin absorption.[32] In another study the impact of psyllium gum, wheat bran, and a combination of the two on the absorption of pharmacological doses of riboflavin (30 mg) was examined with a riboflavin load test. Fractional urine collections were made for 24 h. No effect of wheat bran on riboflavin absorption was detected, but psyllium gum reduced the 24-h apparent absorption of riboflavin from 31.8 to 25.4%.[33]

Pyridoxine (Vitamine B_6)
Experiments on Test Animals

A number of experiments on animals and man using natural and purified forms of dietary fiber suggest that dietary fiber has little effect on the bioavailability of vitamin B_6 in foods.[34] Bioassays on rats and chickens receiving cellulose, pectin, wheat bran, and mixtures of cellulose, pectin, and lignin indicated no inhibitory effect of these test materials on the bioavailability of pyridoxine.[35]

Experiments on Man

In man receiving 15 mg pectin daily, there was no negative effect on plasma pyridoxal-5'-phosphate concentration and urinary 4-pyridoxic-acid excretion. This indicates that dietary pectin supplementation has no effect on the utilization of dietary vitamin B_6.[36] There were no uniform results in experiments on the bioavailability of vitamin B_6 in bread containing varying amounts of wheat bran. Whereas some investigators[37] found similar plasma pyridoxal-5'-phosphate concentrations in man after the intake of white and whole wheat breads, others reported significantly higher fecal B_6 excretion with whole grain bread than with white bread. The plasma vitamin B_6 concentrations were slightly lower subsequent to whole grain bread being ingested.[37] It appears that the significantly higher consumption of dietary fiber by vegetarians has no adverse effect on the availability or metabolism of vitamin B_6.[38,39]

Nicotinic Acid (Niacin, Vitamin PP)

Sina et al.[11] studied the influence of microcrystalline cellulose on the absorption of radioactively labeled nicotinic acid in rats. Serum activity was measured subsequent to the labeled vitamin being administered orally with or without the addition of 5 or 10 g microcrystalline cellulose to the feed. Serum radioactivity was significantly higher when microcrystalline cellulose was added.

Folic Acid

According to the experiments of Luther et al.,[40] DF can bind pteroylmonoglutamates but not polyglutamates. This would suggest that naturally occurring dietary polyglutamates could be split by the normal intestinal conjugase activity, but the product might be bound in the presence of DF. Despite the fact that insoluble dietary residue of various foods was used in this study, other investigators[41] incubated folic acid with defined DF (cellulose, pectin, lignin, sodium alginate, and wheat bran) without observing an absorptive effect. No effects of these DF on plasma or hepatic folate concentrations could be demonstrated in feeding experiments on chickens. Two 6-month studies on patients with diverticulosis, constipation, and irritable colon yielded opposite results. In the patients of one study receiving 3 teaspoons of wheat bran daily, serum folic acid concentration was significantly decreased.[42] In the patients of the other study, administered 10 to 40 g wheat bran daily, there was a significantly higher average folic acid concentration at the end of the observation period than there was at the beginning.[17] These fluctuations of serum folic acid concentrations are probably due to different eating habits during the various seasons, rather than to the ingestion of wheat bran. Results were negative when folic acid monoglutamate was incubated with high fiber bread, like that consumed in Iran. Experiments on healthy subjects showed that there is no change in folate absorption between the low fiber and the high fiber bread meals.[43] After a 21-month treatment of diabetics with a high fiber diet, serum folic acid levels were normal.[30] The results of the investigation show that supply of folic acid requirements is not impaired if a mixed high fiber diet is administered like the one recommended for prophylaxis and therapy of metabolic and GI disorders. Since, however, there are indications that conventional nutrition in Western industrialized countries does not invariably meet folic acid requirements,[44] it cannot be denied that ingestion of bran or isolated DF leads to folic acid requirements being impaired.

As studies on healthy subjects show, maximum postprandial serum folic acid concentrations were obtained subsequent to 200-mg folic acid monoglutamate being ingested together with a standardized test meal. The above-mentioned concentrations were obtained 1 to 2 h later than in the control experiment when 5 g guar, 10 g pectin, or 20 g wheat bran were added to the test meal. The areas under the folic acid concentration curves show that total absorption was significantly decreased up to 7 h after the intake when guar and bran were added to the test meal.[17] Keagy and co-workers[45] have examined the effect of wheat bran or California small white beans in the diet on absorption of monoglutamyl (PteGlu) and heptaglutamyl folic acid (PteGlu7) in healthy men. Relative folate absorption was determined by measuring 24-h urinary folate excretion and serum folate levels at 0, 1, and 2 h after ingestion of a formula meal containing 1.13 μmol PteGlu or PteGlu 7 (500 μg PteGlu equivalent). Addition of 30 g wheat bran accelerated PteGlu absorption whereas PteGlu7 absorption was not significantly affected by either food. Effects of the two foods were qualitatively different. Wheat bran increased the absorption of PteGlu relative to PteGlu7 whereas beans minimized the difference between PteGlu and PteGlu 7 serum areas.

Cobalamin (Vitamin B_{12})
Experiments on Test Animals

Cullen and Oace[46] have examined the effects of cellulose or pectin supplements upon vitamin B_{12} metabolism in rats. The experiments demonstrated that the addition of either 20 to 50% cellulose or 5 to 20% pectin to the semipurified B_{12}-deficient diet enhanced the depletion of body stores of vitamin B_{12}. The authors suggest that both fibers interfere with the recovery of biliary vitamin B_{12} by binding to a residue that is little metabolized until it passes the ileum reabsorption site. Urinary methylmalonic acid excretion was also measured and used as a parameter of vitamin B_{12} deficiency. Compared to the control group, urinary excretion increased significantly subsequent to cellulose and pectin being ingested. However, this occurred much earlier and to a greater extent with pectin than with cellulose. The reason for this is not known. The authors postulate that there may be greater production of propionate during the bacterial decomposition of pectin. In B_{12} deficiencies, methylmalonic acid is produced from propionic acid in the liver. Another explanation would be a change in the intestinal flora with a resulting increase in B_{12} consumption.

Experiments on Man

The influence of DF on vitamin B_{12} has not been studied systematically hitherto. It is only known that there is no change in serum vitamin B_{12} concentrations in patients with diverticulosis on 6-month wheat bran therapy.[42] The serum vitamin B_{12} concentration of diabetics 21 months subsequent to a high fiber diet being administered was also in the normal range.[30] In healthy volunteers and in diabetic patients, vitamin B_{12} absorption was not affected when the glucomannan konjac mannan was added to a test meal.[29]

Ascorbic Acid (Vitamin C)

With 100 mg ascorbic acid being administered daily to healthy subjects, a significant increase in urinary excretion of the vitamin was observed when 14 g hemicellulose was added to the diet. Cellulose and pectin had no effect on urinary ascorbic acid concentration.[47] Postprandial serum concentrations were not measured. Contrary to all expectations, these findings might indicate an increase in intestinal ascorbic acid absorption. Preliminary results of other investigators confirm these findings. They were able to show that 5 g pectin as well as 10 g wheat bran increase serum vitamin C concentration and urinary excretion significantly when they are ingested together with a formula diet containing 400 mg ascorbic acid.[48]

ENTERAL VITAMIN SYNTHESIS

Due to the findings of a large number of experiments on animals it could be definitely demonstrated that those carbohydrates which are hard to digest stimulate the intestinal synthesis of B vitamins and vitamin K. There have been various studies, especially on raw potato starch, inositol, mannitol, sorbitol, pectin, and cellulose. Since the colon is the site of vitamin synthesis, vitamins synthesized in the intestine can probably contribute to the supply of what is required only when coprophagy takes place.[49] For example, rats resist dietary vitamin K deficiency by eating their own feces. Prevention of coprophagy in these animals leads to vitamin K deficiency after a short time.[50] There are findings, however, which indicate that vitamin K requirements even in man are met to a large extent by the intestinal flora.[51] It is not known whether during possible absorption of internally synthesized vitamin K the content of nutritional DF in man determines the amount of synthesized and hence absorbed vitamin K.

Since the human small intestine often harbors considerable microflora,[52] and a free intrinsic factor is often present in the lumen of the small intestine,[53] there has been speculation that vitamin B_{12} synthesized by the small intestinal flora contributes to vitamin B_{12} requirements being met. This might account for the absence of vitamin B_{12} deficiency in some groups of vegetarians.[54] It is not known to what extent bacterial vitamin synthesize in man's small intestine, and thus the requirement in vitamin B_{12} being met can be influenced by those carbohydrates being ingested which are difficult to absorb.

REFERENCES

1. **Vahouny, G. V., Tombes, R., Cassidy, M. M., Kritchevsky, D., and Gallo, L. L.,** Dietary fibers. VI. Binding of fatty acids and monolein from mixed micelles containing bile salts and lecithin, *Proc. Soc. Exp. Biol. Med.,* 166, 12, 1981.
2. **Vahouny, G. V., Roy, R., Gallo, L. L., Story, J. A., and Cassidy, M. M.,** Dietary fibers. III. Effects of chronic intake on cholesterol absorption and metabolism in the rat, *Am. J. Clin. Nutr.,* 33, 2182, 1980.
3. **Dutta, S. K., Bustin, M., and Rubin, J.,** Effect of dietary fiber on pancreatic enzymes and fat malabsorption in pancreatic insufficiency, *Gastroenterology,* 80A, 1939, 1981.
4. **Dunaif, G. and Schneeman, B. O.,** Effects of several sources of dietary fiber on human pancreatic enzymes activity in vitro, *Fed. Proc. Fed. Am. Soc. Exp. Biol.,* 40A, 3500, 1981.
5. **Schneeman, B. O. and Gallaher, D.,** Loss of lipase activity with fiber treatment, *Fed. Proc. Fed. Am. Soc. Exp. Biol.,* 37, 849A, 1978.
6. **Sommer, H. and Kasper, H.,** The effect of dietary fiber on the pancreatic excretory function, *Hepatogastroenterology,* 27, 477, 1980.
7. **Lombardo, D. and Guy, O.,** Studies on the substrate specificity of a carboxyl esterhydrolase from human pancreatic juice. II. Action of cholesterol esters and lipid-soluble vitamin esters, *Biochim. Biophys. Acta,* 611, 147, 1980.
8. **Mathias, P. M., Harries, J. T., Peters, T. J., and Muller, D. P. R.,** Studies on the in vivo absorption of micellar solutions of tocopherol and tocopheryl acetate in the rat, *J. Lipid Res.,* 22, 829, 1981.
9. **Friedman, H. I. and Nylund, B.,** Intestinal fat digestion, absorption, and transport, *Am. J. Clin. Nutr.,* 33, 1108, 1980.
10. **Phillips, W. E. J. and Brien, R. L.,** Effect of pectin, a hypocholesterolemic polysaccharide, on vitamin A utilization in rat, *J. Nutr.,* 100, 289, 1970.
11. **Sina, P. A., Provenghi, R. R., and Cantone, A.,** Dietary cellulose and intestinal absorption of nutrients in rats, *Biochem. Exp. Biol.,* 12, 321, 1976.
12. **Gronowska-Senger, A., Chudy, D., and Smaczny, E.,** Poziom blonnika w diecie a wykorzystanie witaminy. A przez organizm, *Roczn, Pzh.,* 30, 553, 1979.
13. **Mahle, A. E. and Patton, H. M.,** Carotene and vitamin E metabolism in man: the excretion and plasma level as influenced by orally administered mineral oil and a hydrophilic mucilloid, *Gastroenterology,* 9, 44, 1947.
14. **Kelsay, J. L., Behall, K. M., and Prather, E. S.,** Effect of fiber from fruits and vegetables on calcium, magnesium, iron, silicon and vitamin A balances of human subjects, *Fed. Proc. Fed. Am. Soc. Exp. Biol.,* 37, 755, 1978.
15. **Kasper, H., Rabast, U., Fassl, H., and Fehle, F.,** The effect of dietary fiber on the postprandial serum vitamin A concentration in man, *Am. J. Clin. Nutr.,* 32, 1847, 1979.

16. **Barnard, D. L. and Heaton, K. W.**, Bile acids and vitamin A absorption in man: the effects of two bile acid-binding agents, cholestyramine and lignin, *Gut,* 14, 316, 1973.
17. **Kasper, H. and Schrezenmeir, J.**, unpublished data.
18. **Rattan, J., Levin, N. E., Graff, N., Weizer, T., and Gilat, N.**, A high-fiber diet does not cause mineral and nutrient deficiencies, *J. Clin. Gastroenterol.,* 3, 389, 1981.
19. **Wahal, P. K., Singh, R., Kishore, B., Prakash, V., Maheshwari, B. B., Gujral, V. K., and Jain, B. B.**, Effect of high fibre intake on serum vitamin A levels, *J. Assoc. Physicians India,* 34, 269, 1986.
20. **Kratzer, F. H., Rajaguru, R. W., and Vohra, P.**, The effect of polysaccharides on energy utilization, nitrogen retention and fat absorption in chickens, *Poultry Sci.,* 46, 1489, 1967.
21. **Reinhold, J. G.**, Rickets in Asian immigrants, *Lancet,* 2, 1132, 1976.
22. **Zoppi, G., Gobio-Casali, L., Deganello, A., Astolfi, R., Saccomani, F., and Cecchettin, M.**, Potential complications in the use of wheat bran of constipation in infancy, *J. Pediatr. Gastroenterol. Nutr.,* 1, 91, 1982.
23. **Batchelor, A. J. and Compston, J.**, Reduced plasma half-life of radio-labelled 25-hydroxyvitamin D_3 in subjects receiving a high-fibre diet, *Br. J. Nutr.,* 49, 213, 1983.
24. **Dagnelie, P. C., Vergote, F. J.V.R.A., van Staveren, W. A., van den Berg, H., Dingjan, P. G., and Hautvast, J. G.A.J.**, High prevalence of rickets in infants on macrobiotic diets, *Am. J. Clin. Nutr.,* 51, 202, 1990.
25. **Gibson, R. S., Bindra, G. S., Nizan, P., and Draper, H. H.**, The vitamin D status of East Indian Punjabi immigrants to Canada, *Brit. J. Nutr.,* 58, 23, 1987.
26. **deLumen, B. O., Lubin, B., Chiu, D., Reyes, P., and Omaye, S. T.**, Bioavailability of vitamin E in rats fed diets containing pectin, *Nutr. Res.,* 2, 73, 1982.
27. **Omaye, S. T. and Chow, F. I.**, Effect of hard red spring wheat bran on the bioavailability of lipid-voluble vitamins and growth of rats fed for 56 days, *J. Food Sci.,* 49, 504, 1984.
28. **Schaus, E. E., deLumen, B. O., Chow, F. I., Reyes, P., and Omaye, S. T.**, Bioavailability of vitamin B in rats fed graded levels of pectin, *J. Nutr.,* 115, 263, 1985.
29. **Doi, K., Matsuura, M., Kawara, A., Tanaka, T., and Baba, S.**, Influence of dietary fiber (konjac mannan) on absorption of vitamin B_{12} and vitamin E., *Tohoku J. Exp. Med.,* 141 (Suppl.), 677, 1983.
30. **Anderson, J. W., Ferguson, S. K., et al.**, Mineral and vitamin status on high-fiber diets: long-term studies of diabetic patients, *Diabetes Care,* 3, 38, 1980.
31. **Simpson, H. C. R. and Mann, J. I.**, Effect of high-fibre diet on haemostatic variables in diabetes, *Br. Med. J.,* 1, 1608, 1982.
32. **Roe, D. A., Wrick, K., McLain, D., and van Soest, P.**, Effects of dietary fiber sources on riboflavin absorption, *Fed. Proc. Fed. Am. Soc. Exp. Biol.,* 3, 756, 1978.
33. **Roe, D. A., Kalkwarf, H., and Stevens, J.**, Effect of fiber supplements on the apparent absorption of pharmacological doses of riboflavin, *J. Am. Dietetic Assoc.,* 88, 210, 1988.
34. **Gregory, J. F. and Kirk, J. R.**, The bioavailability of vitamin B_6 in foods, *Nutr. Rev.,* 39, 1, 1981.
35. **Nguyen, L. B., Gregory, J. F., and Damron, B. L.**, Effects of selected polysaccharides on the bioavailability of pyridoxine in rat and chickens, *J. Nutr.,* 111, 1403, 1981.
36. **Miller, L. T., Schultz, T. D., and Leklem, J. E.**, Influence of citrus pectin on the bioavailability of vitamin B_6 in man, *Fed. Proc. Fed. Am. Soc. Exp. Biol.,* 39, 797, 1980.
37. **Leklem, J. E., Miller, L. T., Perera, A. D., and Peffer, D. E.**, Bioavailability of vitamin B_6 from wheat bread in humans, *J. Nutr.,* 110, 1819, 1980.
38. **Shultz, T. D. and Leklem, J. E.**, Vitamin B_6 status and bioavailability in vegetarian women, *Am. J. Clin. Nutr.,* 46, 447, 1987.
39. **Lowik, M. R. H., Schrijver, J., van den Berg, H., Hulshof, K. F. A. M., Wedel, M., and Ockhuizen, T.**, Effect of dietary fiber on the vitamin B_6 status among vegetarian and nonvegetarian elderly (Dutch Nutrition Surveillance System), *J. Am. Coll. Nutr.,* 9, 241, 1990.
40. **Luther, L., Santini, R., Brewster, C., Perez-Santiago, E., and Butterworth, C. E.**, Folate binding by insoluble components of American and Puerto Rican diets, *Ala. J. Med. Sci.,* 2, 389, 1965.
41. **Ristow, K. A., Gregory, J. F., and Damron, B. L.**, The effect of dietary fiber on folic acid bioavailability, *Fed. Proc. Fed. Am. Soc. Exp. Biol.,* 40, 854, 1981.
42. **Brodribb, A. J. M. and Humphreys, D. M.**, Metabolic effect of bran in patients with diverticular disease, *Br. Med. J.,* 1, 424, 1976.
43. **Russell, R. M., Ismail-Beig, F., and Reinhold, J. G.**, Folate content of Iranian breads and the effect of their fiber content on the intestinal absorption of folic acid, *Am. J. Clin. Nutr.,* 29, 799, 1976.
44. **Pietrzik, K., Urban, G., and Hötzel, D.**, Biochemische und haematologische Maß stäbe zur Beurteilung des Folatstatus beim Menschen, *Int. Z. Vit. Ern. Forsch.,* 48, 391, 1978.
45. **Keagy, P. M., Shane, B., and Oace, S. M.**, Folate bioavailability in humans: effects of wheat bran and beans, *Am. J. Clin. Nutr.,* 47, 80, 1988.

46. **Cullen, R. W. and Oace, S. M.**, Methylmalonic acid and vitamin B_{12} excretion of rats consuming diets varying in cellulose and pectin, *J. Nutr.*, 108, 640, 1978.
47. **Keltz, F. R., Kies, C., and Fox, H. M.**, Urinary ascorbic acid excretion in the human as affected by dietary fiber and zinc, *Am. J. Clin. Nutr.*, 31, 1167, 1978.
48. **Kasper, H.**, Der Einfluss von Ballastoffen auf die Ausnutzung von Nährstoffen und Pharmaka, in *Pflanzenfasern-Ballastoffe in der menschlichen Ernährung*, Rottka, H., Ed., G. Thieme-Verlag, Stuttgart, 1980.
49. **Hötzel, D. and Barnes, R. H.**, Contributions of the intestinal microflora to the nutrition of the host, *Vit. Horm.*, 24, 115, 1966.
50. **Barnes, R. H., Kwong, E., and Fiala, G.**, Effects of the prevention of coprophagy in the rat, *J. Nutr.*, 68, 603, 1959.
51. Editorial: Intestinal microflora, injury and vitamin K deficiency, *Nutr. Rev.*, 38, 341, 1980.
52. **Bhat, P., Shantakumarie, S., Rajan, D., Mathan, H. I., and Kapadia, C. R.**, Bacterial flora of the gastrointestinal tract in Southern Indian control subjects and patients with tropical sprue, *Gastroenterology*, 62, 11, 1972.
53. **Kapadia, C. R., Mathan, V. J., and Bauer, S. J.**, Free intrinsic factor in the small intestine in man, *Gastroenterology*, 70, 70, 1976.
54. **Albert, M. J., Mathan, V. J., and Baker, S. J.**, Vitamin B_{12} synthesis by human small intestinal bacteria, *Nature*, 283, 781, 1980.

Section 6: Effect of Dietary Fiber on Gastrointestinal Function

Chapter 6.1

THE EFFECT OF DIETARY FIBER ON FECAL WEIGHT AND COMPOSITION

John H. Cummings

HISTORICAL INTRODUCTION

Present-day interest in fiber stems from the middle of the 19th century when the preoccupation of the Victorians with their bowel habits led many physicians to declaim the virtues of bran. John Burne[1] writing in 1840 in *A Treatise on the Causes and Consequences of Habitual Constipation* recommends that "coarse brown and bran bread is very efficacious, the bran acting as a salutory stimulus to the peristaltic action of the intestines". There was little need to convince Burne and his generation that bran stimulated colonic movement and increased fecal output. Nevertheless, each generation of medical scientists seems to have to rediscover this fact for itself, and medical and nutritional literature in the 1970s contained many papers in which little else but the laxative properties of bran were reported.

By 1909, Sir Arthur Hertz (later Sir Arthur Hurst)[2] was writing "One of the most valuable foods for constipation in whole-meal bread . . . white bread, which is made of the endosperm alone and those varieties of brown bread, such as Hovis, which are made from the endosperm and germ, contain only about one-fifth of the cellulose present in wholemeal bread. It is clear, therefore, that the substitution of whole-meal bread for white bread is a very important part of the dietetic treatment of constipation." Thus, 75 years ago fiber was being singled out as the principal component of bran responsible for its colonic effects.

In 1936 Dimock,[3] in his M.D. thesis for the University of Cambridge entitled "Treatment of Habitual Constipation by the Bran Method", was able to review over 50 papers reporting clinical, biochemical, radiological, and physiological studies of the use of fiber in constipation. He discussed various current ideas about the way bran produces its laxative effect, such as the presence of undigestible fiber, its content of vitamin B, phytin, hemicellulose, inorganic salts, and the production of volatile fatty acids from decomposition of cellulose and hemicellulose. As a result of his own observations, he concluded "my view is that bran exerts a mechanical laxative action due to its fibre content. The fibre mixes intimately with the food residues in the colon, even when bran is taken only once a day. I believe that by so doing, it not only retains moisture itself but enables the other residues in the colon to resist dehydration."

The 1930s were a time of vigorous investigation of the laxative properties of dietary fiber. Purified forms of fiber such as ispaghula, various celluloses, agar, karaya, sterculia, and psyllium were all in common use and were a focus of some interesting studies on their mechanism of action. It was widely believed at the time that fiber acted by virtue of its capacity to absorb and retain water in the gut.[4-8] However, the work by Williams and Olmsted,[9] which involved careful metabolic balance studies and fecal analysis of subjects ingesting various fibers prepared from peas, carrots, cabbage, corn bran, wheat bran, etc. concluded that "Contrary to the accepted belief, the effectiveness of indigestible residues is not due primarily to the mechanical stimulus of distention but rather to chemical stimuli which arise from the destruction of hemicelluloses and cellulose by the intestinal bacterial flora. One of these stimulating products is the lower volatile fatty acids." These studies contradicted the experimental data of others and questioned the whole basis of then currently accepted beliefs about fiber. Surprisingly, perhaps because of the international conflict which

TABLE 1
Average Increase in Fecal Output per Gram Fiber Fed

Source	Increase g/g fiber ± SEM	No. of studies (see Tables 2–15)	Comments
Wheat	5.4 (0.7)	41	Mainly bran. Raw 7.2; cooked 4.9 ($p < 0.05$)
Fruit and vegetables	4.7 (0.7)	28	Carrot, peas, cabbage, apple, potato, banana, prunes, and mixed sources
Gums and mucilages	3.7 (0.5)	27	Psyllium/ispaghula, 4.0 (N = 14). Other: traga-canth, xanthan, sterculia, bassara, xylan, agar, gum arabic, 4.0 (N = 9.0)
Cellulose	3.5 (0.8)	7	Also carboxymethylcellu-lose, 4.9 (N = 3); methylcellulose, 8.9 (N = 4)
Oats	3.4 (1.1)	4	Oat bran or oats
Corn	3.3 (0.3)	5	Corn meal or bran
Legumes	2.2 (0.3)	17	Soya products, 2.5 (N = 11)
Pectin	1.2 (0.3)	11	Degree of methoxylation not important

involved many nations at that time, there followed an apparently complete loss of interest in the subject and no significant developments were reported for the next 30 years.

Attention to the effect of dietary fiber on bowel habit returned around 1970, not because of any new insights into the problem of constipation but as a result of epidemiological observations relating bowel habit to disease by Burkitt[10-14] and studies by Painter on the etiology and treatment of diverticular disease.[15-17] In his paper on the etiology of large bowel cancer in 1971,[12] Burkitt suggests that fiber affects bowel function by speeding up transit time, diluting gut contents, and favorably influencing the microbial flora. At the same time, Painter was concluding a series of studies in the U.K. which he interpreted as showing that diverticular disease of the large intestine was due to lack of bulk in colonic contents.[15-17] He surmised from these studies that propulsion of intestinal contents was more difficult if they were dry, inspissated, and of small volume, thus requiring increased intraluminal pressures. He then went on to show that, contrary to current medical opinion, diverticular disease could be satisfactorily treated by increasing the amount of dietary fiber in the form of wheat bran. These studies stimulated new research into the mode of action of fiber in the colon. Since then, much of the early work on fiber has inevitably been repeated and many papers do little if anything to advance our knowledge or understanding of the mode of action of dietary fiber in the colon. However, as a result of better chemical techniques and advancing knowledge of colonic physiology, new concepts have emerged with regard to the mode of action of fiber in the colon and its role in determining colonic function.

MODERN STUDIES

Table 1 is a summary of the result of nearly 100 studies of the effect of the dietary fiber on bowel habit and fecal composition published between 1932 and 1984 and given in detail in Tables 2 to 9. All sources of fiber lead to an increase in fecal output and therefore in the components which make up feces such as fat, nitrogen, water minerals, and trace elements. What is clear from Table 1, hower, is that not all fibers are equal in this respect, pectin for example giving an increase of about 1.3 g of stool per gram of fiber fed while pure cellulose has an effect more than double (3.0 g/g fiber fed), and fruit, vegetables, and bran as sources of fiber being yet more effective (4.9 and 5.7 g/g, respectively).

The reasons for these differences relate to the physicochemical properties of dietary fiber. Two factors, particle size and chemical composition of individual fiber polysaccharides, have already emerged from experimental studies as specifically affecting the mode of action of dietary fiber. Table 10 summarizes studies of the effect of particle size on the efficacy of wheat bran in altering colonic function. In general, these show that if exactly the same source of fiber is fed at two different particle sizes the greater particle size preparation will produce larger changes in stool output. The reason for this is thought to relate to the extent and rate of breakdown of dietary fiber in the large intestine. Large particles are more slowly degraded and so are more likely to survive passage through the gut. In so doing they are able to exert a physical effect on colonic function by providing both bulk to gut contents and a surface for the bacteria which allows for their more efficient metabolism.

Chemical analysis of dietary fiber sources also shows a relation to fecal bulking properties. The more pentose sugars present in the dietary fiber polymers, the greater the increase in stool weight (other factors being equal).[18] This association is an intriguing one and one which is at the present time unexplained. It was initially felt that the response to pentose-containing polysaccharides was simply a reflection of the water-holding capacity of a particular fiber. However, both pentose- and hexose-containing polysaccharides hold water and further research has cast doubt on the water-holding hypothesis[19] as the sole explanation for the action of fiber, although its water-holding properties are still an important component of the explanation of its role in altering gut function.[20-25]

The most telling argument against the water-holding hypothesis is that virtually all fiber is broken down in the gut. Fiber digestion in man has been reported in the literature on many occasions in the past century. Despite this the popular view has persisted that it is not degraded, although there is now ample evidence to the contrary.[26,27] For example, when fiber in mixed diets is fed to healthy subjects, 70 to 80% of it disappears during passage through the gut.[28] The cellulosic fraction tends to survive digestion better than the non-cellulosic polysaccharides and fiber from cereals better survives than that from fruit and vegetables. When the digestion of cabbage and bran fiber were compared in healthy subjects taking equal doses of each material, only 10% of the cabbage fiber could be recovered in feces while 60% of bran fiber was excreted.[25]

Since fiber is extensively degraded, it is not surprising that its water-holding capacity is insufficient alone to explain its physiological effects in the colon. Another mechanism has to be sought whereby fiber can alter colonic metabolism. Williams and Olmsted[9,29] were probably the first to recognize the significance of the extensive breakdown of fiber in the human gut. They suggested that the fecal bulking by fiber could be accounted for by the stimulatory effect on colonic smooth muscle of the major end products of fiber breakdown, the short chain, or volatile fatty acids. Today, however, short chain fatty acids are known to be rapidly absorbed from the human colon and are thought not to control laxation in man.[30] Because of this, little has been learned from the study of their fecal excretion and therefore data from the few studies where they have been measured are not included in the accompanying tables.

A component of normal stools that has been neglected in studies of fiber for many years is the microflora. Bacteria are about 80% water and therefore a potentially important component of stools. Because of their ability to resist dehydration, bacteria are more likely to retain their water against the absorptive forces of the colonic mucosa than are the cellular skeletons of plant material that remain after cooking of food and its subsequent passage through the gut. Stephen and colleagues[31] developed a method for fractionating human feces which allows the contribution from microbial material to be estimated. Using this technique it can be shown that bacteria comprise up to half of the fecal solids in subjects eating typical Western diets. Bacteria are therefore probably an underestimated component of human feces and their role in changes in fecal composition is important. In Tables 2 to 9 it will be seen that fiber almost always brings about an increase in fecal nitrogen excretion. Studies in both man[32] and animals[33-34] have shown that this N is most likely to be bacterial N which increases as the result of microbial growth in the colon through fermentation of fiber. An increase in lipid excretion may in part also be explained this way.

MECHANISM OF ACTION OF DIETARY FIBER

The way in which dietary fiber affects bowel habit cannot be explained on the basis of one simple hypothesis. There are probably at least four distinct effects of fiber by which it brings about an increase in stool weight. Firstly, plant cell walls which resist breakdown by the microflora, e.g., because of lignification as in bran, are able to exert a physical effect on intestinal bulk by retaining water within their cellular structure. Increasing bulk stimulates colonic movement. Secondly, most forms of dietary fiber are extensively degraded by the microflora. The result of this is to stimulate microbial growth and a greater excretion of microbial products in feces. This again contributes to the change in fecal mass. Thirdly, substances which increase bulk in the large intestine often speed up the rate of passage through the bowel. As transit time falls, the efficiency with which the bacterica grows improves. Shortened transit time also leads to reduced water absorption by the colon and therefore wetter stools. Fourthly, dietary fiber is an important source of gas in the colon since the gases H_2, CH_4, and CO_2 are one of the principal end products of fermentation. Gas trapped within gut contents again adds to their bulk. These mechanisms together combine to increase stool weight.

Many workers who have studied the effect of dietary fiber on bowel function have noted the wide range in response among individuals. Table 11 summarizes studies of dietary fiber in subjects with diverticular disease of the colon. In general, it would appear that in response to bran these patients exhibit only about 50% of the response seen in healthy subjects. Whether this is the result or cause of the diverticular disease cannot be said but is worth further study.

Although the literature on dietary fiber and bowel habit contains much that is repetitious, in a small number of papers, evenly distributed over the years, experiments are described which demonstrate new aspects of large bowel physiology hitherto unrecognized. The advent of better carbohydrate chemistry, microbiological techniques, and noninvasive methods of studying colonic function have allowed investigators in recent years to show that dietary fiber has, through its breakdown in the large intestine by the microflora, an important role in maintaining normal digestive function as it does in the ruminant and other hind gut fermenting species.

NOTES TO TABLES

Selection of Papers

These tables summarize essential experimental details from a selection of reports of the effect of dietary fiber, in many forms, on bowel function, fecal weight, and composition published during the past 55 years. It is not a comprehensive survey since such a report would have been very extensive and have contained probably little more useful information than the present one. Studies have been selected for inclusion provided they were conducted on man, were reported as full papers in the English language, and contained numerical data on changes in large bowel function, particularly fecal output and composition. Many early studies from the period 1920 to 1950[35-52] have not been included because they report only qualitative data, percent changes, or results that are otherwise difficult to convert to tabular form. Nevertheless, some of these studies are detailed and thoughtful and well worth consulting.

The series of papers by Fantus and colleagues in 1940 to 1942,[37,40,41] together with the classic work of Williams and Olmsted,[9,29,53-56] that of Cowgill and associates,[58,59] and the comprehensive studies of Tainter et al.[7,8,60,61] on the mode of action of bulk laxatives together laid the foundation for much of present-day thinking about dietary fiber. Unfortunately, only a minority of modern researchers seem to have read or taken note of these early studies. If they had, much that is mundane and repetitious in current nutritional research would have been obviated.

A great deal that is written about fiber and bowel habit concerns constipation. The majority of these papers, however, are worthless, being reports of uncontrolled studies which usually show a beneficial effect of bran or other bulk laxatives. They have not been included in this survey unless they contain clear data on the role of fiber. In general, studies of young children have also been excluded as have those where data are based on a single stool or only 1 day of fecal collection.

Most studies reported are within-subject cross-over type design where each person takes both test and control diets. To say that they are solely experiments to determine the effect of dietary fiber on bowel function is an overstatement, however, since many investigators have used fiber sources such as bran, or foods which contain other nutrients. Nevertheless, there are problems in interpreting and extrapolating to foods as are normally eaten from studies where purified materials such as cellulose are used.[62] So both types of experiments, whole foods and purified materials, are needed to give a full understanding of the effects of fiber. The problem of the purity of fiber sources has been recognized for many years and early studies of bran, such as those reported by Dimock,[3] discuss at length the potential of various components of bran to induce laxation. The answers to some of the questions Dimock posed have not yet been found or even looked for.

Finally, the age-old question "what is fiber" constantly appears when reading the literature. The word "fiber" is used in many different contexts in the papers reported here and clearly means different things to different investigators. All definitions and concepts are included in the tables. Some guide as to the meaning of the word in individual studies is given by an indication of the chemical methods used in the study to measure fiber intake in the experimental subjects.

TABLES 2 to 11

An asterisk in all columns means that the value is significantly different from basal (or other appropriate) control diet.

Column 1: Literature Sources, Diet, Fiber Source

The principal *literature sources* for the data given in the table are recorded in column 1. In recent years the practice has developed in which authors publish the results of a single complete study in several parts, possibly in different journals. Alternatively, and to be decried, is the repeated publication of the same data in several journals. Small alterations may be made to numbers of subjects or details and the work republished. All this conspires to crowd the literature with irrelevant and superfluous information while apparently enhancing the reputation of the authors for industry, science, and original thought. As a means of guiding the reader through this morass, all citations to a single experiment are recorded in this column, insofar as they can be identified.

Diets are either "controlled" — meaning the food is cooked and prepared for the subjects by the investigators and provides a constant background against which to judge the effect of fiber. These are sometimes referred to as "metabolic studies". Commendably, many studies are now carried out in this way. *Ad lib* diets are self-selected by the subjects.

Fiber sources are described as in the paper.

Column 2: Total Number of Subjects in Study, Sex, and Age

The *number of subjects* of each *sex* (M = male, F = female) who took part in the whole study or part of the study are recorded together with the range of ages. A dash indicates that no data are available.

Column 3: Study Period

Study period describes the diet and/or fiber source relevant to the data given on that line. Basal = control diet against which fiber supplements compared.

Column 4: Fiber Intake (g/day) and Fiber Method

Many authors have attempted to measure fiber intake using one of a number of methods, I to XII (see below). Where no method is given in the paper an attempt has been made to calculate dietary fiber intakes using currently available food tables or analytical information. If errors have been committed or wrong assumptions made by me in doing this I apologize in advance to the investigators concerned.

I. Crude fiber[63-64]
II. Williams and Olmsted 1935[56]
III. Southgate[65-70]
IV. Paul and Southgate[71]
V. Van Soest and modifications[72-76]
VI. Crampton and Maynard[77]
VII. O'Shea, Ribiero, and Moran[78]
VIII. McCance, Widdowson, and Shackleton[79]
IX. Katan and von de Bovenkamp[80]
X. Englyst[81-82]
XI. Schweizer[83-84]
XII. Angus, Sutherland, and Farrell[85]

Column 5: Days on Diet

This information appears as in paper. Where this was varied a range is given. (No figure is given for *ad lib* diets since it is assumed to be the subject's usual diet.)

Column 6: Fecal Collection Period (Days)

This is the number of days of fecal collection pooled for analysis. It is the *minimum* included since investigators have used, on occasions, averages of several collection periods for the data.

Column 7: Number of Subjects Collecting Feces

This number may be less than the total number participating in the study either because the subjects were split into groups or some did not collect feces. It is the number which has been used to calculate standard errors in other columns.

Column 8: Fecal Weight (g/day)

Average value (± 1 SE of the mean). Some of these figures are derived by calculation on the basis of data in the original papers. Any errors are therefore not the fault of the original authors, and investigators seeking to follow up these studies should consult the publications themselves. Where data are given in the paper for several periods on the same diet, the information relating to the *final* period has been used in this table.

Column 9: Percent Moisture

If not given in the original paper this has been calculated as:

$$\frac{\text{total fecal weight g/day} - \text{fecal solids g/day}}{\text{total stool weight g/day}} \times 100$$

Column 10: Fecal Solids (g/day)

As given in the paper or calculated from data related to percent moisture of feces (± 1 SE of the mean).

Column 11: Apparent Increase in Fecal Weight Per Gram Dietary Fiber Fed

Calculated as:

$$\frac{\text{fecal output with fiber source g/day} - \text{basal fecal output g/day}}{\text{g fiber fed per day}}$$

Gram of fiber fed per day is always "dietary fiber" as defined in 1972 and 1976.[86-87] Where dietary fiber data are not given in the paper these have been calculated from available knowledge of the food and fiber source used.

Column 12: Transit Time — Hours and Transit Method

Transit time, the time it takes a substance to pass through the gut, can be measured using a number of techniques in the majority of which an oral dose of inert marker is given with food and its appearance in feces is noted. Values for transit time obtained are very dependent on the method used. Colored dyes give short transit times since it is difficult to detect other than the "first appearance" of marker in feces. Methods which measure mean transit time are probably most accurate, while the radio-opaque pellet technique of Hinton et al.[88] gives values which are about 20% greater than the mean transit time methods. Values in this column must be interpreted, therefore, in the light of the method used and are not directly comparable with one another.

Transit Methods

I. Hinton, Lennard-Jones, and Young (1969)[88]
II. Cummings, Jenkins, and Wiggins (1975 and 1976)[89-90]
III. Colored dyes — "first apperance" method[91-93]
IV. ^{51}Cr sodium chromate[94]
V. Cr_2O_6 chromic oxide

Column 13: Fat (g/day)

Note that various methods are used to recover fat, including those which measure total lipid, triglycerides, and fatty acids and fatty acids alone (after hydrolysis); millimoles converted to milligrams by factor × 280.

Column 14: N (g/day)
This is usually measured by the Kjeldahl technique. Note variable conversion factors used by authors to convert fecal N to "protein" (from 5.75 to 6.25).

Column 15: Neutral Steroids (mg/day)
See original papers for methodology which affects results especially in early (pre-1970) papers. Millimoles converted to milligrams by factor $\times$ 386.

Column 16: Acid Steroids (mg/day)
See notes for Column 15. Millimoles converted to milligrams by factor $\times$ 400.

Column 17: Energy (kcal/day)
Total fecal energy excretion usually measured by calorimetry.

Column 18: Comments, Notes, Other Data Available
This column includes special notes about the studies and lists other data available from related publications of the same study.

Other Data Available From Study

A	=	Digestibility (fecal excretion) of fiber
B	=	Volatile fatty acids
C	=	Calcium, magnesium, phosphorus (including phytate)
D	=	Iron, zinc, copper, and other trace elements
E	=	Blood lipids
F	=	Intestinal motility
G	=	Polyethylene glycol, Cr_2O_6 used as markers
H	=	Sodium, potassium, chloride, bicarbonate, ash, or other electrolytes
J	=	Microflora
K	=	Glucose tolerance
L	=	Bile composition and bile acid kinetics
M	=	Breath CH_4 and H_2
N	=	Hematology

TABLES 12 TO 15 (1986–1992)

These additional tables detail papers on the effects of dietary fiber on bowel habit and fecal composition published between 1986 and 1992, and also include one or two additional reports omitted from the earlier survey. As before, the criteria for inclusion are that the studies have been undertaken in adults, contain quantitative data of an experimental, not observational, nature and must include, as a minimum, fecal weights. There may be some publications that do not appear in these tables, but which fit the criteria for inclusion. Such omissions are inadvertent and the author apologizes to anyone whose work has been so excluded.

While in 1985 it appeared that everything that could be said about dietary fiber and bowel habit had been said, papers still continue to appear on this topic at a steady rate. Some of them add little to what is already known, although there is clearly now an increased interest in forms of dietary fiber other than bran. This is seen in the papers on different plant gums and legumes, especially soya. The impetus for these studies is partly commercial since few investigators use these studies to cast light on the unresolved question as to how dietary fiber works. Some progress has been made in this area, by study of the physical properties of fiber in relation to its effect on fecal composition, but a number of important questions remain unanswered.[220,247,248]

The revised version of Table 1 shows average increases in fecal weight (g per day per g fiber fed) for the major sources of dietary fiber, ranked according to their effectiveness. A further 37 papers have been added to the original compilation of about 80 detailing a total of approaching 150 individual dietary studies of assorted fiber sources. These additional data have not made a great deal of difference to the overall rankings and the message remains the same. Dietary fiber is laxative but the significant differences among the results confirm that not all fibers are the same, and one cannot really generalize about the whole group. Therefore, a single number on a food label for fiber is going to give the consumer very little useful information about its laxative effects, without some additional information. Wheat products, usually bran, remain unequivocally top of the league although a small number of studies of methylcellulose suggests it is equally if not more effective as a laxative. With regard to wheat, there are now enough studies of both raw and cooked products to show a statistically significant difference in favor of raw bran (7.2 g/g raw vs. 4.9 cooked, $t = 2.65$, $p = 0.012$). The disadvantage of raw bran, of course, is its high content of phytate.

Fruit and vegetables remain second in the table well ahead of the rest. While many people believe fruit and vegetables contain mainly soluble fiber with little potential to alter bowel habit, in fact this is clearly not the case. Many fruit and vegetables contain significant amounts of insoluble fiber.[253,254] These studies were mostly done with foods rather than purified forms of fiber which means that the subjects are eating intact cell walls, which probably contributes to the effect.

Gums and mucilages have risen up the list to third place although they are well behind wheat, fruit, and vegetables. There is clearly a lot of commercial interest in adding these preparations to food due to their potential cholesterol lowering properties. However, wide differences in the fecal bulking properties of gums are evident. For example, guar is a poor bulker in general giving increases of around 1.0 g/g,[220,225] while tragacanth seems to be the best at 6.4 g/g,[228] although this is only one study.

Cellulose, corn, and oats are all effective laxative substances and give similar effects, with the exceptions of methylcellulose and carboxymethylcellulose, which are better. The legumes, despite being a good source of insoluble fiber,[253] are poor fecal bulkers. Since they also frequently contain resistant starch,[255] this is hard to understand. Finally, pectin remains the least effective along with guar.

How reliable are these rankings? Within each group there is great variability, although despite this the overall differences are statistically significant (by ANOVAR F 4.78 p < 0.001). The variability is due in part to the inherent difference in individual responses and to varying experimental designs, some of which are uncontrolled diets. However, a major problem is lack of consistency in methodology for measurement of dietary fiber. In the earlier part of this chapter, 12 methods were listed as being used to measure fiber in the various studies. A further 7 have been added for the present update as follows:

XIII.   Anderson, Sieling, and Chen[197]
XIV.   Mergenthaler and Scherz[199]
XV.   Meuser et al.[200]
XVI.   Prosky et al.[202-204]
XVII.   Slavin et al.[215]
XVIII. Theander and Westerlund[231]
XIX.   Asp et al.[232]

In addition, a further 7 methods or modifications to methods have been developed over this period.[239-245] Because these methods give widely differing results for the amount of dietary fiber in a food,[256] this creates a problem in comparing data.

What of the future? The emergence of starch as a fecal bulking agent[248-252] is probably the single most important discovery to challenge the role of fiber in the diet. At the very least, the amount and type of starch in experimental diets must be controlled (as must its processing) to eliminate this as a variable. More than likely, we shall have to re-evaluate the whole dietary fiber story in the light of emerging evidence of the importance of resistant starch.

TABLE 2
Effect of Wheat Fiber in Various Forms on Fecal Composition (See Also Table 10)

Literature source	Diet Fiber source	Total number of subjects in study (sex and age)	Study period	Fiber intake (g/day) and fiber method	Days on diet	Fecal collection period (days)	Number of subjects collecting feces	Fecal weight (g/day)	Moisture (%)	Fecal solids (g/day)	Apparent increase in fecal weight per gram dietary fiber fed	Transit time (h) and transit method	Fat (g/day)	N (g/day)	Neutral steroids (mg/day)	Acid steroids (mg/day)	Energy (kcal/day)	Comments Notes Other data available
Cowgill and Anderson (1932)[58] Controlled diet	Low fiber basal	5 M		5.2 —	14	14	5	116 (11)	77	27								Both brans equally effective
	+ Whole bran, 1–1½ oz			—	14	14	5	193* (8)	79	40								
	Low fiber basal		Normal foods	5.2	14	14	5	112 (7)	76	27								A
	+ Acid-washed bran, 1–1½ oz		Low fiber or very low fiber	—	14	14	5	171* (13)	77	39								
	Bran, 1–1½ oz		Bran — whole or with weak acid	—	14	14	4	93 (7)	70	28								
	Very low fiber basal			3.1	14	14	4	189* (22)	74	49								
	+ Whole bran, 1–1½ oz			—	14	14	4	93 (5)	76	22								
	Very low fiber basal			3.1	14	14	4	185* (17)	76	44								
	+ Acid-washed bran, 1–1½ oz			—	14	14												

TABLE 2 (continued)
Effect of Wheat Fiber in Various Forms on Fecal Composition (See Also Table 10)

Literature source	Diet Fiber source	Total number of subjects in study (sex and age)	Study period	Fiber intake (g/day) and fiber method	Days on diet	Fecal collection period (days)	Number of subjects collecting feces	Fecal weight (g/day)	Moisture (%)	Fecal solids (g/day)	Apparent increase in fecal weight per gram dietary fiber fed	Transit time (h) and transit method	Fat (g/day)	N (g/day)	Neutral steroids (mg/day)	Acid steroids (mg/day)	Energy (kcal/day)	Comments	Notes	Other data available
Cowgill and Sullivan (1933)[59] Controlled diet	Basal	6 M		I[a] 30—38	7	7	6	78 (15)										Constipated subjects		
	+ Bran			50	7	7	6	121* (6)										Also studied effect of fruit and vegetables (see Table 8)		
Normal foods	+ High bran			90	7	7	6	187* (18)										Whole bran slightly better than breakfast bran but less palatable		
Bran and breakfast bran (a commercial breakfast cereal)	+ Breakfast bran			90	7	7	6	176* (12)										Noted greater fiber digestibility than in normal subjects A		

Reference	Subjects	Diet/Treatment										Comments
Williams and Olmsted (1936)[9,29,57] Controlled diet Normal foods excluding fruit and vegetables Bran, prepared by washing for 24 h in warm water, extracting with hot ethanol and drying	3 M	Bran	II +24	6	7	3	+79[b]		3.2				Part of a larger study in which 9 other fiber sources fed (see Tables 4, 5, 6, and 7) A, B
McCance and Widdowson (1942)[95] Controlled diet Bread as 40 to 50% of energy intake Bread either white, brown, brown with dephytenized bran, or brown with dephytenized bran and mineral supplement	3 M, 3 F, 21–42	White		10	7	6	116						Laxative properties of brown breads similar C
		Brown		10	7	6	224						
		Brown dephytenized		10	7	6	209						
		Brown dephytenized + minerals		10	7	6	226						
Eastwood et al. (1973)[96] Ad lib diet Bran	8 M, 25–43	Basal	—	7	7	8	107 (15)	76	26 (3)		I 62	216 (46)	Cellulose also studied (see Table 4) E
		+Bran, 16 g	+7[c]	21	7	8	174* (18)	76	41* (3)	9.5	43	207 (34)	

TABLE 2 (continued)
Effect of Wheat Fiber in Various Forms on Fecal Composition (See Also Table 10)

Literature source Diet Fiber source	Total number of subjects in study (sex and age)	Study period	Fiber intake (g/day) and fiber method	Days on diet	Fecal collection period (days)	Number of subjects collecting feces	Fecal weight (g/day)	Moisture (%)	Fecal solids (g/day)	Apparent increase in fecal weight per gram dietary fiber fed	Transit time (h) and transit method	Fat (g/day)	N (g/day)	Neutral steroids (mg/day)	Acid steroids (mg/day)	Energy (kcal/day)	Comments Notes Other data available
Connell and Smith (1974)[97] *Ad lib* diet	10, 25–45	Cornflakes, 1 oz	IV	28	7	8	119 (9)				93 (16)						
		Bran buds, 1 oz	+8	28	7	8	218* (20)			12.3	44* (4)						
Findlay et al. (1974)[98] *Ad lib* diet Bran	6, 28–36	Basal	—	7	7	6	120 (18)	72	33 (4)		66 (18) I, IV					296 (32)	Study included additional group with diverticular disease (see Table 11)
		+Bran, 20 g	+9[c]	35	7	6	183* (22)	74	46* (3)	7.2	50 (11)					352 (45)	See original paper for comments on liquid and solid phases of gut contents F, G

Study	Subjects	Diet														Comments
Walters et al. (1975)[107]	2 M, 3 F, 52-69	Basal	15	12	7	5	93 (10)	75	23 (1)		2.8 (0.2)	1.1 (0.2)	646 (73)	199 (44)	108 (6)	Two separate studies: one of bagasse biscuits in nuns living in a convent (see Table 7); the second an inpatient controlled diet study of wheat bran biscuits
Southgate et al. (1976)[108] McLean Baird et al. (1977)[109] Controlled diet Hospital low fiber Bran crispbread (Energen)		+Bran crispbread	28	12	7	5	166* (15)	77	38* (8)	5.5		3.8 (0.6)	1.6* (0.2)	675 (81)	195 (17)	166* (6)	A, C-E, J
																B, C, E, H
Cummings et al. (1976)[99]	6 M, 21-25	Basal	17	21	7	6	79 (7)	73	21 (1)	II	58 (3)	1.7 (0.2)	1.2 (0.0)	602 (79)	199 (19)	
Jenkins et al. (1975)[100] Controlled diet Normal foods Whole meal bread, All Bran, bran, and bran biscuits		+Fiber	45	21	7	6	228* (30)	80	45* (2)	5.3	40* (4)	2.7* (0.2)	2.0* (0.1)	820 (121)	279* (19)	
Fuchs et al. (1976)[101]	4 M, 2 F, 22-47	Basal		21	3	6	103 (20)	73	28	IV						
Kahaner et al. (1976)[102] Floch and Fuchs (1977/78)[103,104] Ad lib diet All Bran (Kelloggs)		All Bran, 3 oz	+23	21	3	6	226* (45)	74	59	5.3						Eating habits showed reduced eggs, butter, and breakfast meats with increased milk and fruit during bran period Stool pH unchanged

TABLE 2 (continued)
Effect of Wheat Fiber in Various Forms on Fecal Composition (See Also Table 10)

Literature source	Total number of subjects in study (sex and age)	Fiber source Diet	Study period	Fiber intake (g/day) and fiber method	Days on diet	Fecal collection period (days)	Number of subjects collecting feces	Fecal weight (g/day)	Moisture (%)	Fecal solids (g/day)	Apparent increase in fecal weight per gram dietary fiber fed	Transit time (h) and transit method	Fat (g/day)	N (g/day)	Neutral steroids (mg/day)	Acid steroids (mg/day)	Energy (kcal/day)	Comments Notes Other data available
Reinhold et al. (1976)[105] Controlled diet	2 M, 24, 35	White bread, 500 g	V	22[d]	20	—	2	244 (92)	91	21 (5)				2.3 (0.1)				Fecal anaerobe: aerobe ratio increased by bran E, J
		Normal foods, 58 to 62% of energy as bread Bread: white or basari (80 to 90% extraction)		Basari, 500 g 30[d]	20		2	403 (121)	90	40 (8)				2.9 (0.1)				A, C, D
Wyman et al. (1976)[106] Ad lib low fiber avoiding	10 M, 11–41	Basal	IV		5		10	131 (17)	75	30 (3)		65 (8)						Stool weight not significantly increased by
		Raw bran, 12 g		+3.6	14	5	10	183 (21)	76	42* (5)	14.4	53 (17)						

Study	Subjects	Diet		Days	n									Comments
		cereals, bread, fruit, and vegetables												any treatment
		Raw bran, 20 g	+5.9	14	5	10	159 (13)	76	38* (3)	4.7	48* (7)			Cooked bran thought to be less effective than raw bran
		Raw bran or All Bran (Kelloggs)												
		All Bran, 13.2g	+3.6	14	5	10	139 (9)	73	36 (3)	2.2	58 (6)			
		All Bran, 22g	+5.8	14	5	10	164 (20)	77	35 (3)	5.6	50 (9)			
Kay & Truswell (1977)[110]	3 F., 3 M., 22–27	Basal	3.7	14	6	5	125	71	32			288	312	Study design was basal-fiber-basal Steroid output also higher in second basal period
Controlled low fiber Normal foods White bread or coarse bran (Prewetts) made into bread and whole meal bread		+Fiber (23–35 g bran)	8.6	21	6	5	225*	74	53*	5.3^c		256	233	C, E
Cummings et al. (1978)[18]	19 M., 20–38	Basal	III 22	21	7	6	95 (8)	72	27 (1)		II 73 (10)	1.5 (0.1)		Part of a larger study in which fiber from carrot, cabbage, apple (see Table 7), and guar gum (see Table 5) were fed
Stephen and Cummings (1980)[25] Controlled Normal food Bran prepared by extracting with ethanol and acetone		+Bran, 30 g	40	21	7	6	197* (13)	76*	46* (1)	5.7	43* (3)	2.0* (0.1)		J
Farrell et al. (1978)[111]	14 M., 22–46	Basal	V, VI, VII, XII 33	9	4	14	—	—	29 (1)		—	2.9 (0.4)	1.6 (0.1)	151 (6)
Controlled or specified menus		+Fiber	53	9	4	14			50* (1)			3.7* (0.3)	2.0* (0.1)	241* (6) A, C–E, H

TABLE 2 (continued)
Effect of Wheat Fiber in Various Forms on Fecal Composition (See Also Table 10)

Literature source	Diet Fiber source	Total number of subjects in study (sex and age)	Study period	Fiber intake (g/day) and fiber method	Days on diet	Fecal collection period (days)	Number of subjects collecting feces	Fecal weight (g/day)	Moisture (%)	Fecal solids (g/day)	Apparent increase in fecal weight per gram dietary fiber fed	Transit time (h) and transit method	Fat (g/day)	N (g/day)	Neutral steroids (mg/day)	Acid steroids (mg/day)	Energy (Kcal/day)	Comments	Notes	Other data available
	Normal foods All bran, whole meal bread, bran, and bran biscuits											I								
Mathur et al. (1978)[112]		10 M	Basal				10	255 (17)				37 (2)						Significant effect of bran on patients with amoebic dysentery also noted in separate study		
	Ad lib diet Reground bran		+ Bran, 30 g		30		10	295* (14)			3.0ᶜ	32 (2)								
				V								II								
Cummings et al. (1979)[113]		4 M, 20—24	High protein	22	21	7	4	80 (11)	72	22 (2)		70 (6)				221 (19)		No effect of protein intake on stool weight noted in other part of study		
	Controlled diet Normal food Fiber from bran crispbread, whole meal bread,		High protein + fiber	53	21	7	4	210* (9)	73	56* (1)	4.2	50* (7)				444* (27)		C		

Study	Subjects	Diet		Days	n						Comments
All Bran, and fine bran											
Munoz et al. (1979)[114]	10 M, 19–54	Basal	V	28–30	12	6	64 (10)			275 (40)	Part of a larger study of corn bran, soybean hulls, etc. on various aspects of metabolism (see Tables 5 to 7) C–E, K
Bell et al. (1981)[115]		Soft white wheat bran, 26 g	+11	28–30	12	6	99* (7)		3.2	328 (86)	
Sandstead et al. (1978),[116] (1979)[117,118]		Basal		28–30	12	9	81 (6)			530 (21)	
Munoz et al. (1978),[119] (1979),[120] Controlled diet Normal food Hard and soft bran fed as bread		Hard red spring wheat bran, 26 g	+13	28–30	12	9	151* (8)		5.4	477 (107)	
Huijbrechts et al. (1980)[122] Ad lib but semi-controlled Normal food AACC bran	7, x̄ 22.5	Basal	V	56	4	4	194 (32)	74		18.8 (1.1)	Seven subjects studied for 4 weeks then 4 for a further 4 weeks Average weight of 4 subjects: 67.8 kg No change in bile composition or kinetics after bran
		+ Bran 0.5 g/kg (34 g)	45		4		273 (49)	76	5.8	17.3 (3.5) f	
			31					42 (2)		11.9 (2.2) f	L
								62* (11)		10.7 (2.5) f	
Smith et al. (1980)[123] Ad lib hospital diet AACC bran	18 M, 19 F, x̄ 81, 65–96	Basal		28	5	10	27	8	3.6	160	Elderly hospitalized subjects — also studied with ispaghula (see also Table 5)
		+ Fiber, 20 g	+8		5	10	62	17	4.8	216	
									4.4		

TABLE 2 (continued)
Effect of Wheat Fiber in Various Forms on Fecal Composition (See Also Table 10)

Literature source	Diet Fiber source	Total number of subjects in study (sex and age)	Study period	Fiber intake (g/day) and fiber method	Days on diet	Fecal collection period (days)	Number of subjects collecting feces	Fecal weight (g/day)	Moisture (%)	Fecal solids (g/day)	Apparent increase in fecal weight per gram dietary fiber fed	Transit time (h) and transit method	Fat (g/day)	N (g/day)	Neutral steroids (mg/day)	Acid steroids (mg/day)	Energy (kcal/day)	Comments Notes Other data available
Stasse-Wolthuis et al. (1980)[124]	Basal	40 M, 22 F, 18–28		18	35	7	16	89 (12)		22		67 (7) II	1.7		597	288		Also transit studies with radioisotope capsule Colonic pressures unchanged C, F, H
Stasse-Wolthuis (1979)[125,126] Controlled diet Normal food Bran	+Bran, 38 g			VIII[g] IX 37	35	7	16	166*		36*	4.0	48*	(0.3) 2.9		629	254*		Part of a larger study including pectin and the effects of fruit and vegetables (see Tables 3 and 8) Blood pressure unchanged C, E, H

Study	Subjects	Diet		Period (d)	n	Stool wt (g/d)	Transit time (h)	Fecal fiber (g/d)			Nitrogen (g/d)	Comments
			V						III			
Yu & Miller (1981)[127] Controlled diet Normal food AACC bran added to food and cooked	10 M, 20-35	Basal		18	6	10	143 (11)	74 (1)	36 (1)	32 (2)	4.5 (0.4)	1.9 (0.1)	179 (5)	Nitrogen balances A, H
		+Bran, 15 g	+6	18	6	10	172* (12)	75 (1)	43* (1) 4.8	29 (2)	5.4 (0.6)	2.1* (0.1)	211* (5)	
			V						I			
Van Dokkum et al. (1982),[128] (1983)[129] Controlled diet Normal food Breads containing coarse and fine bran	12 M, x̄ 23	Basal		20	4	12	77	21		88		1.1	374	Mainly a study of mineral balance and fiber digestibility
		+Coarse bran	22	20	4	12	140*	34*		52*		1.6*	322	Also studied coarse and fine brans (see Table 10) A-E
		Coarse bran, low dose	22	20	4	12	137	34	4.8	77		1.3	324	
		Coarse bran, high dose	35	20	4	4	202*	46	5.0	45*		1.8	355	
		Coarse bran	22	20	4	4	158	35		35		1.8	316	
		Whole meal bread	22		4	4	143	34		45		1.5	258	
			X									
Graham et al, (1982)[130] Ad lib low fiber diet AACC bran	11 F, 20-40	Basal		14	7	5	31 (9)	67	10					Constipated subjects; also studied with corn bran (see Table 6) which was more effective per gram material fed H
		+Bran, 20 g	+8	14	7	5	58*	72*	16*	3.4				
			X						II			
Andersson et al. (1983)[131] Controlled diet Normal food Bread either white, brown, or whole meal with added phytic acid	5 M, 1 F	White bread	16	24	6	6	137 (38)	79	29 (5)	46 (17)				Principally a study of the effect of fiber on mineral balance, and which showed no effect C, D
		Brown bread	24	24	6	6	175* (50)	79	37* (6) 5.0	41 (13)				
		Whole meal bread	31	24	6	6	236* (51)	80	47* (6) 6.4	39 (12)				

TABLE 2 (continued)
Effect of Wheat Fiber in Various Forms on Fecal Composition (See Also Table 10)

Literature source	Total number of subjects in study (sex and age)	Diet Fiber source	Study period	Fiber intake (g/day) and fiber method	Days on diet	Fecal collection period (days)	Number of subjects collecting feces	Fecal weight (g/day)	Moisture (%)	Fecal solids (g/day)	Apparent increase in fecal weight per gram dietary fiber fed	Transit time (h) and transit method	Fat (g/day)	N (g/day)	Neutral steroids (mg/day)	Acid steroids (mg/day)	Energy (kcal/day)	Comments Notes Other data available
Eastwood et al. (1983)[24]	9 M, 26–44	*Ad lib* diet Basal	XI	19	7	7	8	120 (6)	72	33 (1)		—				220 (17)		A study comparing *in vitro* and *in vivo* properties of potato and bran fiber (see Table 7) E
		Coarse bran Bran, 16 g		27	21	7	8	183* (8)	75	46* (1)	7.9	55 49				212 (35)		
Stephen et al. (1986)[132] Controlled Normal food Bran-enriched breads	19 M, 11 F	Basal	X	20	21	6	7	114 (20)	75	28 (3)		66 (17)	2.3 (0.3)	1.5 (0.2)			125 (12)	A dose-response study showing a linear increase in stool output with increasing doses of bran-enriched bread A, C–E
		+ Bran bread, 30 g		22	21	6	7	128* (22)	76	30* (2)	6.4	53 (12)	2.4 (0.3)	1.6 (0.2)			136* (12)	
		Basal		21	21	6	8	130 (28)	78	29 (3)		68 (14)	2.8 (0.3)	1.5 (0.2)			135 (14)	
		+ Bran bread, 60 g		25	21	6	8	163* (27)	78	36* (3)	7.7	54* (10)	2.9 (0.5)	1.7* (0.2)			162* (14)	
		Basal		21	21	6	7	110 (15)	74	28 (3)		73 (15)	3.5 (0.7)	1.5 (0.2)			133 (18)	
		+ Bran bread, 110 g		30	21	6	7	145* (13)	75	36* (2)	4.4	59 (7)	3.7 (0.8)	1.6 (0.2)			163* (14)	

Basal	24	21	6	8	173 (15)	79	37 (2)		39 (4)	4.3 (0.3)	2.1 (0.1)	178 (9)
+ Bran bread, 170 g	36	21	6	8	240* (14)	77	54* (2)	5.4	34 (3)	4.7 (0.3)	2.4* (0.1)	263*(9)

a Milligrams of crude fiber per kilogram body weight per day.
b Figures are increases over basal diet period — fiber remaining in stool.
c Assumes bran is about 44% dietary fiber.
d Acid detergent fiber.
e Per gram of dietary fiber.
f Micromole per kilogram per day.
g A variety of fiber methods used (see paper).

TABLE 3
Effect of Purified Pectin on Fecal Composition

Literature source	Diet Fiber source	Total number of subjects in study (sex and age)	Study period	Fiber intake (g/day) and fiber method	Days on diet	Fecal collection period (days)	Number of subjects collecting feces	Fecal weight (g/day)	Moisture (%)	Fecal solids (g/day)	Apparent increase in fecal weight per gram dietary fiber fed	Transit time (h) and transit method	Fat (g/day)	N (g/day)	Neutral steroids (mg/day)	Acid steroids (mg/day)	Energy (kcal/day)	Comments	Notes Other data available
Drasar and Jenkins (1976)[133]	Ad lib diets Pectin — Bulmers NF	10 M, 22—25	Basal	— III	14	7	4	119 (22)										Also studied were guar gum and bananas (see Tables 5 and 8) Serum cholesterol lowered by pectin but fecal microflora unchanged	E, J
			+Pectin 35 g	+32	14	7	4	148 (13)			0.9								
Durrington et al. (1976)[134]	Ad lib diet Pectin — Bulmers NF	12 M, 22—45	Basal	— III	7	5	12	150 (10)				59 (9) I						Serum cholesterol fell but not triglycerides	E
			+Pectin, 12 g	+10	21	5	12	186* (15)			3.6	44 (6)							

Study	Subjects	Diet	Period (days)	n	Days	Stool wt (g/d)	% H₂O	Fat (g/d)	N	Energy	Transit time (h)	Comments
Kay and Truswell (1977)[135] Controlled diet Normal food Pectin — Bulmers NF	4 M, 5 F, 21–28	Basal +Pectin, 15 g	III 14 21	6 6	9 9	140 168	71 68*	40 52*	2.3	III 34 37	3.8 8.6	335 390*	265 371*	Study design was control-test-control; data from first control period reported here Serum cholesterol fell but not triglycerides E
Miettinen and Tarpila (1977)[136] Controlled diet Normal food Pectin-Firmagel Buenes Ltd.	5 F, 4 M, 33–60	Basal +Pectin, 40–50 g	III 14 +37 g 14	3 3	9 9	200 (89) 269 (49)	36 (3) 46* (6)	1.9	3.1 (0.4) 3.9 (0.4)	585 (62) 642 (87)	342 (8) 537* (93)	2 Normal subjects, 6 hyperlipidemics, 1 diabetic, 1 diverticular disease Serum cholesterol decreased but not triglycerides Bile composition unchanged E,L
Cummings et al. (1979)[137] Controlled diet Normal food Pectin-Bulmers NF	5 M, 21–24	Basal +Pectin, 36 g	III 15 42	7 7	5 5	21 48	107 (25) 123* (25)	73 72	27 (3) 31* (3)	0.5	II 77 (18) 70 (16)	1.5 (0.1) 2.7* (0.2)	1.3 (0.2) 1.6* (0.2)	239 (42) 322* (37)	After 3 weeks on pectin, changes in bowel habit somewhat greater than at 6 weeks Serum glutamyl transpeptidase unchanged A, C

TABLE 3 (continued)
Effect of Purified Pectin on Fecal Composition

Literature source Diet Fiber source	Total number of subjects in study (sex and age)	Study period	Fiber intake (g/day) and fiber method	Days on diet	Fecal collection period (days)	Number of subjects collecting feces	Fecal weight (g/day)	Moisture (%)	Fecal solids (g/day)	Apparent increase in fecal weight per gram dietary fiber fed	Transit time (h) and transit method	Fat (g/day)	N (g/day)	Neutral steroids (mg/day)	Acid steroids (mg/day)	Energy (Kcal/day)	Comments Notes Other data available
Strasse-Wolthuis et al. (1980)[124] Controlled diet Normal food Pectin-Bulmers NF	40 M, 25 F, 18–28	Basal +Pectin, 10 g	18 VIII[a] 27 IX	35 35	7 7	15 15	89 (9) 99	75 74	22 (5) 26	— 1.0	II 59 (6) 63	1.6 (0.5) 2.8*		617 669	263 398		Part of a larger study including wheat bran and the effect of fruit and vegetables (see Tables 2 and 8) Blood pressure unchanged Serum cholesterol reduced C, E, H
Strasse-Wolthuis (1979)[125,126]																	
Spiller et al. (1980)[138] Ad lib diet but excluding certain high fiber foods Pectin-Sunkist	42, 23–60	Basal +Pectin, 6g	III +6	14 21	7 7	12 12	55 (5) 54 (8)			0	I 118 (13) 120 (17)						Subjects selected for low stool weight and slow transit Cellulose also given (see Table 4) B

Study	Subjects	Diet													Comments
Ross and Leklem (1981)[139] Controlled diet Normal food Low fiber Pectin "slow set grade 200"	8 M, 20–27	Basal	III	22	6	8	105	70	31		32	5.1	866	425	No significant changes in fecal excretions, but fecal β-glucuronidase activity increased 35% while 7-α-dehydroxylase activity was unchanged
		+Pectin, 15 g +12		22	6	8	126	74	33	1.5	34	4.9	863	464	
Judd and Truswell (1982)[140] Ad lib diets Pectin-Bulmers NF Either 37% (low) methoxy or 71% (high) methoxy	5 M, 5 F, 23–38	Low methoxy, 15 g	IV	21	7	10	124 (8)	72	34 (2)		III 25 (3)	6.2 (0.5)	399 (71)	412 (31)	Both pectins reduced blood cholesterol to a similar extent; triglycerides unchanged. High methoxy pectin produced greater fecal bulk E
		High methoxy, 15 g		21	7	10	161* (21)	74	39* (2)		23 (3)	6.8 (0.8)	452 (60)	436 (51)	
Fleming et al. (1983)[141] Marthinsen and Fleming (1982)[142]	5 M, 21–32	Basal	V	9	3	5	54		14						Part of a study including cellulose, corn bran, and xylose (see Tables 4 to 6)
		+Pectin, 0.5 g/kg	+32b	9	3	5	86		22	1.0					
Fleming and Rodriguez (1983)[143] Pectin — Sigma															Fecal pH unchanged. Fecal mutagenic activity negligible in all diets A, B, M

TABLE 3 (continued)
Effect of Purified Pectin on Fecal Composition

Literature source	Diet Fiber source	Total number of subjects in study (sex and age)	Study period	Fiber intake (g/day) and fiber method	Days on diet	Fecal collection period (days)	Number of subjects collecting feces	Fecal weight (g/day)	Moisture (%)	Fecal solids (g/day)	Apparent increase in fecal weight per gram dietary fiber fed	Transit time (h) and transit method	Fat (g/day)	N (g/day)	Neutral steroids (mg/day)	Acid steroids (mg/day)	Energy (kcal/day)	Comments Notes Other data available
Hillman et al. (1983)[144]	Ad lib diet Pectin, 9.3 g/kg, methoxyl	10 M, 20 F, 21—43	Basal +Pectin, 12 g	III +11	28 28	2 2	10 10	135 (21) 119 (25)			0	51 (7) 57 (4)						Cellulose and lignin also studied (see Tables 4 and 7) Stool pH unchanged

[a] A variety of fiber methods used.
[b] Assumes average weight of subjects 70.0 kg and pectin 91% dietary fiber.

TABLE 4
Effect of Cellulose and Cellulose Derivatives on Fecal Composition

Literature source	Diet Fiber source	Total number of subjects in study (sex and age)	Study period	Fiber intake (g/day) and fiber method	Days on diet	Fecal collection period (days)	Number of subjects collecting feces	Fecal weight (g/day)	Moisture (%)	Fecal solids (g/day)	Apparent increase in fecal weight per gram dietary fiber fed	Transit time (h) and transit method	Fat (g/day)	N (g/day)	Neutral steroids (mg/day)	Acid steroids (mg/day)	Energy (kcal/day)	Comments	Notes Other data available
Williams and Olmsted (1936)[9,29,57] Controlled diet Cellulose — celluflour commercially available	Normal food	3 M	Celluflour	+12[a] II	6	7	3	+15			1.2							Part of a larger study in which 9 other fiber sources fed (see Tables 2, 5, 6, and 7)	A, B
Tainter (1943)[60] "Constant" diet Methylcellulose	Normal food	—	Basal +Methylcellulose, 10 g	+10	7-14 7-14	7-14 7-14	—	127 232	81 82	24 41	10.5							Part of a study in which a variety of combinations of methylcellulose, magnesium oxide, and bran were tested for their laxative effect (see Table 9)	

TABLE 4 (continued)
Effect of Cellulose and Cellulose Derivatives on Fecal Composition

Literature source	Diet Fiber source	Total number of subjects in study (sex and age)	Study period	Fiber intake (g/day) and fiber method	Days on diet	Fecal collection period (days)	Number of subjects collecting feces	Fecal weight (g/day)	Moisture (%)	Fecal solids (g/day)	Apparent increase in fecal weight per gram dietary fiber fed	Transit time (h) and transit method	Fat (g/day)	N (g/day)	Neutral steroids (mg/day)	Acid steroids (mg/day)	Energy (kcal/day)	Comments Notes Other data available
Berberian et al. (1952)[61] *Ad lib* diet Methylcellulose tablets		8	Control	—	—	7	8	163	80	32	6.0							Further studies were undertaken in the same subjects with a combination of psyllium and methylcellulose (see Table 9)
			+Methylcellulose 4.5 g	+45	7	7	8	190	80	38								
Marks (1949)[145] *Ad lib* diet Sodium carboxymethylcellulose (CMC)		38	Basal		7	7	—	100										An early study briefly described
			+CMC, 10 g	+10	7	7		140			4.0							
			+CMC, 20 g	+20	7	7		180			4.0							
Eastwood et al. (1973)[96] *Ad lib* diet Cellulose (Whatman CF1)		8 M, 25—43	Basal		7	7	4	152 (16)	81	29 (4)		55					396	Bran also studied (see Table 2)
			+Cellulose, 16 g	+16	21	7	4	221* (29)	74	57* (6)	4.3	36					478 (122)	E

Study	Subjects	Diet										Comments
Ismail-Beigi et al. (1977)[146] Controlled diet	3 M	Basal white bread	V	9–20	—	3	141 (24)	20 (1.5)				
60% of energy from bread Cellulose — Whatman No. 3 taken with either white bread or Basari (80 to 90% extraction brown bread)		+Cellulose[b] 12 g		9–20	—	3	223	32	6.8			Cellulose caused increased fecal excretion of calcium, magnesium, and zinc and negative balances of all three C, D
		Basal Basari bread		14		2	280 (112)					
		+Cellulose, 12 g		14		2	482 (225)		16.8			
Slavin and Marlett (1980)[147,148] Controlled diet	7 F, 20–39	Basal	V 9	20–30	5	7	75 (9)	19 (1.6)		I 102 (22)	2.8 (0.2)	1.3 (0.1)	Fecal calcium, and magnesium excretion increased
		+Cellulose, 16 g	24	20–30	5	7	130* (11)	39* (3)	3.5	63 (10)	3.4 (0.3)	1.4 (0.1)	Fat, nitrogen, and energy digestibilities unaffected A, C
Spiller et al. (1980)[138] Ad lib diet but excluding certain high fiber foods Cellulose — Solka floc®	42, 23–60	Basal	—	14	7	13	64 (7)			I 122 (12)			Subjects selected for low stool weight and slow transit
		+Cellulose, 14 g	+14	21	7	13	97 (11)		2.3	62 (8)			Pectin also given (see Table 3) B
Fleming et al. (1983)[141]	5 M, 21–32	Basal	V 0	9	3	5	54	14					Part of a study including pectin,

TABLE 4 (continued)
Effect of Cellulose and Cellulose Derivatives on Fecal Composition

Literature source	Fiber source Diet	Total number of subjects in study (sex and age)	Study period	Fiber intake (g/day) and fiber method	Days on diet	Fecal collection period (days)	Number of subjects collecting feces	Fecal weight (g/day)	Moisture (%)	Fecal solids (g/day)	Apparent increase in fecal weight per gram dietary fiber fed	Transit time (h) and transit method	Fat (g/day)	N (g/day)	Neutral steroids (mg/day)	Acid steroids (mg/day)	Energy (Kcal/day)	Comments	Notes Other data available
Marthinsen and Fleming (1982)[142]	+Cellulose 0.5 g/kg			+35 g[e]	9	3	5	106		42	1.5								corn bran and xylan (see Tables 3, 5, and 6)
Fleming and Rodriguez (1983)[143]	Controlled semipurified diets Cellulose — Alphacell from ICN																		Fecal pH Fecal-mutagenic activity negligible on all diets A, B, M
Hillman et al. (1983)[144] Ad lib diet Cellulose — α-cellulose from Sigma	Basal +Cellulose, 15 g			— +15	28 28	2 2	10 10	133 (21) 208* (30)			5.0	II 55 (6) 40* (4)						Pectin and lignin also fed (see Tables 3 and 7) Stool pH fell
Wrick et al. (1983)[149] Van Soest et al. (1978)[150]	Basal +Cellulose, 13—18 g day	24	V		24 24	7 7	12 12	102 137		25 33		56[d] 47						Part of a larger study in which coarse and fine bran and cabbage fi-
Ehle et al. (1982)[151]																			

Heller et al. (1980)[152] — ber were fed (see Tables 7 and 10) A, B
Van Soest (1981)[153] (1984)[154]
Van Soest et al. (1983)[155] Controlled diet Normal food Low fiber Cellulose — Solka floc® baked into bread

[a] Figures are increases over basal diet period — fiber remaining in stool.
[b] Cellulose taken with 150 g apple compote (90 g apple + 60 g syrup).
[c] Assumes average weight of subjects of 70 kg.
[d] Various transit methods used (see Van Soest et al. [1983]).[156]

TABLE 5
Effect of Plant Gums, Mucilages, and Other Polysaccharides on Fecal Composition

Literature source	Diet Fiber source	Total number of subjects in study (sex and age)	Study period	Fiber intake (g/day) and fiber method	Days on diet	Fecal collection period (days)	Number of subjects collecting feces	Fecal weight (g/day)	Percent moisture	Fecal solids (g/day)	Apparent increase in fecal weight per gram dietary fiber fed	Transit time (h) and transit method	Fat (g/day)	N (g/day)	Neutral steroids (mg/day)	Acid steroids (mg/day)	Energy (kcal/day)	Comments Notes Other data available
Williams and Olmsted (1936)[9,29,57] Controlled diet Normal food Agar-agar		3M	Agar-agar	+16 II	6	7	3	+111[a]			8.7							Part of a larger study in which 9 other fiber sources were fed (see Tables 2, 4, 6, and 7) A,B
Gray and Tainter (1941)[7] Ad lib diet Karaya gum — sterculia urens Bassora gum (Imbicoll) Psyllium seed (black psyllium NF) Ispaghula — from Plantago ovata (Konsyl Siblin)		5M	Basal +Karaya, 5 g Basal +Imbicoll, 5 g Basal	+5 +5	7 7 7 7 7	3 3 3 3 3	5 5 5 5 5	68 83 (17) 84 135 (24) 96		18(2) 20 (40) 21 (2) 31 (5) 20 (2)	3.0 10.2							A major early study of the laxative effects of plant gums including animal data and extensive in vitro studies

Study	Subjects	Diet	Fiber (g)	Days	a	b	Fecal wt (SD)	c (d)	Ratio	Comments
Psyllium — from Plantago loeflingii (mucilose)		+Psyllium seed, 5 g	+5	7	3	5	118 (24)	26 (6)	4.4	
		Basal		7	3	5	96	20 (2)		
		+Konsyl, 5 g	+5	7	3	5	122 (30)	22 (6)	5.2	
		Basal		7	3	5	96	22 (2)		
		+Mucilose, 5 g	+5	7	3	5	110 (25)	17 (4)	2.8	
		Basal		7	3	5	90	19 (2)		
		+Siblin, 5 g	+5	7	3	5	99 (37)	16 (4)	1.8	
Block (1947)[157] *Ad lib* diet Psyllium (Metamucil)	22 M, 18 F	Basal		7	1	14	52 (6)			Mental hospital patients Includes one of the earliest observations of the moderating effect of fiber on blood glucose K
		+Psyllium, 12 g	+12	7	1	14	63 (23)		0.9	
		III								
Drasar and Jenkins (1976)[133] *Ad lib* diets Guar gum (clear gum, Hercules Powder Co.)	10 M, 22–25	Basal		14	7	3	100			Also studied were pectin and banana (see Tables 3 and 8) Guar lowered blood cholesterol but did not produce a detectable change in the fecal microflora E,J
		+Guar gum, 35 g	+30	14	7	3	204 (21)		3.5	

TABLE 5 (continued)
Effect of Plant Gums, Mucilages, and Other Polysaccharides on Fecal Composition

Literature source	Diet Fiber source	Total number of subjects in study (sex and age)	Study period	Fiber intake (g/day) and fiber method	Days on diet	Fecal collection period (days)	Number of subjects collecting feces	Fecal weight (g/day)	Percent moisture	Fecal solids (g/day)	Apparent increase in fecal weight per gram dietary fiber fed	Transit time (h) and transit method	Fat (g/day)	N (g/day)	Neutral steroids (mg/day)	Acid steroids (mg/day)	Energy (kcal/day)	Comments	Notes Other data available
Cummings et al. (1978)[18] Controlled Normal food Guar gum (clear gum, Hercules Powder Co.)		19 M, 20–38	Basal	22 III	21	7	3	120 (20)	74	30 (3)								Part of a larger study in which fiber from bran, carrot, cabbage, and apple were studied (see Tables 2 and 7)	
			+Guar, 20 g	39	21	7	3	139 (17)	74	35 (1)	1.1								
Prynne and Southgate (1979)[158] Controlled diet Normal food Ispaghula husk (Isogel)		2 M, 2 F, 28–31	Basal	20 III	21	5	4	162 (22)	77	37 (5)								Data also given for apparent digestibilities of N, fat, energy, and ash, none of which changed significantly Great detail of nonstarch polysaccharide intakes and outputs A	
			+Ispaghula, 25 g	44	21	5	4	242* (188)	82	43* (14)	3.2								

Study	Subjects	Diet								I			Notes
Spiller et al. (1979)[159]	50, 25–65	Basal	—	21	7	10	58	19		101		1.0 (0.1)	Subjects selected for low stool weight and slow transit, "double blind parallel repeated measures" design. A cellulose-pectin biscuit also studied (see Table 9) C, H, N
Ad lib low fiber-restricted diet Psyllium seed hydrocolloid		+Psyllium powder, 20 g	+10	21	7	10	107	29	4.9	92		1.1 (0.2)	
Smith et al. (1980)[123]	18 M, 29 F, 65–96	Basal	—		5	15	37	10			4.2		Elderly hospitalized subjects. Also studied with bran (see Table 2). Colonic motility (pressures) unchanged. Both ispaghula and bran equally effective per gram of fiber fed C, F, H
Ad lib hospital diet Ispaghula (Fybogel)		+Ispaghula, 10 g	+8	28	5	15	75	20	4.7		7.9		
Eastwood et al. (1983)[160]	5 M	Basal	—	7	5	5	135	36		63	4.2		The gum had no discernable effect on anything. A "toxicity" study B, E, H, K, M, N
Ad lib diet Gum Karaya (Sterculia urens from Nargina)		+Karaya, 10.5 g	+8	21	5	5	139	38	0.5	68	3.9		
Fleming et al. (1983)[141]	5 M, 21–32	Basal	V 0	9	3	5	54	14					Part of a study including cel-

TABLE 5 (continued)
Effect of Plant Gums, Mucilages, and Other Polysaccharides on Fecal Composition

Literature source	Diet Fiber source	Total number of subjects in study (sex and age)	Study period	Fiber intake (g/day) and fiber method	Days on diet	Fecal collection period (days)	Number of subjects collecting feces	Fecal weight (g/day)	Percent moisture	Fecal solids (g/day)	Apparent increase in fecal weight per gram dietary fiber fed	Transit time (h) and transit method	Fat (g/day)	N (g/day)	Neutral steroids (mg/day)	Acid steroids (mg/day)	Energy (kcal/day)	Comments Notes Other data available
Marthinsen and Fleming (1982)[142] Fleming and Rodriguez (1983)[143] Controlled semi-purified diets Xylan (ICN)	+Xylan, 0.5 g/kg			+35[b]	9	3	5	65		16	0.3							lulose, corn bran, and pectin (see Tables 3, 4, and 6); fecal pH unchanged A, B, M
Ross et al.(1983)[161] Ad lib diet Gum Arabic	Basal +Gum Arabic, 25 25 g	5 M, 30—55		—	21	5 5	5 5	147 161		37 52	0.6	51 71				699 779	472 424	Serum cholesterol reduced and some changes in breath H_2 excretion Extensive breakdown of gum in gut A, B, E, H, K, M, N

[a] Figures are increases over basal diet period — fiber remaining in stool.
[b] Assumes average weight of subjects of 70 kg and also that xylan was 100% dietary fiber.

TABLE 6
Effect of Oats and Corn Products on Fecal Composition

Literature source	Diet Fiber source	Total number of subjects in study (sex and age)	Study period	Fiber intake (g/day) and fiber method	Days on diet	Fecal collection period (days)	Number of subjects collecting feces	Fecal weight (g/day)	Moisture (%)	Fecal solids (g/day)	Apparent increase in fecal weight per gram dietary fiber fed	Transit time (h) and transit method	Fat (g/day)	N (g/day)	Neutral steroids (mg/day)	Acid steroids (mg/day)	Energy (Kcal/day)	Comments	Notes Other data available
Williams and Olmsted (1936)[9,29,57] Controlled diet	Corn germ meal, 55 g Normal food but excluding fruit and vegetables Corn germ meal prepared by washing for 24 h in warm water extracting with hot ethanol and drying	3 M		+26 II	6	7	3	+96[a]			4.6							Part of a larger study in which 9 other fiber sources fed (see Tables 2, 4, 5, and 7)	A, B
Calloway and Kretsch (1978)[162]	Formula diet	6 M, 28–42		4 V	15	6	6	68 (10)	79	14 (1)		28 (10) III	1.2 (0.3)	1.0 (0.1)		238 (24)	98 (16)	Subjects average weight, 72.8 kg	
Kretsch et al. (1979)[163] Controlled egg-based high protein formula diet	Oat bran (toasted)			12	15	6	6	112* (16)	75	28* (3)	5.5	31 (7)	2.0* (0.4)	1.5* (0.2)		504* (37)	184* (27)	No difference between toasted and plain bran for any parameter Principally a	
	Oat brain (plain)			12	15	6	6	128* (29)	77	29* (2)	5.0	27 (6)	1.9* (0.3)	1.6* (0.2)		501 (62)	189* (41)		

TABLE 6 (continued)
Effect of Oats and Corn Products on Fecal Composition

Literature source	Diet Fiber source	Total number of subjects in study (sex and age)	Study period	Fiber intake (g/day) and fiber method	Days on diet	Fecal collection period (days)	Number of subjects collecting feces	Fecal weight (g/day)	Moisture (%)	Fecal solids (g/day)	Apparent increase in fecal weight per gram dietary fiber fed	Transit time (h) and transit method	Fat (g/day)	N (g/day)	Neutral steroids (mg/day)	Acid steroids (mg/day)	Energy (kcal/day)	Comments	Notes Other data available
Cooked oat bran either plain or toasted																		study of N balance which was not affected by oat bran Blood lipids unchanged Guatemalan diet also fed (See Table 8)	A, E
Munoz et al. (1979)[114,120] Controlled diet Dry milled corn bran baked into bread		10 M 19—54	Basal +Corn bran, 26 g	V +24	28—30 28—30	12 12	7 7	72 (10) 144* (10)			3.0					337 (68) 483 (52)		Part of a larger study including wheat bran and soybean hulls (see Tables 2 and 7) No effect on serum cholesterol	C, D, E, K

Reference	Subjects	Diet									III					Comments
Judd and Truswell (1982)[164] Controlled diet Normal food Rolled oats — served as porridge and substituted for flour in bread, cakes, and biscuits	6 M, 4 F, 24–37	Basal +Oats, 110–160 g	23 25c	21 21	6 6	10 10	114 125	74 73	29 34*		36 30	3.4 5.1*	282 315	230 372*	230 (33)	Study design was control-oats-control; data from first control period presented here Blood cholesterol fell significantly E
		V														
Kirby et al. (1981)[165] Controlled diet Normal food Oat bran — served as muffins or hot cereal	8 M, 35–62	Basal +Oat bran, 100 g	20 43	10 10	3 3	8 8	147 (14) 169* (16)			35 (2) 43* (2)	1.0			862 (68) 819 (61)	230 (33) 354* (28)	Serum cholesterol lowered Glucose tolerance unaffected E, K
		X														
Graham et al. (1982)[130] Ad lib low fiber diet Corn bran (G-60 grade Staley Mfg. Co.) fine particle size	11 F, 20–40	Basal +Corn bran, 20 g	17	14 14	7 7	6 6	31 (2) 82* (18)		65 66	11 28*	3.0					Constipated subjects also studied with wheat bran which was less effective per gram material fed (see Table 2) H
Fleming et al. (1983)[141] Marthinsen and Fleming (1982)[142]	5 M, 21–32	Basal	0	9	3	5	54		14							

TABLE 6 (continued)
Effect of Oats and Corn Products on Fecal Composition

Literature source	Diet Fiber source	Total number of subjects in study (sex and age)	Study period	Fiber intake (g/day) and fiber method	Days on diet	Fecal collection period (days)	Number of subjects collecting feces	Fecal weight (g/day)	Moisture (%)	Fecal solids (g/day)	Apparent increase in fecal weight per gram dietary fiber fed	Transit time (h) and transit method	Fat (g/day)	N (g/day)	Neutral steroids (mg/day)	Acid steroids (mg/day)	Energy (kcal/day)	Comments Notes Other data available
Fleming and Rodriguez (1983)[143] Controlled semi-purified diets Corn bran (Quaker Oats)			+Corn bran, 0.6 g/kg	+29[d]	9	3	5	139*		46	2.9							Part of a study including cellulose, pectin, and xylose (see Tables 3 to 5) Fecal pH unchanged A, B, M

[a] Figures are increases over basal diet period — fiber remaining in stool.
[b] Oat bran fed at 0.6 g/kg/day.
[c] Oatmeal diet contained only 2 g more dietary fiber because of substitutions — according to the authors.
[d] Assumes average weight of subjects of 70 kg.

TABLE 7
Effect of Miscellaneous Purified Forms of Fiber on Fecal Composition

Literature source	Diet fiber source	Total number of subjects in study (sex and age)	Study period	Fiber intake (g/day) and fiber method	Days on diet	Fecal collection period (days)	Number of subjects collecting feces	Fecal weight (g/day)	Moisture (%)	Fecal solids (g/day)	Apparent increase in fecal weight per gram dietary fiber fed	Transit time (h) and transit method	Fat (g/day)	N (g/day)	Neutral steroids (mg/day)	Acid steroids (mg/day)	Energy (kcal/day)	Comments Notes Other data available
Williams and Olmsted (1936)[9,29,57]	Controlled diet Normal food, excluding vegetables and fruit Carrots, cabbage, and peas obtained on the open market, chopped and washed in warm water for 24 h, then extracted with hot ethanol and dried Alfalfa leaf meal, cotton seed hull meal, and sugar beet pulp from Ralston Purina	3 M	Alfalfa leaf meal, 21 g	+13	6	7	3	+40 a			3.0							Also studied: cellulose, wheat bran, agar-agar, and corn germ meal (see Tables 2, 4, 5, and 6) A
			Carrot, 38 g	+18	6	7	3	+90			5.6							
			Cotton seed hulls, 25 g	+18	6	7	3	+16			2.1							
			Sugar beet pulp, 27 g	+15	6	7	3	+67			4.9							
			Canned peas, 27 g	+12	6	7	3	+28			3.3							
			Cabbage, 35 g	+17	6	7	3	104			6.9							

TABLE 7 (continued)
Effect of Miscellaneous Purified Forms of Fiber on Fecal Composition

Literature source	Fiber source Diet Co. then processed as other materials	Total number of subjects in study (sex and age)	Study period	Fiber intake (g/day) and fiber method	Days on diet	Fecal collection period (days)	Number of subjects collecting feces	Fecal weight (g/day)	Moisture (%)	Fecal solids (g/day)	Apparent increase in fecal weight per gram dietary fiber fed	Transit time (h) and transit method	Fat (g/day)	N (g/day)	Neutral steroids (mg/day)	Acid steroids (mg/day)	Energy (kcal/day)	Comments Notes Other data available
Walters et al. (1975)[107]	Basal	20 F, 25—72		18	—	7	9	88 (6)	75	22 (2)		I 47 (6)	4.3 (0.5)		420 (51)	156 (20)		Blood lipids and fecal microflora unchanged A separate study of bran also reported (see Table 2) E, J
McLean Baird (1977)[109] Ad lib diet in convent	+ Bagasse, 10.5 g			27	84	7	9	140* (10)	76	33* (1)	5.8	37 (3)	6.7* (0.5)		377 (13)	234* (16)		
Bagasse (sugar cane residue from Tate and Lyle) made into biscuits			III									II						
Cummings et al. (1978)[18]	Basal	19 M, 20—38		22	21	7	6	88 (9)	70	26 (1)		80 (11)						Bran and guar gum also studied (see Tables 2 and 5) J
Stephen and Cummings (1980)[25]	+Cabbage, 30 g			40	21	7	6	143* (16)	75*	35 (6)	3.0	64* (8)						

Study	Subjects	Diet										Comments
Controlled diet Cabbage, carrot, and apple obtained commercially, dried, extracted with hot ethanol and acetone, then dried and ground		Basal	22	21	7	6	117 (7)	74	30 (1)		60 (9)	
		+Carrot, 30 g	42	21	7	6	189* (16)	79*	39* (2)	3.6	50 (6)	
		Basal	22	21	7	6	141 (20)	77	30 (2)		50 (9)	
		+Apple, 25 g	44	21	7	6	203* (29)	80*	37* (3)	2.8	43* (6)	
		+Apple, 25 g	44	21	7	6	203* (29)	80*	37* 3	2.8	43* (6)	
Munoz et al. (1979)[114,120] Controlled diet Soybean hulls (SBH) and textured vegetable protein (TVP) fed as bread	10 M, 19–54	Basal	V	28–30	12	5	68 (9)				388 (51)	Also studied on bran and corn bran (see Tables 2 and 6) Plasma cholesterol unchanged but triglycerides fell with SBH C, D, E, K
		+SBH, 26 g	+23	28–30	12	5	128* (16)			2.6	330 (87)	
		Basal		28–30	12	3	92 (10)					
		+TVP, 26 g	+4	28–30	12	3	102 (21)					
Eastwood et al. (1983)[24] Ad lib diet Potato concentrate purified by commercial company and either air- or roller-dried or boiled; fed with either milk or soup	9 M, 26–44	Basal	XI 20	7	7	7	161 (26)	75 (1)	39 (5)		I 50 (11)	4.9 (0.9)	Also studied on bran (see Table 2) No significant effect on fecal composition or blood lipids A, E
		+Roller-dried potato, 20 g	33	21	7	7	215 (44)	76 (2)	47 (6)	4.1	33 (5)	6.9 (1.3)	
		Basal	18	7	7	7	170 (32)	74 (1)	42 (6)		48 (8)	4.2 (0.8)	
		+Air-dried potato, 20 g	28	21	7	7	207 (42)	75 (2)	47 (6)	3.7	42 (6)	4.7 (0.8)	
		Basal		—	7	5	204 (50)	78 (3)	39 (7)		35 (7)	3.5 (0.7)	
		+Boiled potato, 20 g		—	7	5	231 (51)	78 (2)	47 (7)	2.7[b]	32 (10)	4.5 (0.7)	

TABLE 7 (continued)
Effect of Miscellaneous Purified Forms of Fiber on Fecal Composition

Literature source	Diet Fiber source	Total number of subjects (sex and age)	Study period	Fiber intake (g/day) and fiber method	Days on diet	Fecal collection period (days)	Number of subjects collecting feces	Fecal weight (g/day)	Moisture (%)	Fecal solids (g/day)	Apparent increase in fecal weight per gram dietary fiber fed	Transit time (h) and transit method	Fat (g/day)	N (g/day)	Neutral steroids (mg/day)	Acid steroids (mg/day)	Energy (kcal/day)	Comments / Notes / Other data available
Hillman et al. (1983)[144]	Basal	10 M, 20 F, 21–43		III	28	2	10	139 (17)				50 (5) II						Cellulose and pectin also studied (see Tables 3 and 4) Stool pH unchanged
	Lignin — pure Aspen autohydrolyzed from Stake Technology Ltd.		+Lignin, 12 g	+12	28	2	10	177 (25)			3.2	40 (5)						
Schweizer et al. (1983)[166]	Basal	2 M, 4 F, 20–30		14 V, XI	14	7	6	129 (16)	77	28		62 (4) I			735 (49)	242 (19)		Never-dried soya increased fecal deoxycholate while purified soya increased low-density lipoprotein cholesterol and altered glucose tolerance A, C, D, E, K
	Soya: a never-dried pulp obtained as a by-product of milk production; purified soya fiber obtained from soya flour by extraction		+Never-dried soya pulp, 54 g	33	21	7	6	153* (14)	77	34* (3)	1.3	44 (9)			726 (28)	294 (23)		
			+Purified soya pulp, 26.5 g	34	21	7	6	178* (28)	77	39* (4)	2.4	59 (11)			764 (66)	215 (17)		

Study	n	Diet				III								Notes
Tsai et al. (1983)[167] Controlled diet Normal food but low fiber Soy polysaccharide[c]	14 M, 20—30	Basal +Soy, 25 g	— —	17 17		14 14		140 (11) 176* (16)	76 78	34 (3) 39 (4)	26 (3) 29 (3)	7.2 (0.8) 5.7* (1.0)	1.6 (0.2) 1.9 (0.2)	246 (59) 289 (49)	109 (8) 118 (16)	263 (32) 279 (23)	Fasting blood glucose fell but lipids unchanged C, D, E, H, K
Wrick et al. (1983)[149,156] Controlled diet Normal food Cabbage — ethanol-extracted and incorporated into bread	24	Basal +Cabbage	— —	24 24	V 7 7	12 12		102 110		25 24	56[d] 58						12 g cell wall material daily at first but increased later up to 24 g/day Bran and cellulose also fed (see Tables 4 and 10) A, B

[a] Stool weights are increased over basal period — fiber remaining.
[b] Assumes fiber intake increased by about 10 g.
[c] Soy polysaccharides "a fiber-rich product purified from soy bean cotyledon".
[d] Various transit methods used (see Van Soest et al., 1983).

TABLE 8
Effect of Foods Containing Fiber on Fecal Composition

Literature source	Diet Fiber source	Total number of subjects in study (sex and age)	Study period	Fiber intake (g/day) and fiber method	Days on diet	Fecal collection period (days)	Number of subjects collecting feces	Fecal weight (g/day)	Moisture (%)	Fecal solids (g/day)	Apparent increase in fecal weight per gram dietary fiber fed	Transit time (h) and transit method	Fat (g/day)	N (g/day)	Neutral steroids (mg/day)	Acid steroids (mg/day)	Energy (kcal/day)	Comments	Notes Other data available
Cowgill and Sullivan (1933)[59] Controlled diet Normal food Fruits and vegetables		6 M	Basal		7	7	6	78 (15)										Constipated subjects Also studied effect of various brans (see Table 2) Noted greater digestibility of fiber than in healthy subjects	A
			+Fruit and vegetables	30–38[a]	7	7	5	165[a] (27)											
			+Fruit and vegetables and bran	90	7	7	3	193[a] (10)											
				108–113															
McCance and Widdowson (1942)[168] Controlled diet Normal food Fruit — plums, greengages, pears, and damsons		2 M, 2 F, 27–41	Basal	14–28	7	7	4	155										A chance observation in a study of mineral balance on various breads Fruit had no effect	C
			+Fruit, 31–183 g		7	7	4	156											

Study	Subjects	Diet	I	Age		Group							Notes
Antonis and Bersohn (1962)[169,170] Controlled diets Normal prison foods	58 M: 29 white, 29 black	High fat, high fiber	15	22–29[b]	7	22 Wh	236 (13)			2.1 (0.1)	479 (10)	463 (29)	Prisoners in South Africa A very large study of the effect of diet, especially fat and fiber, on fecal lipids, blood lipids, and bile acids E
		High fat, low fiber	4	22–29	7	22 Wh	85* (6)			1.2* (0.1)	324* (31)	450 (38)	
		High fat, high fiber	15	22–29	7	21 Bl	259 (16)			4.4 (0.3)	590 (62)	517 (31)	
		High fat, low fiber	4	22–29	7	21 Bl	99* (6)			2.1* (0.2)	310* (27)	521 (31)	
		Low fat, high fiber	15	15–17	7	18 Wh	209 (13)			2.2 (0.1)	537 (35)	459 (28)	
		Low fat, low fiber	4	15–17	7	18 Wh	100* (9)			1.5* (0.1)	297* (25)	320* (25)	
		Low fat, high fiber	15	15–17	7	13 Bl	240 (10)			2.6 (0.1)	543 (51)	393 (18)	
		Low fat, low fiber	4	15–17	7	13 Bl	97* (7)			1.6* (0.1)	277* (24)	316* (20)	
Southgate and Durnin (1970)[28] Controlled diet Normal food	23 M, 26 W, 18–78	Diet 1	III 9.7	10–14	7	c 12 YM	82 (6)	75	21 (1)	4.1 (0.3)		117 (6)	A large and detailed study of the energy value of the diet as influenced by fiber A
		Diet 2	21.5	10–14	7	12 YM	163* (8)	76	38* (1)	8.3	6.4* (0.3)		206* (6)
											1.8 (0.1)		
											2.2* (0.1)		
		Diet 1	6.2	10–14	7	14 YW	47 (3)	68	15 (0.8)		3.0 (0.2)		83 (4)
		Diet 2: contains fruit and vegetables and whole meal bread	16.2	10–14	7	14 YW	91* (5)	73	24* (1.0)	4.4	3.7* (0.2)	1.0 (0.1)	127* (5)	
											1.3* (0.1)		
		Diet 3: contains larger amounts of fruit and vegetables	31.9	10–14	7	14 YW	181* (8)	78	40* (1.1)	5.2	6.2* (0.3)	2.2 (0.1)	210* (7)	
Diet 1: no fruit or vegetables except potato														

TABLE 8 (continued)
Effect of Foods Containing Fiber on Fecal Composition

Literature source	Total number of subjects in study (sex and age)	Study period	Fiber intake (g/day) and fiber method	Days on diet	Fecal collection period (days)	Number of subjects collecting feces	Fecal weight (g/day)	Moisture (%)	Fecal solids (g/day)	Apparent increase in fecal weight per gram dietary fiber fed	Transit time (h) and transit method	Fat (g/day)	N (g/day)	Neutral steroids (mg/day)	Acid steroids (mg/day)	Energy (kcal/day)	Comments Notes Other data available
Drasar and Jenkins (1976)[133] Ad lib diet Bananas and Plantain banana	10 M, 22–25	Diet 1	9.6	10–14	7	11 EM	79 (11)	77	18 (1.0)			5.1 (0.3)	1.4 (0.1)			103 (5)	
		Diet 2	28.3	10–14	7	11 EM	140* (12)	77	32* (1.7)	3.3		5.4 (0.4)	2.0* (0.2)			164* (8)	
		Diet 1	7.4	10–14	7	12 EW	60 (5)	75	15 (0.8)			4.5 (0.3)	0.9 (0.1)			90 (5)	
		Diet 2	20.9	10–14	7	12 EW	130* (7)	79	28* (1.0)	5.1		4.8 (0.0)	1.4* (0.1)			150* (6)	
		Basal	IV	14	7	5	121 (15)										Also studied pectin and guar (see Tables 3 and 5) Blood lipids and fecal microflora unaffected E, J
		+Banana, 1000 g	+34	14	7	5	170 (23)			1.4							
		+Plantain, 1000 g	+58	14	7	4	208 (46)			1.5							
Flynn, Beirn, and Burkitt (1977)[171]	48 M, 20–56	Basal[d]	5.6	—	—	5	149 (20)				I 46 (20)						No change in blood lipids E, F
		+Potato,	7.3	—	—	5	249*			11.6	33						

Study	Subjects	Diet	Fiber intake	Days	n	Fecal wt (g/d)	Transit (h)	Frequency	Fecal fiber	Fat	N	Energy	Notes
		Ad lib diet Cooked potato	860 g	(+8.6)^e		(39)		(21)					
		Basal^d (low fiber)	3.5		18	125 (15)		62 (18)					
		+Potato, 860 g	6.6 (+8.6)^e		18	294* (24)		35* (24)					
Beyer and Flynn (1978)^{172}	6 M, 21–29	Controlled diet	I					III				63	
		Normal food	Low fiber	1.1	5	51		48	2.5	1.1		140*	
		Mixed sources	Increased fiber	8.7	5	157		12	6.1*	2.2*			
Calloway and Kretsch (1978)^{162}	6 M, 28–42	Formula diet	V 0	19.6	3	68 (26)	79	14 (3.2)	1.2 (0.7)	1.0 (0.3)		238 (58)	98 (40)
Kretsch et al. (1979)^{163}		Guatemalan diet	89	3.5^f	3	327* (89)	81	62* (10)	1.9* (0.1)	3.4* (0.3)		502* (160)	348* (64)
		Controlled egg-based high protein formula diet		2.9									Also studied with oat bran (see Table 6) A, E
		Guatemalan diet contained mainly black beans and corn tortilla together with rice, bread, cheese, pumpkin, squash, and banana												
Robertson et al. (1979)^{173}	5	Ad lib diet Basal	V 21 (14–33)		7	142 (37)	75	35 (6)	2.7 (0.4)		I 72 (12)	602 (73)	271 (29)
		Raw carrot +Carrot	+6	5.8	7	177* (33)	76	42 (6)	3.5 (0.7)		55 (14)	645 (96)	389 (33)	Serum cholesterol fell Breath hydrogen excretion increased C, E, H, M

TABLE 8 (continued)
Effect of Foods Containing Fiber on Fecal Composition

Literature source	Diet / Fiber source	Total number of subjects in study (sex and age)	Study period	Fiber intake (g/day) and fiber method	Days on diet	Fecal collection period (days)	Number of subjects collecting feces	Fecal weight (g/day)	Moisture (%)	Fecal solids (g/day)	Apparent increase in fecal weight per gram dietary fiber fed	Transit time (h) and transit method	Fat (g/day)	N (g/day)	Neutral steroids (mg/day)	Acid steroids (mg/day)	Energy (Kcal/day)	Comments	Notes Other data available
Stasse-Wolthuis et al. (1979)[174] Controlled diet Normal food Mixed fiber sources	Low fiber	23 M, 23 F, 20—27		12 III[g], VIII, IX	21	3—5	43	69 (8)	74	18 (2)		55 (3) II	1.2 (0.1)					Diets were fed at either high or low cholesterol (about 200 and 600 mg/day). Serum cholesterol fell in both groups with fiber but results confounded by changes in fat intake	C, E, H
	High fiber			33	21	3—5	43	184* (11)	76	44* (7)	3.5	37* (2)	2.5* (0.1)						
Stasse-Wolthuis et al. (1979)[124-126] Controlled diet Normal food	Low fiber	40 M, 22 F, 18—28		18 g	35	7	15	89 (10)		23		66 (10) I	2.2 (0.5)			682	364	Also studied with pectin and wheat bran (see Tables 2 and 3)	
	+ Fruit and vegetables, 1065 g			43	35	7	15	138*		32*	2.0	53*	2.9			888	290		

Study	Subjects	Diet	V							III			Comments
Fruit and vegetables													Serum cholesterol changes not significant. No change in blood pressure C, E, H
Kelsay et al. (1978)[175-178] Controlled diet	12 M, 37-58	Low fiber	4	26	7	12	89 (9)	73	23 (2)	6.0	52 (4)	4.9 (0.5)	1.3 (0.1)	117
Low fiber with fruit and vegetable juices then with whole fruit and vegetables (no cereals)		High fiber	24	26	7	12	209* (9)	75	52* (2)		38* (4)	6.4* (0.4)	2.6* (0.2)	255* Blood pressure unchanged except in those in whom diastolic was 80 mm+ Mineral balances became "lower" A, C, D
Kelsay et al. (1981)[179] Controlled diet	12 M, 35-49	Low fiber	2	21	7	12	87 (5)	74	23 (1)	4.9	30 (3)	4.8 (0.4)	1.4 (0.1)	113 (6) Latin square design
Low fiber with fruit and vegetable juice then with increasing amounts of fruit and vegetables		+Fruit and vegetables	10	21	7	12	127* (8)	75	32* (2)		27 (2)	5.4 (0.4)	1.8 (0.1)	162* (10) Blood pressure unchanged Calcium, magnesium, and copper balance unchanged
		+Fruit and vegetables	19	21	7	12	171* (12)	75	42* (2)	2.5	27 (2)	6.0 (0.4)	2.3 (0.1)	209* (11) Zinc balance "decreased"
		+Fruit and vegetables	26	21	7	12	274* (26)	78	50* (3)	5.8	31 (4)	6.2 (0.1)	2.6 (0.2)	255* (16) A, C, D

TABLE 8 (continued)
Effect of Foods Containing Fiber on Fecal Composition

Literature source	Diet Fiber source	Total number of subjects in study (sex and age)	Study period	Fiber intake (g/day) and fiber method	Days on diet	Fecal collection period (days)	Number of subjects collecting feces	Fecal weight (g/day)	Moisture (%)	Fecal solids (g/day)	Apparent increase in fecal weight per gram dietary fiber fed	Transit time (h) and transit method	Fat (g/day)	N (g/day)	Neutral steroids (mg/day)	Acid steroids (mg/day)	Energy (kcal/day)	Comments Notes Other data available
Leeds et al. (1982)[180]	Basal	8 F, 21—36		22 IV	14	14	6—8	115 (15)		31		53 (8) III						All subjects noted marked increase in flatulence
	Ad lib diet with substitution of meat and vegetables by canned baked beans (Haricot)		+Haricot beans, 450 g	49	14	14	6—8	150* (14)		38	1.3	45 (6)						Noticeable effect of menstruation on transit time

a Milligrams of crude fiber per kilogram body weight per day.
b Weeks on diet (data are from Table 5).
c YM, young men; YW, young women; EM, elderly men; EW, elderly women.
d Subjects divided into those consuming more than 5 g crude fiber per day (average 5.6 g/day) and those consuming less (average 3.5 g/day).
e Dietary fiber equivalent.
f Dietary fiber values calculated from food tables (IV).
g A variety of fiber methods used (see paper).

TABLE 9
Effect of Mixed Sources of Fiber on Fecal Composition

Literature source	Diet Fiber source	Total number of subjects in study (sex and age)	Study period	Fiber intake (g/day) and fiber method	Days on diet	Fecal collection period (days)	Number of subjects collecting feces	Fecal weight (g/day)	Moisture (%)	Fecal solids (g/day)	Apparent increase in fecal weight per gram dietary fiber fed	Transit time (h) and transit method	Fat (g/day)	N (g/day)	Neutral steroids (mg/day)	Acid steroids (mg/day)	Energy (kcal/day)	Comments	Notes Other data available
Berberian et al. (1952)[61]	Ad lib diet Tablets containing 0.4 g methylcellulose and 0.1 g psyllium	8	Basal +6 Tablets +9 Tablets	+3 +4½	— 7 7	7 7 7	8 8 8	163 184 213	80 81 82	32 35 38	7 11.1							Also studied with pure methylcellulose (see Table 4)	
Tainter (1943)[60]	"Constant" diets, normal foods Various combinations of methylcellulose (MC), bran (B), and magnesium oxide (MO)	—	Basal 35% MC 65% B 5 g 10 g 3.5% MO 35% MC 61.5% B 10 g 10% MO 45% MC 45% B 10 g 10% MO 90% MC 10 g	3.2* 6.4 6.2 6.5 9	7–14 7–14 7–14 7–14 7–14 7–14	7–14 7–14 7–14 7–14 7–14 7–14	—	127 145 160 179 177 231	81 78 81 81 83 84	24 31 31 35 30 36	5.6 5.2 8.4 7.7 11.6							Also studied with pure methylcellulose (see Table 4) Magnesium oxide providing significant additional laxation	

TABLE 9 (continued)
Effect of Mixed Sources of Fiber on Fecal Composition

Literature source	Diet Fiber source	Total number of subjects in study (sex and age)	Study period	Fiber intake (g/day) and fiber method	Days on diet	Fecal collection period (days)	Number of subjects collecting feces	Fecal weight (g/day)	Moisture (%)	Fecal solids (g/day)	Apparent increase in fecal weight per gram dietary fiber fed	Transit time (h) and transit method	Fat (g/day)	N (g/day)	Neutral steroids (mg/day)	Acid steroids (mg/day)	Energy (kcal/day)	Comments Notes Other data available
Raymond et al. (1977)[181] Controlled formula diets	Low cholesterol basal	3 F, 5 M, 19–67	Low cholesterol basal	0	28	7	6	177 (46)	82	32 (2)		I			505 (41)	194 (23)		Hospitalized subjects, 5 with lipid disorders, 3 normals
			+Fiber	60	28	7	6	239* (35)	77	54* (9)	1.0	60 (9)			656 (75)	266 (47)		No decrease in plasma cholesterol
	Either high (1000 mg) or low (<50 mg) cholesterol Fiber muffins containing corn pericarp, soybean hulls, wheat bran, hydroxyethylcellulose, and pectin		High cholesterol basal	0	28	7	6	192 (41)	89	22 (2)		35* (8)			1189 (84)	423 (122)		E
			+Fiber	60	28	7	6	286* (21)	77	66* (4)	1.6	66 (11)			1152 (57)	401 (89)		
												46* (9)						
Spiller et al. (1979)[159] Ad lib but low fiber-restricted diets	Basal	50, 25–65	Basal		21	7	16	62		17		I		0.9 (0.1)				Subjects selected for low stool weight and slow transit. "Dou-
	+Cellulose-pectin		+Cellulose-pectin	+20	21	7	16	106		31	2.2	95		1.1 (0.1)				
												69						

Study	Subjects, age	Diet	V				(SD)	I (SD)	Notes
Cellulose-pectin biscuit									ble-blind parallel repeated measures" design Also studied with psyllium (see Table 5) C, H, N
Spiller et al. (1982)[121]	22, 24–57	Basal		28	5	11	100 (16)	77 (12)	Considerable individual variation in responses noted
		Ad lib low fiber normal food diet	+2	28	5	11	114 (18)	70 (12)	
		Low fiber bar containing mainly oats and rice							
		High fiber bar containing soy and corn bran, peanut butter, oats, carrots, prunes, pectin, rice, etc.	+10	28	5	11	146* (25)	70 (14)	

* Assumes bran about 44% fiber.

TABLE 10
Effect of Particle Size on Fecal Composition

Literature source	Fiber source Diet	Total number of subjects in study (sex and age)	Study period	Fiber intake (g/day) and fiber method	Days on diet	Fecal collection period (days)	Number of subjects collecting feces	Fecal weight (g/day)	Moisture (%)	Fecal solids (g/day)	Apparent increase in fecal weight per gram dietary fiber fed	Transit time (h) and transit method	Fat (g/day)	N (g/day)	Neutral steroids (mg/day)	Acid steroids (mg/day)	Energy (kcal/day)	Comments Notes Other data available
Macrae et al. (1942)[182]	Semicontrolled diet; mainly bread (74% of energy intake) White bread and whole meal bread made from either medium or fine-ground flour	6	I White bread (530–630 g)	0.9	10	7	6	62		18			2.7	1.4			99	A study of the digestibility of the nutrients in bread. Fineness of grinding made no significant difference to energy or nitrogen utilization but medium flour produced significantly greater stool bulk than fine flour
			Medium whole meal	11.7	10	7	6	283*		69*			4.9*	2.3*			325*	
			Fine whole meal	12.0	10	7	6	232*		69*			4.5*	2.3*			317*	
Brodribb and Groves (1978)[183]	Ad lib diet with either coarse	9 M, 12 F	III Basal		7	7	21	140										Coarse bran increased stool weight significantly more than fine bran
			+Coarse bran, +20 g	+10	14	7	21	219			8.0							

Study		Diet		Days		n						Comments
		bran or same bran finely milled	+Fine bran, 20 g	+9	14	7	21		199		6.6	
Heller et al. (1980)[152]	24	Basal				4	8					Also studied with cabbage and cellulose (see Tables 4 and 7)
Controlled diet		Coarse bran, 32 g	+12	V	14	4	8	74	123	31		Coarse bran produced greater fecal bulk, high moisture content, and faster transit than fine bran; fiber digestibility less in coarse bran; dietary changes during the study made comparisons with basal diet difficult
Normal food AACC white wheat bran fed whole and after fine grinding, in bread		Fine bran	+12		14	4	8	72	108	29		
										a		
										37		
										56		
Smith et al. (1981)[184]	24[b]	Basal	—	III	7	7	6		80			Coarse brans both produced significantly greater effects on bowel habit
									(6)			
Ad lib diet		+Fine CRSW, 20 g	+58		28	7	6		92		2.1	I 56 (11) 51
									(11)			
Canadian red spring wheat bran (CRSW)		Basal	—		7	7	6		96			(12) 61 (6)
									(6)			
or French soft wheat bran (FSW) in		+Coarse CRSW	+7.5		28	7	6		123*		3.6	21* (9) 54
									(11)			
either coarse or fine form		Basal	—		7	7	6		81			(8) 41
									(11)			
		+Fine FSW, 20 g	+59		28	7	6		102		3.6	(5) 48
									(6)			
		Basal	—		7	7	6		68			Effects on motility not great F

TABLE 10 (continued)
Effect of Particle Size on Fecal Composition

Literature source	Diet Fiber source	Total number of subjects in study (sex and age)	Study period	Fiber intake (g/day) and fiber method	Days on diet	Fecal collection period (days)	Number of subjects collecting feces	Fecal weight (g/day)	Moisture (%)	Fecal solids (g/day)	Apparent increase in fecal weight per gram dietary fiber fed	Transit time (h) and transit method	Fat (g/day)	N (g/day)	Neutral steroids (mg/day)	Acid steroids (mg/day)	Energy (kcal/day)	Comments Notes Other data available
Van Dokkum et al. (1982),[128] (1983)[129] Controlled diet Normal food Breads containing coarse and fine bran		12 M 23	+Coarse FSW, 20 g	+6.9	28	7	6	(9) 106* (6)			5.5	(8) 20* (7)						(See also Table 2) Fecal weight significantly lower with fine bran than coarse bran A, B, C, D, E, N
			Coarse bran	22	20	4	12	126		33		44	1.7				327	
			Fine bran	22	20	4	4	102*		29		62	1.6				315	

a Various transit methods used (see papers).
b Patients with diverticular disease.

TABLE 11
Effect of Fiber on Fecal Composition in Patients With Diverticular Disease (See Also Table 10)

Literature source Diet Fiber source	Total number of subjects in study (sex and age)	Study period	Fiber intake (g/day) and fiber method	Days on diet	Fecal collection period (days)	Number of subjects collecting feces	Fecal weight (g/day)	Moisture (%)	Fecal solids (g/day)	Apparent increase in fecal weight per gram dietary fiber fed	Transit time (h) and transit method	Fat (g/day)	N (g/day)	Neutral steroids (mg/day)	Acid steroids (mg/day)	Energy (kcal/day)	Comments Notes Other data available
Findlay et al. (1974)[98] Ad lib diet Coarse bran	7 30–84	Basal +Bran, 20 g	— 9[a]	7 35	7 7	7 7	84 101 (19)	70 74	23 24 (3)	1.9	I, IV 93 58* (8)				273 241 (85)		Study included a control group of healthy subjects (see Table 2) Effect of bran on fecal weight only one third that seen in controls Intraluminal pressure in response to food reduced by bran. F, G
Parks (1974)[185,186] Out-patient semicontrolled diet	11 M, 10 F	Low fiber High fiber	III — +12	4 4	6 6	21 21	96 176*	77 78	20 34	6.7	I, IV 44 37*	2.0 2.0					Similar value for transit by both methods

TABLE 11 (continued)
Effect of Fiber on Fecal Composition in Patients With Diverticular Disease (See Also Table 10)

Literature source	Diet Fiber source	Total number of subjects in study (sex and age)	Study period	Fiber intake (g/day) and fiber method	Days on diet	Fecal collection period (days)	Number of subjects collecting feces	Fecal weight (g/day)	Moisture (%)	Fecal solids (g/day)	Apparent increase in fecal weight per gram dietary fiber fed	Transit time (h) and transit method	Fat (g/day)	N (g/day)	Neutral steroids (mg/day)	Acid steroids (mg/day)	Energy (kcal/day)	Comments Notes Other data available
	Low residue than with addition of 40 g bran, fruit, vegetables, and whole meal bread																	Increased abdominal discomfort noted in early weeks
Brodribb and Humphreys (1976)[187] *Ad lib* diet Coarse bran		10 M, 30 F, 25—85	Basal			4	40	66				I						Colonic motility in response to eating reduced Patients had lower basal fiber intakes than healthy controls F, K
			+Bran, 24 g	+10	8[b]	4	40	89*			2.3							
Taylor and Duthie (1976)[188] *Ad lib* diet High fiber diet		20	Basal			5	20	79 (7)				I 97 (7)						Bran was the most effective of the three treatments
			High fiber diet		28	5	5	102 (16)				76* (7)						

Study	Treatment									Comments
	Normacol (an ispaghula derivative)		28	5	5	105* (13)	72* (11)		268	Bran reduced postprandial motility while ispaghula increased basal pressures
	Bran tablets	~8	28	5	10	121* (7)	56* (4)		164	
	Bran tablets (9)						I, IV			
Eastwood et al. (1978)[189]	Basal			7	7	82	88		145	C, F, H
Ad lib diet	+ Bran, 20 g	+9	28	7	7	103	50*	2.4	226	
Coarse bran	Basal			7	7	75	62		206	
Ispaghula (Fybogel)	+Ispaghula, 7 g	+7	28	7	7	108	72	4.7	218	
	Basal			7	7	95	48			
Lactulose	Lactulose, 20–40 ml	+20	28	7	10	160*	40	3.2		
Tarpila et al. (1978)[190]	Time zero control	—	c	3	11	167 (20)		5.3 (1.1)	733 (106)	No effect on biliary cholesterol saturation
Ad lib diet	High fiber			3	11	215 (28)	33 (4)	4.2 (0.7)	330 (48)	
Bran rusks 6 per day	6 Months control			3	11	155 (19)	38 (4)	4.2 (0.5)	816 (133)	Biliary deoxycholate decreased by bran. No consistent cholesterol-lowering effect
	High fiber			3	11	272* (24)	29 (2)	6.9* (1.4)	475 (82)	E, L
	12 Months control			3	11	179 (35)	55* (5)	5.5 (1.4)	697 (93)	
	High fiber			3	11	265 (44)	37 (6)	5.0 (0.9)	320 (49)	
							47 (7)		883 (147)	
									384 (61)	
									709 (91)	
									346 (89)	
									541 (46)	
									240 (39)	
Ornstein et al. (1981)[191]	Placebo	III 17.5	d 4	7	57	119 (6)	II 50 (4)			Fiber supplement conferred no benefit on symptoms but did relieve constipation
Ad lib diet	Bran	22.2	4	7	57	137* (7)	45 (4)	3.9		
Bran crisp bread										
Ispaghula (Fybogel)	Ispaghula	24.2	4	7	57	161 (8)	47 (4)	6.3		
Placebo										

a Assumes bran about 44% fiber.
b After 8-month treatment, patients showed satisfactory clinical response.
c Some 22 patients allocated to control or high fiber diet and followed for 12 months.
d Four months on each diet; 58 patients divided into 3 groups, each of which took all 3 treatments in random order.

TABLE 12
Effect of Cereal Products on Fecal Composition

Literature source	Fiber source Diet	Total number of subjects (sex and age)	Study period	Fiber intake (g/day) and fiber method	Days on diet	Fecal collection period (days)	Number of subjects collecting feces	Fecal weight (g/day)	Moisture (%)	Fecal solids (g/day)	Apparent increase in fecal weight per gram dietary fiber fed	Transit time (h) and transit method	Fat (g/day)	N (g/day)	Neutral steroids (mg/day)	Acid steroids (mg/day)	Energy (kcal/day)	Comments Notes Other data available
Fedail et al. (1984)[192] Controlled diet Wheat bran Sorghum bran	Basal Sorghum Wheat	10M 23 (22–24)		X 20 +2.5 +7.9	21 21 21	3 3 2	10 10 10	138 (14) 173 (15) 221[a] (31)			14.0 10.5	II 31 (2) 30 (1) 26[a] (1)						Sudan medical students Symptom diary Stool consistency
Eastwood et al. (1986)[193] Ad lib diet White or Wholemeal bread	Ad lib + White bread + Wholemeal bread	14M 14F 69 (50–82)		IV 13–14 12–14 22–23	182 182	7 7 7	28 28 28	74 (5) 80 (4.8) 101[a] (5.9)	72 75 73	21 (1.4) 20 (1) 27[a] (1.3)	3.4	I 80 (5.8) 76 (6.4) 74 (5.9)	2.5 (0.2) 3.1 (0.3) 3.6 (0.3)		640 (60) 640 (48) 720 (84)	266 (31) 243 (23) 232 (19)		Long term study in the community
Marlett et al. (1986)[194] Ad lib diet AACC wheat bran	Ad lib + Bran	5F 2M 59–76		V 8.5 20.9	11 22	9 9	7 7	122 (44) 170[a] (52)	76 74	29 (5) 44[a] (6)	3.9							Dietary compliance study
Mallet et al. (1987)[195]	Ad lib	3M 3F		IV 16–21	21	5	6	44 (12)										Study of fecal flora and en-

Study	Diet	n	Age	Period (d)	Tables	Fiber (g)	Wet wt (SE)	% H2O	Dry wt (SE)	pH	Transit (h) (SE)	BA (mg/d) (SE)	Notes
	Ad lib Wheat bran	22–26	Bran Ad lib	+13	21 21	5 5	6 6	137 (30) 92 (27)			4.4			zymes. J, Ammonia Also pectin (see T14) g fecal weight/g fiber based on average of 3 control periods
Reddy et al. (1987)[196]	Ad lib Mixed grain bread	8M 7F	Ad lib +Bread	+11g	28	2 2	15 15	151 (18) 228 (21)	75 77	38 (4) 52 (5)	7.0			Fecal mutagenesis pH
Wisker et al. (1988)[198]	Low High	6F 23–27	Controlled diet Wheat/Rye	19.7 48.3	XIV, XV and X 21 21	5 5	6 6	144 (17) 329a (39)			6.5		2.4 (0.2) 4.2 (0.2) 1.7 (0.2) 2.9 (0.3) 144 (17) 307 (41)	Study of energy metabolism Body weight A
Spiller et al. (1986)[201]	Basal B C D	36F 19.8 18–32	Semi-controlled Wheat bread	15 (3) +5.7 +17.1 +28.5	V, XVI 13 13 13 13	5 5 5 5	36 12 12 12	73 (6) 95a (10) 139a (12) 212 (17)	73 74 76 77	20 (1.5) 25a (2.2) 34a (2.6) 49a (3.2)	3.8 3.8 4.9	I 77 (8) 58 (5) 58 (10) 50 (5)	641 (86) 568 (72) 550 (93) 492 (65)	58 (7.9) 80 (13) 96 (14) 92 (9)	Dose response study H, L
Stevens et al. (1988)[205]	Basal Bran	12F 29 22–38	Semi-controlled AACC Bran	21 40	V, XVI 7 14	7 7	12 12	79 (8) 135a (9)	75 75	20 (1) 34a (2)	2.9	I–V 70 (6.3) 47a (3.2)			Also psyllium (Table 14) Stool consistency
Villaume et al. (1988)[206]	Basal	5			21	5	5	77	62	29					Letter 2 diet periods

TABLE 12 (continued)
Effect of Cereal Products on Fecal Composition

Literature source	Diet Fiber source	Total number of subjects in study (sex and age)	Study period	Fiber intake (g/day) and fiber method	Days on diet	Fecal collection period (days)	Number of subjects collecting feces	Fecal weight (g/day)	Moisture (%)	Fecal solids (g/day)	Apparent increase in fecal weight per gram dietary fiber fed	Transit time (h) and transit method	Fat (g/day)	N (g/day)	Neutral steroids (mg/day)	Acid steroids (mg/day)	Energy (kcal/day)	Comments	Notes	Other data available
Controlled diet Wheat bran			+Bran	+8.8	49		5	95	65	33	2.0							at 1 year interval	A, K	
Melcher et al. (1991)[207]		14M 10F	Ad lib	XVI	7	7	24	155 (18)	74	40 (4.1)								Consistency	M	
Ad lib Fiber-One (Wheat and corn bran)		20–36	+Fiber-One	+240	13	13	24	287ª (21)	74	74 (4.3)	5.5	II								
Jenkins et al. (1987)[208]		34M 39F	Ad lib	XVI	14	3		124 (12)										Dose-response study		
Ad lib diet Bran Flakes and All Bran		29	Bran Flakes 30g	5.6	14	3		136 (13)										Fecal weight on control periods varied (see original paper)		
		18–61	60	9.5	14	3		137 (5)												
			All Bran 30	11.2	14	3		138 (11)												
			60	19.0	14	3		168 (7)												

Study	Subjects	Age	Diet	Fiber (g)	Days	n	Wet wt	% H₂O	Dry wt	Transit	Section	Value 1	Value 2	SCFA	Other	Notes
Anderson et al. (1984)[209] Controlled diet Oats and (Beans)	20M	34–66	Control	19	3		212 (14)	80	27 (4)	2.7						Also beans (see T13) Hypercholesterolemic volunteers E, K
			Oats	47	3			78	42a (4)	2.0				719 (140) 829 (9)	109 (37) 180 (43)	
Miyoshi et al. (1987)[210] Controlled diet Rice	5M	21.4	Polished rice	6.2	14	5	125 (19)	80	25 (1.3)		III	26 (5.2)	2.3 (0.3)	1.5 (0.1)			C, E, H, N Blood urea
			Brown rice	15.0	8	5	192a (23)	73	51a (9)	7.6		24a (1.9)	10.6a (2.1)	2.4a (0.4)			
Miyoshi et al. (1986)[211] Controlled diet	5M	20.2	Brown rice	30.1	14	5	238a (20)	77	54a (4)	5.5	III	27 (0.2)	12a (1.1)	2.5 (0.2)		278 (30)	A, E, N Blood urea Proteins
			Polished rice	14.8	14	5	154 (22)	81	29 (3)			28 (0.3)	2.5 (0.2)	2.0 (0.2)		140 (12)	
Kaneko et al. (1986)[212] Controlled diet Rice (Agar)	5F	18–20	A	18.2	5	5	276 (27)		44 (4.4)	8.6	V	21 (3.5)	1.7 (0.3)				Diets A: High fiber, low protein brown rice B: Semi-purified low protein agar C: Low fiber, normal protein white rice D: High fiber, normal protein brown rice
			B		5	5	120 (9.4)		19 (1.5)			6.3 (0.7)	0.7 (0.1)				
			C	11.8	5	5	126 (14)		25 (2.9)	7.5		7.8 (0.6)	1.0 (0.1)				
			D	16.2	5	5	242 (15)		41 (2.5)			24 (1.2)	1.8 (0.3)				

TABLE 12 (continued)
Effect of Cereal Products on Fecal Composition

Literature source	Diet / Fiber source	Total number of subjects in study (sex and age)	Study period	Fiber intake (g/day) and fiber method	Days on diet	Fecal collection period (days)	Number of subjects collecting feces	Fecal weight (g/day)	Moisture (%)	Fecal solids (g/day)	Apparent increase in fecal weight per gram dietary fiber fed	Transit time (h) and transit method	Fat (g/day)	N (g/day)	Neutral steroids (mg/day)	Acid steroids (mg/day)	Energy (kcal/day)	Comments / Notes / Other data available
Sugawara et al. (1991)[213]		6 26–32	Basal	V, XVI	10	6	6	115 (4.5)	79 (1.3)	24								pH, fecal cholesterol C, A.
	Controlled diet		Corn	+4.2	10	6	6	128 (7.3)	79 (1.8)	26	2.8							pH Fecal ammonia and enzymes
	Corn residue		Basal		10	6	6	117 (4.0)	78 (1.4)	26								J

[a] significantly different from control

TABLE 13
Effect of Legumes on Fecal Composition

Literature source	Diet Fiber source	Total number of subjects in study (sex and age)	Study period	Fiber intake (g/day) and fiber method	Days on diet	Fecal collection period (days)	Number of subjects collecting feces	Fecal weight (g/day)	Moisture (%)	Fecal solids (g/day)	Apparent increase in fecal weight per gram dietary fiber fed	Transit time (h) and transit method	Fat (g/day)	N (g/day)	Neutral steroids (mg/day)	Acid steroids (mg/day)	Energy (kcal/day)	Comments / Notes / Other data available
Slavin et al. (1985)[214]	Controlled diets Soya	16 M, 20–34	Ensure	V, XVII	10	5		67 (5)				72						Liquid diets with added soya fiber. Fecal consistency. See also Reference 216
			Enrich 30 g soya	+25	10	5		115 (13)		19	1.9	48						
			Ensure	+25	10	5		100 (10)		29	1.3	57						
			Ensure 30 g soya	+50	10	5		150 (20)		25	1.7	51						
			Ensure 60 g soya			5		145 (13)		30		55						
			Ad lib															
Kurpad et al. (1988)[217]	Ad lib diet	6M	Ad lib	II		3	6	196 (23)	87	25 (5.8)		27 (5.9)		3.5 (0.7)				A, H
	Beans (haricot)		Beans	+18	7	3	6	216 (31)	86	29 (3.1)	1.1	33 (6.6)		3.3 (0.4)				
Anderson et al. (1984)[209]	Controlled diet	20M, 34–66	Control	XIII	19		3		132 (23)	80	31 (7)					878 (206)	154 (37)		See also T12 (Oats)
	Beans (Oats)		Beans	47		3		140 (14)	77	32 (3)	0.3				894 (184)	108[a] (20)		E, K

TABLE 13 (continued)
Effect of Legumes on Fecal Composition

Literature source	Total number of subjects (sex and age)	Study period	Fiber intake (g/day) and fiber method	Days on diet	Fecal collection period (days)	Number of subjects collecting feces	Fecal weight (g/day)	Moisture (%)	Fecal solids (g/day)	Apparent increase in fecal weight per gram dietary fiber fed	Transit time (h) and transit method	Fat (g/day)	N (g/day)	Neutral steroids (mg/day)	Acid steroids (mg/day)	Energy (kcal/day)	Comments	Notes	Other data available
Fleming et al. (1985)[218]	12M 21–35	Ad lib	III	23	3		172 (12)	78	38 (21)		42 (3)						B, M		
Ad lib Red kidney beans		Beans	+8.4	23	3		198[a] (12)	78	44 (12)	3.1	41 (3)						pH		

[a] significantly different from control

TABLE 14
Effect of Gums and Mucilages and Other Purified Sources on Fecal Composition

Literature source Diet Fiber source	Total number of subjects (sex and age)	Study period	Fiber intake (g/day) and fiber method	Days on diet	Fecal collection period (days)	Number of subjects collecting feces	Fecal weight (g/day)	Percent moisture	Fecal solids (g/day)	Apparent increase in fecal weight per gram dietary fiber fed	Transit time (h) and transit method	Fat (g/day)	N (g/day)	Neutral steroids (mg/day)	Acid steroids (mg/day)	Energy (kcal/day)	Comments Notes Other data available
Abraham and Mehta (1988)[219] Controlled diet Psyllium	7M 31.8 26–38	Basal	V	21	5	7	104 (24)	75	26 (3)					556 (44)	289 (93)		Fiber from psyllium measured by Englyst method[82] E, K, Retinyl esters Glucagon
		Psyllium	+18	21	5	7	223 (39)	84	36 (5)	6.6				732 (100)	320 (89)		
Tomlin and Read (1988)[220] Semi-controlled Guar Ispaghula Xanthan gum	6M 1F	Control	X	7	7	7	160				51						In vitro fermentation
		Ispaghula	+12.8	7	7	7	214a			4.2	46						Data read from graphs Fiber data by Englyst[82]
		Control		7	7	7	160				51						
		Guar	+13.5	7	7	7	173			1.0	40						
		Control		7	7	7	159				51						
		Xanthan	+14.0	7	7	7	186			1.9	53						
Rasmussen et al. (1987)[221] Ad lib Ispaghula	6M 3F 30.3 25–38	Ad lib	X		3		178 (20)										In vitro fermentation B
		Ispaghula	+25	14	3		276a (15)			3.9							Fiber by Englyst[82]
		Lactulose	+30	14	3		200 (26)			0.7							

TABLE 14 (continued)
Effect of Gums and Mucilages and Other Purified Sources on Fecal Composition

Literature source	Fiber source Diet	Total number of subjects in study (sex and age)	Study period	Fiber intake (g/day) and fiber method	Days on diet	Fecal collection period (days)	Number of subjects collecting feces	Fecal weight (g/day)	Percent moisture	Fecal solids (g/day)	Apparent increase in fecal weight per gram dietary fiber fed	Transit time (h) and transit method	Fat (g/day)	N (g/day)	Neutral steroids (mg/day)	Acid steroids (mg/day)	Energy (kcal/day)	Comments	Notes	Other data available
Miettenen et al. (1989)[222] Controlled diet	Lactulose	9	Basal			3		159 (26)	78	35 (4)			3 (1)		787 (103)	346 (64)		Patients with lipid disorders		
	Plantago ovata		Plantago	+25	11	3		251[a] (39)	84	39 (4)	3.7		4[a] (1)		759 (96)	468[a] (72)		Also guar study with diverticular disease patients	E	
Hamilton et al. (1988)[223] Ad lib	Methylcellulose	44F 6M 27 18–70	Placebo	X		7	9	101										Data read from graphs Also constipated subjects studied with psyllium and methyl cellulose See also Reference 224		
			M-C 2g	+2		7	20	115			7.0									
			M-C 4g	+4		7	21	154[a]			12.2									
Perragini et al. (1986)[225]		6M 21–28	Basal	22	14		6	68 (6)				46 (3.5) II							E, M, A	

Study	Subjects	Age	Diet	Fiber (g)	Days	n	Wet wt (g)	% H₂O	Dry wt (g)	Freq	pH	Transit (h)	Energy	Other
Controlled diet Guar			Guar	+10	14			76 (14)		6		54 (7.2)		
Anderson et al. (1986)[226] Ad lib diet Carboxyme-thylcellulose	5M 38 24–58		Ad lib CMC	+15	7 23	5 5	5 5	140 (33) 242 (20)	73 75	38 (7) 60 (5)	0.8 6.8	I 53 (10) 46 (10)	5.3 (0.8) 7.8 (0.8)	672 (120) 728 (160)	364 (77) 664 (116)	B, E, K, M, N Blood bio-chemistry
Eastwood et al. (1987)[227] Ad lib Xanthan gum	5M 35 26–50		Ad lib Xanthan	10.4 to 12.9	7 23	5 5	5 5	187 (27) 242 (39)	76 79	44 (3) 51 (6)	4.8	56 (12) 45 (10)	7.8 (2.2) 8.1 (1.4)	560 (80) 600 (40)	347 (39) 656 (116)	B, E, K, M, N Blood bio-chemistry Immuno-globulins
Eastwood et al. (1984)[228] Ad lib Tragacanth	5M 36 21–57		Control Gum	9.9	7 21	5 5	5 5	125 (18) 188ᵃ (26)	74 75	32 (5) 46ᵃ (6)	6.4	46 36	3.9 (1) 7.0 (1.4)	386 (66) 521 (111)	368 (36) 752 (112)	B, E, K, M, N, Blood bio-chemistry
Tomlin and Read (1988)[229] Ad lib Ispaghula (I) Polydextrose (P)	12M 20–30		Basal I 7g P 30g I 2g and P 30 g Basal I 7g I 2g and P 10 g	+6 +30 +32 +6 +12	10 10 10 10 10 10 10	10 10 10 10 10 10 10		171 180ᵃ 174ᵃ 183ᵃ 220 254ᵃ 236ᵃ			1.5 5.7	II 54 59 59 59 33 35 36				Stool consist-ency Medians not means
Stevens et al. (1988)[205] Semi-controlled Psyllium	12F 29 22–38		Basal Psyllium	V, XVI 21 40	7 14	7 7	12 12	79 (8) 163ᵃ (11)	75 80	20 (1) 33ᵃ (1)	4.4	I-V 70 (6.3) 59ᵃ (3)				Also bran (see Table 12)

TABLE 14 (continued)
Effect of Gums and Mucilages and Other Purified Sources on Fecal Composition

Literature source	Total number of subjects in study (sex and age)	Study period	Fiber intake (g/day) and fiber method	Days on diet	Fecal collection period (days)	Number of subjects collecting feces	Fecal weight (g/day)	Percent moisture	Fecal solids (g/day)	Apparent increase in fecal weight per gram dietary fiber fed	Transit time (h) and transit method	Fat (g/day)	N (g/day)	Neutral steroids (mg/day)	Acid steroids (mg/day)	Energy (kcal/day)	Comments Notes Other data available
Mallet et al. (1987)[195]	3M 3F 22—26	Ad Lib Pectin	IV 16—21 +16	21 21	5 5	6 6	103 (18) 93ᵃ (36)			6.8							Also bran (see Table 12) Mainly study of fecal flora See notes to T. 12
Ad lib Pectin																	

ᵃ significantly different from control

TABLE 15
Effect of Foods and Mixed Diets on Fecal Composition

Literature source Fiber source Diet	Total number of subjects in study (sex and age)	Study period	Fiber intake (g/day) and fiber method	Days on diet	Fecal collection period (days)	Number of subjects collecting feces	Fecal weight (g/day)	Moisture (%)	Fecal solids (g/day)	Apparent increase in fecal weight per gram dietary fiber fed	Transit time (h) and transit method	Fat (g/day)	N (g/day)	Neutral steroids (mg/day)	Acid steroids (mg/day)	Energy (kcal/day)	Comments Notes Other data available
Allinger et al. (1989)[230,246] Ad lib Vegetarian	6M 20F 44 27–61	Ad lib Vegetarian	XVIII XIX 20 30	91 91	2 2		118 176[a]	72 78	33 38[a]	5.8							Fecal pH L Urinary N, K, Na
Kesaniemi et al. (1990)[233] Semi-controlled Mixed foods	34M 50 47–55	Basal High fiber	IV 12 26	56 56	3 3		144 (18) 197[a] (10)	71 78	33 (1) 43[a] (2)	3.6				2268 (115) 2088 (102)	1351 (83) 1391[a] (91)		E Biliary lipids Cholesterol kinetics
Tinker et al. (1991)[234] Ad lib (grape juice) Prunes	41M	Grape Prunes	XVI 18 24	28 28	3 3		171 (5) 209[a] (7)	77 78	40 (1) 47[a] (1)	6.3					501 (54) 518 (67)		E
Forsum et al. (1990)[235] Controlled diet	21	A B₁	XVII 57.6 71.4	20 20	5 5	5 5	288 (62) 179	80 80	58 (8.9) 36	4.7 1.8							A Fecal biomass A = Cereals

TABLE 15 (continued)
Effect of Foods and Mixed Diets on Fecal Composition

Literature source Diet Fiber source	Total number of subjects in study (sex and age)	Study period	Fiber intake (g/day) and fiber method	Days on diet	Fecal collection period (days)	Number of subjects collecting feces	Fecal weight (g/day)	Moisture (%)	Fecal solids (g/day)	Apparent increase in fecal weight per gram dietary fiber fed	Transit time (h) and transit method	Fat (g/day)	N (g/day)	Neutral steroids (mg/day)	Acid steroids (mg/day)	Energy (kcal/day)	Comments Notes Other data available
Mixed sources		B_2	55.0	20	5	5	108 (19) (21)	77	25 (1.7) (1.5)	0.8							B_1, B_2 = digestible fibers C = low fiber
		C	12.0	20	5	6	74 (9)	72	21 (2.4)								
Ghoos et al. (1988)[236] Semi-controlled Mixed sources	11F 14M 45.8 47.8	Low High	I 13.2 23.2	3 3	25 26	136 (15) 288a (25)	85 86	20 (1.7) 39 (3.5)						115 (18) 393 (44)		E, L Monastery
Miles et al. (1988)[237] Controlled Fruit and vegetables	12M 41	High Low	37 26	42 42	7 7							4.3 (0.4) 3.5 (0.3)	2.6 (0.2) 1.6 (0.1)			249 (18) 134 (9)	A Digestible energy Metabolisable energy Week 5 values used

| Reddy et al. (1988)[238] | 11F 46–67 | Ad lib | XIII 17 | | 2 | 86 (26) | | Also follow up at one year Fecal steroids pH E |
| | | Low fat/high fiber | 37 | 26 | 2 | 145[a] (18) | 3.0 | |

Low fat/ high fiber

[a] significantly different from control

REFERENCES

1. **Burne, J.,** *A Treatise on the Causes and Consequence of Habitual Constipation,* Longman, Orme, Brown, Green & Longmans, London, 1840.
2. **Hertz, A. F.,** *Constipation and Allied Intestinal Disorders,* Oxford Medical Publ., 1909.
3. **Dimock, E. M.,** The Treatment of Habitual Constipation by the Bran Method, M.D. thesis, University of Cambridge, Cambridge, U.K., 1936.
4. **Porges, M.,** Treatment of constipation with Normacol, *Med. J. Rec.,* 128, 87, 1928.
5. **Morgan, H.,** The laxative effect of a regenerated cellulose in the diet, *JAMA,* 102, 995, 1934.
6. **Ivy, A. C. and Isaacs, B. L.,** Karaya gum as a mechanical laxative: an experimental study on animals and man, *Am. J. Dig. Dis.,* 5, 315, 1938.
7. **Gray, H. and Tainter, M. L.,** Colloid laxatives available for clinical use, *Am. J. Dig. Dis.,* 8, 130, 1941.
8. **Tainter, M. L. and Buchanan, O. H.,** Quantitative comparisons of colloidal laxatives, *Ann. N.Y. Acad. Sci.,* 58, 438, 1954.
9. **Williams, R. D. and Olmsted, W. H.,** The effect of cellulose, hemicellulose and lignin on the weight of the stool: a contribution to the study of laxation in man, *J. Nutr.,* 11, 433, 1936.
10. **Burkitt, D. P.,** Related disease — related causes, *Lancet,* ii, 1229, 1969.
11. **Burkitt, D. P.,** The aetiology of appendicitis, *Br. J. Surg.,* 58, 595, 1971.
12. **Burkitt, D. P.,** Epidemiology of cancer of the colon and rectum, *Cancer,* 28, 3, 1971.
13. **Burkitt, D. P.,** Varicose veins, deep vein thrombosis and haemorrhoids: epidemiology and suggested aetiology, *Br. Med. J.,* 2, 556, 1972.
14. **Burkitt, D. P., Walker, A. R. P., and Painter, N. S.,** Effect of dietary fibre on stools and transit times, and its role in the causation of disease, *Lancet,* ii, 1408, 1972.
15. **Painter, N. S.,** Diverticular disease of the colon, *Br. Med. J.,* ii, 475, 1968.
16. **Painter, N. S.,** Diverticular disease of the colon: a disease of this century, *Lancet,* 2, 586, 1969.
17. **Painter, N. S., Almeida, A. L., and Colebourne, K. W.,** Unprocessed bran in the treatment of diverticular disease of the colon, *Br. Med. J.,* 2, 137, 1972.
18. **Cummings, J. H., Southgate, D. A. T., Branch, W., Houston, H., Jenkins, D. J. A., and James, W. P. T.,** Colonic response to dietary fibre from carrot, cabbage, apple, bran and guar gum, *Lancet,* i, 5, 1978.
19. **Stephen, A. M. and Cummings, J. H.,** Water holding by dietary fibre in vitro and its relationship to faecal output in man, *Gut,* 20, 722, 1979.
20. **Eastwood, M. A., Brydon, W. G., and Tadesse, K.,** Effect of fiber on colonic function, in *Medical Aspects of Dietary Fiber,* Spiller, G. A. and Kay, R. M., Eds., Plenum Press, New York, 1980, 1.
21. **Robertson, J. A. and Eastwood, M. A.,** An examination of factors which may affect the water holding capacity of dietary fibre, *Br. J. Nutr.,* 45, 83, 1981.
22. **Robertson, J. A. and Eastwood, M. A.,** A method to measure the water-holding properties of dietary fibre using suction pressure, *Br. J. Nutr.,* 46, 247, 1981.
23. **Robertson, J. A. and Eastwood, M. A.,** An investigation of the experimental conditions which could affect water-holding capacity of dietary fibre, *J. Sci. Food Agric.,* 32, 819, 1981.
24. **Eastwood, M. A., Robertson, J. A., Brydon, W. G., and MacDonald, D.,** Measurement of water-holding properties of fibre and their faecal bulking ability in man, *Br. J. Nutr.,* 50, 539, 1983.
25. **Stephen, A. M. and Cummings, J. H.,** Mechanisms of action of dietary fibre in the human colon, *Nature (London),* 284, 283, 1980.
26. **Cummings, J. H.,** Dietary fibre, *Br. Med. Bull.,* 37, 65, 1981.
27. **Cummings, J. H.,** Polysaccharide fermentation in the human colon, in *Colon and Nutrition,* Kasper, H. and Goebell, Eds., MTP Press, Lancaster, 1982, 91.
28. **Southgate, D. A. T. and Durnin, J. V. G. A.,** Calorie conversion factors. An experimental measurement of the factors used in the calculation of the energy value of human diets, *Br. J. Nutr.,* 24, 517, 1970.
29. **Williams, R. D. and Olmsted, W. H.,** The manner in which food controls the bulk of the feces, *Ann. Intern. Med.,* 10, 717, 1936.
30. **Cummings, J. H.,** Short chain fatty acids in the human colon, *Gut,* 22, 763, 1981.
31. **Stephen, A. M. and Cummings, J. H.,** The microbial contribution to human faecal mass, *J. Med. Microbiol.,* 13, 45, 1980.
32. **Stephen, A. M.,** Dietary Fibre and Human Colonic Function, Ph.D. thesis, University of Cambridge, Cambridge, U.K., 1980.
33. **Mason, V. C.,** Some observations on the distribution and origin of nitrogen in sheep faeces, *J. Agric. Sci. Camb.,* 73, 99, 1969.

34. **Mason, V. C. and Palmer, R.**, The influence of bacterial activity in the alimentary canal of rats on faecal nitrogen excretion, *Acta Agric. Scand.*, 23, 141, 1973.
35. **Bastedo, W. A.**, Food and bulk producing drugs in constipation, *Rev. Gastroenterol. N.Y.*, 2, 279, 1935.
36. **Stein, D. and Gelehrter, J.**, Effects of hydrogels on the configuration and function of the colon, *Rev. Gastroenterol. N.Y.*, 7, 39, 1940.
37. **Fantus, B., Kopstein, G., and Schmidt, H. R.**, Roentgen study of intestinal motility as influenced by bran, *JAMA*, 114, 404, 1940.
38. **Fantus, B., Wozasek, O., and Steigmann, F.**, Studies on colonic irritation. Examination of feces, *Am. J. Dig. Dis.*, 8, 296, 1941.
39. **Fantus, B., Wozasek, O., and Steigmann, F.**, Studies on colonic irritation. Effect of bran, *Am. J. Dig. Dis.*, 8, 298, 1941.
40. **Fantus, B. and Frankl, W.**, The mode of action of bran. I. Effect of bran upon composition of stools, *J. Lab. Clin. Med.*, 26, 1774, 1941.
41. **Fantus, B. and Frankl, W.**, The mode of action of bran. II. Influence of size and shape of bran particles and of crude fiber isolated from bran. A preliminary report, *Rev. Gastroenterol.*, 8, 277, 1941.
42. **Werch, S. C. and Ivy, A. C.**, On the fate of ingested pectin, *Am. J. Dig. Dis.*, 8, 101, 1941.
43. **Wozasek, O. and Steigmann, F.**, Studies on colon irritation. III. Bulk of feces, *Am. J. Dig. Dis.*, 9, 423, 1942.
44. **Streicher, M. H. and Quirk, L.**, Constipation: clinical and roentgenologic evaluation of the use of bran, *Am. J. Dig. Dis.*, 10, 179, 1943.
45. **Machle, W., Heyroth, F. F., and Witherup, S.**, The fate of methyl-cellulose in the human digestive tract, *J. Biol. Chem.*, 153, 551, 1944.
46. **Streicher, M. H. and Quirk, L.**, Constipation: further clinical evidence of the use of bran as a dietary laxative agent, *Am. J. Dig. Dis.*, 11, 259, 1944.
47. **Hoppert, C. A. and Clark, A. J.**, Digestibility and effect on laxatives of crude fibre and cellulose in certain common foods, *J. Am. Dietet. Assoc.*, 21, 157, 1945.
48. **Blake, A. D.**, Clinical evaluation of a new laxative, *Am. J. Dig. Dis.*, 15, 336, 1948.
49. **Schweis, K.**, The use of methylcellulose as a bulk laxative, *N.Y. State J. Med.*, 48, 1822, 1948.
50. **Schultz, J.**, Carboxymethylcellulose as a colloid laxative, *Am. J. Dig. Dis.*, 16, 319, 1949.
51. **Bargen, J. A.**, A method of improving function of the bowel: the use of methylcellulose, *Gastroenterology*, 13, 275, 1949.
52. **Cass, L. J. and Wolf, L. P.**, A clinical evaluation of certain bulk and irritant laxatives, *Gastroenterology*, 20, 149, 1952.
53. **Olmsted, W. H., Duden, C. W., Whitaker, W. M., and Parker, R. F.**, A method for the rapid distillation of the lower volatile fatty acids from stools, *J. Biol. Chem.*, 85, 115, 1929–1930.
54. **Olmsted, W. H., Curtis, G., and Timm, O. K.**, Cause of laxative effect of feeding bran pentosan and cellulose to man, *Proc. Soc. Exp. Biol. Med.*, 32, 141, 1934.
55. **Olmsted, W. H., Curtis, G., and Timm, O. K.**, Stool VFA. IV. The influence of feeding bran, pentosan, and fiber to man, *J. Biol. Chem.*, 108, 645, 1935.
56. **Williams, R. D. and Olmsted, W. H.**, A biochemical method for determining indigestible residue (crude fiber) in faeces. Lignin, cellulose and non-water soluble hemicellulose, *J. Biol. Chem.*, 108, 653, 1935.
57. **Olmsted, W. H., Williams, R. D., and Bauerlein, T.**, Constipation: the laxative value of bulky foods, *Med. Clin. N. Am.*, 20, 449, 1936.
58. **Cowgill, G. R. and Anderson, W. E.**, Laxative effects of wheat bran and washed bran in healthy men. A comparative study, *JAMA*, 98, 1866, 1932.
59. **Cowgill, G. R. and Sullivan, A. J.**, Further studies on the use of wheat bran as a laxative, *JAMA*, 100, 795, 1933.
60. **Tainter, M. L.**, Methyl cellulose as a colloid laxative, *Proc. Soc. Exp. Biol. Med.*, 54, 77, 1943.
61. **Berberian, D. A., Pauly, R. J., and Tainter, M. L.**, Comparison of a plain methyl cellulose with a compound bulk laxative tablet, *Gastroenterology*, 20, 143, 1952.
62. **Cummings, J. H.**, Cellulose and the human gut, *Gut*, 25, 805, 1984.
63. Analytical Methods Committee, Determination of the crude fibre in national flour, *Analyst*, 68, 276, 1943.
64. AOAC, *Official Methods of Analysis of the Association of Official Analytical Chemists*, 11th ed., Horwitz, W., Ed., AOAC, Washington, D.C., 1970, 129.
65. **Southgate, D. A. T.**, Determination of carbohydrates in foods. II. Unavailable carbohydrates, *J. Sci. Food Agric.*, 20, 331, 1969.
66. **Southgate, D. A. T.**, The analysis of dietary fibre, in *Fiber in Human Nutrition*, Spiller, G. A. and Amen, R. J., Eds., Plenum Press, New York, 1976, 73.
67. **Southgate, D. A. T.**, *Determination of Food Carbohydrates*, Applied Science, London, 1976.
68. **Southgate, D. A. T., Bailey, B., Collinson, E., and Walker, A. F.**, A guide to calculating intakes of dietary fibre, *J. Hum. Nutr.*, 30, 303, 1976.

69. **Southgate, D. A. T., Bailey, B., Collinson, E., and Walker, A. F.,** Dietary fiber analysis tables, *Am. J. Clin. Nutr.,* 31, S281, 1978.
70. **Southgate, D. A. T.,** Use of the Southgate method for unavailable carbohydrates in the measurement of dietary fiber, in *The Analysis of Dietary Fiber in Food,* James, W. P. T. and Theander, O., Eds., Marcel Dekker, New York, 1981, 1.
71. **Paul, A. A. and Southgate, D. A. T.,** *McCance and Widdowson's The Composition of Foods,* Her Majesty's Stationery Office, London, 1978.
72. **Van Soest, P. J.,** Use of detergents in the analysis of fibrous feeds. II. A rapid method for the determination of fiber and lignin, *J. Assoc. Off. Agric. Chem.,* 46, 829, 1963.
73. **Van Soest, P. J.,** Non-nutritive residues. A system for the replacement of crude fibre, *J. Assoc. Off. Agric. Chem.,* 49, 546, 1966.
74. **Van Soest, P. J.,** Development of comprehensive system of feed analyses and its application to forages, *J. Anim. Sci.,* 26, 119, 1967.
75. **Van Soest, P. J. and Wine, R. H.,** Use of detergents in the analysis of fibrous feeds. IV. Determination of plant cell wall constituents, *J. Assoc. Off. Agric. Chem.,* 50, 50, 1967.
76. **Goering, H. K. and Van Soest, P. J.,** Forage Fiber Analysis: Apparatus, Reagents, Procedures and some Applications, Agriculture Handbook No. 379, Agriculture Research Service, U.S. Department of Agriculture, Washington, D.C., 1970, 1.
77. **Crampton, E. W. and Maynard, L. A.,** The relation of cellulose and lignin content to the nutritive value of animal feeds, *J. Nutr.,* 15, 383, 1938.
78. **O'Shea, J., Ribiero, M. A. do V., and Moran, M. A.,** Relationships between digestibility (in vitro), crude fibre and cellulose content of some animal feeds, *Ir. J. Agric. Res.,* 7, 173, 1968.
79. **McCance, R. A., Widdowson, E. M., and Shackleton, L. R. B.,** *The Nutritive Value of Fruits, Vegetables and Nuts,* His Majesty's Stationery Office, London, 1936.
80. **Katan, M. B. and von de Bovenkamp, P.,** Determination of total dietary fiber by difference and of pectin by calorimetry or copper titration, in *Analysis of Dietary Fiber in Human Foods,* James, W. P. T. and Theander, O., Eds., Marcel Dekker, New York, 1981.
81. **Englyst, H., Wiggins, H. S., and Cummings, J. H.,** Determination of the non-starch polysaccharides in plant foods by gas-liquid chromatography of constituent sugars as alditol acetates, *Analyst,* 107, 307, 1982.
82. **Englyst, H. N. and Cummings, J. H.,** Simplified method for measurement of total non-starch polysaccharides by gas-liquid chromatography of constituent sugars as alditol acetates, *Analyst,* 109, 937, 1984.
83. **Schweitzer, T. F. and Wursch, P.,** Analysis of dietary fiber, in *Analysis of Dietary Fiber in Foods,* James, W. P. T. and Theander, O., Eds., Marcel Dekker, New York, 1981, 203.
84. **Schweitzer, T. F. and Wursch, P.,** Analysis of dietary fibre, *J. Sci. Food Agric.,* 30, 613, 1979.
85. **Angus, R., Sutherland, T. M., and Farrell, D. J.,** A simplified method for determining fibre in foods, *Proc. Nutr. Soc. Aust.,* 2, 90, 1977.
86. **Trowell, H.,** Crude fibre, dietary fibre and atherosclerosis, *Atherosclerosis,* 16, 138, 1972.
87. **Trowell, H., Southgate, D. A. T., Wolever, T. M. S., Leeds, A. R., Gassull, M. A., and Jenkins, D. J. A.,** Dietary fibre redefined, *Lancet,* i, 967, 1976.
88. **Hinton, J. M., Lennard-Jones, J. E., and Young, A. C.,** A new method of studying gut transit times using radio-opaque markers, *Gut,* 10, 842, 1969.
89. **Cummings, J. H. and Wiggins, H. S.,** Transit through the gut measured by analysis of a single stool, *Gut,* 17, 219, 1975.
90. **Cummings, J. H., Jenkins, D. J. A., and Wiggins, H. S.,** Measurement of the mean transit time of dietary residue through the human gut, *Gut,* 17, 210, 1976.
91. **Mulinos, M. G.,** The value of elective drugs in the treatment of constipation, *Rev. Gastroenterol.,* 2, 292, 1935.
92. **Davignon, J., Simmonds, W. S., and Ahrens, E. H.,** Usefulness of chromic oxide as an internal standard for balance studies in formula-fed patients and for assessment of colonic function, *J. Clin. Invest.,* 47, 127, 1968.
93. **Sharpe, S. J. and Robinson, M. F.,** Intermittent and continuous faecal markers in short-term metabolic balance studies in young women, *Br. J. Nutr.,* 24, 489, 1970.
94. **Hansky, J. and Connell, A. M.,** Measurement of gastrointestinal transit using radioactive chromium, *Gut,* 3, 187, 1962.
95. **McCance, R. A. and Widdowson, E. M.,** Mineral metabolism on dephytenized bread, *J. Physiol.,* 101, 304, 1942.
96. **Eastwood, M. A., Kirkpatrick, J. R., Mitchell, W. D., Bone, A., and Hamilton, T.,** Effects of dietary supplements of wheat bran and cellulose on faeces and bowel function, *Br. Med. J.,* iv, 392, 1973.
97. **Connell, A. M. and Smith, C. L.,** The effect of dietary fibre on transit time, in *Proc. 4th Int. Symp. GI Motility,* Mitchell Press, Vancouver, Canada 1974, pp. 365.

98. **Findlay, J. M., Mitchell, W. D., Smith, A. N., Anderson, A. J. B., and Eastwood, M. A.,** Effects of unprocessed bran on colon function in normal subjects and in diverticular disease, *Lancet,* i, 146, 1974.
99. **Cummings, J. H., Hill, M. J., Jenkins, D. J. A., Pearson, J. R., and Wiggins, H. S.,** Changes in fecal composition and colonic function due to cereal fiber, *Am. J. Clin. Nutr.,* 29, 1468, 1976.
100. **Jenkins, D. J. A., Hill, M. J., and Cummings, J. H.,** Effect of wheat fiber on blood lipids, fecal steroid excretion and serum iron, *Am. J. Clin. Nutr.,* 28, 1408, 1975.
101. **Fuchs, H.-M., Dorfman, S., and Floch, M. H.,** The effect of dietary fiber supplementation in man. II. Alteration in fecal physiology and bacterial flora, *Am. J. Clin. Nutr.,* 29, 1443, 1976.
102. **Kahaner, N., Fuchs, H., and Floch, M. H.,** The effect of dietary fiber supplementation in man. I. Modification of eating habits, *Am. J. Clin. Nutr.,* 29, 1437, 1976.
103. **Floch, M. H. and Fuchs, H.-M.,** Effect of dietary fiber supplementation in man, *Am. J. Clin. Nutr.,* 30, 833, 1977.
104. **Floch, M. H. and Fuchs, H.-M.,** Modifications of stool content by increased bran intake, *Am. J. Clin. Nutr.,* 31, S185, 1978.
105. **Reinhold, J. G., Faradji, B., Abadi, P., and Ismail-Beigi, F.,** Decreased absorption of calcium, magnesium, zinc and phosphorus by humans due to increased fiber and phosphorus consumption as wheat bread, *J. Nutr.,* 106, 493, 1976.
106. **Wyman, J. B., Heaton, K. W., Manning, A. P., and Wicks, A. C. B.,** The effect of intestinal transit and the feces of raw and cooked bran in different doses, *Am. J. Clin. Nutr.,* 29, 1474, 1976.
107. **Walters, R. L., Baird, I. M., Davies, P. S., Hill, M. J., Drasar, B. S., Southgate, D. A. T., Green, J., and Morgan, B.,** Effects of two types of dietary fibre on faecal steroid and lipid excretion, *Br. Med. J.,* 2, 536, 1975.
108. **Southgate, D. A. T., Branch, W. J., Hill, M. J., Drasar, B. S., Walters, R. L., Davies, P. S., and Baird, I. M.,** Metabolic responses to dietary supplements of bran, *Metabolism,* 25, 1129, 1976.
109. **Baird, I. M., Walters, R. L., Davies, P. S., Hill, M. J., Drasar, B. S., and Southgate, D. A. T.,** The effects of two dietary fiber supplements on gastrointestinal transit, stool weight and frequency, and bacterial flora, and fecal bile acids in normal subjects, *Metabolism,* 26, 117, 1977.
110. **Kay, R. M. and Truswell, A. S.,** The effect of wheat fibre on plasma lipids and faecal steroid excretion in man, *Br. J. Nutr.,* 37, 227, 1977.
111. **Farrell, D. J., Girle, L., and Arthur, J.,** Effects of dietary fibre on the apparent digestibility of major food components and on blood lipids in men, *Aust. J. Exp. Biol. Med. Sci.,* 56, 469, 1978.
112. **Mathur, M. S., Ram, H., and Chadda, V. S.,** Effect of bran on intestinal transit time in normal Indians and in intestinal amoebiasis, *Am. J. Proct. Gastroent. Colon Rect. Surg.,* 29, 30, 1978.
113. **Cummings, J. H., Hill, M. J., Jivraj, T., Houston, H., Branch, W. J., and Jenkins, D. J. A.,** The effect of meat protein and dietary fiber on colonic function and metabolism. I. Changes in bowel habit, bile acid excretion and calcium absorption, *Am. J. Clin. Nutr.,* 32, 2086, 1979.
114. **Munoz, J. M., Sandstead, H. H., Jacob, R. A., Logan, G. M., Reck, S. J., Klevay, L. M., Dintzis, F. R., Inglett, G. E., and Shuey, W. C.,** Effects of some cereal brans and textured vegetable protein on plasma lipids, *Am. J. Clin. Nutr.,* 32, 580, 1979.
115. **Bell, E. W., Emken, E. A., Klevay, L. M., and Sandstead, H. H.,** Effects of dietary fiber from wheat, corn and soy hull bran on excretion of fecal bile acids in humans, *Am. J. Clin. Nutr.,* 34, 1071, 1981.
116. **Sandstead, H. H., Munoz, J. M., Jacob, R. A., Klevay, L. M., Reck, S. J., Logan, G. M., Dintzis, F. R., Inglett, G. E., and Shuey, W. C.,** Influence of dietary fiber on trace element balance, *Am. J. Clin. Nutr.,* 31, S180, 1978.
117. **Sandstead, H. H., Klevay, L. M., Jacob, R. A., Munoz, J. M., Logan, G. M., Reck, S. J., Dintzis, F. R., Inglett, G. E., and Shuey, W. C.,** Effects of dietary fiber and protein level on mineral element metabolism, in *Dietary Fibers: Chemistry and Nutrition,* Inglett, G. E. and Falkehag, S. I., Eds., Academic Press, New York, 1979, 147.
118. **Sandstead, H., Klevay, L., Jacob, R., Munoz, J., Johnson, L., Dintzis, F., and Inglett, G.,** Mineral requirements: influence of fiber and protein, *Am. J. Clin. Nutr.,* 32, 933, 1979.
119. **Munoz, J. M., Sandstead, H. H., Jacob, R. A., Logan, G. M., Jr., and Kelvay, L. M.,** Effects of dietary fiber on plasma lipids of normal men, *Am. J. Clin. Nutr.,* 31, 696, 1978.
120. **Munoz, J. M., Sandstead, H. H., and Jacob, R. A.,** Effect of dietary fiber on glucose tolerance of normal men, *Diabetes,* 28, 496, 1979.
121. **Spiller, G. A., Wong, L. G., Whittam, J. H., and Scala, J.,** Correlation of gastrointestinal transit time to fecal weight in adult humans and the levels of fiber intake, *Nutr. Rep. Int.,* 25, 23, 1982.
122. **Huijbregts, A. W. M., van Berge-Henegouwen, G. P., Hectors, M. P. C., von Schaik, A., and van der Werf, S. D. J.,** Effects of a standard wheat bran preparation on biliary lipid composition and bile acid metabolism in young healthy males, *Eur. J. Clin. Invest.,* 10, 451, 1980.
123. **Smith, R. G., Rowe, M. J., Smith, A. N., Eastwood, M. A., Drummond, E., and Brydon, W. G.,** A study of bulking agents in elderly patients, *Age Aging,* 9, 267, 1980.

124. **Stasse-Wolthuis, M., Albers, H. F. F., van Jeveren, J. C. C., Wil de Jong, J., Hautvast, J. G. A. J., Hermus, R. J. J., Katan, M. B., Brydon, W. G., and Eastwood, M. A.**, Influence of dietary fiber from vegetables and fruits, bran or citrus pectin on serum lipids, fecal lipids, and colonic function, *Am. J. Clin. Nutr.*, 33, 1745, 1980.
125. **Stasse-Wolthuis, M., Katan, M. B., Hermus, R. J. J., and Hautvast, J. G. A. J.**, Increase of serum cholesterol in man fed a bran diet, *Atherosclerosis*, 34, 87, 1979.
126. **Stasse-Wolthuis, M.**, Effect of a natural high fibre diet on blood lipids and intestinal transit in man, *Qual. Plant.*, 29, 31, 1979.
127. **Yu, M. H. M. and Miller, L. T.**, Influence of cooked wheat bran on bowel function and fecal excretion of nutrients, *J. Food Sci.*, 216, 720, 1981.
128. **Van Dokkum, W., Wesstra, A., and Schippers, F. A.**, Physiological effects of fibre-rich types of bread. I. The effect of dietary fibre from bread on the mineral balance of young men, *Br. J. Nutr.*, 47, 451, 1982.
129. **Van Dokkum, W., Pikaar, N. A., and Thissen, J. T. N. M.**, Physiological effects of fibre-rich types of bread. II. Dietary fibre from bread: digestibility by the intestinal microflora and water-holding capacity in the colon of human subjects, *Br. J. Nutr.*, 50, 61, 1983.
130. **Graham, D., Moser, S. E., and Estes, M. K.**, The effect of bran on bowel function in constipation, *Am. J. Gastroenterol.*, 77, 599, 1982.
131. **Andersson, H., Navert, B., Bingham, S. A., Englyst, H. N., and Cummings, J. H.**, The effects of breads containing similar amounts of phytate but different amounts of wheat bran on calcium, zinc and iron balance in man, *Br. J. Nutr.*, 50, 503, 1983.
132. **Cummings, J. H., Stephen, A. M., Wayman, B., Englyst, H. N., and Wiggins, H. S.**, The effect of age, sex and level of intake on the colonic response in man to wholemeal bread with added wheat bran, *Br. J. Nutr.*, 56, 349, 1986.
133. **Drasar, B. S. and Jenkins, D. J. A.**, Bacteria, diet and large bowel cancer, *Am. J. Clin. Nutr.*, 29, 1410, 1976.
134. **Durrington, P. N., Manning, A. P., Bolton, C. H., and Hartog, M.**, Effect of pectin on serum lipids and lipoproteins, whole-gut transit-time, and stool weight, *Lancet*, 2, 394, 1976.
135. **Kay, R. M. and Truswell, A. S.**, Effect of citrus pectin on blood lipids and fecal steroid excretion in man, *Am. J. Clin. Nutr.*, 30, 171, 1977.
136. **Miettinen, T. A. and Tarpila, S.**, Effect of pectin on serum cholesterol, fecal bile acids and biliary lipids in normolipidemic and hyperlipidemic individuals, *Clin. Chim. Acta*, 79, 471, 1977.
137. **Cummings, J. H., Southgate, D. A. T., Branch, W. J., Wiggins, H. S., Houston, H., Jenkins, D. J. A., Jivraj, T., and Hill, M. J.**, The digestion of pectin in the human gut and its effect on calcium absorption and large bowel function, *Br. J. Nutr.*, 41, 477, 1979.
138. **Spiller, G. A., Chernoff, M. C., Hill, R. A., Gates, J. E., Nassar, J. J., and Shipley, E. A.**, Effect of purified cellulose, pectin, and a low-residue diet on fecal volatile fatty acids, transit time, and fecal weight in humans, *Am. J. Clin. Nutr.*, 33, 754, 1980.
139. **Ross, J. K. and Leklem, J. E.**, The effect of dietary citrus pectin on the excretion of human fecal neutral and acid steroids and the activity of 7 α-dehydroxylase and β-glucuronidase, *Am. J. Clin. Nutr.*, 34, 2068, 1981.
140. **Judd, P. A. and Truswell, A. S.**, Comparison of the effects of high- and low-methoxyl pectins on blood and faecal lipids in man, *Br. J. Nutr.*, 48, 451, 1982.
141. **Fleming, S. E., Marthinsen, D., and Kuhnlein, H.**, Colonic function and fermentation in men consuming high fiber diets, *J. Nutr.*, 113, 2535, 1983.
142. **Marthinsen, D. and Fleming, S. E.**, Excretion of breath and flatus gases by humans consuming high-fiber diets, *J. Nutr.*, 112, 1133, 1982.
143. **Fleming, S. E. and Rodriguez, M. A.**, Influence of dietary fiber on fecal excretion of volatile fatty acids by human adults, *J. Nutr.*, 113, 1613, 1983.
144. **Hillman, L., Peters, S., Fisher, A., and Pomare, E. W.**, Differing effects of pectin, cellulose and lignin on stool pH, transit time and weight, *Br. J. Nutr.*, 50, 189, 1983.
145. **Marks, M. M.**, Cellulose esters in the treatment of constipation, *Am. J. Dig. Dis.*, 16, 215, 1949.
146. **Ismail-Beigi, F., Reinhold, J. G., Faraji, B., and Abadi, P.**, Effects of cellulose added to diets of low and high fiber content upon the metabolism of calcium, magnesium, zinc and phosphorus by man, *J. Nutr.*, 107, 510, 1977.
147. **Slavin, J. L. and Marlett, J. A.**, Influence of refined cellulose on human bowel function and calcium and magnesium balances, *Am. J. Clin. Nutr.*, 33, 1932, 1980.
148. **Slavin, J. C. and Marlett, J. A.**, Effect of refined cellulose on apparent energy, fat and nitrogen digestibilities, *J. Nutr.*, 110, 2020, 1980.
149. **Wrick, K. L., Robertson, J. B., Van Soest, P. J., Lewis, B. A., Rivers, J. M., Roe, D. A., and Hackler, L. R.**, The influence of dietary fiber source on human intestinal transit and stool output, *J. Nutr.*, 113, 1464, 1983.

150. **Van Soest, P. J., Robertson, J. B., Roe, D. A., Rivers, J., Lewis, B. A., and Hackler, L. R.,** The role of dietary fiber in human nutrition, in *Proc. Cornell Nutrition Conference for Feed Manufacturers,* Canada, 1978, 5.
151. **Ehle, F. R., Robertson, J. B., and Van Soest, P. J.,** Influence of dietary fibers on fermentation in the human large intestine, *J. Nutr.,* 112, 158, 1982.
152. **Heller, S. N., Hackler, L. R., Rivers, J. M., Van Soest, P. J., Roe, D. A., Lewis, B. A., and Robertson, J.,** Dietary fiber: the effect of particle size of wheat bran on colonic function in young adult men, *Am. J. Clin. Nutr.,* 33, 1734, 1980.
153. **Van Soest, P. J.,** Some factors influencing the ecology of gut fermentation in man, in *Banbury Report No. 7: Gastrointestinal Cancer: Endogenous Factors,* Bruce, W. R., Correa, P., Lipkin, M., Tannenbaum, S. R., and Wilkins, T. D., Eds., Cold Spring Harbor Laboratory, Cold Spring Harbor, N.Y., 1981, 61.
154. **Van Soest, P. J.,** Some physical characteristics of dietary fibre and their influence on the microbial ecology of the human colon, *Proc. Nutr. Soc.,* 43, 25, 1984.
155. **Van Soest, P. J., Horrath, P. J., McBurney, M. I., and Allen, M. S.,** *Unconventional Sources of Dietary Fiber, Symposium Series 214,* Furda, I., Ed., American Chemical Society, Washington, D.C., 1983, 135.
156. **Van Soest, P. J., Uden, P., and Wrick, K. L.,** Critique and evaluation of markers for use in humans and farm and laboratory animals, *Nutr. Rep. Int.,* 27, 17, 1983.
157. **Block, L. H.,** Management of constipation with a refined psyllium combined with dextrose, *Am. J. Dig. Dis.,* 14, 64, 1947.
158. **Prynne, C. J. and Southgate, D. A. T.,** The effects of a supplement of dietary fibre on faecal excretion by human subjects, *Br. J. Nutr.,* 41, 495, 1979.
159. **Spiller, G. A., Shipley, E. A., Chernoff, M. C., and Cooper, W. C.,** Bulk laxative efficacy of a psyllium seed hydrocolloid and of a mixture of cellulose and pectin, *J. Clin. Pharmacol.,* 19, 313, 1979.
160. **Eastwood, M. A., Brydon, W. G., and Anderson, D. M. W.,** The effects of dietary gum karaya (sterculia) in man, *Toxicol. Lett.,* 17, 159, 1983.
161. **Ross, A. H., McLean, Eastwood, M. A., Brydon, W. G., Anderson, J. R., and Anderson, D. M. W.,** A study of the effects of dietary gum arabic in humans, *Am. J. Clin. Nutr.,* 37, 268, 1983.
162. **Calloway, D. H. and Kretsch, M. J.,** Protein and energy utilization in men given a rural Guatemalan diet and egg formulas with and without added oat bran, *Am. J. Clin. Nutr.,* 31, 1118, 1978.
163. **Kretsch, M. J., Crawford, L., and Calloway, D. H.,** Some aspects of bile acid and urobilinogen excretion and fecal elimination in men given a rural Guatemalan diet and egg formulas with and without added oat bran, *Am. J. Clin. Nutr.,* 32, 1492, 1979.
164. **Judd, P. A. and Truswell, A. S.,** The effect of rolled oats on blood lipids and fecal steroid excretion in man, *Am. J. Clin. Nutr.,* 34, 2061, 1982.
165. **Kirby, R. W., Anderson, J. W., Sieling, B., Rees, E. D., Lin Chen, W.-J., Miller, R. E., and Kay, R. M.,** Oat-bran intake selectively lowers serum low-density lipoprotein cholesterol concentrations of hypercholesterolemic men, *Am. J. Clin. Nutr.,* 34, 824, 1981.
166. **Schweizer, T. F., Bekhechi, A. R., Koellreutter, B., Reimann, S., Pometta, D., and Bron, B. A.,** Metabolic effects of dietary fiber from dehulled soybeans in humans, *Am. J. Clin. Nutr.,* 38, 1, 1983.
167. **Tsai, A. C., Mott, E. L., Owen, G. M., Bennick, M. R., Lo, G. S., and Steinke, F. H.,** Effects of soy polysaccharide on gastrointestinal functions, nutrient balance, steroid excretions, glucose tolerance, serum lipids, and other parameters in humans, *Am. J. Clin. Nutr.,* 38, 504, 1983.
168. **McCance, R. A. and Widdowson, E. M.,** Mineral metabolism of healthy adults on white and brown bread dietaries, *J. Physiol.,* 101, 44, 1942.
169. **Antonis, A. and Bersohn, I.,** The influence of diet on serum lipids in South African white and Bantu prisoners, *Am. J. Clin. Nutr.,* 10, 485, 1962.
170. **Antonis, A. and Bersohn, I.,** The influence of diet on fecal lipids in South African white and Bantu prisoners, *Am. J. Clin. Nutr.,* 11, 143, 1962.
171. **Flynn, J. F., Beirn, S. F. O., and Burkitt, D. P.,** The potato as a source of fiber in the diet, *Ir. J. Med. Sci.,* 146, 285, 1977.
172. **Beyer, P. L. and Flynn, M. A.,** Effects of high- and low-fiber diets on human feces, *J. Am. Dietet. Assoc.,* 72, 271, 1978.
173. **Robertson, J., Brydon, W. G., Tadesse, K., Wenham, P., Walls, A., and Eastwood, M. A.,** The effect of raw carrot on serum lipids and colon function, *Am. J. Clin. Nutr.,* 32, 1889, 1979.
174. **Stasse-Wolthuis, M., Hautvast, J. G. A. J., Hermus, R. J. J., Katan, M. B., Bausch, E., Rietberg-Brussard, J. H., Velema, J. P., Zondervan, J. H., Eastwood, M. A., and Brydon, W. G.,** The effect of a natural high-fiber diet on serum lipids, fecal lipids, and colonic function, *Am. J. Clin. Nutr.,* 32, 1881, 1979.

175. **Kelsay, J. L., Behall, K. M., and Prather, E. S.,** Effect of fiber from fruits and vegetables on metabolic responses of human subjects. I. Bowel transit time, number of defecations, fecal weight, urinary excretions of energy and nitrogen and apparent digestibilities of energy, nitrogen and fat, *Am. J. Clin. Nutr.*, 31, 1149, 1978.
176. **Kelsay, J. L., Behall, K. M., and Prather, E. S.,** Effect of fiber from fruits and vegetables on metabolic responses of human subjects. II. Calcium, magnesium, iron and silicon balances, *Am. J. Clin. Nutr.*, 32, 1876, 1979.
177. **Kelsay, J. L., Jacob, R. A., and Prather, E. S.,** Effect of fiber from fruits and vegetables on metabolic responses of human subjects. III. Zinc, copper and phosphorus balances, *Am. J. Clin. Nutr.*, 32, 2307, 1979.
178. **Kelsay, J. L., Goering, H. K., Behall, K. M., and Prather, E. S.,** Effect of fiber from fruit and vegetables on metabolic responses of human subjects: fiber intakes, fecal excretions and apparent digestibilities, *Am. J. Clin. Nutr.*, 34, 1849, 1981.
179. **Kelsay, J. L., Clark, W. M., Herbst, B. J., and Prather, E. S.,** Nutrient utilization by human subjects consuming fruits and vegetables as sources of fiber, *J. Agric. Food Chem.*, 29, 461, 1981.
180. **Leeds, A. R., Khumalo, T. D., Ndaba, G., and Lincoln, D.,** Haricot beans, transit time and stool weight, *J. Plant Foods*, 4, 33, 1982.
181. **Raymond, T. L., Connor, W. E., Lin, D. S., Warner, S., Fry, M. M., and Connor, S. L.,** The interaction of dietary fibers and cholesterol upon the plasma lipids and lipoproteins, sterol balance, and bowel function in human subjects, *J. Clin. Invest.*, 60, 1429, 1977.
182. **Macrae, T. F., Hutchinson, J. C. D., Irwin, J. O., Bacon, J. S. D., and McDougall, E. I.,** Comparative digestibility of wholemeal and white breads and the effect of the degree of fineness and grinding on the former, *J. Hyg. Camb.*, 42, 423, 1942.
183. **Brodribb, A. J. M. and Groves, C.,** Effect of bran particle size on stool weight, *Gut*, 19, 60, 1978.
184. **Smith, A. N., Drummond, E., and Eastwood, M. A.,** The effect of coarse and fine Canadian Red Spring Wheat and French Soft Wheat bran on colonic motility in patients with diverticular disease, *Am. J. Clin. Nutr.*, 34, 2460, 1981.
185. **Parks, T. G.,** The effect of low and high residue diet on the rate of transit and composition of the feces, in *Proc. 4th Int. Symp. GI Motility,* Mitchell Press, Vancouver, Canada, 1974.
186. **Parks, T. G.,** Diet and diverticular disease, *Proc. R. Soc. Med.*, 67, 1037, 1974.
187. **Brodribb, A. J. M. and Humphreys, D. M.,** Diverticular disease: three studies. I. Relation to other disorders and fibre intake. II. Treatment with bran. III. Metabolic effects of bran in patients with diverticular disease, *Br. Med. J.*, 1, 424, 1976.
188. **Taylor, I. and Duthie, H. L.,** Bran tablets and diverticular disease, *Br. Med. J.*, 1, 988, 1976.
189. **Eastwood, M. A., Smith, A. N., Brydon, W. G., and Pritchard, J.,** Comparison of bran, ispaghula and lactulose on colon function in diverticular disease, *Gut*, 19, 1144, 1978.
190. **Tarpila, S., Miettinen, T. A., and Metsaranta, L.,** Effects of bran on serum cholesterol, faecal mass, fat, bile acids and neutral sterols, and biliary lipids in patients with diverticular disease, *Gut*, 19, 137, 1978.
191. **Ornstein, M. H., Littlewood, E. R., Baird, I., McLean, Fowler, J., North, W. R. S., and Cox, A. G.,** Are fibre supplements really necessary in diverticular disease of the colon? A controlled clinical trial, *Br. Med. J.*, 282, 1353, 1981.
192. **Fedail, S. S., Badi, S. E. M., and Musa, A. R. M.,** The effects of sorghum and wheat bran on the colonic functions of healthy Sudanese subjects, *Am. J. Clin. Nutr.*, 40, 776, 1984.
193. **Eastwood, M. A., Elton, R. A., and Smith, J. H.,** Long term effect of whole meal bread on stool weight, transit time, fecal bile acids, fats, and neutral sterols, *Am. J. Clin. Nutr.*, 43, 343, 1986.
194. **Marlett, J. A., Balasubramanian, R., Johnson, E. J., and Draper, N. R.,** Determining compliance with a dietary fiber supplement, *J. Natl. Cancer Inst.*, 76, 1065, 1986.
195. **Mallett, A. K., Rowland, I. R., and Farthing, M. J.,** Dietary modification of intestinal bacterial enzyme activities — potential formation of toxic agents in the gut, *Scand. J. Gastroenterol.*, 129(Suppl. 22), 251, 1987.
196. **Reddy, B. S., Sharma, C., Simi, B., Engle, A., Laakso, K., Puska, P., and Korpela, R.,** Metabolic epidemiology of colon cancer: effect of dietary fiber on fecal mutagens and bile acids in healthy subjects, *Cancer Res.*, 47, 644, 1987.
197. **Anderson, J. W., Sieling, B., and Chen, W.-J. L.,** *Plant Fiber and Food,* University of Kentucky, Lexington, 1980.
198. **Wisker, E., Maltz, A., and Feldheim, W.,** Metabolizable energy of diets low or high in dietary fiber from cereals when eaten by humans, *J. Nutr.*, 118, 945, 1988.
199. **Mergenthaler, E. and Scherz, H.,** Beitrage zur Analytik von als Lebensmittelzusatzstoffen verwendeten Polysacchariden, *Z. Lebens. Unter. Forsch.*, 162, 25, 1976.

200. **Meuser, F., Suckow, P., and Kulikowski, W.,** Verfahren zur Bestimmung von unloslichen und loslichen Ballaststoffen in Lebensmitteln, *Z. Lebens. Unters. Forsch.*, 181, 101, 1985.
201. **Spiller, G. A., Story, J. A., Wong, L. G., Nunes, J. D., Alton, M., Petro, M. S., Furumoto, E. J., Whittam, J. H., and Scala, J.,** Effect of increasing levels of hard wheat fiber on fecal weight, minerals and steroids and gastrointestinal transit time in healthy young women, *J. Nutr.*, 116, 778, 1986.
202. **Prosky, L., Asp, N.-G., Furda, I., Devries, J. W., Schweizer, T. F., and Harland, B. F.,** Vitamins and other nutrients. Determination of total dietary fiber in foods, food products, and total diets: interlaboratory study, *J. Assoc. Off. Anal. Chem.*, 67, 1044, 1984.
203. **Prosky, L., Asp, N.-G., Furda, I., Devries, J. W., Schweizer, T. F., and Harland, B. F.,** Vitamins and other nutrients. Determination of total dietary fiber in foods and food products: collaborative study, *J. Assoc. Off. Anal. Chem.*, 68, 677, 1985.
204. **Prosky, L., Asp, N.-G., Schweizer, T. F., Devries, J. W., and Furda, I.,** Determination of insoluble, soluble and total dietary fiber in foods and food products: interlaboratory study, *J. Assoc. Off. Anal. Chem.*, 71, 1017, 1988.
205. **Stevens, J., Van Soest, P. J., Robertson, J. B., and Levitsky, D. A.,** Comparison of the effects of psyllium and wheat bran on gastrointestinal transit time and stool characteristics, *J. Am. Diet. Assoc.*, 88, 323, 1988.
206. **Villaume, C., Bam, H. W., and Mejean, L.,** Physico-chemical properties of wheat bran and long term physiological effects in healthy man, *Diabete Metab.*, 14, 664, 1988.
207. **Melcher, E. A., Levitt, M. D., and Slavin, J. L.,** Methane production and bowel function parameters in healthy subjects on low and high fiber diets, *Nutr. Cancer*, 16, 85, 1991.
208. **Jenkins, D. J. A., Peterson, R. D., Thorne, M. J., et al.,** Wheat fiber and laxation: dose response and equilibration time, *Am. J. Gastroenterol.*, 82, 1259, 1987.
209. **Anderson, J. W., Story, L., Sieling, B., Chen, W.-J. L., Petro, M. S., and Story, J.,** Hypocholesterolemic effects of oat-bran or bean intake for hypercholesterolemic men, *Am. J. Clin. Nutr.*, 40, 1146, 1984.
210. **Miyoshi, H., Okuda, T., Okuda, K., and Koishi, H.,** Effects of brown rice on apparent digestibility and balance of nutrients in young men on low protein diets, *J. Nutr. Sci. Vitaminol.* (Tokyo), 33, 207, 1987.
211. **Miyoshi, H., Okuda, T., Oi, Y., and Koishi, H.,** Effects of rice fiber on fecal weight, apparent digestibility of energy, nitrogen and fat, and degradation of neutral detergent fiber in young men, *J. Nutr. Sci. Vitaminol.* (Tokyo), 32, 581, 1986.
212. **Kaneko, K., Nishida, K., Yatsuda, J., Osa, S., and Koike, G.,** Effect of fiber on protein, fat and calcium digestibilities and fecal cholesterol excretion, *J. Nutr. Vitaminol.* (Tokyo), 32, 317, 1986.
213. **Sugawara, M., Sato, Y., Yokoyama, S., and Mitsuoka, T.,** Effect of corn fiber residue supplementation on fecal properties, flora, ammonia and bacterial enzyme activities in healthy humans, *J. Nutr. Sci. Vitaminol.* (Tokyo), 37, 109, 1991.
214. **Slavin, J. L., Nelson, N. L., McNamara, E. A., et al.,** Bowel function of healthy men consuming liquid diets with and without dietary fiber, *J. Parent. Entr. Nutr.*, 9, 317, 1985.
215. **Slavin, J. L., Marlett, J. A., and Neilson, M. J.,** Determination and apparent digestibility of neutral detergent fiber monosaccharides in women, *J. Nutr.*, 113, 2353, 1983.
216. **Fischer, M., Adkins, W., Hall, L., et al.,** The effects of dietary fibre in a liquid diet on bowel function of mentally retarded individuals, *J. Ment. Defic. Res.*, 29, 373, 1985.
217. **Kurpad, A. V., Holmes, J., and Shetty, P. S.,** Effect of fibre supplementation and activated charcoal on faecal parameters and transits in the tropics, *Indian J. Gastroenterol.*, 7, 199, 1988.
218. **Fleming, S. E., O'Donnell, A. U., and Perman, J. A.,** Influence of frequent and long-term bean consumption on colonic function and fermentation, *Am. J. Clin. Nutr.*, 41, 909, 1985.
219. **Abraham, Z. D. and Mehta, T.,** Three-week psyllium husk supplementation: effect of plasma cholesterol concentrations, fecal steroid excretion, and carbohydrate absorption in men, *Am. J. Clin. Nutr.*, 47, 67, 1988.
220. **Tomlin, J. and Read, N. W.,** The relation between bacterial degradation of viscous polysaccharides and stool output in human beings, *Br. J. Nutr.*, 60, 467, 1988.
221. **Rasmussen, H. S., Holtug, K., Andersen, J. R., Krag, E., and Mortensen, P. B.,** The influence of ispaghula husk and lactulose on the in vivo and the in vitro production capacity of short-chain fatty acids in humans, *Scand. J. Gastroenterol.*, 22, 406, 1987.
222. **Miettinen, T. A. and Tarpila, S.,** Serum lipids and cholesterol metabolism during guar gum, plantago ovata and high fibre treatments, *Clin. Chem. Acta*, 183, 253, 1989.
223. **Hamilton, J. W., Wagner, J., Burdick, M. A., and Bass, P.,** Clinical evaluation of methylcellulose as a bulk laxative, *Dig. Dis. Sci.*, 33, 993, 1988.

224. **Marlett, J. A., Li, B. U. K., Patrow, C. J., and Bass, P.**, Comparative laxation of psyllium with and without senna in an ambulatory constipated population, *Am. J. Gastroent.*, 82, 333, 1987.
225. **Penagini, R., Velio, P., Vigorelli, R., Bozzani, A., Castagnone, D., Ranzi, T., and Bianchi, P. A.**, The effect of dietary guar on serum cholesterol, intestinal transit, and fecal output in man, *Am. J. Gastroent.*, 81, 123, 1986.
226. **Anderson, D. M. W., Eastwood, M. A., and Brydon, W. G.**, The dietary effects of sodium carboxymethylcellulose in man, *Food Hydrocolloids*, 1, 37, 1986.
227. **Eastwood, M. A., Brydon, W. G., and Anderson, D. M. W.**, The dietary effects of xanthan gum in man, *Food Add. Contam.*, 4, 17, 1987.
228. **Eastwood, M. A., Brydon, W. G., and Anderson, D. M. W.**, The effects of dietary gum tragacanth in man, *Toxicol. Lett.*, 21, 73, 1984.
229. **Tomlin, J. and Read, N. W.**, A comparative study of the effects on colon function caused by feeding ispaghula husk and polydextrose, *Aliment. Pharmacol. Therap.*, 2, 513, 1988.
230. **Allinger, U. G., Johansson, G. K., Gustafsson, J. A., and Rafter, J. J.**, Shift from a mixed to a lactovegetarian diet: influence on acidic lipids in fecal water — a potential risk factor for colon cancer, *Am. J. Clin. Nutr.*, 50, 992, 1989.
231. **Theander, O. and Westerlund, E.**, Studies on dietary fiber. 3. Improved procedures for analysis of dietary fiber, *J. Agric. Food Chem.*, 34, 330, 1986.
232. **Asp, N.-G., Johansson, C.-G., Hallmer, H., and Siljestrom, M.**, Rapid enzymatic assay of insoluble and soluble dietary fiber, *J. Agric. Food Chem.*, 31, 476, 1983.
233. **Kesaniemi, Y. A., Tarpila, S., and Miettinen, T. A.**, Low vs high dietary fiber and serum, biliary, and fecal lipids in middle aged men, *Am. J. Clin. Nutr.*, 51, 1007, 1990.
234. **Tinker, L. F., Schneeman, B. O., Davis, P. A., Gallaher, D. D., and Waggoner, C. R.**, Consumption of prunes as a source of dietary fiber in men with mild hypercholesterolemia, *Am. J. Clin. Nutr.*, 53, 1259, 1991.
235. **Forsum, E., Eriksson, C., Goranzon, H., and Sohlstrom, A.**, Composition of faeces from human subjects consuming diets based on conventional foods containing different kinds and amounts of dietary fibre, *Br. J. Nutr.*, 64, 171, 1990.
236. **Ghoos, Y., Rutgeerts, P., Vantrappen, G., Hiele, M., and Schurmans, P.**, The effect of long-term fibre and starch intake by man on faecal bile acid excretion, *Eur. J. Clin. Invest.*, 18, 128, 1988.
237. **Miles, C. W., Kelsay, J. L., and Wong, N. P.**, Effect of dietary fiber on the metabolizable energy of human diets, *J. Nutr.*, 118, 1075, 1988.
238. **Reddy, B. S., Engle, A., Simi, B., O'Brien, L. T., Barnard, R. J., Pritikin, N., and Wynder, E. L.**, Effect of low fat, high carbohydrate, high fiber diet on fecal bile acids and neutral sterols, *Prev. Med.*, 17, 432, 1988.
239. **Mongeau, R. and Brassard, R.**, A rapid method for the determination of soluble and insoluble dietary fiber: comparison with AOAC total dietary fiber procedure and Englyst's method, *J. Food Sci.*, 51, 1333, 1986.
240. **Neilson, M. J. and Marlett, J. A.**, A comparison between detergent and nondetergent analyses of dietary fiber in human foodstuffs, using high-performance liquid chromatography to measure neutral sugar composition, *J. Agric. Food Chem.*, 31, 1342, 1983.
241. **Englyst, H. N. and Hudson, G. J.**, Colorimetric method for routine measurement of dietary fibre as nonstarch polysaccharides. A comparison with gas-liquid chromatography, *Food Chem.*, 24, 63, 1987.
242. **Marlett, J. A.**, Analysis of dietary fiber, *Animal Feed Sci. Tech.*, 23, 1, 1989.
243. **Li, B. W. and Cardozo, M. S.**, Simplified method for the determination of total dietary fiber and its soluble and insoluble fractions in foods, in *New Developments in Dietary Fiber*, Furda, I. and Brine, C. J., Eds., Plenum Press, New York, 1990, 283.
244. **Jeraci, J. L. and Van Soest, P. J.**, Improved methods for analysis and biological characterization of fiber, in *New Developments in Dietary Fiber*, Furda, I. and Brine, C. J., Eds., Plenum Press, New York, 1990, 245.
245. **Lee, S. C. and Hicks, V. A.**, Modifications of the AOAC total dietary fiber method, in *New Developments in Dietary Fiber*, Furda, I. and Brine, C. J., Eds., Plenum Press, New York, 1990, 237.
246. **Johansson, G. K., Ottova, L., and Gustafsson, J. A.**, Shift from a mixed diet to a lactovegetarian diet: influence on some cancer-associated intestinal bacterial enzyme activities, *Nutr. Cancer.*, 14, 239, 1990.
247. **Adiotomre, J., Eastwood, M. A., Edwards, C. A., and Brydon, W. G.**, Dietary fiber: in vitro methods that anticipate nutrition and metabolic activity in humans, *Am. J. Clin. Nutr.*, 52, 128, 1990.
248. **Kurpad, A. V. and Shetty, P. S.**, Effects of antimicrobial therapy on faecal bulking, *Gut*, 27, 55, 1986.
249. **Shetty, P. S. and Kurpad, A. V.**, Increasing starch intake in the human diet increases fecal bulking, *Am. J. Clin. Nutr.*, 43, 210, 1986.

250. **Tomlin, J. and Read, N. W.,** The effect of resistant starch on colon function in humans, *Br. J. Nutr.,* 64, 589, 1990.
251. **Cummings, J. H., Beatty, E. R., Kingman, S., Bingham, S. A., and Englyst, H. N.,** Laxative properties of resistant starches, *Gastroenterology,* 102, A548, 1992.
252. **Flourie, B., Florent, C., Jouany, J. P., Thivend, P., Etanchaud, F., and Rambaud, J. C.,** Colonic metabolism of wheat starch in healthy humans. Effects on fecal outputs and clinical symptoms, *Gastroenterology,* 90, 111, 1986.
253. **Englyst, H. N., Bingham, S. A., Runswick, S. A., Collinson, E., and Cummings, J. H.,** Dietary fibre (non-starch polysaccharides) in fruit, vegetables and nuts, *J. Hum. Nutr. Dietet.,* 1, 247, 1988.
254. **Englyst, H. N., Bingham, S. A., Runswick, S. A., Collinson, E., and Cummings, J. H.,** Dietary fibre (non-starch polysaccharides) in cereal products, *J. Hum. Nutr. Dietet.,* 2, 253, 1989.
255. **Englyst, H. N., Kingman, S. M., and Cummings, J. H.,** Classification and measurement of nutritionally important starch fractions, *European J. Clin. Nutr.,* 1992 (in press).
256. **Wood, R., Englyst, H. N., Southgate, D. A. T., and Cummings, J. H.,** Determination of dietary fibre — collaborative trials Part IV. A comparison of the Englyst and Prosky procedures for measurement of soluble, insoluble and total dietary fibre, *J. Assoc. Publ. Analysts,* 1992 (in press).

Chapter 6.2

SUGGESTIONS FOR A BASIS ON WHICH TO DETERMINE A DESIRABLE INTAKE OF DIETARY FIBER

Gene A. Spiller

In the period 1986 to 1991, various suggestions have been made on fiber intake. In the United States, the National Research Council[1] in its 1989 10th edition of the *Recommended Dietary Allowances* recommends that *a desirable fiber intake* be achieved by consumption of sufficient amounts of fruits, vegetables, legumes, and whole grain cereals, but does not recommend any optimal or minimum level. The same council[2] in its *Diet and Health* also published in 1989 does not arrive at any definite recommendation on fiber intake, just stating that "it is reasonable to recommend a diet containing high levels of fiber-rich foods . . . ".

The Surgeon General of the United States[3] in his *Report on Nutrition and Health* (1988) underlines "the prudence of increasing consumption of whole grain foods and cereals, vegetables (including dried beans and peas) and fruits". Again there is no statement as to a recommended daily intake of dietary fiber.

The aforementioned publications do not arrive at a specific recommendation for fiber intake while supporting the role of fiber in the diet. In view of this lack of consensus on the desirable daily fiber intake, the following suggestions made in the first edition of this Handbook are presented here again as a possible basis to determine a desirable level of fiber intake for people living in industrialized societies.

CORRELATION OF TRANSIT TIME TO FECAL WEIGHT

The basis of the method suggested here is the correlation of transit time (TT) to fecal wet weight. This is a simple and practical method that could allow some immediate recommendations.

Several studies have shown that: (1) TT decreases rapidly as FWW increases to 160 to 200 g/d and (2) beyond FWWs of 160 to 200 g/d there is little change in TT as FWW increases. The line correlating TT to FWW becomes practically asymptotic to the abscissa for this FWW.[4-9] Figures 1 and 2 summarize these concepts. When data correlating TT to FWW are presented for individual subjects (Figure 2) one finds a wide scatter of points correlating TT to FWW below FWW values of 160 to 180 g/d; many values for TT are as high as 4 or 5 days.[4-8] This indicates that as FWW values increase, there is a *critical fecal wet weight* (CFW) to 160 to 200 g/d, beyond which practically no TT is greater than 2 days. While we do not know the *ideal* transit time for humans, it may be reasonable to assume that extremely long transit times are not desirable, and that a more *predictable* colon function is preferable.

EPIDEMIOLOGICAL CORRELATIONS

A well-executed epidemiological study on two Scandinavian populations showed lower colon cancer incidence in the population with an average FWW of 200 g/d compared to the group with an average of 150 g/d.[10] This supports the concept that there is a CFW, that its value is in the range of 200 g/d for adults, and that the CFW is a basic physiological concept.

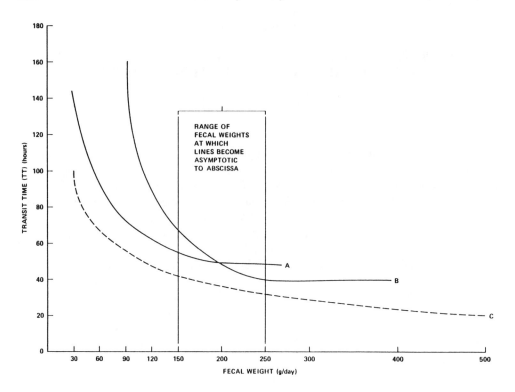

FIGURE 1. Correlation of transit time to fecal weight in three different studies. Curve A is from Spiller et al.,[5] curve B is from Connell,[9] and curve C is from Burkitt et al.[4]

CORRELATION TO LEVELS OF DIETARY FIBER

The amount of fiber needed to achieve the CFW appears to be in the range of 35 to 45 g/d,[8] as long as enough cereal fiber is included (probably 60 to 70%) especially wheat-type fiber. Wheat-type fibers are high in water-insoluble fractions (see definition by Asp, Chapter 3.1). The question of how much of the water-soluble fibers we need in relation to their effect on lipid and carbohydrate metabolism has not yet been answered, but it is certainly logical to assume that a fraction of the fiber should be of the water-soluble type, perhaps 30 to 40%. Pharmacological uses of dietary fiber and their effective levels are not part of these considerations.

OVERALL DIETARY PATTERN

Part of any recommendation on the intake of dietary fiber should include the importance of eating a variety of dietary fibers. In this way, both water-insoluble and water-soluble components would be represented.

The data on dietary fiber content of various foods, as presented in the Appendix of this Handbook, indicate that it is difficult to obtain sufficient dietary fiber from a single food (except for concentrated sources) and that the easiest way to obtain a reasonable amount of dietary fiber in the daily diet is to consume a diversity of unrefined plant foods, such as whole grain products, in the form of breads and cereals, beans, nuts, vegetables, and fruits. Whole grain wheat deserves a special mention as a high source of insoluble dietary fiber, while beans and oats deserve a special mention as a source of good mixtures of water-soluble

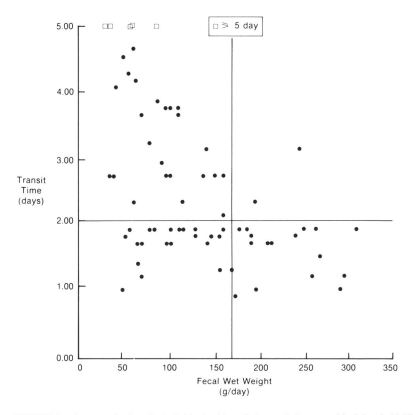

FIGURE 2. Scatter of points for individual subjects below and above a critical threshold (CFW).

and water-insoluble fiber. The use of concentrated sources such as wheat bran (for the wheat-type fiber portion) or oat bran offer additional assurance of a sufficient daily intake of particular fiber types. In bread selection great care should be taken, as there is a tremendous diversity of breads on the market: the amount and type of dietary fiber may vary greatly according to the level of extraction and type of flours used.

A RECOMMENDED INTAKE OF DIETARY FIBER

In summary, it appears reasonable to recommend, to adults living in industrialized societies, 35 to 45 g/d total dietary fiber as measured by one of the all-encompassing methods which include water-soluble and water-insoluble fiber. Using other analytical methods, this is approximately equivalent to the neutral detergent residue (NDR) of Van Soest plus pectins, gums, and mucilages, or to the sum of cellulose, noncellulosic polysaccharides, and lignin of Southgate. The sum of each individual polymer of dietary fiber may also be used. The reader is referred to Section 3 for details. Wheat-type fibers, the sources of which probably include whole wheat, rye, and related whole grains high in water-insoluble fiber, should probably be 50 to 70% of the total fiber, with the rest made up of dietary fibers from beans, oats, fruits, and vegetables, most of which are high in water-soluble fiber.

REFERENCES

1. **National Research Council,** *Recommended Dietary Allowances,* National Academy Press, Washington, D.C., 1989.
2. **National Research Council,** *Diet and Health,* Natinal Academy Press, Washington, D.C., 1989.
3. *The Surgeon General's Report on Nutrition and Health,* U.S. Department of Health and Human Services, U.S. Government Printing Office, Washington, D.C., 1988.
4. **Burkitt, D. P., Walker, A. R. P., and Painter, N. S.,** Dietary fiber and disease, *JAMA,* 229, 1068, 1974.
5. **Spiller, G. A., Chernoff, M. C., Shipley, E. A., Beigler, M. A., and Briggs, G. M.,** Can fecal weight be used to establish a recommended intake of dietary fiber (plantix)?, *Am. J. Clin. Nutr.,* 39, 659, 1977.
6. **Spiller, G. A., Shipley, E. A., and Blake, J. A.,** Recent progress in dietary fiber (plantix) in human nutrition, *CRC Crit. Rev. Food Sci. Nutr.,* 10, 31, 1978.
7. **Spiller, G. A., Wong, L. G., Whittam, J. H., and Scala, J.,** Correlation of gastrointestinal transit time to fecal weight in adult humans at two levels of fiber intake, *Nutr. Rep. Int.,* 25, 23, 1982.
8. **Spiller, G. A., Story, J. A., Wong, L. G., Nunes, J. D., Alton, M., Petro, M. S., Furamoto, E. J., Whittam, J. H., and Scala, J.,** Effect of increasing levels of hard wheat fiber on fecal weight, minerals and steroids and gastrointestinal transit time in healthy young women, *J. Nutr.,* 116, 778, 1986.
9. **Connell, A. H.,** Fiber, bulk and colonic activity, in *Fiber Deficiency and Colonic Disorders,* Reilly, R. W. and Kirsner, J. B., Eds., Plenum Press, New York, 1975, 81.
10. International Agency for Cancer Research, Dietary fiber, transit time, fecal bacteria and colon cancer in two Scandinavian populations, *Lancet,* i, 207, 1977.

Chapter 6.3

EFFECT OF DIETARY FIBER AND FIBER-RICH FOODS ON STRUCTURE OF THE UPPER GASTROINTESTINAL TRACT

Clifford Tasman-Jones

INTRODUCTION

A diet low in dietary fiber is associated with a spectrum of degenerative diseases. These include atherosclerotic vascular disease, diverticular disease, gallstones, diabetes mellitus, cancer, etc. These associations arising from analysis of population data, have stimulated interest in determining mechanisms which may explain how dietary fiber and its metabolites may induce functional and structural intestinal changes. The chemical heterogenicity, complexity, and differing physicochemical properties of the individual members of the carbohydrate components that are represented by the inclusive term "dietary fiber" have presented major problems in unraveling and explaining the effects of dietary fiber on the hollow gut.

Dietary fiber is accepted to represent plant cell wall. The best chemically defined and analyzable component of the plant cell wall is nonstarch polysaccharide (NSP) which has a water-soluble or fermentable component and an insoluble component. Separately defined and chemically measurable are the starches of which the starch resistant to normal luminal digestion is important. It is associated with plant cell wall and is metabolized in the colon in a manner similar to nonstarch polysaccharide. Some gravimetric analyses of dietary fiber include a variable amount of starch.

The metabolic and growth function of all tissues, including the mucosa of the gastrointestinal tract, are under the control of a variety of hormones. In addition, the gastrointestinal tract is influenced by hormones and active peptides which are released locally in the gut lumen and are formed in response to the presence of food. NSP affects some of the general hormones, such as insulin, which have known trophic effects.[1] Fermentable NSP and resistant starch are associated with an increased production of the polyamines: putrescine, spermadine, and spermine, substances associated with increased ornithine decarboxylase activity and mucosal trophic activity.

STOMACH

The effects of NSP and starch on the gastric mucosal structure have not been adequately studied. Rat stomachs stimulated to secrete acid show ultrastructural changes of the surface epithelial cells.[2] Feeding, which also stimulates acid production, increases in gastric cell kinetics.[3] Excess acid production can cause damage to the gastric surface cells. The effects of NSP and resistant starch on acid production in the stomach have not been reported. Some gel dietary fibers, such as pectin and guar gum, effectively increase the gastric mucus barrier, forming a cytoprotective layer to the epithelial cells. The effects of NSP and starch on acid production and the secretion of cytoprotective polypeptides, including prostaglandin and epidermal growth factor, in the production of the mucus coat are worthy of further investigation. Clinical studies in the human suggest that an increased dietary NSP may reduce the incidence of duodenal ulcer.[4]

SMALL INTESTINE

Nutritional, hormonal, pharmacological, and intraluminal digestive products influence cell replacement by the continual renewal of the epithelium of both the small and large intestine.[1] Inert bulk (kaolin) in the rat small intestine does not alter mucosal growth of the rat small bowel, but both guar and pectin promote growth. Pectin appears to delay the maturation of the normal rate of small intestinal mucosa[5] and pectin, but not cellulose-accelerated cell turnover in the jejunum of conventional rats.[6]

In the dog, maturation leads to a more regular villus pattern,[7] whereas in the rat, maturation leads to a more leaf-shaped, broad villi.[8] In the human there are significant differences in the structure of the small bowel mucosa of those brought up on a western diet compared with those in third world countries. Jejunal villi, on the Western diet, are long and regular, while those in the developing world tend to be broad, leaf-shaped, and variable.[9] Differences in diet provide a possible explanation for these geographic differences in structure. A Western diet has a high proportion of fat and carbohydrate and a low dietary fiber compared with the diet of the developing countries in which fat is relatively low but the proportion of fiber high. From the evidence available, it seems that those fibers which are most readily fermentable are the ones associated with a significant influence in growth of the small bowel mucosa.

Arising from the salivary and Brunner's glands of the duodenum, the hormone epidermal growth factor (EGF) increases DNA and ornithine decarboxylase activity in the gut. The effects of fiber in stimulating epidermal growth factor secretion is not clear.

The proximal/distal gradient of decreasing intestinal diameter, villus density, means villus length and crypt cell production may be explained by EGF and other hormonal factors, possibly arising as a result of fermentation products in the colon.

NSP has a varying influence on the length of the small gut.[5,10] When bran and cellulose are fed, there is little effect on the surface morphology of the small intestine,[5,10] but pectin gives irregular villi in both the jejunum and the ileum.[5,10,11] Alfalfa and pectin are associated with cellular swelling, loss of microvilli, and sometimes hemorrhage on the jejunal surface. Oat bran reduces the crypt cell population by decreasing cell replication, pectin increases villus cell exfoliation causing a faster cell migration along the villi, and guar gum gives a marked increased growth, without alteration in crypt villus morphometrics but with increased crypt cell production.[12]

When animals and man are maintained solely with intravenous feeding, there is atrophy of the small bowel mucosa. In rats, if short chain fatty acids are infused intravenously or intracellularly, there is a significant reduction in mucosal atrophy.[13] The liver is the major site of short chain fatty acid metabolism with the production of some ketone bodies and amino acids including β hydroxybutyrate and glutamine. Glutamine added to intravenous feeding formulas increases the jejunal mucosal weight, DNA content, stimulates mucosal growth,[14] and improves gut immune function.[15] Further, glutamine may be important in the prevention and management of small bowel injury such as occurs in irradiation.[16]

REFERENCES

1. **Johnson, L. R.,** Regulation of gastrointestinal mucosal growth, *Physiol. Rev.,* 68, 456, 1988.
2. **Wood, L. R., and Dubois, A.,** Scanning electron microscopy of the stomach during modification of acid secretion, *Am. J. Physiol.,* 244, G475, 1983.
3. **Hunt, T. E.,** Mitotic activity in the gastric mucosa of the rat after fasting and refeeding, *Anat. Res.,* 127, 529, 1965.

4. **Rydning, G. A., Berstead, A., Aadlund, E., and Ødengaard, V.**, Prophylactic effect of high fiber diet and duodenal ulcer disease, *Lancet,* 2, 736, 1982.
5. **Tasman-Jones, C., Owen, R. L., and Jones, A. L.**, Semipurified dietary fiber and small bowel morphology in rats, *Dig. Dis. Sci.,* 27, 519, 1982.
6. **Komai, M., Takehisa, F., and Kimura, S.**, Effect of dietary fiber on intestinal epithelial cell kinetics of germ-free and conventional mice, *Nutr. Rep. Int.,* 26, 255, 1982.
7. **Hoskins, J. D., Henk, W. G., and Abdelbaki, Y. Z.**, Scanning electron microscopic study of the small intestine of dogs from birth to 337 days of age, *Am. J. Vet. Res.,* 43, 1715, 1982.
8. **Baker, S. J., Mathan, V. I., and Cherian, V.**, The nature of the villi in the small intestine of the rat, *Lancet,* 1, 860, 1963.
9. **Baker, S. J.**, Geographical variations in the morphology of the small intestinal mucosa in apparently healthy individuals, *Pathol. Microbiol.,* 39, 222, 1973.
10. **Cassidy, M. M., Lightfoot, F. G., and Vahouny, G. V.**, Morphological aspects of dietary fibers in the intestine, *Adv. Lipid Res.,* 19, 203, 1982.
11. **Bollard, J. E., Tasman-Jones, C., Thomsen, L. L., and Maher, K.**, Dietary fiber and small intestinal morphometrics, unpublished work.
12. **Jacobs, L. R.**, Effect of dietary fiber on mucosal growth and cell proliferation in the small intestine of the rat: a comparison of oat bran, pectin and guar with total fiber deprivation, *Am. J. Clin. Nutr.,* 37, 954, 1983.
13. **Koruda, M. J., Rolandelli, R. H., Bliss, D. Z., Hastings, J., Rombear, J. L., and Settle, R. G.**, Parenteral nutrition supplemented with short-chain fatty acids: effect on the small bowel mucosa in normal rats, *Am. J. Clin. Nutr.,* 51, 685, 1991.
14. **O'Dwyer, S. T., Smith, R. J., Hwang, T. L., and Wilmore, D. W.**, Maintenance of small bowel mucosa with glutamine-enriched parenteral nutrition, *J. Parenter. Enteral Nutr.,* 13, 517, 1989.
15. **Burke, D., Alverdy, J. C., Aoys, E., and Moss, G. S.**, Glutamine supplemented TPN improves gut immune function, *Arch. Surg.,* 124, 1396, 1989.
16. **Klimberg, V. S., Salloum, R. M., Kasper, M., Plumley, D. A., Dolson, D. J., Hautamaki, R. D., Mendenhall, W. R., Bova, F. C., Bland, K. I., Copeland, E. B., and Souba, W. W.**, Oral glutamine accelerates healing of the small intestine and improves outcome after whole body radiation, *Arch. Surg.,* 125, 1040, 1990.

Chapter 6.4

EFFECT OF DIETARY FIBER (NONSTARCH POLYSACCHARIDE) ON THE STRUCTURE OF THE COLON

Clifford Tasman-Jones

The normal colon shows differences of function along its length.[1,2] Associated with these functional differences are differences in the rate of epithelial cell proliferation.[3] The rat colon has an overall proximal to distal decrease in the intestinal circumference, number of crypts per unit area, and in the diameter of the midproportion of the crypts.[4] These structural changes coincide with significant changes in the number and metabolic activity of the resident gut flora, the important factor in fermentation with the colon. The cecum is the major area of fermentation of the soluble nonstarch polysaccharides and of food starch resistant to small intestinal digestion. Colonic bacteria ferment nonstarch polysaccharides (NSP) and resistant starch, as well as degrade mucus produced by the colonic mucosa.[5]

There is increasing interest in the fermentation products of NSP and resistant starch and their influences on colonic mucosa, as well as their potential for inhibition of premalignant and malignant mucosal changes. When dietary fiber is added to the rat diet, the proportion of replicating epithelial cells increases and there are modifications of goblet cell mucin production.

A number of studies have shown a variety of structural changes which are related to dietary fiber. Berry and Ebers[6] noted that "bulbous nodular projections" of the rat colon were larger and more frequent in rats fed a commercial diet than when fed a whole grain diet. Wheat bran fed rats have an increased proximal and distal total colonic weight compared with those fed a fiber free diet but with the mucosal weight increased only in the distal colon.[7] Using DNA and RNA as a measure of mucosal hyperplasia, the changes are most marked in the distal colon.[7] Increased colonic weight has been confirmed by feeding other diets which give high fecal residue.[8,9] Rats which are fed parenterally[10] or on oral elemental diets[11,12] show marked hypoplastic changes. Guar in the rat diet increases cecal and colonic mucosal weight, DNA, and RNA; pectin increases the DNA only and oat bran has no effect. The effect of guar is greatest in the cecum. Those NSP components which are most readily fermented have the greatest effect in the proximal colon. The effects of less readily fermentable NSP components are most marked in the distal colon.

Bile salts alter the kinetics of rat colonic mucosa.[13] Some soluble NSPs modify bile secretion, while insoluble NSPs bind bile salts. Other possible influences on the structure could be through alterations induced by bacterial floral degradation to form short chain fatty acids.[14]

Short chain fatty acids are produced by the metabolism of NSP, starch, and mucus within the gut[15] and these are trophic to the colonic mucosa.[16] An increase in ornithine decarboxylase activity is associated with trophic factors. The inhibitor DL-alpha-difluoromethylornithine inhibits OCD in the upper gut but not in the colon. There is increased bacterial ornithine decarboxylase activity and production of the polyamines putrescine, spermadine, and spermine during the fermentation of NSP.

Of particular importance is butyrate which appears to have a stabilizing effect on colonocytes.[17]

Little is known of the effects of NSP on the mucus layer, which is an essential component of the structure of the colon. It is suggested that this may be modified in premalignant and malignant conditions of the large bowel.[18]

REFERENCES

1. **Davis, G. R., Santa Ani, C. A., Morawsky, S. G., and Fordtran, J. S.**, Permeability characteristics of the human jejunum, ileum, proximal colon and distal colon. Results of potential difference measurements and unidirectional fluxes, *Gastroenterology,* 83, 844, 1982.
2. **Fromm, M. and Hegel, U.**, Segmental heterogenicity of epithelial transport in rat large intestine, *Pfluegers Arch.,* 71, 378, 1978.
3. **Sunter, J. P., Watson, A. J., Weight, N. A., and Appleton, D. R.**, Cell proliferation at different sites along the length of the rat colon, *Virchows Arch. (Cell Pathol.),* 32, 75, 1979.
4. **Grutschmidt, S., Sandforth, F., and Riecken, E. R.**, Segmental variations in the surface architecture of the normal rat colonic mucosa, *Virchows Arch. (Cell Pathol.),* 43, 349, 1983.
5. **Cummings, J. H. and Englyst, H. N.**, Fermentation in the human large intestine and the available substances, *Am. J. Clin. Nutr.,* 45, 1243, 1987.
6. **Berry, C. S. and Ebers, A. D.**, Scanning electron microscopy of Wistar rat colon, *Scand. J. Gastroenterol.,* 187 (Suppl.), 70, 1981.
7. **Jacobs, L. R. and Schneeman, V. O.**, Effects of wheat bran on rat colonic structure and mucosal growth, *J. Nutr.,* 798, 111, 1981.
8. **Fischer, J. E.**, Effects of feeding diets containing lactose, agar, cellulose, raw potato starch or arabinose on the dry weight of cleaned gastrointestinal tract organs in the rat, *Am. J. Physiol.,* 550, 183, 1957.
9. **Dowling, R. H., Riecken, E. O., Laws, J. W., and Booth, C. C.**, The intestinal response to high bulk feeding in the rat, *Clin. Sci.,* 1, 32, 1967.
10. **Morin, C. L., Ling, V., and Bourassi, D.**, Small intestinal and colonic changes induced by a chemically defined diet, *Dig. Dis. Sci.,* 123, 25, 1980.
11. **Janna, P., Carpenter, Y., and Williams, G.**, Colonic mucosal atrophy induced by a liquid elemental diet in rats, *Am. J. Dig. Dis.,* 808, 22, 1977.
12. **Storme, G. and Williams, G.**, The effect of a liquid elemental diet on cell proliferation in the colon of rats, *Cell Tissue Res.,* 221, 216, 1981.
13. **Deschner, E. E. and Raicht, R. F.**, Influence of bile on kinetic behaviour of colonic epithelial cells of the rat, *Digestion,* 322, 19, 1979.
14. **Thomsen, L. L. and Tasman-Jones, C.**, Dietary factors in the control of pH and volatile fatty acid production in the rat cecum, *Coll. Nutr. Falk Symp.,* 47, 32, 1982.
15. **Smith, C. G. and Briant, M. P.**, Introduction to metabolic activities of intestinal bacteria, *Am. J. Clin. Nutr.,* 149, 33, 1979.
16. **Sakata, T.**, Stimulatory effect of short-chain fatty acids on epithelial cells proliferation in the rat intestine: a possible explanation for trophic effects of fermentable fibre, gut microbes and luminal trophic factors, *Br. J. Nutr.,* 58, 95, 1987.
17. **Kruz, H. J.**, Effects of sodium butyrate, a new pharmacological agent on cells in culture, *Mol. Cell. Biochem.,* 65, 42, 1984.
18. **Traynor, O. J., Costa, N. L., Blumgart, L. H., and Wood, C. B.**, A scanning electron microscopy study of ultrastructural changes in the colonic mucosa of patients with large bowel tumours, *Br. J. Surg.,* 791, 68, 1981.

Chapter 6.5

INFLUENCES OF FIBER ON THE ECOLOGY OF THE INTESTINAL FLORA

Margo N. Woods and Sherwood L. Gorbach

INTRODUCTION

A variety of environmental and physiological conditions are known to influence microbial composition and metabolic activities of the intestinal microflora.[1,2] Among the recognized factors within the bowel lumen are

1. Temperature
2. Gas composition
3. Acidity or pH
4. Osmotic and ionic effects
5. Diet and availability of nutrients
6. Surface tension and liquid flow
7. Endogenous and exogenous substances that may inhibit bacterial growth (bile salts, volatile and nonvolatile fatty acids, bacteriocides, intestinal antibodies, and drugs)
8. Bacterial interactions and competition
9. Intestinal motility

Individual microbial species vary in their sensitivity to changes in these parameters. The composition of the flora itself can affect many of these factors. Fiber has the potential of influencing most of the factors listed above. This complex interactive system is only just being explored and only fragmentary data are available in humans.

INTESTINAL BACTERIA

Bacteria are distributed throughout the intestine, but the major concentration reside in the large bowel. The upper bowel, including the stomach, duodenum, and jejunum, has a sparse microflora derived largely from the oral cavity. The bacteria are washed down in a wave-like fashion along with saliva. The organisms are found in the upper bowel in relatively low concentrations, up to 10^5 colony-forming units (CFU) per milliliter. The ileum is a transitional zone, with a flora containing elements from the upper intestine, along with some coliforms and anaerobes from the colon. Across the ileocecal valve there is a marked increase in numbers and types of bacteria, which remains fairly consistent throughout the large bowel. Total concentrations are 10^{11} to 10^{12} CFU per gram, approaching the theoretical limit of forms that can be accommodated in that mass.

Although over 400 species of anaerobic bacteria are present in the large intestine of a human being, five genera account for the majority of the viable forms: *Bacteroides, Eubacterium, Bifidobacterium, Peptostreptococcus,* and *Fusobacterium*. The first four are saccharolytic, indicating that they can break down various complex carbohydrates present in the intestine and colon. Various facultative and aerobic microorganisms also exist in the colonic flora. Bacteria account for 35 to 50% of volume of the contents of the human colon or 41 to 57% of the dry weight.[3,4]

TABLE 1
Morphologic Characteristics of Human Intestinal Microflora

Gram-negative anaerobic nonsporing rods
  Bacteroides
  Fusobacterium
Gram-negative facultative rods
  Enterobacteriaceae
Gram-positive cocci
  Streptococcus — facultative bacteria
  Peptostreptococcus — anaerobic bacteria
Gram-negative anaerobic cocci — minor contribution to flora in man
Gram-positive nonsporing rods
  Bifidobacterium — anaerobic bacteria
  Lactobacillus — facultative or anaerobic bacteria
  Eubacterium — anaerobic bacteria
Spore-forming anaerobic rods
  Clostridium

Another way of describing the intestinal flora is by morphological characteristics. Six major categories are listed in Table 1, including an example of typical species found in the human intestine.

DIETARY FIBER

Dietary fiber is a heterogeneous material. Its physiological effects depend on specific properties, some of which can influence the intestinal flora. Among these properties are

1. Particle size: particle size determines the surface area of the fiber and alters it susceptibility to digestion, its binding properties, water-holding properties, and transit time in the bowel.
2. Cation-exchange characteristics: the ability to bind endogenous and exogenous materials in the intestine is related to ionic binding properties of the fiber, which appears to be influenced by the amount of lignin present. The binding capacity of the fiber may determine its availability for metabolism by the flora.
3. Water-holding capacity: the swelling and permeability properties can influence the ability of bacteria to infiltrate and digest the fiber by changing the surface area available for digestion and the speed of transport through the intestine.
4. Digestibility or degradability: this depends on the composition of the fiber.
    A. Lignin — not digested by the flora
    B. Cellulose — 30 to 50% digested by the flora
    C. Hemicellulose — 50 to 80% digested by the flora
    D. Pectin and gums — 90 to 100% digested by the flora

Typical food sources of dietary fiber include wheat bran, corn bran, oat bran, vegetables, fruit, legumes, and nuts. The total fiber content of these food items, as well as the proportion of the various fiber components, varies greatly. Different amounts of cellulose, hemicellulose, lignin, and pectin influence various microbial characteristics in the intestinal flora.

Most human experiments have been performed with fiber sources such as wheat bran. Thus there is more information on the effect of wheat bran on the intestinal flora than is known about the individual fiber components such as hemicellulose, cellulose, lignin, and pectin which are difficult to obtain in their pure form and are less palatable in an experimental diet.

Two approaches have been taken in studies of fiber and its effect on the intestinal microflora. In the first approach, the intestinal flora has been measured in people eating customary diets with different levels of fiber intakes (Table 2). For example, vegetarians and nonvegetarians, or Western and Japanese people eating their customary diet, have been studied. The second approach involves a defined diet in a study population to which changes are made in the type and composition of the dietary fiber (Table 3).

The results shown in Table 2 and 3 reveal a confusing and inconsistent pattern. Much of the variability in these studies reflects a lack of standardization in the basal diet and the fiber source, as well as great diversity in the parameters measured and the methods used in the determinations. The most useful approach to evaluate the impact of dietary fiber on health appears to be the evaluation of the effect of exact fiber sources added to a defined basal diet on selected bacterial enzymes.[19,37,38-40] In the few studies that have measured bacterial enzymes, bran and wheat germ were reported to decrease 7α-dehydroxylase[19] while pectin had no effect on this enzyme.[37,38] The effect of pectin on β-glucuronidase is in conflict with reports of increased[38] and decreased[40] activity. Additional human studies are needed before an evaluation of the effect of individual fibers on enzymes of the bacterial flora can be carried out.

TABLE 2
Fecal Microflora in Different Human Populations

Western diet	Non-Western diet	Fecal microflora (major organisms or characteristics compared)	Ref.
Western	Vegetarian	No change in predominant fecal flora	5
English	Ugandans (48)	English had 30-fold more Bacteroides and 4-fold more Bifidobacterium; Ugandans had significantly greater numbers of Streptococci, Enterococci, Lactobacilli, and yeasts	6
British (91) American (34)	Ugandans, South India, Japanese	British and Americans had a greater numbers of Bacteroides and a higher ratio of anaerobes	7
British	Strict vegetarians	Vegetarians had fewer isolates of Bacteroides that could dehydrogenate bile acids	8
Western (17)	Japanese, Seventh Day Adventists (11), American vegetarians (12), Chinese (11)	Westerners had greater conversion of bile acids to secondary bile acids and 2.5 times β-glucuronidase activity	9
American diet in Japanese (1)	Japanese diet in Japanese (1)	Western diet resulted in disappearance of Fusobacterium (10-month study)	10
High risk	Low risk	High risk populations had higher levels of Clostridium paraputrificum which was able to dehydrogenate steroids	11
Western Japanese (18)	Traditional Japanese (15)	Tradiational diets have more aerobes and facultative bacteria, higher Streptococcus faecalis, and fewer Bifidobacterium; Western diet eliminated Eubacterium contortum	12
North American	Japanese, Hawaiian (20)	No consistent pattern between types or numbers in fecal samples; great differences between individuals	13
High risk colon cancer	Low risk colon cancer	High risk group had more anaerobes (Bacteroides and Fusobacterium); low risk and more Eubacterium	14
Non-Seventh Day Adventists	Seventh Day Adventists	Seventh Day Adventists had higher Lactobacillus and lower Clostridium perfringens than the U.S. population. Clostridium septum, C. tertim, and Fusobacterium were lower in the Adventist group	15
	Nonvegetarian-Seventh Day Adventists	Adhering and nonadhering Seventh Day Adventists showed little differences	
High risk colon cancer, urban Danes, Copenhagen	Low risk colon cancer, rural Finns	High risk group had higher ratio of anaerobes due to decrease in aerobes (Enterococcus, Streptococcus, and Lactobacillus)	16
England (36), Scotland (11), Wales (65), U.S. (8)	Japan, Hong Kong, Uganda	Western population had greater numbers of Clostridium paraputrificum than non-Western groups	17
High risk, U.S.	Low risk, Africa	Western population had higher levels of Bacteroides and Bifidobacterium	18
U.S. (15)	Lacto-ovo vegetarians (13), Vegetarians (17)	Fecal bacterial enzymes. β-Glucuronidase, nitroreductase, and azo-reductase were higher in the omnivores compared to the vegetarian groups; 7α-dehydroxylase was higher in omnivores compared to lacto-ovo vegetarians	19

Note: Number of subjects in parentheses.

TABLE 3
Effect of Various Fiber on Fecal Microflora

Diet and fiber	Amount	Duration	No. of subjects	Fecal microflora (major organisms of characteristics compared)	Ref.
Low Residue Diets					
Low residue diet		21–56 days	6 astronauts	No significant change in fecal flora; decrease in *Enterococci* in low residue diet	20
Low residue diet (glucose-base)		15 days	11	Diverse microbial population reduced to bacteroids, coliforms, and *Enterococci*	21
Vivonex low residue diet		9 days	3	Disappearance of *Bifidobacterium* and increase in *E. coli*; decrease in very oxygen-sensitive anaerobes	22
Chemically defined diet		10 days	3	*Enterobacteria* increased, *Enterococci* and other lactic acid bacteria decreased in number	23
Elemental-low residue		12 days	14	Decrease in *Enterococci*; no change in total anaerobes, aerobes, or coliforms	24
Low residue diet		7 days	10	No change in fecal flora	25
Usual Diet with Fiber Supplement					
American diet plus			*In vitro* incubation of colon flora	Plant sources cited resulted in induction of enzymes in Bacteroides species that were capable of degrading the polysaccharides	32
Laminarin	—				
Xylan	—				
Guar gum	—				
Psyllium hydrocolloid	—				
American diet plus					
All Bran	1 oz	3 weeks	6	No significant difference in qualitative or quantitative count of bacteria; ratio of anaerobes to aerobes appeared to increase	31

TABLE 3 (continued)
Effect of Various Fiber on Fecal Microflora

Diet and fiber	Amount	Duration	No. of subjects	Fecal microflora (major organisms of characteristics compared)	Ref.
British diet plus Carrots	200 g, raw	3 weeks	5	Total breath hydrogen increased two-fold by the 3rd week; no change was seen until 10 days after the start of eating carrots; this suggests an increase in bacteria capable of digesting carrots or an induction of enzymes present in the flora	33
British diet plus Wheat bran	18 g DF	3 weeks	6	Cabbage stimulated growth of intestinal flora	34
Cabbage	18 g DF				
Western diet plus Bran	30 g	1–2 months	4	Addition of fiber led to a reduction of fecal 7α-dehydroxylase activity	19
Wheat germ	30 g		5		
British diet plus Coarse bran	12–26 g	14–70 days	24	Fecal samples from persons on fiber-supplemented diets showed no difference in the *in vitro* digestibility of the individual fiber; this might suggest that endogenous sources of nutrients and not diet are the energy source of flora; however, increased volatile fatty acids were observed in fecal samples of persons on the fiber diets for more than 2 weeks	35
Western diet plus Wheat bran	1 oz	3–14 days	7	No change in flora; no change in ability to digest bran	26

British diet plus Pectin Guar Plantains Bananas	35 g/day 35 g/day 1000 g/day 1000 g/day	2 weeks	4 3 5 4	No significant difference in composition of flora	27
American diet plus All Bran	3 oz/day (27 g dietary fiber)	3 weeks	6	Increase in anaerobes in high fat diet; no change in aerobes; slight increase in *Streptococcus* during fiber supplement; slight decrease in *Lactobacillus* during fiber supplementation	28
British diet plus Wheat bran	11.7 g of crude fiber	3 weeks	4	No change in relative number of the following: *Enterobacteria, Enterococcus, Lactobacillus, Clostridium, Bacteroides, Bifidobacterium, Eubacterium,* or *Streptococcus*	29
Western diet plus Bran Bagasse	39 g 10.5 g	12 weeks	20 20	No change in composition of the bacteria; increase in total bacteria excreted associated with increase in stool weight	30
British diet plus Gum arabic (GA)	25 g	7-day control; 21-day test diet	5	Flora not tested — effect on metabolism tested; GA caused a significant increase in breath hydrogen after chronic but not acute treatment with GA; this suggests increases in number of flora capable of metabolizing GA or induction of bacterial enzymes	36
American diet plus Pectin	15 g	21 days	6	Pectin caused a decrease in anaerobic/aerobic ratio from 3.6 to 2.6 ($p < .01$) 7α-dehydroxylase increased and cholesterol dehydrogenase decreased but neither reached significance	37

TABLE 3 (continued)
Effect of Various Fiber on Fecal Microflora

Diet and fiber	Amount	Duration	No. of subjects	Fecal microflora (major organisms of characteristics compared)	Ref.
Basal diet 12% protein 33% fat 260 mg cholesterol 5 g NDF plus Pectin	 15 g	18-day cycles	8 (M)	35% increase of β-glucuronidase on pectin diet No effect of pectin or 7α-dehydroxylase (question of adequacy of fiber supplementation and wash out times) Only pectin decreased fecal pH	38
Basal diet 0.8 g kg wgt of egg albumin 30% fat 0 gm DF plus Cellulose Pectin Xylan Corn Bran	(30—40 g 1 day) .5 g/kg wgt .5 g/kg wgt .5 g/kg wgt .6 g/kg wgt	9-day cycles	5 (M)	Indirect effect on flora via changes of pH which can affect species and enzymatic activity Pectin Decreased fecal pH	39

REFERENCES

1. **Simon, G. L. and Gorbach, S. L.**, Intestinal flora in health and disease, *Gastroenterology,* 86, 174, 1984.
2. **Goldin, B. R., Lichtenstein, A. H., and Gorbach, S. L.**, The role of intestinal flora, in *Modern Nutrition in Health and Disease,* 7th ed., Shils, M. and Young, V., Eds., Lea & Febiger, Philadelphia, 1985.
3. **Salyer, A. A.**, Energy sources of major intestinal fermentative anaerobes, *Am. J. Clin. Nutr.,* 32, 158, 1979.
4. **Stephen, A. N. and Cummings, J. H.**, The microbial contribution to human fecal mass, *J. Med. Microbiol.,* 13, 45, 1980.
5. **Moore, W. E. C., Cato, E. P., and Holdeman, L. V.**, Anaerobic bacteria of the gastrointestinal flora and their occurrence in clinical infections, *J. Infect. Dis.,* 119, 641, 1969.
6. **Aries, V., Crowther, J. S., Drasar, B. S., Hill, M. J., and Williams, R. E. O.**, Bacteria and aetiology of cancer of the large bowel, *Gut,* 10, 334, 1969.
7. **Hill, M. J., Drasar, B. S., Aries, V., Crowther, J. S., Hawksinth, G., and Williams, R. E. O.**, Bacteria and aetiology of cancer of the large bowel, *Lancet,* 1, 95, 1971.
8. **Aries, V. C., Crowther, J. S., Drasar, B. S., Hill, M. J., and Ellis, F. R.**, The effect of a strict vegetarian diet on the faecal flora and faecal steroid concentration, *J. Pathol. Bacteriol.,* 103, 54, 1971.
9. **Reddy, B. S. and Wynder, E. L.**, Large bowel carcinogenesis: fecal constituents of populations with diverse incidence rates of colon cancer, *J. Natl. Cancer Inst.,* 40, 1437, 1973.
10. **Ueno, K. et al.**, in *Anaerobic Bacteria: Role in Disease,* Balowz, A., DeHaan, R. M., Dowell, V. R., Jr., and Gage, L. B., Eds., Charles C. Thomas, Springfield, IL, 1974, 135.
11. **Hill, M. J.**, Steroid nuclear dehydrogenation and colon cancer, *Am. J. Clin. Nutr.,* 27, 1475, 1974.
12. **Finegold, S. M., Atteberg, H. R., and Sutter, V. L.**, Effect of diet on human fecal flora: comparison of Japanese and American diets, *Am. J. Clin. Nutr.,* 27, 1456, 1974.
13. **Moore, W. E. C. and Holdeman, L. V.**, Human fecal flora: the normal flora of 20 Japanese-Hawaiians, *Appl. Microbiol.,* 27, 961, 1974.
14. **Peach, S., Fernandez, F., Johnson, K., and Drasar, B. S.**, The non-sporing anaerobic bacteria in human faeces, *J. Med. Microbiol.,* 7, 213, 1974.
15. **Finegold, S. M., Sutter, V. L., Sugihara, P. T., Elder, H. A., Lehmann, S. M., and Phillips, R. L.**, Fecal microbial flora in Seventh Day Adventist population and control subjects, *Am. J. Clin. Nutr.,* 30, 1781, 1977.
16. **International Agency for Research of Cancer, Intestinal Microbiology Group**, Dietary fibre, transit-time, faecal bacteria, steroids, and colon cancer in two Scandinavian populations, *Lancet,* 2, 207, 1977.
17. **Draser, B. S., Goddard, P., Heaton, S., Peach, S., and West, B.**, Clostridia isolated from faeces, *J. Med. Microbiol.,* 9, 63, 1976.
18. **Moore, W. E. C., Cato, E. P., and Holdeman, L. V.**, Some current concepts in intestinal bacteriology, *Am. J. Clin. Nutr.,* 31, 533, 1978.
19. **Goldin, B. R., Swenson, L., Dwyer, J., Sexton, M., and Gorbach, S. L.**, Effect of diet and Lactobacillus acidophilus supplements on human fecal bacterial enzymes, *J. Natl. Cancer Inst.,* 64, 255, 1980.
20. **Cordaro, J. T., Sellers, W. M., Bull, R. J., and Schmidt, J. P.**, Study of man during a 56-day exposure to an oxygen-helium atmosphere at 258 mmHg total pressure, *Aerospace Med.,* 37, 594, 1966.
21. **Winitz, M., Adams, R. F., Seedman, D. A., Davis, P. N., Jayko, L. G., and Hamilton, J. A.**, Studies in metabolic nutrition employing chemically defined diets. II. Effects on gut microflora populations, *Am. J. Clin. Nutr.,* 23, 546, 1970.
22. **Attebery, W. R., Sutter, V. L., and Finegold, S. M.**, Effect of a partially chemically defined diet on normal human fecal flora, *Am. J. Clin. Nutr.,* 25, 1391, 1972.
23. **Crowther, J. S., Drasar, B. S., Goddard, P., Hill, M. J., and Johnson, K.**, The effect of a chemically defined diet of the faecal flora and faecal steroid concentrations, *Gut,* 14, 790, 1973.
24. **Burnside, G. and Deurode, G. J.**, Effects of an elemental diet of human fecal flora, *Gastroenterology,* 66, 210, 1974.
25. **Bounous, G. N. and Cohn, I.**, Stability of normal human fecal flora during a chemically defined, low residue liquid diet, *Ann. Surg.,* 181, 58, 1975.
26. **Hirschberg, N. and Fantus, B.**, *Rev. Gastroenterology,* 9, 370, 1942.
27. **Drasar, B. S. and Jenkins, D. J. A.**, Bacteria, diet and large bowel cancer, *Am. J. Clin. Nutr.,* 29, 1410, 1976.
28. **Fuchs, H. M., Dorfman, S., and Floch, M. H.**, The effect of dietary fiber supplementation in man. II. Alteration in fecal physiology and bacterial flora, *Am. J. Clin. Nutr.,* 29, 1443, 1976.
29. **Drasar, B. S., Jenkins, D. J. A., and Cummings, J. H.**, The influence of a diet rich in wheat fibre on the human faecal flora, *J. Med. Microbiol.,* 9, 423, 1976.

30. **McLean-Baird, I., Walters, R. L., Davies, P. S., Hill, M. J., Drasar, B. S., and Southgate, D. A. T.**, The effect of two dietary fiber supplements on gastrointestinal transit, stool weight, and frequency, and bacterial flora, and fecal bile acids in normal subjects, *Metabolism*, 26, 117, 1977.
31. **Floch, M. J. and Fuchs, H. M.**, Modification of stool content by increased bran intake, *Am. J. Clin. Nutr.*, 31, S185, 1978.,
32. **Salyer, A. A., Palmer, J. K., and Wilkins, T. D.**, Degradation of polysaccharides by intestinal bacterial enzymes, *Am. J. Clin. Nutr.*, 31, S128, 1978.
33. **Robertson, J., Brydon, W. G., Tadesse, K., Wenhan, P., Walls, A., and Eastwood, M. A.**, The effect of raw carrot on serum lipids and colon function, *Am. J. Clin. Nutr.*, 32, 1889, 1979.
34. **Stephen, A. M. and Cummings, J. H.**, Mechanism of action of dietary fiber in the human colon, *Nature (London)*, 284, 283, 1980.
35. **Ehle, F. R., Robertson, J. B., and Van Soest, P. J.**, Influence of dietary fiber on fermentation in the human large intestine, *J. Nutr.*, 112, 158, 1982.
36. **McLean Ross, A. W., Eastwood, M. A., Anderson, J. R., and Anderson, D. M. W.**, A study of the effects of dietary gum arabic in humans, *Am. J. Clin. Nutr.*, 37, 368, 1983.
37. **Doyle, R. B., Wolfman, M., Vargo, D., and Floch, M. H.**, Alteration in bacterial flora induced by dietary pectin, *Am. J. Clin. Nutr.*, 34, 635, 1981.
38. **Ross, J. K. and Leklem, J. E.**, The effect of dietary citrus pectin on the excretion of human fecal neutral and acid steroids and the activity of 7α-dehydroxylase and β-glucuronidase, *Am. J. Clin. Nutr.*, 34, 2068, 1981.
39. **Fleming, S. E., Marthinsen, D., and Kuhnlein, H.**, Colonic function and fermentation in men consuming high fiber diets, *J. Nutr.*, 113, 2535, 1983.
40. **Mallett, A. K., Rowland, I. R., and Farthing, M. J. G.**, Dietary modification of intestinal bacterial enzymes activities — potential formation of toxic agents in the gut, *Scand. J. Gastroenterol.*, 129, S251, 1987.
41. **Benno, Y., Endo, K., Miyoshi, H., Okuda, T., Koishi, H., and Mitsuoka, T.**, Effect of rice fiber on human fecal microflora, *Microbiol. Immunol.*, 33, 435, 1989.

Chapter 6.6

INTERACTION BETWEEN HUMAN GUT BACTERIA AND FIBROUS SUBSTRATES

Joseph L. Jeraci, Betty A. Lewis, and Peter J. Van Soest

Dietary fiber is now recognized as playing an important physiological and nutritional role in human diets. Dietary fibers demonstrate a wide range in their chemical composition and physical characteristics.[1,2] Each source of dietary fiber has an intrinsic property that is based on its chemical composition and physical characteristics which determines the biological and fermentive properties, i.e., the maximum limit for the rate and extent of fermentation for a particular substrate under optimal environmental conditions.[3,4] The effects of different dietary fibers on human intestinal bacteria are further complicated since these dietary fibers also affect environmental conditions throughout the GI tract.[4-7] Attempts to understand interactions between dietary fibers and intestinal bacteria also have to take into account how possible responses of the GI tract will affect the fermentation.[7] The presence of dietary fibers in the human diet could affect intestinal bacteria directly through catabolite regulation and indirectly through physical changes in the GI tract environment. The amount of fiber fermented, the amount of microbial organic matter produced, and the amount of water held by each fraction must be considered in order to predict the effect of fiber on colonic contents.[8] References 9 and 10 give more detailed information concerning the bacteria and the intestinal environment.

Intrinsic properties of cereal brans have received considerable attention, but other sources of dietary fiber, which include vegetables, gums, wood products, and synthetic polymers, offer a variety of properties.[11-13] Mucopolysaccharides from sloughed epithelial cells and secreted mucins are carbohydrates supplied by the host that are available to intestinal bacteria.[14,15] *In vitro* studies with *Bacteroides* species suggest that these host substances are not an important energy source for the bacteria.[16,17] The *Bacteroides* may be utilizing low levels of a variety of polysaccharides *in vivo* rather than a single source. Some of the predominant anaerobic bacterial species and carbohydrates found in the human intestine which have been studied in pure culture are summarized in Table 1. The type of enzymatic mechanism used to ferment a particular polysaccharide usually depends upon the type of polysaccharide being fermented rather than the isolated bacterial species present.[18] Based on DNA homologies of fecal bacteria, the colon of each person evaluated had a bacterial population specific for that individual.[19] Recent developments concerning the mechanisms by which colonic bacteria degrade polysaccharides have been reviewed.[20]

Person-to-person variation in the microbial fermentation of dietary fiber as shown in Table 2 was the most consistent result reported when mixed cultures of human fecal bacteria were incubated with various dietary fibers.[21,22] The variation from person to person has been found to be dramatic with Solka floc® as the source of dietary fiber[21-23] with fermentation ranging from 0 to 40%. Solka floc® is a commercially processed wood cellulose, which is used as a source of dietary fiber for human and animal diets. The chemical and biological properties of Solka floc® have been found to be different from native vegetable and forage celluloses.[24] Mixed rumen bacteria incubated with Solka floc® usually demonstrate an 18- to 24-h lag before significant fermentation can be observed.[3,4]

TABLE 1
Some of the Predominant Anaerobic Bacterial Species which have been Studied in Pure Cultures and Carbohydrates Found in the Human Intestine

Component	Degradability	Bacterial species
Cellulose	Partially fermentable	1[a]
Methyl and carboxy methyl cellulose	Partially fermentable or unfermentable	N.K.
Hemicellulose	Partially fermentable	3,4,5,8,11,13
Pectin	Highly fermentable	4,5,6,8,10,15
Cereal gums	Highly fermentable	2,6,7,9
Guar gum, locust bean gum	Highly fermentable	5,7,11,16
Arabinogalactans	Partially fermentable	5,6,7,8,9,10,14
Lignin	Unfermentable	N.K.
Maillard polymer	Unfermentable	N.K.
Algal gum	Unfermentable	N.K.
Mucopolysaccharide	Highly fermentable	4,5,6,10
Mucin glycoprotein	Partially fermentable	Few bacteroides strains: 12, 17

Note: N.K., not known.

[a] Adapted from Reference 18: 1, *Bacteroides* sp.; 2, *B. distansnis;* 3, *B. eggerthii;* 4, *B. fragilis* subspecies; 5, *B. ovatus;* 6, *B. thetaiotaomicron;* 7, *B. uniformis;* 8, *B. vulgatus;* 9, *B.* "T4-1''; 10, *B.* "3452A''; 11, *Bifidobacterium adolescentis;* 12, *B. bifidum;* 13, *B. infantis;* 14, *B. longum;* 15, *Eubacterium eligens;* 16, *Ruminococcus albus;* and 17, *R. torques.*

TABLE 2
Concentration (g/g) of Various Neutral Detergent Fibers Remaining after Being Incubated with Inoculum from Different Human Donors at Various Times in Batch Culture

Substrate[a]	Hours	Human donor					
		1	SD	2	SD	3	SD
Cabbage	6	0.58[b]	0.03	0.56	0.02	0.39	0.05
Wheat bran	6	0.69	0.02	0.86	0.01	0.72	0.02
Alfalfa	6	0.85	0.01	0.83	0.02	0.89	0.02
Cabbage	24	0.10	0.01	0.20	0.03	0.17	0.02
Wheat bran	24	0.56	0.04	0.53	0.03	0.53	0.04
Alfalfa	24	0.61	0.03	0.65	0.02	0.59	0.05
Cabbage	48	0.05	0.02	0.07	0.01	0.14	0.05
Wheat bran	48	0.56	0.02	0.53	0.03	0.53	0.01
Alfalfa	48	0.59	0.04	0.60	0.04	0.54	0.03
Solka floc®	48	1.00	0.01	0.99	0.03	0.77	0.02

[a] Ethanol-extracted cabbage, coarse white wheat bran (AACC Certified ROT 3691), Solka floc® (food grade cellulose), and alfalfa hay.
[b] n = 3.

TABLE 3
Effect of Inoculum Source on the Fermentation of Neutral Detergent Fibers in Various Substrates[3]

Inoculum source (substrate)	Fermentation (%)				
		Bovine		Equine	
	Human	Concentrate-fed rumen	Hay-fed rumen	Hay-fed cecum	Hay- and grain-fed cecum
Alfalfa	38	53	57	49	50
Timothy	1	40	50	32	27
Wheat bran	53	56	71	—	—
Cabbage	91	91	91	—	—
Wheat straw	0	31	42	—	—

Rumen bacteria and human fecal bacteria that ferment dietary fiber have many similarities in respect to nutritional requirements, volatile fatty acid production, and fermentation balances.[25-28] However, human fecal bacteria were more sensitive to certain dietary fibers than bovine rumen or equine cecum bacteria (Table 3).[3] Also, some humans produce methane gas.[28]

Ehle et al.[22] reported that the source of dietary fiber (coarse white wheat bran, fine white wheat bran, cabbage, and Solka floc®) in the diet was a significant factor influencing the *in vitro* fermentation of coarse white wheat bran,* ethanol-extracted cabbage,** Solka floc®,*** and alfalfa hay when incubated with the respective human fecal bacteria. No long-term microbial adaptation to these fiber-supplemented diets was observed since fermentation values obtained from 12 individuals that received a single fiber supplement for an extended period of time (approximately 70 days) were not significantly different from fermentation values obtained in another 12 individuals who received a different fiber supplement every 2 weeks. In the same study, the apparent *in vivo* fermentation of neutral detergent fiber (NDF) was significantly affected by the source of dietary fiber in the fiber-supplemented diets.[29] Estimates of the apparent *in vivo* fermentation were confounded by the quantity of microbial organic matter and the presence or lack (for cabbage) of unfermented residue from the diet in the feces. Except for the coarseness of the wheat bran, the source of dietary fiber in the diet significantly affected the true calculated *in vivo* fermentation of NDF. Regardless of the dietary fiber source, ingestion of Solka floc® in any 2-week period depressed the fermentation of NDF in all future periods.[29] This depression of fermentation resulted from a carryover effect by the Solka floc®.

The observation that previous exposure to Solka floc® depresses the fermentation of other fibrous substrates was confirmed with *in vitro* techniques.[7,30] Human fecal bacteria were incubated in continuous culture (high fiber chemostat system) and batch culture. These bacteria received Solka floc® or pectin as the substrate. The bacteria were maintained in continuous culture vessels for 17 days, then incubated in batch culture flasks that had Solka floc® or pectin as the substrate. A 36-h depression of pectin fermentation in the batch culture flasks was observed only when bacteria received Solka floc® as the continuous culture substrate (Table 4). A selective depression of Solka floc® fermentation in the batch culture flasks was not observed when bacteria received Solka floc® or pectin as the continuous culture substrate.

* Coarse white wheat bran AACC certified food grade RO7-3691 (American Association of Cereal Chemists, St. Paul, MN).
** Ethanol-extracted cabbage, see Reference 22.
*** Solka floc® (Brown Co., Berlin, NH).

TABLE 4
Concentration (g/g) of Batch *In Vitro* Substrates Remaining after Being Incubated with Different Inoculum Sources at Various Times[a]

Batch *in vitro* substrate	Inoculum from continuous-fed cultures	Time (h)					
		0	3	12	24	36	48
Pectin	Solka floc®	1.00	1.07	1.00	0.28	0.07	0.06
	SD	0.02	0.01	0.01	0.07	0.03	0.01
Pectin	Pectin	1.00	0.88	0.16	0.09	0.07	0.04
	SD	0.03	0.07	0.04	0.04	0.03	0.01
Solka floc®	Solka floc®	1.00	1.00	1.00	0.96	0.84	0.61
	SD	0.04	0.03	0.01	0.02	0.06	0.07
Solka floc®	Pectin	1.00	1.00	0.97	0.92	0.83	0.61
	SD	0.02	0.01	0.03	0.05	0.01	0.08

[a] The experiment was conducted with replicate incubations of both continuous and batch cultures. In the continuous cultures there was a single fermentation vessel for each substrate per replicate, while in the batch cultures there were triplicate observations for each inoculum, substrate, and time per replicate.

TABLE 5
Isolation of Cellulolytic Bacteria from Human Feces from Five Subjects[a]

Strain	Isolation substrate[b]	Tentative genus
HS7	Wheat straw	*Ruminococcus*
W8	Wheat straw	*Ruminococcus*
W9	Wheat straw	Unknown
W10	Wheat straw	*Clostridium*
W11	Wheat straw	*Ruminococcus*
F12	Filter paper[c]	Unknown

[a] Adapted from Reference 32. One subject yielded two cellulolytic isolates (HS7 and F12).
[b] Wheat straw was delignified with alkaline hydrogen peroxide and pebble milled prior to use.
[c] Whatman no. 1 filter paper was pebble milled prior to use.

Although colonic fermentation of the hydrated and less lignified cellulose of plant foods has been well established for humans,[24,31] fermentation of the more crystalline isolated celluloses (Solka floc®, filter paper) by fecal bacteria has been demonstrated for only 20 to 30% of the subjects studied.[22-24] With alkaline hydrogen peroxide-delignified wheat straw as substrate (Table 5), cellulolytic bacteria were isolated from four of five individuals.[32] These isolates were then able to ferment filter paper cellulose in pure cultures. Five of the isolates also showed hemicellulolytic activity.

Variation in the microbial fermentation of different sources of dietary fiber among people reflects responses by the bacteria and responses by the intestinal tract in a particular individual.

Significant amounts of starch (20%) may survive digestion and absorption in the small intestine.[33] The proportion of dietary starch passing the ileum is related to the plant source, food processing effects, diet portion, and individual variation. This resistant or malabsorbed starch, like other nondigestible polysaccharides, is fermented to short chain fatty acids (SCFA) and the gases hydrogen, methane, and carbon dioxide. Recent studies have shown differences among human subjects in the rate at which the fecal bacteria ferment the starch and in the relative proportions of the individual SCFA formed.[34,35] Weaver et al.[36] observed significantly higher proportions of acetate and lower proportions of butyrate to total SCFA in subjects with polyps or colon cancer. Butyrate, the predominant energy source for colonocytes, may play a regulatory role in the pathogenesis of colon cancer.

In vitro systems have been evaluated as models for fermentation of fiber in the large intestine.[3] Human feces afford an adequate and representative inoculum for *in vitro* systems and have been used in many studies of colonic fermentation.[8,37,38] In an *in vitro* system, SCFA production from fermentation of ileal effluents was significantly correlated with SCFA production from dietary fiber isolates but not with the SCFA production from whole foods.[39]

REFERENCES

1. **Eastwood, M. A.,** Dietary fibre in human nutrition, *J. Sci. Food Agric.*, 25, 1523, 1974.
2. **Van Soest, P. J. and Robertson, J. B.,** Chemical and physical properties of dietary fibre, in *Proc. Miles Symp. Nutr. Soc. Canada,* Hawkins, W. W., Ed., Halifax, Nova Scotia, 1976, 13.
3. **Jeraci, J. L.,** *Interactions Between Rumen or Human Fecal Inocula and Fiber Substrates,* Master's thesis, Cornell University, Ithaca, NY, 1981.
4. **Van Soest, P. J.,** *Nutritional Ecology of the Ruminant,* O & B Books, Corvallis, OR, 1982; Comstock Pub. Assoc., Ithaca, NY, 1987.
5. **Stevens, C. E.,** Physiological implications of microbial digestion in the large intestine of mammals: relation to dietary factors, *Am. J. Clin. Nutr.*, 31, S161, 1978.
6. **Spiller, G. A., Chernoff, M. C., Hill, R. A., Gates, J. E., Nassar, J. J., and Shipley, E. A.,** Effect of purified cellulose, pectin, and a low-residue diet on fecal volatile fatty acids, transit-time, and fecal weight in humans, *Am. J. Clin. Nutr.*, 33, 754, 1980.
7. **Jeraci, J. L.,** Use of the High Fiber Chemostat System to Study Interactions Among Gut Microflora, Ph.D. thesis, Cornell University, Ithaca, NY, 1984.
8. **McBurney, M. I., Horvath, P. J., Jeraci, J. L., and Van Soest, P. J.,** Effect of in vitro fermentation using human faecal inoculum on the water-holding capacity of dietary fibre, *Br. J. Nutr.*, 53, 17, 1985.
9. **Roth, H. P. and Mehlman, M. A., Eds.,** Symposium on role of dietary fiber in health, *Am. J. Clin. Nutr.*, 31 (Suppl.), 1978.
10. **Hentges, D. J., Ed.,** *Human Intestinal Microflora in Health and Disease,* Academic Press, New York, 1983.
11. **Cummings, J. H., Hill, M. J., Jenkins, P. J. A., Pearson, J. R., and Wiggins, H. S.,** Changes in fecal composition and colonic function due to cereal fiber, *J. Food Sci.*, 47, 125, 1976.
12. **Van Soest, P. J., Horvath, P. J., McBurney, M. I., Jeraci, J. L., and Allen, M.,** Some in vitro and in vivo properties of dietary fibers from noncereal sources, in *Unconventional Sources of Dietary Fiber,* Series 214, Furda, I., Ed., American Chemical Society, Washington, D.C., 1983.
13. **Horvath, P. J.,** The Measurement of Dietary Fiber and the Effects of Fermentation, Ph.D. thesis, Cornell University, Ithaca, NY, 1984.
14. **Savage, D. C.,** Factors involved in colonization of the gut epithelial surface, in Symp. on Role of Dietary Fiber in Health, Roth, H. P. and Mehlman, M. A., Eds., *Am. J. Clin. Nutr.*, 31 (Suppl.), S131, 1978.
15. **Salyers, A. A., O'Brien, M., and Schmetter, B.,** Catabolism of mucopolysaccharides, plant gums, and Maillard products by human colonic *Bacteroides,* in *Unconventional Sources of Dietary Fiber,* Series 214, Furda, I., Ed., American Chemical Society, Washington, D.C., 1983.

16. **Salyers, A. A. and McCarthy, R. E.**, Assessing the importance of host-derived polysaccharides as carbon sources for bacteria growing in the human colon, *Anim. Feed Sci. Tech.*, 23, 109, 1989.
17. **Salyers, A. A.**, Activities of polysaccharide-degrading bacteria in the human colon, in *Dietary Fiber, Chemistry, Physiology, and Health Effects*, Kritchevsky, D., Bonfield, C., and Anderson, J. W., Eds., Plenum Press, New York, 1990, 187.
18. **Salyers, A. A.**, Energy sources of major intestinal fermentative anaerobes, in 5th Int. Symp. on Intestinal Microecology, Luckey, T. D., Ed., *Am. J. Clin. Nutr.*, 32, 158, 1979.
19. **Johnson, J. L.**, Specific strains of *Bacteroides* species in human fecal flora as measured by deoxyribonucleic acid homology, *Appl. Environ. Microbiol.*, 39, 407, 1980.
20. **Salyers, A. A.**, Polysaccharide utilization by human colonic bacteria, in *New Developments in Dietary Fiber*, Furda, I. and Brine, C. J., Eds., Plenum Press, New York, 1990, 151.
21. **Jeraci, J. L., Robertson, J. B., and Van Soest, P. J.**, A human fecal inoculum in the in vitro fermentation procedure, *J. Anim. Sci. Suppl.*, 51, 206, 1980.
22. **Ehle, F. R., Robertson, J. B., and Van Soest, P. J.**, Influence of dietary fibers on fermentation in the human large intestine, *J. Nutr.*, 112, 158, 1982.
23. **Betian, H. G., Linehan, B. A., Bryant, M. P., and Holdeman, L. V.**, Isolation of a cellulolytic *Bacteroides* sp. from human feces, *Appl. Environ. Microbiol.*, 33, 1009, 1977.
24. **Van Soest, P. J., Jeraci, J. L., Foose, T., Wrick, K., and Ehle, F. R.**, Comparative fermentation of fibre in man and other animals, in *Proc. Dietary Fibre in Human and Animal Nutrition Symp.*, Wallace, G. and Bell, L., Eds., The Royal Society of New Zealand, Palmerston North, N.Z., 1982.
25. **Bryant, M. P.**, Nutritional features and ecology of predominant anaerobic bacteria for the intestinal tract, *Am. J. Clin. Nutr.*, 27, 1313, 1974.
26. **Miller, T. L. and Wolin, M. J.**, Fermentations by saccharolytic intestinal bacteria, in 5th Int. Symp. on Intestinal Microecology, Luckey, T. D., Ed., *Am. J. Clin. Nutr.*, 32, 164, 1979.
27. **Smith, C. J. and Bryant, J. P.**, Introduction to metabolic activities of intestinal bacteria, in 5th Int. Symp. Intestinal Microecology, Luckey, T. D., Ed., *Am. J. Clin. Nutr.*, 32, 149, 1979.
28. **Wolin, M. J. and Miller, T. L.**, Carbohydrate fermentation, in *Human Intestinal Microflora in Health and Disease*, Hentges, D. J., Ed., Academic Press, New York, 1983, 147.
29. **Stevens, J.**, personal communication, 1984.
30. **Jeraci, J. L. and Horvath, P. J.**, In vitro fermentation of dietary fiber by human fecal organisms, *Anim. Feed Sci. Tech.*, 23, 121, 1989.
31. **Cummings, J. H.**, Microbial digestion of complex carbohydrates in man, *Proc. Nutr. Soc.*, 43, 35, 1984.
32. **Wedekind, K. J., Mansfield, H. R., and Montgomery, L.**, Enumeration and isolation of cellulolytic and hemicellulolytic bacteria from human feces, *Appl. Environ. Microbiol.*, 54, 1530, 1988.
33. **Stephen, A. M., Haddad, A. C., and Phillips, S. F.**, Passage of carbohydrates into the colon, *Gastroenterology*, 85, 589, 1983.
34. **Weaver, G. A., Krause, J. A., Miller, T. L., and Wolin, M. J.**, Constancy of glucose and starch fermentations by two different human faecal microbial communities, *Gut*, 30, 19, 1989.
35. **Scheppach, W., Fabian, C., Sachs, M., and Kasper, H.**, *Scand. J. Gastroenterol.*, 23, 755, 1988.
36. **Weaver, G. A., Krause, J. A., Miller, T. L., and Wolin, M.J.**, Short chain fatty acid distributions of enema samples from a sigmoidoscopy population: an association of high acetate and low butyrate ratios with adenomatous polyps and colon cancer, *Gut*, 29, 1539, 1988.
37. **McBurney, M. I. and Thompson, L. U.**, Effect of human faecal inoculum on in vitro fermentation variables, *Br. J. Nutr.*, 58, 233, 1987.
38. **McBurney, M. I. and Thompson, L. U.**, Dietary fiber and energy balance: integration of the human ileostomy and in vitro fermentation models, *Anim. Feed Sci. Tech.*, 23, 261, 1989.
39. **McBurney, M. I., Thompson, L. U., Cuff, D. J., and Jenkins, D. J. A.**, Comparison of ileal effluents, dietary fibers, and whole foods in predicting the physiological importance of colonic fermentation, *Am. J. Gastroenterol.*, 83, 536, 1988.

Chapter 6.7

EFFECTS OF DIETARY FIBER ON DIGESTIVE ENZYMES

Barbara O. Schneeman and Daniel Gallaher

Dietary fibers affect the functioning of the GI tract as indicated by a lower digestibility and availability of nutrients from high fiber diets. Assimilation of nutrients from diets requires the movement of the bolus of food through the gut, the enzymatic hydrolysis of complex nutrients to simpler compounds, and absorption of these compounds into and through the small intestinal cells. The presence of dietary fibers can alter these processes, resulting in a slower rate of nutrient absorption and a shift in the site of absorption to the more distal areas of the small intestine. In this chapter, the effects of dietary fibers on digestive enzyme activity and on the intestinal contents are reviewed.

Table 1 presents the effects of various fiber sources on amylase, lipase, trypsin, chymotrypsin, or pepsin activity *in vitro*. The enzymes were derived from human samples or from commercial enzyme preparations. In general, commercial lipase or amylase is of porcine origin, and trypsin and chymotrypsin are of bovine origin. Discrepancies are most likely due to the enzyme source or to the method of incubating the fiber and enzyme and reporting values. As shown in Table 2, lipase inhibitory activity is associated with several cereals.

Addition of fiber sources to an *in vitro* protein digestibility test can lead to reductions in the percentage of digestible casein (Table 3), indicating that fibers can interfere with proteolytic enzyme activity. Other *in vitro* data indicate that certain foods which contain fiber may slow starch or carbohydrate hydrolysis (Table 4). For both carbohydrates and protein the change in *in vitro* digestibility was dependent on the source of fiber (Tables 3 and 4). The data in Table 4 indicate that the physical state of the plant cell wall rather than simply the presence of dietary fiber may be important in slowing the rate of carbohydrate hydrolysis. Grinding brown rice or lentil samples significantly increased the percentage of starch hydrolyzed in a 30-minute period.[11] These results indicate that the physical state of the food or of the cell wall layers can slow the penetration of digestive enzymes.[11,13] Tinker and Schneeman[14] demonstrated *in vivo* that the consumption of the viscous polysaccharide, guar gum, slows the disappearance of starch from the small intestine of rats. An interference with starch hydrolysis by amylase may contribute to this effect. These studies suggest that slowing enzymatic hydrolysis in the intestine could contribute to the apparent slower rate of nutrient assimilation associated with certain fiber-rich foods or diets.

The activity of digestive enzymes *in vivo* has been estimated (Table 5). Both rat studies, collecting total intestinal contents, and human studies based on a sample of duodenal aspirate indicate that within the intestinal contents pancreatic enzyme activities are either similar or significantly higher when a fiber supplement is added to a basal diet. In pancreatic duct cannulated rats, instillation of a pectin test diet reduced amylase and chymotrypsin secretion; however, infusion of a pectin alone (i.e., not in a test diet) did not change basal pancreatic protein secretion from basal values.[17] In contrast, two viscous polysaccharides, konjac mannan and Na alginate, have been reported to increase pancreatic output,[18] although this response could be due to long-term adaptation to continual feeding and not a change in the acute response. The data in Table 5 illustrate an interesting point: although various fibers may interfere with digestive enzyme activity based on *in vitro* evidence, they do not reduce the total amount of measurable digestive enzyme activity in the gut contents. The only reported significant decrease in enzyme activity occurred in pancreatectomy or pancreatitis patients, who cannot respond effectively by increasing secretion.[20] Enzyme activity from

TABLE 1
Percent of Control Enzyme Activity *In Vitro*

Fiber source	Amylase	Lipase	Trypsin	Chymotrypsin	Pepsin	Ref.
Alfalfa		48.6	63.0*	93.9		1[c]
Alfalfa	87.3	72.8	29.0*	51.6*		2[d]
Oat bran	72.6	83.83	94.9	71.3		2
Wheat bran	8.0					1
Wheat bran		82.1	96.1	90.8		1
Wheat bran	66.9*	85.9	93.8	76.2		2
Rice bran		70.0	92.1	90.1		1
Safflower meal		44.6*	56.3*	90.1		1
Xylan	32.7*	31.0*	11.2*	20.0*		2
Xylan		20.8*	91.8	98.5		1
Cellulose	20.4*	4.6*	55.3*	52.9*		2
Cellulose		9.9*	87.5	78.3*		1
Pectin		113.0	105.0	105.0		1
Pectin	148.0*	123.0	100.0	129.0*		2
Pectin-HM[a]	50.0	20.0	40.0	20.0		4+[e]
Pectin-LM[b]	0.0	5.0	12.0	25.0		4+
Pectin					98.0	5+[c]
Guar gum	54.0					3+[e]
Guar gum	60.0	45.0	90.0	95.0		4+
Guar gum		74.0				6+[c]
Carob bean Gum		121.0				6+
Na-alginate		89.0				6+
Agar-agar		101.0				6+
Carrageenan					74.0	5+
Carrageenan		Inhibits				7+[c]
Carrageenan					Inhibits	8+[c]
Carrageenan		59.0				6+
Psyllium	59.0					3+
Lignin	100.0					3+

Note: An asterisk means that there was a significant change from control. A plus sign in the reference column indicates that a statistical analysis was not reported in these studies.

[a] High methoxy.
[b] Low methoxy.
[c] Commercial enzyme source was used.
[d] Human pancreatic juice was used.
[e] Human duodenal juice was used.

intestinal contents is typically measured under *in vitro* conditions that optimize activity and thus may not reflect the physiologically available activity within the gut contents. To answer the question of whether fiber sources can slow the rate of substrate hydrolysis, *in vivo* studies have been conducted that estimate the rate or extent of lipid and carbohydrate disappearance from the gastrointestinal tract.

Table 6 summarizes several studies conducted in humans and rats to determine if fiber supplements will delay the absorption of lipid. The physiological importance of *in vitro* lipase inhibition by wheat bran and wheat germ has been studied extensively.[9,25] Borel et al.[25] reported that feeding wheat bran or wheat germ decreases gastrointestinal lipolysis of fats, resulting in lower intestinal absorption of cholesterol and fatty acids. Experimental

TABLE 2
Pancreatic Lipase Inhibition by Cereals, *In Vitro*

Cereal source	Lipase inhibitory activity[a] (IU/g)
French soft wheat	25.6 ± 1.1
French durum wheat	33.6 ± 1.0
Scandinavian soft wheat	43.3 ± 4.1
North American hard wheat	37.9 ± 1.1
Barley (8 varieties)	23.5 ± 2.0
White sorghum (5 varieties)	22.4 ± 4.8
Red sorghum (4 varieties)	3.3 ± 1.5
Millet (6 varieties)	37.3 ± 3.3

Note: Adapted from Cara et al. (Reference 9).

[a] Defined by Borel et al. (1989) as the mg of material that decreases lipase activity by 50% under their experimental conditions.

TABLE 3
Decrease in *In Vitro* Casein Digestibility[a] Due to Fiber Addition

Fiber source	Decrease digestibility of casein	Fiber: protein (wt:wt)
Holocellulose	1.66	0.4
Lignin	1.36	0.4
Citrus pectin	4.03	0.4
Xylan	5.34	0.4
Karaya gum	4.42	0.4
Wheat bran	0.15	0.5
Brown rice	7.64	0.5
Cooked broccoli	8.93	0.5
Cooked blackeyed peas	9.35	0.5
Canned corn	14.86	0.5

Note: Adapted from Gagne, C. M. and Acton, J. C., *J. Food Sci.*, 48, 734, 1983. With permission.

[a] Enzyme mixture was trypsin, chymotrypsin, and peptidase followed by a bacterial protease.

evidence suggests that *in vitro* inhibition of lipase by cereal fractions may be due to a protein fraction.[9] However, *in vivo* reductions of lipid digestion may be due to interference with micelle formation as well as direct inhibition of lipolytic activity. The results summarized in Table 6 indicate that sources of viscous polysaccharides reduce the overall rate of lipid digestion.

The change in the activity of small intestinal brush order enzymes with fiber treatments in animals is shown in Table 7. Two of the studies tend to report increases in enzyme activity due to the fiber supplement where a change in activity was observed, and two studies reported decreases with pectin treatment. One study reported that thymidine kinase activity was higher in rats fed alfalfa, guar gum, or psyllium but not in those fed cellulose or pectin than the fiber-free control. This apparent discrepancy is most likely due to factors such as feeding very high levels of fiber, use of weanling animals that may be unable to adapt to high fiber intakes, not fasting the animals prior to killing them for collection of intestinal

TABLE 4
In Vitro Carbohydrate Hydrolysis of Foods

Product	% Starch hydrolyzed in 30 min	% Carbohydrate released in 3 h	Ref.
Wheat			
Rolled	5.1		11[a]
Cooked, rolled	45.8		11[a]
White bread	77.6		11[a]
Whole meal bread	80.1		11[a]
Whole meal bread		27	12[b]
Rice			
Cooked, brown	17.6		11[a]
Cooked, ground brown	68.2		11[a]
Cooked, white	30.8		11[a]
Cooked, ground white	71.8		11[a]
Rye, rolled	11.9		11[a]
Barley, rolled	13.5		11[a]
Oats, rolled cooked	68.0		11[a]
Maize, cooked meal	71.5		11[a]
Brown lentils			
Whole	12.1		13[a]
Ground	60.9		13[a]
Lentils, ground cooked		15	12[b]
Soybeans, ground cooked		6	12[b]

[a] Enzyme source is commercial α-amylase and amyloglucosidase.
[b] Enzyme source is human saliva and jejunal juice.

mucosa, or differences in the site of tissue sampling. In Table 8, we have summarized a variety of reasons that will lead to different observations when examining digestive enzyme adaptation and activity.

In altering digestion and absorption in the small intestine, another effect of dietary fiber could be to alter the composition of the intestinal contents. Table 9 gives the effect of several fibers on viscosity of human duodenal juice and Figure 1 presents the viscosity of gastric and intestinal contents of rats fed different fiber sources. In addition, it has been reported that addition of fiber to a basal diet will increase the volume and weight of intestinal content in rats.[15,31,32] Sandberg et al.[21,22] reported that the wet weight of ileostomy fluid was increased by 94 g/d due to wheat bran and by 314 g/d due to pectin. The greater volume or viscosity of intestinal contents will have an impact on the interaction of substrates and enzymes as well as on the movement of nutrients to sites for absorption.

TABLE 5
In Vivo Pancreatic Enzyme Activity: Values Expressed as Percentage of Fiber-Free Treated Controls

Fiber source	Amylase	Lipase	Trypsin	Chymotrypsin	Protease	Species	Ref.
Total Units in Intestinal Contents (% Control)							
Apple pectin	119	193*			142*	Rat	18
Carrageenan	121	203*			140*		
Na-alginate	111	208*			136*		
Locust gum	104	167*			134*		
Xanthan gum	109	303*			142*		
Guar gum	115	321*			161*		
Cellulose	142	89.5	114	69.6		Rat	15
Wheat bran	71.0	172*	101	80.4			
Pectin	152*	216*	240*	138*			
Guar gum	141*	218*			159*		
Total Units in Ileostomy Fluid (% Control)							
Pectin	883	359*	151			Rat	19
Wheat bran	488	187	180*				
Units per ml of Intestinal Fluid (% Control)							
Pectin	175*	144	154	130		Human	16
Carob flour	179*	218*	228	163*			
Pectin[a]	53*	37*	37*			Human	20
Wheat bran[b]	48*	45	65				
Rate of Pancreatic Secretion (% Control)							
Pectin	47.8*	61.5			44.9*	Rat	16
Carob flour	91.4	108			63.6		
Carrageenan	56.8	51.4			51.3		
Guar gum	67.2	114			102		
Pectin	122	125			185	Rat	18
Carrageenan	115	132			217*		
Na-alginate	155*	109			170		
Locust gum	153*	160			208*		
Xanthan gum	173*	155			205*		
Guar gum	232*	186*			250*		
Cellulose	No change in pancreatic protein secretion from baseline					Rat	17
Pectin							

Note: *The value was reported as different from the fiber-free treated control.

[a] Pancreatectomized patients who received a pancreatic enzyme supplement.
[b] Chronic pancreatitis patients who did not receive an enzyme supplement.

TABLE 6
Effect of Fiber Sources on Lipid Digestion and Absorption

Fiber source	Dose	Results	Ref.
		Human Studies	
Pectin	5 g	Triolein breath test indicated a 30% reduction in lipid digestibility in pancreatectomized patients receiving enzyme replacement	20
Pectin	15 g/day	Fat excretion in ileostomy fluid increased by 36%	21
Wheat bran	20 g	Triolein breath test indicated up to a 30% reduction in lipid digestibility in pancreatitis patients	20
Wheat bran	16 g/day	No change in fat excretion in ileostomy fluid	22
		Animal studies	
Cellulose	20%	Intestinal disappearance of triolein reduced by 20–30% for 5-h period after meal compared to fiber-free group	23
Cellulose	10%	Lymphatic appearance of triolein was not lower than fiber-free adapted rats; appearance of cholesterol was lower at 4 h but not at 24 h after lipid infusion	33
Wheat bran	10%	Delayed the disappearance of triglyceride from the gastrointestinal tract	25
Wheat bran	20%	1.6-fold nonsignificant increase in the excretion of fat in ileostomy fluid	19
Wheat germ	10%	Delayed the disappearance of triglyceride from the gastrointestinal tract	25
Guar gum	5%	Lymphatic appearance of triolein and cholesterol was lower than fiber-free adapted rats at 4 h after lipid infusion; only cholesterol appearance was lower at 24 h	33
Guar gum	5%	Intestinal disappearance of cholesterol and triolein was 20–25% lower than cellulose at 2 h after meal	24
Pectin	5%	Lymphatic appearance of triolein and cholesterol was lower than fiber-free adapted rats at 4 h after lipid infusion; only cholesterol appearance was lower at 24 h	33
Pectin	5%	Threefold significant increase in the excretion of fat in ileostomy fluid	19
Konjac mannan	5%	Intestinal disappearance of cholesterol and triolein was 40% lower than cellulose at 2 h after meal	24
Chitosan	5%	Intestinal disappearance of cholesterol and triolein did not differ from cellulose at 2 h after meal	24
Psyllium husk	5%	Lymphatic appearance of triolein and cholesterol was lower than fiber-free treatment at 4 and 24 h after lipid infusion	33

TABLE 7
Small Intestinal Enzyme Activity: Change in Enzyme Activity

Fiber source	Peptidase	Sucrase	Lactase	Maltase	Thymidine kinase	Ref.
Pectin	↑	NC	—	—	—	26
Pectin	—	↓	↓	NC	—	27
Pectin	—	↑	↑	↑	—	28
Pectin	↓[a]	—	—	—	—	29
Pectin	—	NC	—	—	NC	30
Cellulose	↑	NC	—	—	—	26
Cellulose	—	NC	NC	NC	—	27
Cellulose	—	NC	NC	NC	—	28
Cellulose	—	NC	—	—	NC	30
Oat bran	NC	NC	—	—	—	26
Wheat bran	NC	NC	—	NC	—	31
Alfalfa	—	—	—	—	↑[b]	30
Guar gum	—	↑[a]	—	—	↑[a,b]	30
Psyllium	—	↑[a]	—	—	↑[a,b]	30

Note: ↑, ↓ = direction of change from control; NC = no change; — = not determined.

[a] Proximal intestine.
[b] Distal intestine.

TABLE 8
Reasons for Differences in Enzyme Values

Use of weanling vs. adult animals
Level and type of fiber added
Protein content of the diet
Fasting or fed state at time of killing
Methodology differences relative to sample preparation and analysis
Method of expressing units relative to volume of sample, milligrams of tissue, protein, or DNA

TABLE 9
Effect of Dietary Fiber on Viscosity of Duodenal Juice (mPa)

Duodenal juice	30
LM-pectin (2.5 g%)	40
HM-pectin (1.5%)	200
Guar gum (0.15 g%)	500
Wheat bran (1.5 g%)	90

Adapted from Isaksson, G., et al., *Gastroenterology*, 82, 918, 1982.

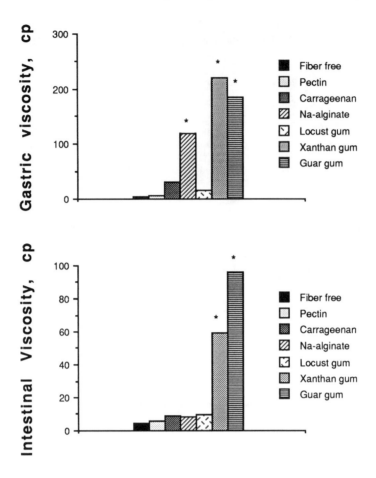

FIGURE 1. Gastric and intestinal viscosity in rats fed different fiber sources. *Value differs significantly from the fiber-free control group (p < 0.05). Data adapted from Ikegami et al., 1990.[18]

REFERENCES

1. **Schneeman, B. O.,** Effect of plant fiber on lipase, trypsin, and chymotrypsin activity, *J. Food Sci.*, 43, 634, 1978.
2. **Dunaif, G. and Schneeman, B. O.,** The effect of dietary fiber on human pancreatic enzyme activity in vitro, *Am. J. Clin. Nutr.*, 34, 1034, 1981.
3. **Hansen, W. E. and Schulz, G.,** The effect of dietary fiber on pancreatic amylase activity in vitro, *Hepato-Gastroenterology*, 29, 157, 1982.
4. **Isaksson, G., Lundquist, I., and Ihse, I.,** Effect of dietary fiber on pancreatic enzyme activity in vitro, *Gastroenterology*, 82, 918, 1982.
5. **Houck, J. C., Bhayana, J., and Lee, T.,** The inhibition of pepsin and peptic ulcers, *Gastroenterology*, 39, 196, 1960.
6. **Harmuth-Hoene, A. E. and Schwerdtfeger, E.,** Effect of indigestible polysaccharides on protein digestibility and nitrogen retention in growing rats, *Nutr. Metab.*, 23, 399, 1979.
7. **Gatfield, I. L. and Stute, R.,** Enzymatic reactions in the presence of polymers. The competitive inhibition of trypsin by A-carrageenan, *FEBS Lett.*, 28, 29, 1972.
8. **Anderson, W., Baille, A. J., and Harthill, J. E.,** Peptic inhibition by macroanions, *J. Pharm. Pharmacol.*, 20, 715, 1968.

9. **Cara, R., Borel, P., Armaud, M., Lafont, H., Lesgards, G., and Lairon, D.,** Milling and processing of wheat and other cereals affect their capacity to inhibit lipase in vitro, *J. Food Sci.,* in press.
10. **Gagne, C. M. and Acton, J. C.,** Fiber constituents and fibrous food residues effects on the in vitro enzymatic digestion of protein, *J. Food Sci.,* 48, 734, 1983.
11. **Snow, P. and O'Dea, K.,** Factors affecting the rate of hydrolysis of starch in food, *Am. J. Clin. Nutr.,* 34, 2721, 1981.
12. **Jenkins, D. J. A.,** Rate of digestion of foods and postprandial glycaemia in normal and diabetic subjects, *Br. Med. J.,* 281, 14, 1980.
13. **Wong, S. and O'Dea, K.,** Importance of physical form rather than viscosity in determining the rate of starch hydrolysis in legumes, *Am. J. Clin. Nutr.,* 37, 66, 1983.
14. **Tinker, L. F. and Schneeman, B. O.,** The effect of guar gum or wheat bran on the disappearance of ^{14}C-labelled starch from the rat gastrointestinal tract, *J. Nutr.,* 119, 403, 1989.
15. **Schneeman, B. O., Forman, L. P., and Gallaher, D.,** Pancreatic and intestinal enzyme activity in rats fed various fiber sources, in *Fiber in Human and Animal Nutrition,* Wallace, G. and Bell, L., Eds., Bulletin 20, The Royal Society of New Zealand, 1983, 139.
16. **Sommer, H. and Kasper, H.,** The effect of dietary fiber on the pancreatic excretory function, *Hepato-Gastroenterology,* 27, 477, 1980.
17. **Schneeman, B. O.,** Acute pancreatic and biliary response to protein, cellulose and pectin, *Nutr. Rep. Int.,* 20, 45, 1979.
18. **Ikegami, S., Tsuchihashi, N., Harada, H., and Innami, S.,** Effects of viscous indigestible polysaccharides on pancreatic biliary secretion and digestive organs in rats, *J. Nutr.,* 120, 353, 1990.
19. **Isaksson, G., Asp, N.-G., and Ihse, I.,** Effects of dietary fiber on pancreatic enzyme activities of ileostomy evacuates and on excretion of fat and nitrogen in the rat, *Scand. J. Gastroenterol.,* 18, 417, 1983.
20. **Isaksson, G., Lundquist, I., Akesson, B., and Ihse, I.,** Effects of pectin and wheat bran on intraluminal pancreatic enzyme activities and on fat absorption as examined with the triolein breath test in patients with pancreatic insufficiency, *Scand. J. Gastroenterol.,* 19, 467, 1984.
21. **Sandberg, A.-S., Ahderinne, R., Andersson, H., Hallgren, B., Hasselblad, K., Isaksson, B., and Hultén, L.,** The effects of citrus pectin on the absorption of nutrients in the small intestine, *Human Nutrition: Clinical Nutrition,* 37C, 171, 1983.
22. **Sandberg, A.-S., Andersson, H., Hallgren, B., Hasselblad, K., Isaksson, B., and Hultén, L.,** Experimental model for in vivo determination of dietary fibre and its effects on the absorption of nutrients in the small intestine, *Br. J. Nutr.,* 45, 283, 1981.
23. **Gallaher, D. and Schneeman, B. O.,** Effect of dietary cellulose on site of lipid absorption, *Am. J. Physiol.,* 249, G184, 1985.
24. **Ebihara, K. and Schneeman, B. O.,** Interaction of bile acids, phospholipids, cholesterol, and triglycerides with dietary fibers in the small intestine of rats, *J. Nutr.,* 119, 1100, 1989.
25. **Borel, P., Lairon, D., Senft, M., Chantan, M., and Lafont, H.,** Wheat bran and wheat germ: effect on digestion and intestinal absorption of dietary lipids in the rat, *Am. J. Clin. Nutr.,* 49, 1192, 1989.
26. **Farness, P. L. and Schneeman, B. O.,** Effects of dietary cellulose, pectin and oat bran on the small intestine in the rat, *J. Nutr.,* 112, 1315, 1982.
27. **Thomsen, L. L. and Tasmen-Jones, C.,** Disaccharide levels of the rat jejunum are altered by dietary fibre, *Digestion,* 23, 252, 1982.
28. **Schwartz, S. E., Starr, C., Backman, S., and Holtzapple, P. G.,** Dietary fiber decreases cholesterol and phospholipid synthesis in rat intestine, *J. Lipid Res.,* 24, 746, 1983.
29. **Brown, R. C., Kelleher, J., and Losowsky, M. S.,** The effect of pectin on the structure and function of the rat small intestine, *Br. J. Nutr.,* 42, 357, 1979.
30. **Calvert, R., Schneeman, B. O., Satchithanandam, S., Cassidy, M., and Vahouny, G. V.,** Dietary fiber and intestinal adaptation: effects on intestinal and pancreatic digestive enzyme activities, *Am. J. Clin. Nutr.,* 41, 1249, 1985.
31. **Stock-Damgé, C., Aprahamian, M., Raul, F., Humbert, W., and Bouchet, P.,** Effects of wheat bran on the exocrine pancreas and the small intestinal mucosa in the dog, *J. Nutr.,* 114, 1076, 1984.
32. **Poksay, K. S. and Schneeman, B. O.,** Pancreatic and intestinal response to dietary guar gum in rats, *J. Nutr.,* 113, 1544, 1983.
33. **Vahouny, G. V., Satchithanandam, S., Chen, I., Tepper, S. A., Kritchevsky, D., Lightfoot, F. G., and Cassidy, M. M.,** Dietary fiber and intestinal adaptation: effects on lipid absorption and lymphatic transport in the rat, *Am. J. Clin. Nutr.,* 47, 201, 1988.

Chapter 6.8

INFLUENCE OF DIETARY FIBER ON THE PRODUCTION, ABSORPTION, OR EXCRETION OF SHORT CHAIN FATTY ACIDS IN HUMANS

Sharon E. Fleming

Short chain fatty acids (SCFA), also referred to as volatile fatty acids (VFA), primarily include acetate, propionate, butyrate, and valerate. These compounds are produced via microbial fermentation of carbohydrates or dietary fiber in the cecum or colon of nonruminant animals including humans. The importance of the microflora in the production of SCFA is clearly illustrated by the data presented in Table 1, and further background information has been reviewed elsewhere.[43] SCFA also may include iso-butyrate and iso-valerate but, as these compounds are produced primarily from proteins, this review will not focus on these isomers. Data from laboratory rodents (mice and rats), pigs (both conventional and miniature), and nonhuman primates will be included in this chapter because of the similarities these animals show to humans in intestinal physiology and functions. Data from dogs, rabbits, and ruminant animals will be excluded, however, even though these data provide valuable insights regarding the fermentability of dietary constituents and regarding the absorption and physiological roles of SCFA. Interspecies comparisons and further data regarding the production of SCFA throughout the intestinal tract have been provided previously.[3,10,14] Although this chapter is not claimed to be exhaustive, data spanning the years of 1921 to the present are included. Data regarding the influence of dietary fiber on the production, absorption, and excretion of SCFA are included from 18 manuscripts using laboratory rodents, 11 manuscripts using pigs, 2 manuscripts using nonhuman primates, and from 11 manuscripts using humans. The influence of dietary fiber on the production or absorption of SCFA has most frequently been measured indirectly. For example, data regarding the "production" of SCFAs include measures of the concentration or pool size of SCFA in digesta in the cecum or large intestine. Data regarding the "absorption" of SCFA frequently includes measurements of concentrations in portal, hepatic venous or arterial plasma, or flux across the intestine. These data are supplemented with more direct measures of production or absorption when possible. Data regarding "excretion" are derived from fecal analyses.

The studies which are reported differ in many respects other than in the source or quantity of dietary fiber, or in the animal model that was used. For example, several strains of rats, breeds of pigs, and species of nonhuman primates have been used; animal ages and body weights have varied considerably; the length of time animals or humans were exposed to test diets ranged from 1 day to 3 years; and both males and females have been studied. These descriptors have been included in the tables when possible, and efforts have been made to identify the effects of some of these variables. In two studies, the effect of gender was evaluated using laboratory rats (Table 2). In both studies the effect of gender had a significant influence on SCFA production, absorption, and excretion. The effects were not consistent, however, and in many cases the differences between males and females were not significantly different. Perhaps these data only emphasize the importance of having internal consistency within each experiment in the distribution of animals by gender among diet groups. The influence of the duration of exposure to the test diets has been systematically measured in several experiments. The available data from three of the four studies reviewed suggest that increasing the exposure time increases production, absorption, and excretion of

TABLE 1
Influence of the Microflora on Production, Absorption, or Excretion of SCFA

Animal model	Diet	Specimen/Data	Germ-free	Conventional	Conclusions regarding the influence of the microflora	Ref.
Mice, male, NMRI (Norwegian), 22–30 g body wt	Non-purified	Cecal digesta (μmol/kg, x̄ ± SD) Acetate Propionate Butyrate Total SCFA	(n = 10) 990 ± 380 17 ± 5.8 7.1 ± 3.6 1,020 ± 390	(n = 6) 73,700 ± 21,500 13,300 ± 4,490 35,900 ± 10,200 124,600 ± 32,900	Higher conc. with microflora Higher conc. with microflora Higher conc. with microflora Higher conc. with microflora	44
Mice, male, NMRI (Swedish), 35 g body wt		Cecal digesta (μmol/kg, x̄) Acetate Propionate Butyrate Total SCFA	(n = 2) 340 7.4 2.0 360		Conc. are very low in germ-free animals, and conc. in serum parallel conc. in cecal digesta	
		Serum (μmol/L, x̄) Acetate Propionate Butyrate Total SCFA	270 4.2 5.0 290			
Rats, male and female, AGUS, 340–390 g body wt		Cecal digesta (μmol/kg, x̄ ± SD) Acetate Propionate Butyrate Total SCFA	(n = 5) 450 ± 120 10 ± 7.2 2.5 ± 0.5 490 ± 130			
		Serum (μmol/L, x̄ ± SD) Acetate Propionate Butyrate Total SCFA	(n = 5) 350 ± 50 4.2 ± 6.6 2.9 ± 1.8 370 ± 45			

Rats, male, Wistar, 180 g body wt. Fed 21 days	FF[a]	Cecal digesta ($\bar{x}$ ± SEM, n = 10)			
		Acetate, μmol/ml	<5mM	54.9 ± 3.2	Higher conc. with microflora
		Propionate, μmol/ml	~0	18.9 ± 1.5	Higher conc. with microflora
		Butyrate, μmol/ml	~0	6.1 ± 0.7	Higher conc. with microflora
		Total VFA, mM	<5mM	79.9 ± 4.9	Higher conc. with microflora
		VFA Pool, μmol	~0	136 ± 8	Larger pool with microflora
		VFA Flux, μmol/min	~0	+1.08 ± 0.22	Greater flux with microflora

[a] FF represents a fiber-free diet.

TABLE 2
Influence of Gender on Production, Absorption, or Excretion of SCFA

Animal model	Fiber	Specimen/Data	Gender Male	Gender Female	Conclusion regarding influence of gender	Ref.
Rats, Wistar, 3-week old; fed 14 weeks	None	Feces: ($\bar{x} \pm$ SD, n = 6)				31
		Acetate (μmol/g)	32.3 ± 7.5	34 ± 4.16	No difference	
		Propionate (μmol/g)	1.62 ± 1.62	4.86 ± 2.56[a]	Conc. greater in female rats	
		Butyrate (μmol/g)	0.68 ± 0.79	3.18 ± 2.27[a]	Conc. greater in female rats	
		Total SCFA (mg/g)	2.12 ± 0.46	2.87 ± 0.98	No difference	
		Weight (g/24 h)	0.49 ± 0.12	0.56 ± 0.10	No difference	
Bran (wheat)		Data not presented, but authors stated "differences were no longer apparent in 14-week old rats" fed control, bran, or meat diets.			No difference in 14-week old rats	
Rats, Hooded Wistar, males at 190 g, females at 130 g, fed 14 days	Cellulose Gum arabic	Cecal Fluid ($\bar{x} \pm$ SEM, n = 5)				34
		Cellulose				
		Acetate (μmol/ml)	66.1 ± 4.2	46.0 ± 1.9[a]	Conc. greater in male rats	
		Propionate (μmol/ml)	18.5 ± 3.9	11.3 ± 1.3[a]	Conc. greater in male rats	
		Butyrate (μmol/ml)	15.3 ± 1.0	17.5 ± 1.2	No difference	
		Total VFA (μmol/ml)	103.0 ± 5.5	78.1 ± 4.0[a]	Conc. greater in male rats	
		Gum arabic				
		Acetate (μmol/ml)	154.6 ± 7.4	149.0 ± 3.1	No difference	
		Propionate (μmol/ml)	35.4 ± 1.4	39.5 ± 1.4[a]	Conc. greater in female rats	
		Butyrate (μmol/ml)	15.9 ± 1.6	19.5 ± 2.0	No difference	
		Total VFA (μmol/ml)	206.7 ± 12.0	210.1 ± 5.8	No difference	
		Hepatic portal venous blood ($\bar{x} \pm$ SEM, n = 5, μmol/ml)				
		Cellulose				
		Acetate	0.67 ± 0.04	0.60 ± 0.06	No difference	
		Propionate	0.14 ± 0.02	0.09 ± 0.02	No difference	
		Butyrate	0.07 ± 0.01	0.09 ± 0.01	No difference	

Total VFA	0.88 ± 0.06	0.86 ± 0.07	No difference
Gum arabic			
Acetate	1.45 ± 0.05	1.09 ± 0.06[a]	Conc. greater in male rats
Propionate	0.24 ± 0.05	0.21 ± 0.02	No difference
Butyrate	0.08 ± 0.02	0.09 ± 0.02	No difference
Total VFA	1.78 ± 0.10	1.45 ± 0.08[a]	Conc. greater in male rats

[a] Denotes significant difference ($p < 0.05$) between male and female.

SCFA in laboratory rats (Table 3). It should be noted, however, that mature adult animals were used in the one study which did not show this increasing effect with duration of exposure, whereas young growing animals were used in the other three studies. The covariance of animal growth with duration of exposure must be considered in these studies.

The influence of the amount ingested of a given fiber has been evaluated commonly by feeding diets with increasing concentrations of fiber. This approach is valid when feed intakes are unchanged, but these data were not always available. Based on the studies reviewed (Table 4), increasing cellulose intakes did not consistently influence SCFA production (SCFA concentrations in cecal digesta were variably influenced in one study and increased in another study) or absorption (in the one study available, absorption of acetate and of total VFA were unaffected; absorption of propionate and butyrate were increased). Excretion of VFA in feces increased with increasing cellulose intakes in the one study that was available. Fewer studies are available using other sources of dietary fiber. In at least one study, however, the luminal pool of individual or total SCFA was increased with increasing dietary concentrations of pectin, wheat bran, maize cobs, or lucerne stems. By contrast, digesta concentrations of individual or total SCFA were not influenced by increasing dietary concentrations of alfalfa or wheat bran.

The influence of the presence or absence of a dietary fiber has been evaluated by comparing responses to a fiber-free diet with responses to a fiber-containing diet. The validity of this approach is determined by feed intakes as the concentrations of all other nutrients are diluted by the fiber. Of the studies reviewed, pectin quite consistently increased digesta concentrations of SCFA, the luminal pool of SCFA, and SCFA flux across the cecum (Table 5). The luminal pool of SCFA was increased consistently also when gum arabic was consumed, although the SCFA concentrations of digesta were often not changed. The data regarding wheat bran were less consistent, but this may be accounted for in part by the range of fiber intakes among these studies (wheat bran diets ranged from 4 to 18% fiber).

Comparisons among sources of dietary fibers have been made most commonly by feeding diets of equivalent fiber concentrations. In some cases, however, fiber concentrations covaried with the source of fiber. In comparison to cellulose, fibers including pectin, oat bran, wheat bran, and psyllium seemed to result in higher concentrations and luminal pools of SCFA (Table 6). In comparison to wheat bran, gum arabic and beans increased SCFA luminal pools, but concentrations were relatively unaffected. Hepatic portal plasma concentrations of SCFA were usually greater when animals consumed pectin, oat bran, wheat bran, and gum arabic than when they consumed cellulose (Table 7). Excretion of SCFA in feces may be determined primarily by fecal output as the source of fiber seemed to have little influence on SCFA concentrations in feces, but altered daily SCFA excretion in some studies (Table 8). Alternatively, experimental error regarding collection and processing of feces to ensure against losses prior to analyses may account for the inconsistencies noted among studies.

It is now evident that by altering the quantity or source of fiber in the diet, that changes may be induced in the production of SCFA, the quantity of SCFA available to intestinal cells, the quantity of SCFA absorbed, and, thus, the quantity of SCFA available to the liver or peripheral cells. The water-solubility of a fiber is undoubtedly one of the major factors which determine the extent to which SCFA are produced from a specific dietary fiber. Other factors may include the residence time in the intestinal lumen and the extent to which the particles provide suitable attachments for the microflora.

Basic studies strongly suggest that SCFA are absorbed via passive transport along the length of the intestine, but evidence of carrier-mediated transport exists only for the proximal small intestine.[4,6,11-13,21,56] Absorption of SCFA seems to be stimulated by increases in enteric blood flow,[36] and this suggests that the absorption of SCFA from fiber-containing diets may

TABLE 3
Influence of the Duration of Feeding on Production, Absorption, or Excretion of SCFA

Animal model	Fiber	Specimen/Data		0 weeks	1 weeks	2 weeks	3 weeks	4 weeks	6 weeks	Conclusions regarding influence of duration of feeding	Ref.
Rats, male and female, Dark Agouti, 21 weeks old	Pectin (5%)	Cecal contents ($\bar{x} \pm$ SD, n = 5) Dry:wet wt	Pellet diet	0.32 ± 0.07	0.33 ± 0.04	0.28 ± 0.02	0.32 ± 0.03	0.29 ± 0.03	0.28 ± 0.01		35
			Pellet + pectin	—	0.23 ± 0.10*,1	0.27 ± 0.02	0.21 ± 0.03*	0.21 ± 0.02*	0.23 ± 0.04*	No effect	
		VFA Conc, μmol/g wet[b]									
		Acetate	Pectin	—	27	34	38	34	41	↑ duration may ↑ conc	
		Propionate	Pectin	—	7.2	9.6	7.2	7.6	9.2	No effect	
		Butyrate	Pectin	—	4.8	4.0	4.0	2.4	3.2	↑ duration may ↓ conc	

Animal model	Fiber	Specimen/Data		4 (n = 3) wk	8 (n = 5) wk	16 (n = 3) wk	Conclusions	Ref.
Rats, male and female, Wistar		Cecal contents, μmol/g wet[b]						
		Acetate	ED	36	37	28	↑ duration may exaggerate differences from ED	
			Pectin	37	49	44[a]		
		Propionate	ED	18	16	13	No effect	
			Pectin	17	14	12		
		Butyrate	ED	7.7	9.0	5.8	↑ duration may exaggerate differences from ED	
			Pectin	8.3	10.2	10.9[a]		

Animal model	Fiber	Specimen/Data		4 weeks		8 weeks		12 weeks		Conclusions	Ref.
				Ref. 45	Ref. 48	Ref. 45	Ref. 48	Ref. 45	Ref. 48		
Rats, male, Wistar, 420 g body wt	Gum arabic, Wheat bran (100 g/kg diet)	Cecal contents ($\bar{x} \pm$ SE, n = 5) SCFA, μmol/rat	Control	328	332 ± 50	234	182 ± 24	172	276 ± 42		
			Gum arabic	859	449 ± 90	719	432 ± 39	688	622 ± 102	No effect for either study	
			Wheat bran	219	270 ± 30	250	263 ± 36	266	243 ± 21	No effect for either study	
		SCFA, μmol/g dry	Control	611	664[c]	356	433	369	587	Conclusions are not clear	
			Gum arabic	433	449	535	444	636	523	Conclusions are not clear	
			Wheat bran	356	644	407	453	420	412		

Animal model	Fiber	Specimen/Data		0 days	5 days	14 days	21 days	Conclusions	Ref.
Rats, male, Wistar, 200 g body wt	Guar gum Gum arabic	Cecal digesta ($\bar{x}$, n = 5)[b] VFA Pool, μmol	Guar	125	575	850	1025	↑ Duration → ↑ pool	47
			Gum arabic	125	425	775	1025	↑ Duration → ↑ pool	
				3 days	7 days	21 days			
		Acetate Conc, mM	Guar	89	91	100		No effect	
			Gum arabic	41	70	85		↑ Duration → ↑ concentration	

TABLE 3 (continued)
Influence of the Duration of Feeding on Production, Absorption, or Excretion of SCFA

Animal model	Fiber	Specimen/Data		Duration of feeding					Conclusions regarding influence of duration of feeding	Ref.
			0 days	5 days	14 days	21 days				
Rats, male, Wistar, 3 months old	Gum arabic Wheat bran	Absorption from cecum (µmol/L)								48
		Acetate Guar	0.6	3.4	5.5	5.5			↑ Duration → ↑ absorption, then plateau	
		Gum arabic	0.6	1.0	4.2	6.4			↑ Duration → ↑ absorption	
		Propionate Guar	0.3	1.3	3.8	3.9			↑ Duration → ↑ absorption, then plateau	
		Gum arabic	0.3	0.3	1.5	2.7			↑ Duration → ↑ absorption	
		Butyrate Guar	0.1	0.3	0.4	0.4			↑ Duration → ↑ absorption, then plateau	
		Gum arabic	0.1	0.2	0.6	1.0			↑ Duration → ↑ absorption	
			4 weeks		8 weeks		12 weeks			
		Feces ($\bar{x}$ ± SE, n = 5) SCFA, µmol/day Control	42 ± 6		39 ± 9		109 ± 40		↑ Duration may ↑ excretion	
		Gum arabic	68 ± 16		169 ± 22		102 ± 14		↑ Duration may ↑ excretion	
		Wheat bran	104 ± 23		156 ± 25		142 ± 32		↑ Duration may ↑ excretion	
			0 day	5 days	8 days	16 days	22 days			57
Rats, male, Wistar, 180 g	Soybean fiber	Cecal digesta ($\bar{x}$, n = 6)[b] VFA pool, µmol FF	122	—	122	—	203		↑ duration may ↑ pool	
		Soy	122	324	730	1054	1338		↑ duration may ↑ conc.	
		Acetate, µmol/l Soy	54	51	68	81	89		↑ duration may ↑ conc.	
		Propionate, µmol/l Soy	19	24	32	51	54		↑ duration may ↑ conc.	
		Butyrate, µmol/l Soy	11	27	19	8	11		Variable effects	

Absorption from cecum ($\bar{x}$, µmol/L, n = 6)[b]						
Acetate	Soy	0.9	2.9	3.8	7.9	9.7	↑ duration may ↑ absorption
Propionate	Soy	0.6	1.2	2.9	4.7	6.2	↑ duration may ↑ absorption
Butyrate	Soy	0.3	1.2	1.5	0.6	0.3	No effect

[a] Indicates value for pectin diet is significantly ($p \leq 0.05$) different from values for pellet or ED (experimental diet) diets.
[b] Values extrapolated from data presented in figures in original manuscript.
[c] Values calculated from other data presented in original manuscript. In this study there was a significant effect of time on total SCFA (µmol/g dry), but the differences were not clearly defined in the original manuscript.

TABLE 4
Influence of the Dietary Fiber Concentration on Production, Absorption, or Excretion of SCFA

Animal model	Fiber	Specimen/Data	Level of fiber in diet				Conclusion regarding influence of dietary fiber concentration	Ref.
Rats, male, Sprague Dawley, 320 g body wt, fed 9 weeks	Cellulose	Cecal Digesta	0%	5%		10%		7
		Wt, g/rat ($\bar{x}$ ± SD, n = 8)	9.06 ± 1.54	9.64 ± 1.28		11.13 ± 1.90	↑ % cellulose → ↑ weight cecal contents	
		Acetate, mg/rat ($\bar{x}$ ± SD)	43.1 ± 10.8	41.5 ± 8.9		49.7 ± 14.9	No significant effect	
		Acetate, μmol/g ($\bar{x}$)[a]	79	72		74	No effect	
		Propionate, μmol/g ($\bar{x}$)[a]	13	9		8	↑ % cellulose may ↓ propionate conc.	
		Butyrate, μmol/g ($\bar{x}$)[a]	16	28		23	↑ % cellulose may ↑ butyrate conc.	
		Feces: ($\bar{x}$ ± SD)						
		Acetate, mg/rat/day	54.4 ± 10	55.6 ± 13		60.0 ± 16	No significant effect	
		Propionate, mg/rat/day	4.71 ± 1.5	4.61 ± 1.5		5.28 ± 1.4	No significant effect	
		Butyrate, mg/rat/day	5.37 ± 1.7	5.40 ± 10		7.25 ± 2.3	No significant effect	
Rats, male, Sprague Dawley, 50 g body wt, fed 4 weeks	Cellulose	Cecal digesta ($\bar{x}$ ± SEM, n = 5)	0%	2.5%	5.0%	10%		16
		VFA/rat, μmol						
		8.5% casein	68 ± 3	104 ± 4	102 ± 5	121 ± 3	↑ % cellulose → significant ↑ VFA/rat	
		22% casein	170 ± 7	206 ± 9	208 ± 11	332 ± 12	↑ % cellulose → significant ↑ VFA/rat	
	Pectin	Cecal digesta ($\bar{x}$ ± SEM, n = 5)	0%	2.5%	5%	7.5%	10%	
		VFA/rat, μmol						
		8.5% casein	65 ± 4	101 ± 4	148 ± 6	286 ± 5	420 ± 8	↑ % pectin → significant ↑ VFA/rat
		22% casein	190 ± 10	160 ± 15	304 ± 14	342 ± 18	724 ± 38	↑ % pectin → significant ↑ VFA/rat
Pigs, male, Yorkshire, 150–200 lb body wt, fed 15 weeks	Bran (wheat?)	Cecal digesta ($\bar{x}$, n = 4)	Control	Bran (33 lb per 100 lb of control)				5
		Total acids, meq/100ml	22.2	17.6[b]			Conc. lower for bran diet	
		Acetate, meq/100ml	10.5	10.5			No difference	
		Propionate, meq/100ml[c]	6.9	5.7			Likely no difference	
		Butyrate, meq/100ml[c]	1.1	1.3			No difference	
		Total acid pool, g	4.6	6.4			Pool larger for bran diet	

Animal	Diet	Measurement					Comments	Ref
Pigs, male, large white, 40 kg body wt, fed 2–3 weeks		Acetate pool, meq	30.3				Pool larger for bran diet	17
		Propionate pool, meq	20.2				Pool larger for bran diet	
		Butyrate pool, meq	3.3				Pool larger for bran diet	
Pigs, male, Yorkshire, 17 kg initial body wt; 48–89 kg final body wt		Fecal excretion	Control (3.1%) (n = 6)	Cereal (7.2%) (n = 5)	Groundnut (10.2%)[d] (n = 6)		Difference appears to be due more to fiber source than to level of fiber in diet	18
		Total VFA, mmol/day	3.3 ± 0.58	34.9 ± 4.09	24.3 ± 5.81			
Pigs, male, Yorkshire × Lacombe, 50 kg body wt, (Fed 2 weeks)	Alfalfa	Cecal digesta ($\bar{x}$, n = 4)[e]	\% alfalfa meal in diet					24
			0	20	40	60		
		Acetate, mM	16.4	14.5	20.9	14.5	No effect	
		Propionate, mM	7.3	5.5	4.5	2.7	No effect	
		Butyrate, mM	2.7	1.8	2.7	0.9	No effect	
(Fed 1 week)	Alfalfa	Cecal digesta ($\bar{x}$, n = 3)	\% of alfalfa meal in diet					
		VFA Conc, mmol/l	0(4.78)	27.3(9.85)		52.2(15.01)[f]		
		Acetate	55.7[a]	63.9[g]		59.8[a,b,g]	No consistant change	
		Propionate	30.1[a]	25.3[g]		18.4[c]	Decrease conc. with increased intake	
		Butyrate	9.0[a]	7.5[a,g]		6.2[b]	Decrease conc. with increased intake	
		Net production in cecum[h] (mmol/h, $\bar{x}$ ± SEM, n = 4)						
		Acetate	22.5 ± 4.5	37.3 ± 5.5		28.3 ± 4.6	No consistent change	
		Propionate	8.4 ± 1.1	11.2 ± 1.3		7.1 ± 1.1	No consistent change	
		Butyrate	1.6 ± 0.5	1.8 ± 0.6		1.7 ± 0.6	No effect	
		Total	32.5[a]	50.3[b]		37.1[a,b,g]	No consistent change	
Pigs, large white, 45 kg body wt, fed 30 days	Lupin	Proximal colon digesta	7.5%	15.0%	22.5%	30.0%[i]		40
		Total VFA, mmol/g dry, $\bar{x}$, n = 3						
	Lupin	Lupin	0.27	0.27	0.31	0.27	No effect	
	Bran	Wheat bran	0.18	0.36	0.43	0.46	Increase conc. with increase NDF	
	Maize	Maize cobs	0.14	0.14	0.21	0.25	Increase conc. with increase NDF	
	Lucerne	Lucerne stems	0.23	0.28	0.31	0.31	Increase conc. with increase NDF	

TABLE 4 (continued)
Influence of the Dietary Fiber Concentration on Production, Absorption, or Excretion of SCFA

Animal model	Fiber	Specimen/Data	Level of fiber in diet		Conclusion regarding influence of dietary fiber concentration	Ref.
Pigs, male, large white, 58 kg body wt, fed 2 weeks	Cellulose	Portal vein conc ($\bar{x}$, n = 5)[c]	6%	16%		52
		Total VFA, μmol/L, 10 h	500	613	No effect	
		Absorption (mmol/d, $\bar{x}$, n = 5)			No effect	
		Acetate[c]	899	987		
		Propionate[c]	213	324	Absorption may increase with increased DF	
		Butyrate[c]	45	84	Absorption may increase with increased DF	
		Total VFA	1184 ± 85	1428 ± 216	No effect	

[a] Calculated from data in original reference.
[b] Indicates significant difference between diets.
[c] Values calculated from other data presented in original manuscript.
[d] Dietary fiber measured as acid detergent fiber.
[e] Values extrapolated from data presented in figures in the original manuscript.
[f] Value in brackets refers to dietary fiber measured as crude fiber.
[g] Values in the same row and with different superscripts are significantly different at p ≤0.05.
[h] Determined using radiolabeled SCFA.
[i] Dietary fiber measured as neutral detergent fiber (% dry weight).

TABLE 5
Influence of the Presence or Absence of Fiber on Production, Absorption, or Excretion of SCFA

Animal model	Specimen/Data		Source of DF (level in brackets)		Comments	Ref.
			Production			
Rats, male, Sprague Dawley, 50 g body wt., fed 4 weeks	Cecal digesta (n = 5, x̄ ± SEM) VFA, μmol/rat 8.5% casein 22% casein		FF 68 ± 3 65 ± 4 170 ± 7 190 ± 10	Cellulose (10%) 119 ± 5 252 ± 9	Pectin (10%) 420 ± 8 724 ± 38	Pool greater for cellulose than FF Pool greater for pectin than FF Pool greater for cellulose than FF Pool greater for pectin than FF	16
Rats, male and female, Wistar, 3 weeks old, fed 11 weeks	Cecal digesta (x̄ ± SD) VFA conc, μmol/g dry weight Acetate Propionate Butyrate		Meat (0%) (n = 4) 138 ± 12.5 63.5 ± 10.4 26.9 ± 9.1	Bran (17.7%) (n = 6) 235 ± 50.5 43.8 ± 5.8 114.4 ± 21.9		Conc. may be greater for bran than FF No difference Conc. greater for bran than FF	31
Rats, male and female, Wistar, 3 weeks old, fed 4 or 16 weeks	Cecal digesta (x̄, n = 3)[a] SCFA conc, μmol/g wet weight Acetate Propionate Butyrate	4 weeks 16 weeks 4 weeks 16 weeks 4 weeks 16 weeks	FF 36 28 18 13 7.7 5.8	Pectin (5%) 37 44 17 12 8.3 10.9		No difference No difference (SD bars overlap) No difference No difference No difference No difference (SD bars overlap)	35
Rats, male, Wistar, 250 g body wt, fed 2 weeks	Cecal digesta (x̄ ± SD, n = 10) Total VFA, μg/g dry wt Colonic digesta (x̄ ± SD, n = 10) Total VFA, μg/g dry wt		Elemental (0%) 26.4 ± 6.3 Negligible[b]	Gum arabic (13%) 13.7 ± 7.7 Negligible		No effect No effect	58
Rats, male, Wistar, 190 g body wt, fed 3 weeks	Cecal digesta (x̄ ± SEM, n = 12) Total VFA, mM Acetate, mM[d] Butyrate, mM[d]		FF 126.5 ± 7.3 90.2 3.3	Mixed fibers (ca. 24%) 149.5 ± 6.5[c] 89.8 22.0		Conc. greater for mixed fiber diet than FF No effect No effect	36

TABLE 5 (continued)
Influence of the Presence or Absence of Fiber on Production, Absorption, or Excretion of SCFA

Animal model	Specimen/Data		Source of DF (level in brackets)		Comments	Ref.
Rats, male, Wistar, 420 g body wt, fed 4 or 12 weeks	Cecal digesta ($\bar{x}$, n = 5)[a]			Wheat bran (ca. 4%)		45
	SCFA conc, µmol/g	4 weeks	Control (0.8%) 611	356	Conc. lower for wheat bran than FF	
		12 weeks	369	420	No effect	
	SCFA pool, µmol	4 weeks	328	219	No effect	
		12 weeks	172	266	Pool greater for wheat bran than FF	
				Gum arabic (10%)		
	SCFA conc, µmol/g	4 weeks	611	433	Conc. may be lower for gum arabic than FF	
		12 weeks	369	636	Conc. greater for gum arabic than FF	
	SCFA pool, µmol	4 weeks	328	859	Pool greater for gum arabic than FF	
		12 weeks	172	688	Pool greater for gum arabic than FF	
Rats, male, Wistar, 380 g body wt, fed 4 or 12 weeks	Cecal digesta ($\bar{x}$, n = 5)		Elemental (0%)	Wheat bran (ca. 4%[d])		48
	SCFA pool, µmol	4 weeks	322 ± 50	270 ± 30	No effect	
		12 weeks	276 ± 42	243 ± 21	No effect	
	Acetate pool, µmol	12 weeks	195	151	Pool may be smaller for bran than FF	
	Butyrate pool, µmol	12 weeks	23	35	Pool may be greater for bran than FF	
			Elemental (0%)	Gum arabic (10%)		
	SCFA Pool, µmol	4 weeks	332 ± 50	449 ± 90	No effect	
		12 weeks	276 ± 42	622 ± 103	Pool greater for gum arabic than FF	
	Acetate Pool, µmol[a]	12 weeks	195	346	Pool greater for gum arabic than FF	
	Butyrate Pool, µmol[a]	12 weeks	23	78	Pool greater for gum arabic than FF	
Rats, male, Wistar, 180 g body wt, fed 3 weeks	Cecal digesta ($\bar{x}$ ± SEM, n = 10)		FF	Pectin (10%)		50
	Acetate, µmol/ml		55 ± 3.2	99 ± 5.0[c]	Conc. greater for pectin than FF	
	Propionate, µmol/ml		19 ± 1.5	36.0 ± 2.2[c]	Conc. greater for pectin than FF	
	Butyrate, µmol/ml		6.1 ± 0.7	9.1 ± 1.0	No effect	
	Total SCFA, µmol/ml		80 ± 4.9	144 ± 7.7[c]	Conc. greater for pectin than FF	
	SCFA Pool, µmol		136 ± 8	605 ± 24[c]	Pool greater for pectin than FF	
Rat, male, Wistar, 6 weeks old, fed 3 weeks	Cecal digesta ($\bar{x}$)[a]		FF (n = 12)	Soy Fiber (ca. 22%) (n = 30)		57
	VFA Pool, µmol		203	1338	Pool greater for soy fiber than FF	

Animal	Measurement	Control	Test	Result	Ref.
Pigs, large white, 90 kg body wt, fed 20 days	Fecal VFA (x̄ ± SEM, n = 4) mmol/day mmol/g[d]	Milk (0) 4.3 ± 0.2 2.36	Milk + Bran[e] 11.5 ± 0.9[a,c] 3.95	Excretion higher for bran than FF Conc. may be higher for bran than FF	28
Pigs	Fecal VFA 7 days old, mmol/l Fed 28 d, mmol/l	Milk (0) 2.7 ± 0.4 2.7 ± 0.4[c]	Oats, Casein (1.75) Corn, Soybean (2.9)[f] 3.9 ± 1.1 8.2 ± 1.1[c]	No effect Excretion for corn/soy diet greater than FF	33

Absorption

Animal	Measurement	Control	Test	Result	Ref.
Rats, male, Wistar, 190 g body wt, fed 20 days	Flux across cecum[g] (μmol/min, x̄ ± SEM, n = 12) Acetate Propionate Butyrate	FF +0.74 ± 0.09 +0.24 ± 0.02 +0.05 ± 0.01	Mixed fibers (ca. 24%) +10.35 ± 0.91[c] +4.64 ± 0.61[c] +2.54 ± 0.34[c]	Flux greater for mixed fiber diet than FF Flux greater for mixed fiber diet than FF Flux greater for mixed fiber diet than FF	36
Rats, male, Wistar, 200 g body wt, fed 3 weeks	Digestive balance[h] (μmol/min, x̄ ± SEM, n = 12) Acetate Butyrate	FF +2.25 ± 0.17 —	Mixed Fibers +15.10 ± 1.98[c] +3.25 ± 0.33[c]	Net absorption greater for fiber than FF Net absorption greater for fiber than FF	42
Rats, male, Wistar, 180 g body wt, fed 3 weeks	Flux across cecum of VFA (μmol/min, x̄ ± SEM, n = 10)	FF +1.08 ± 0.22	Pectin (10%) +6.65 ± 0.73[c]	Flux greater for pectin than FF	50

Excretion

Animal	Measurement	Control	Test	Result	Ref.
Rats, male and female, Wistar, 3 weeks old, fed 11 weeks	Feces (x̄ ± SD) VFA conc, μmol/g dry wt Acetate Propionate Butyrate	Meat 10% (n = 4) 70 ± 10.8 19.2 ± 5.4 9.4 ± 2.6	Bran (17.7%) (n = 6) 87 ± 12.6 9.6 ± 3.4 14.5 ± 3.8	No difference Conc. lower for bran than FF Conc. may be greater for bran than FF	31
Rats, male, Wistar, 250 g body wt, fed 2 weeks	Feces (x̄ ± SD) VFA conc, mg/g dry wt	Elemental (0%) 4.4 ± 2.7	Gum arabic (13%) 8.6 ± 2.7[c]	Conc. greater for gum arabic than FF	58

TABLE 5 (continued)
Influence of the Presence or Absence of Fiber on Production, Absorption, or Excretion of SCFA

Animal model	Specimen/Data		Source of DF (level in brackets)		Comments	Ref.
Rats, male, Wistar, 420 g body wt, fed 12 weeks	Feces ($\bar{x} \pm$ SEM, n = 5) SCFA, μmol/day	4 weeks 12 weeks	Elemental (0%) 42 ± 6 109 ± 40	Bran (ca. 4%^{c,d}) 104 ± 23 142 ± 32	Excretion greater for bran than FF Excretion greater for bran than FF	45
	SCFA, μmol/day	4 weeks 12 weeks	Elemental (0%) 42 ± 6 109 ± 40	Gum arabic (10%) 68 ± 16 102 ± 14	No effect No effect	

[a] Values extrapolated from data presented in figures in original manuscript.
[b] Denotes negligible.
[c] Indicates significant difference between diets.
[d] Values calculated from other data presented in original manuscript.
[e] 100 g wheat bran + 180 g powdered milk per day for a 90-kg pig.
[f] Dietary fiber measured as crude fiber.
[g] Flux = Arteriovenous difference (μmol/ml) × cecal blood flow (ml/min) × % of plasma water in the blood.
[h] Digestive balance = Portal vein − artery difference (μmol/ml) × portal blood flow (ml/min).

TABLE 6
Influence of the Source of Dietary Fiber on SCFA Production

Animal model	Specimen/Data	Source of DF (level in brackets)			Comments	Ref.
Rats, male, Sprague-Dawley, 50 g body wt, fed 4 weeks	Cecal digesta ($\bar{x}$ ± SEM, n = 5) VFA, μmol/rat	Cellulose (5%) 102 ± 5		Pectin (5%) 148 ± 6	Cellulose and pectin were evaluated in separate experiments, but it appears that the pool of VFA is greater with pectin than cellulose	16
	VFA, μmol/rat	Cellulose (10%) 119 ± 5		Pectin (10%) 420 ± 8		
Rats, male, Hooded Wistar 210 g body wt, fed 2 weeks	Cecal digesta fluid ($\bar{x}$ ± SEM, n = 5, 10:00h) Acetate, μmol/ml Propionate, μmol/ml Butyrate, μmol/ml Total VFA, μmol/ml	Cellulose (10%) 50.0 ± 2.4 17.0 ± 1.5 7.2 ± 0.7 77.2 ± 1.2		Oat bran (36.5% or 10% fiber in diet) 65.6 ± 4.4*,a 34.4 ± 5.9* 39.2 ± 3.5* 147.2 ± 3.9*	Conc greater for oat bran than for cell. Conc greater for oat bran than for cell. Conc greater for oat bran than for cell. Conc greater for oat bran than for cell.	32
Rats, male Hooded Wistar 190 g body wt, fed 2 weeks	Cecal digesta fluid ($\bar{x}$ ± SEM, n = 5) Acetate, μmol/ml Propionate, μmol/ml Butyrate, μmol/ml Total VFA, μmol/ml	Cellulose (10%) 66.1 ± 4.2 18.5 ± 3.9 15.3 ± 1.0 103.1 ± 5.5		Gum arabic (10%) 154.6 ± 7.4*,a 35.4 ± 1.4* 15.9 ± 1.6 206.7 ± 12.0*	Conc greater for gum arabic than cell. Conc greater for gum arabic than cell. No difference Conc greater for gum arabic than cell.	34
Rats, male Hooded Wistar 250 g body wt, fed 2 weeks	Cecal digesta fluid ($\bar{x}$ ± SEM, n = 6) Acetate, μmol/ml Propionate, μmol/ml Butyrate, μmol/ml Total VFA, μmol/ml	Cellulose (10%) 113 ± 8 33 ± 2 32 ± 4 157 ± 12		Gum arabic (10%) 95 ± 7*,a 30 ± 2 22 ± 2* 171 ± 11	Conc greater for cellulose than gum arabic No effect Conc greater for cellulose than gum arabic No effect	41
Rats, male, Wistar, 420 g body wt	Cecal digesta fluid ($\bar{x}$, n = 5)[b] Total SCFA, μmol/g (4 weeks) (12 weeks) Total SCFA, μmol (4 weeks) (12 weeks)	Control (0.8%) 611 369 328 172	Gum arabic (100 g/kg) 433 636 859 688	Wheat bran (100 g/kg) 356 420 219 266	(Data difficult to interpret since the fiber content of gum arabic and wheat bran differ) Conc may be greatest for control Conc may be greatest for gum arabic Conc is greatest for gum arabic Conc is greatest for gum arabic	45
Rats, male, Wistar, 200 g body wt, fed 3 weeks	Cecal digesta ($\bar{x}$, n = 5)[b] VFA Pool, μmol/rat VFA Conc. mM Acetate Propionate Butyrate	Guar gum (15%) 1000 100 61 12	Gum arabic (15%) 1000 85 38 23		No effect Conc may be greater for guar gum Conc may be greater for guar gum Conc may be greater for gum arabic	47
Rats, male Hooded Wistar, 200 g body wt, fed 10 days	Cecal digesta ($\bar{x}$ ± SE, n = 6) VFA Conc, μmol/ml Acetate Propionate	Cellulose (10%) 77 ± 6[a,c] 27 ± 2[a]	Bran (10%) 144 ± 4[c] 33 ± 2[a]	Wheat fractions Aleurone (10%) Seed coat (10%) 199 ± 12[d] 107 ± 4[b] 62 ± 3[b] 28 ± 1[a]	Aleurone > bran > seed coat > cellulose Aleurone > bran, seed coat, cellulose	46

TABLE 6 (continued)
Influence of the Source of Dietary Fiber on SCFA Production

Animal model	Specimen/Data	Source of DF (level in brackets)				Comments	Ref.
	Butyrate		20 ± 1[a]	54 ± 6[c]	24 ± 2[b]	52 ± 5[c]	Bran, seed coat > aleurone, cellulose
	Total		128 ± 7[a]	235 ± 9[c]	289 ± 15[d]	192 ± 5[b]	Aleurone > bran > seed coat > cellulose	
	Total VFA Pool, μmol		264 ± 15[a]	564 ± 50[b]	1088 ± 110[c]	302 ± 34[a]	Aleurone > bran > seed coat, cellulose	
Rats, male, Wistar, 420 g body wt	Cecal digesta (x̄ ± SEM, n = 5)		Elemental	Gum arabic (100 g/kg)		Wheat bran (100 g/kg)	(Data difficult to interpret since fiber content of gum arabic and wheat bran differ)	48
	Total SCFA, μmol	4 weeks	332 ± 50	449 ± 90		270 ± 30	Pool may be greatest for gum arabic
		8 weeks	182 ± 24	431 ± 39		263 ± 36	Pool may be greatest for gum arabic
		12 weeks	276 ± 42	622 ± 103		243 ± 21	Pool may be greatest for gum arabic
Rats, male, Hooded Wistar, 200 g body wt, fed 10 days	Cecal digesta (x̄ ± SEM, n = 6)		Wheat bran (70 g/kg) (Diet with corn oil)	Rice bran (70 g/kg)				55
	SCFA Conc, μmol/ml						
	Acetate		56 ± 6	67 ± 4			No effect
	Propionate		15 ± 2	21 ± 1*,a			Conc greater for rice bran
	Butyrate		21 ± 2	18 ± 1			No effect
	Total		95 ± 9	110 ± 6			No effect
	SCFA Pool, μmol		122 ± 14	192 ± 14*			Pool greater for rice bran
	SCFA Conc, μmol/ml		(Diets with fish oil)				
	Acetate		62 ± 5	67 ± 3			No effect
	Propionate		16 ± 1	17 ± 1			No effect
	Butyrate		27 ± 3	16 ± 1*			Conc greater for wheat bran
	Total		109 ± 5	102 ± 5			No effect
	SCFA Pool, μmol		113 ± 4	171 ± 11*			Pool greater for rice bran
Pigs, mature, Yorkshire, ca. 70 kg body wt, fed 12 weeks	Cecal digesta (x̄, n = 5)		Cellulose (16.1)	Coarse bran (15.8)	Fine bran (17.3)	Alfalfa (16.3)[d]		26
	VFA Conc, mM						
	Acetate		99	104	99	120	No difference
	Propionate		33[a]	42[a,b]	48[b]	36[a,c]	Fine bran > cellulose, alfalfa
	Butyrate		13[a]	23[b]	29[b]	14[a]	Fine bran, coarse bran > cellulose, alfalfa
Pigs, female, mature, crossbred, fed 10 days	Cecal digesta (x̄, n = 4)		Corn, Hay (38.3)	Corn, Soy (11.1)			(Both source and level of NDF varied)	38
	VFA Conc, mM		70.5	134.3*,a			Corn soy diet > corn hay diet
	Acetate, mM[c]		54.6	83.7			Corn soy diet > corn hay diet
	Butyrate, mM[c]		3.5	13.3			Corn soy diet > corn hay diet
Pigs, male, Hanford miniature, 5-month old, 40 kg body wt, fed 2 weeks	Cecal digesta (x̄ ± SD, n = 6)		Wheat Bran (7)	Red kidney beans (7)[f]				51
	SCFA Conc, mmol/l						
	Acetate		70 ± 10	86 ± 16			No effect
	Propionate		28 ± 3.5	42 ± 6.6			Conc for bean diet greater than bran
	Butyrate		11 ± 2.3	8.5 ± 2.2			No effect
	Total SCFA		110 ± 15	140 ± 8.4			Conc for bean diet greater than bran

	Cellulose (9.7)	Psyllium husk (9.7)		
SCFA Pool, mmol/animal				49
Acetate	35 ± 2.5	80 ± 29	Pool greater for bean diet than bran	
Propionate	14 ± 1.4	36 ± 10	Pool greater for bean diet than bran	
Butyrate	5.4 ± 0.7	7.3 ± 3.2	No effect	
Total SCFA	55 ± 4.1	126 ± 36	Pool greater for bean diet than bran	
Monkeys, male, adult, African green, fed 3 years	Colonic digesta (n = 3 or 2, x̄ ± SD)			
	Acetate, μmol/g	48 ± 4.5	105 ± 0.4*,a	Conc greater for psyllium than cellulose
	Propionate, μmol/g	17 ± 5.6	37 ± 14.1*	Conc greater for psyllium than cellulose
	Butyrate, μmol/g	6 ± 1.7	10 ± 7.4	No effect
	Total VFA, μmol/g	81 ± 8.0	162 ± 31.2*	Conc greater for psyllium than cellulose

a   Asterisk indicates significant difference between diets.
b   Values extrapolated from data presented in figures in original manuscripts. Significance of differences among diet groups not always clearly identified.
c   Values in a row with different superscripts are significantly different at P ≤ 0.05.
d   Value in brackets indicate % of cell wall material in the diet.
e   Values calculated from other data presented in original manuscript.
f   Dietary fiber measured as total dietary fiber.

TABLE 7
Influence of the Source of Dietary Fiber on SCFA Absorption

Animal model	Specimen/Data	Source of DF (level in brackets)				Comments	Ref.
		Control	Wheat Bran[a]		Pectin[a]		
Rats, male, Hooded Wistar, 200 g body wt	Hepatic portal plasma (n = 6) Acetate at 10:00h, μmol/ml Total VFA at 10:00h, μmol/ml Acetate at 20:00h, μmol/ml Total VFA 20:00h, μmol/ml	0.32 ± 0.03^c 0.33 ± 0.02^c 0.12 ± 0.01^b 0.15 ± 0.01^b	0.16 ± 0.02^a 0.17 ± 0.02^a 0.08 ± 0.01^a 0.10 ± 0.01^a		$0.24 \pm 0.04^{b,2}$ 0.25 ± 0.03^b $0.09 \pm 0.02^{a,b,c}$ $0.11 \pm 0.02^{a,b,c}$	Significant effect of fiber, but conclusions are compromised since the fiber contents of wheat bran and pectin differ	27
		Cellulose (10%)	Oat Bran (36.5% or 10% fiber in diet)				
Rat, male, Hooded Wistar, 210 g body wt, fed 2 weeks	Hepatic portal venous plasma ($\bar{x} \pm$ SEM, n = 5 at 10:00 h) Acetate, μmol/ml Propionate, μmol/ml Butyrate, μmol/ml Total VFA, μmol/ml	0.58 ± 0.02 0.11 ± 0.01 0.04 ± 0.01 0.75 ± 0.02	0.67 ± 0.07 $0.22 \pm 0.04^{*,d}$ $0.24 \pm 0.05^*$ $1.18 \pm 0.15^*$			No effect Conc greater for oat bran than for cellulose Conc greater for oat bran than for cellulose Conc greater for oat bran than for cellulose	32
		Cellulose (10%)	Gum arabic (10%)				
Rats, male, Hooded Wistar, 190 g body wt, fed 2 weeks	Hepatic portal venous plasma ($\bar{x} \pm$ SEM, n = 5) Acetate, μmol/ml Propionate, μmol/ml Butyrate, μmol/ml Total VFA, μmol/ml	0.67 ± 0.04 0.14 ± 0.02 0.07 ± 0.01 0.88 ± 0.06	$1.45 \pm 0.05^{*,d}$ $0.24 \pm 0.05^*$ 0.08 ± 0.02 $1.78 \pm 0.1^*$			Conc greater for gum arabic than for cellulose Conc greater for gum arabic than for cellulose No effect Conc greater for gum arabic than for cellulose	34
		Cellulose (10%)	Gum arabic (10%)				
Rats, male, Hooded Wistar, 250 g body wt, fed 2 weeks	Hepatic portal venous plasma ($\bar{x} \pm$ SEM, n = 6) Acetate, μmol/ml Propionate, μmol/ml Butyrate, μmol/ml Total VFA, μmol/ml	0.72 ± 0.04 0.15 ± 0.01 0.08 ± 0.01 0.99 ± 0.05	$1.11 \pm 0.15^{*,d}$ 0.22 ± 0.04 $0.14 \pm 0.02^*$ $1.47 \pm 0.19^*$			Conc greater for gum arabic than for cell No effect Conc greater for gum arabic than for cell Conc greater for gum arabic than for cell	41
		Guar gum (15%)	Gum arabic (15%)				
Rats, male, Wistar, 200 g body wt, fed 3 weeks	Cecal absorption[e] Acetate, μmol/min Propionate, μmol/min Butyrate, μmol/min	5.5 3.9 0.42	6.4 2.7 0.96			No effect Absorption may be greater for guar gum Absorption may be greater for gum arabic	47
		Cellulose (10%)	Bran (10%)	Wheat Fractions Aleurone (10%)	Seed Coat (10%)		
Rats, male, Wistar 200 g body wt Fed 10 days	Hepatic portal venous plasma ($\bar{x} \pm$ SEM, n = 6) Acetate, μmol/ml Propionate, μmol/ml Butyrate, μmol/ml Total VFA, μmol/ml	$0.73 \pm 0.03^{a,2}$ 0.16 ± 0.01^a 0.10 ± 0.01^a 1.09 ± 0.04^a	1.16 ± 0.13^b 0.23 ± 0.03^b 0.29 ± 0.04^c 1.83 ± 0.17^c	2.25 ± 0.15^c 0.64 ± 0.05^c 0.18 ± 0.03^b 3.18 ± 0.21^c	1.05 ± 0.08^b 0.22 ± 0.03^b $0.23 \pm 0.04^{b,c}$ 1.66 ± 0.10^b	Aleurone > Bran, Seed coat > Cellulose Aleurone > Bran, Seed coat > Cellulose Bran ≥ Seed coat > Aleurone > Cellulose Aleurone > Bran, Seed coat > Cellulose	46
		Polysaccharide free diet		Pectin (20 g)			
Humans, male & female, 19–41 yr old. Fed 1 day	Plasma venous, forearm Acetate, μmol/L, 12 hr pp[5]	31.9		$92.6^{*,4}$			39

1 Diets contained 10% wheat bran or 10% pectin which differ in fiber concentrations.
2 Values in a row with common superscripts are significantly different (P ≤ 0.05).
3 Superscripts for the 20:00 h data in original paper seemed to be in error and the more logical superscripts are used here.
4 Asterisk indicates significant difference (P ≤ 0.05) between fiber sources.
5 Values extrapolated from data presented in figures in the original manuscript.

TABLE 8
Influence of the Source of Dietary Fiber on Excretion of SCFA in Feces

Animal model	Specimen/Data		Source of DF (level in brackets)						Comments	Ref.
Rats, male, Wistar, 420 g body wt	Fecal excretion of SCFA (μmol/day, $\bar{x}$, n = 5)[a]		Control (0.8%)		Gum arabic (100 g/kg)		Wheat bran (100 g/kg)		(Data difficult to interpret since the fiber contents of gum arabic and wheat bran differ) Excretion may be greatest for gum arabic Excretion may be least for control	45
	4 weeks		186		407		166			
	12 weeks		55		214		193			
Rats, male, Wistar, 420 g body wt	Fecal excretion of SCFA (μmol/day, $\bar{x} \pm$ SEM, n = 5)		Elemental		Gum arabic (100 g/kg)		Wheat bran (100 g/kg)		(Data difficult to interpret since the fiber contents of gum arabic and wheat bran differ) Excretion may be greater for wheat bran No difference No difference	48
	4 weeks		42 ± 6		68 ± 16		104 ± 23			
	8 weeks		39 ± 9		169 ± 22		156 ± 25			
	12 weeks		109 ± 40		102 ± 14		142 ± 32			
Pigs, mature, Yorkshire, ca. 70 kg body wt, fed 12 weeks	Fecal VFA conc, mM, $\bar{x}$ Acetate Propionate Butyrate		Cellulose (16.1) 24 12 5[a]		Coarse bran (15.8) 29 15 8[b]		Fine bran (17.3) 26 15 8[b]		Alfalfa (16.3)[b] 30 13 6[ab,2]	No effect No effect Coarse and fine bran > cellulose	25
Monkeys, male, adult, African green, fed 3 years	Fecal VFA, (μmol/g, n = 5, $\bar{x} \pm$ SD) Acetate Propionate Butyrate Total VFA		Cellulose (9.7) 27 ± 7.6 11 ± 4.7 5 ± 2.0 50 ± 12.1				Psyllium husk (9.7) 33 ± 10.1 14 ± 5.1 6 ± 2.2 58 ± 16.9			No effect No effect No effect No effect	49
Humans	Feces — total acid output									Quantitative data not available; diets high in protein and fat caused low VFA output, diets high in cereals caused high VFA output	1
Humans, male, adult, fed 1 week	Feces — titratable acidity, $\bar{x}$, n = 3 (1N alkali, cc)	Cellu flour (72)[b] 5[c]	Cottonseed hull meal (106) 28	Corn germ meal (115) 110	Alfalfa leaf meal (86) 28	Canned peas (75) 45	Agar-agar (80) 90	Carrots (107) 97		Acid excretion influenced by DF	2
		Sugar beet pulp (93) 98				Cabbage (102) 135		Wheat bran (146) 301			
Humans, male, 21–25 years old, fed 3 weeks	Feces, $\bar{x}$, n = 6 VFA, mmol/kg VFA, mmol/day	Mixed sources (17 g/day) 93 7						Mixed + wheat bran (45 g/day) 87 20[d]		No effect Excretion for high bran diet greater than low fiber diet	9

TABLE 8 (continued)
Influence of the Source of Dietary Fiber on Excretion of SCFA in Feces

Animal model	Specimen/Data	Source of DF (level in brackets)			Comments	Ref.
Humans, male adults, fed 2 weeks	Feces, dialysate (mmol/l, x̄ ± SEM, n = 4)	Control (21.8 g/day)		Control + wheat fiber (53.2 g/day)		15
	Acetate	31.7 ± 2.8		39.5 ± 2.5	No effect	
	Propionate	13.2 ± 1.3		12.3 ± 0.9	No effect	
	Butyrate	12.8 ± 1.0		14.3 ± 1.2	No effect	
	Total SCFA	57.7 ± 4.7		66.1 ± 4.2	No effect	
Humans, males and females, 23—60 years, fed 3 weeks	Feces (n = 12—14/group, x̄ ± SD)	Placebo (low)		Pectin (5%)		22
	Acetate, g/7 days	1.2 ± 0.7		1.7 ± 1.9	No effect	
	Propionate, g/7 days	0.5 ± 0.3		0.6 ± 0.7	No effect	
	Butyrate, g/7 days	0.4 ± 0.2		0.6 ± 0.7	No effect	
	Total VFA, g/7 days	2.4 ± 1.4		3.3 ± 3.7	No effect	
		Placebo (low)		Cellulose		
	Acetate, g/7 days	1.2 ± 0.7		2.1 ± 1.6	Excretion may be higher for cellulose	
	Propionate, g/7 days	0.5 ± 0.3		0.9 ± 0.7	Excretion may be higher for cellulose	
	Butyrate, g/7 days	0.4 ± 0.2		0.7 ± 0.8	Excretion may be higher for cellulose	
	Total VFA, g/7 days	2.4 ± 1.4		4.3 ± 3.4	Excretion may be higher for cellulose	
Humans, male, young adult, fed 2 weeks	Feces (x̄, n = 3)	Cellulose[c]	Fine bran	Coarse bran	Cabbage	
	Acetate, mM	53	51	69	78	25
	Propionate, mM	22	22	29	28	No effect
	Butyrate, mM	16	25	27	25	No effect
	Total VFA, mM	107[a]	118[a,b]	145[a,b]	166[b,f]	Conc greater for cabbage than cellulose
Humans, men, 21—35 years, fed 9 days	Fecal Excretion (x̄, n = 5) VFA Excretion, g/3 days	FF	Cellulose[g]	Pectin	Xylan	Corn bran	30
	Acetate	0.57[b]	0.61[b]	0.67[b]	0.38[b]	1.29[a]	Corn bran highest
	Propionate	0.39	0.49	0.56	0.37	0.52	No difference
	Butyrate	0.22[b]	0.33[a,b]	0.40[a]	0.20[b]	0.41[a]	Corn bran and pectin higher than FF and xylan
	Total VFA	1.47[b,c]	1.80[b,c]	2.02[b]	1.16[c]	2.68[a]	Corn bran highest, FF and xylan lowest
	VFA Conc, % wet wt						
	Acetate	0.31	0.18	0.25	0.22	0.32	No difference
	Propionate	0.21[a]	0.14[b,c]	0.20[a]	0.17[a,b]	0.11[c]	Corn bran lowest, FF and pectin highest
	Butyrate	0.14[a,b]	0.10[b,c]	0.14[a,b]	0.08[c]	0.09[b,c]	Xylan lowest, FF and pectin highest
	Total VFA	0.85[a]	0.52[b]	0.75[a,b]	0.57[b]	0.63[a,b]	Xylan and cellulose lower than FF
Humans, male, 21—35 years old, fed 23 days	Feces (x̄, n = 12)	Control (33 g DF/day)		Bean diet (42 g DF/day)			37
	Acetate, mg/3 days	1428		1721		No effect	
	mg/g wet	2.75		3.05		No effect	

Propionate,	mg/g dry	11.49	12.94	No effect
	mg/3 days	688	761	No effect
	mg/g wet	1.22	1.33	No effect
	mg/g dry	5.16	5.71	No effect
Butyrate,	mg/3 days	900	989	No effect
	mg/g wet	1.64	1.74	No effect
	mg/g dry	6.91	7.33	No effect
Total VFA,	mg/3 days	3354	3887	Conc greater for bean diet
	mg/g wet	6.32	6.87[d]	
	mg/g dry	26.4	29.0	No effect

[a] Values calculated from data in original manuscript.
[b] Value in brackets refers to total insoluble residue (lignin + cellulose + hemicellulose).
[c] Data referred to in Grove et al., 1929 (see Ref. 1).
[d] Indicates a significant difference at $p \leq 0.05$.
[e] Fiber sources added to fiber-free basal diet in sufficient quantity to provide 12 g cell wall per day.
[f] Values in a row with common superscripts are significantly different at $p \leq 0.05$.
[g] Fiber sources provided 0.5 g DF/kg body wt daily.

exceed the rate which would be predicted solely from the change in luminal SCFA concentrations (e.g., by using the absorption equations of Fleming et al.[56]). Absorption does not seem to be influenced significantly by changes in pH within the range of 5.4 and 7.4[56] which is commonly reported for digesta in the cecum or proximal colon. Thus, SCFA absorption may not be stimulated by the presence of an acidic luminal milieu. Based on these data, the dynamic nature of SCFA production and absorption must be emphasized. The presence of fermentable substrate will stimulate SCFA production, causing an increase in luminal SCFA concentration and an increase in concentration-dependent SCFA absorption. This increased absorption will attenuate the rise in luminal concentrations of SCFA. This must be considered when luminal concentration data are the sole means used to assess the influence of a dietary treatment on the "production", or availability to the host, of SCFA.

Much interest has been focused recently on the physiological roles of SCFA, and the scope of this topic exceeds the intent of this chapter. The reader may wish, however, to refer elsewhere for this information,[8,23,43,53] as SCFA influence water and electrolyte movements in the colon, provide energy, and stimulate cellular proliferation. Of the three major SCFA, butyrate may be unique as it has been proposed to be a preferable energy source to glucose or ketone bodies for colonocytes, to reduce cellular proliferation, and to stimulate differentiation of cells including colon carcinoma cells. The energy value of unavailable carbohydrates,[54] including dietary fibers,[19] may be determined primarily by the extent to which the fiber has been fermented to produce SCFA and by their oxidation.

REFERENCES

1. **Roux, J. C. and Goiffon, R.,** (1921) Arch. mal app. digestif. 11:25, in Grove, E. W., Olmsted, W. H., and Koenig, K., The effect of diet and catharsis on the lower volatile fatty acids in the stools of normal men, *J. Biol. Chem.*, 85, 127, 1929.
2. **Williams, R. D. and Olmsted, W. H.,** The effect of cellulose, hemicellulose and lignin on the weight of the stool: a contribution to the study of laxation in man, *J. Nutr.*, 11, 433, 1936.
3. **Elsden, S. R., Hitchcock, M. W. S., Marshall, R. A., and Phillipson, A. T.,** Volatile acid in the digesta of ruminants and other animals, *J. Exp. Biol.*, 22, 191, 1946.
4. **Smyth, D. H. and Taylor, C. B.,** Intestinal transfer of short chain fatty acids in vitro, *J. Physiol. (London)*, 141, 73, 1958.
5. **Friend, D. W., Cunningham, H. M., and Nicholson, J. W. G.,** The production of organic acids in the pig. II. The effect of diet on the levels of volatile fatty acids and lactic acid in sections of the alimentary tract, *Can. J. Anim. Sci.*, 43, 156, 1963.
6. **Dawson, A. M., Holdsworth, C. D., and Webb, J.,** Absorption of short chain fatty acids in man, *J. Proc. Exp. Biol. Med.*, 117, 97, 1964.
7. **Yang, M. G., Manoharan, K., and Young, A. K.,** Influence and degradation of dietary cellulose in cecum of rats, *J. Nutr.*, 97, 260, 1969.
8. **Ballard, F. J.,** Supply and utilization of acetate in mammals, *Am. J. Clin. Nutr.*, 25, 773, 1972.
9. **Cummings, J. H., Hill, M. J., Jenkins, D. J. A., Pearson, J. R., and Wiggins, H. S.,** Changes in fecal composition and colonic function due to cereal fiber, *Am. J. Clin. Nutr.*, 29, 1468, 1976.
10. **Remsey, C. and Demigne, C.,** Partition and absorption of volatile fatty acids in the alimentary canal of the rat, *Ann. Rech. Veter.*, 7, 39, 1976.
11. **Schmitt, M. G., Soergel, K. H., and Wood, C. M.,** Absorption of short chain fatty acids from the human jejunum, *Gastroenterology*, 70, 211, 1976.
12. **Schmitt, M. G., Soergel, K. H., and Wood, C. M.,** Absorption of short chain fatty acids from the human ileum, *Dig. Dis.*, 22, 340, 1977.
13. **McNeil, N. I., Cummings, J. H., and James, W. P. T.,** Short chain fatty acid absorption by the human large intestine, *Gut*, 19, 819, 1978.
14. **Stevens, C. E.,** Physiological implications of microbial digestion in the large intestine of mammals: relation to dietary factors, *Am. J. Clin. Nutr.*, 31, S161, 1978.

15. **Cummings, J. H., Hill, M. J., Bone, E. S., Branch, W. J., and Jenkins, D. J. A.**, The effect of meat protein and dietary fiber on colonic function and metabolism. II. Bacterial metabolites in feces and urine, *Am. J. Clin. Nutr.*, 32, 2094, 1979.
16. **Hove, E. L. and King, S.**, Effects of pectin and cellulose on growth, feed efficiency, and protein utilization, and their contribution to energy requirement and cecal VFA in rats, *J. Nutr.*, 109, 1274, 1979.
17. **Sambrook, I. E.**, Studies on digestion and absorption in the intestines of growing pigs. VIII. Measurements of the flow of total lipid, acid-detergent fibre and volatile fatty acids, *Br. J. Nutr.*, 42, 279, 1979.
18. **Kass, M. L., Van Soest, P. J., and Pond, W. G.**, Utilization of dietary fiber from alfalfa by growing swine. II. Volatile fatty acid concentrations in and disappearance from the gastrointestinal tract, *J. Anim. Sci.*, 50, 192, 1980.
19. **Lockhart, H. B., Lee, H. S., O'Mahony, S. P., Hensley, G. W., and Houlihan, E. J.**, Caloric value of fiber-containing cereal fractions and breakfast cereals, *J. Food Sci.*, 45, 372, 1980.
20. **Milton, K., Van Soest, P. J., and Robertson, J. B.**, Digestive efficiencies of wild howler monkeys, *Physiol. Zool.*, 53, 402, 1980.
21. **Ruppin, H., Bar-Meir, S., Soergel, H., Wood, C. M., and Schmitt, M. G.**, Absorption of short chain fatty acids by the colon, *Gastroenterology*, 78, 1500, 1980.
22. **Spiller, G. A., Chernoff, M. C., Hill, R. A., Gates, J. E., Nassar, J. J., and Shipley, E. A.**, Effect of purified cellulose, pectin, and a low-residue diet on fecal volatile fatty acids, transit time, and fecal weight in humans, *Am. J. Clin. Nutr.*, 33, 754, 1980.
23. **Cummings, J. H.**, Short chain fatty acids in the human colon, *Gut*, 22, 763, 1981.
24. **Kennelly, J. J., Aherne, F. X., and Sauer, W. C.**, Volatile fatty acid production in the hindgut of swine, *Can. J. Anim. Sci.*, 61, 349, 1981.
25. **Ehle, F. R., Jeraci, J. L., Robertson, J. B., and Van Soest, P. J.**, The influence of dietary fiber on digestibility, rate of passage and gastrointestinal fermentation in pigs, *J. Anim. Sci.*, 55, 1071, 1982.
26. **Ehle, F. R., Robertson, J. B., and Van Soest, P. J.**, The influence of dietary fibers on fermentation in the human large intestine, *J. Nutr.*, 112, 158, 1982.
27. **Illman, R. J., Trimble, R. P., Snoswell, A. M., and Topping, D. L.**, Daily variations in the concentrations of volatile fatty acids in the splanchnic blood vessels of rats fed diets high in pectin and bran, *Nutr. Rep. Int.*, 26, 439, 1982.
28. **Bardon, T. and Fioramonti, J.**, Nature of the effects of bran on digestive transit time in pigs, *Br. J. Nutr.*, 50, 685, 1983.
29. **Fleming, S. E., Marthinsen, D., and Kuhnlein, H.**, Colonic function and fermentation in men consuming high fiber diets, *J. Nutr.*, 113, 2535, 1983.
30. **Fleming, S. E. and Rodriquez, M. A.**, Influence of dietary fiber on fecal excretion of volatile fatty acids by human adults, *J. Nutr.*, 113, 1613, 1983.
31. **McKay, L. F. and Eastwood, M. A.**, The influence of dietary fibre on caecal metabolism in the rat, *Br. J. Nutr.*, 50, 679, 1983.
32. **Storer, G. B., Trimble, R. P., Illman, R. J., Snoswell, A. M., and Topping, D. L.**, Effects of dietary oat bran and diabetes on plasma and caecal volatile fatty acids in the rat, *Nutr. Res.*, 3, 519, 1983.
33. **Etheridge, R. D., Seerley, R. W., and Huber, T. L.**, The effect of diet on fecal moisture, osmolarity of fecal extracts, products or bacterial fermentation and loss of minerals in feces of weaned pigs, *J. Anim. Sci.*, 58, 1403, 1984.
34. **Storer, G. B., Illman, R. J., Trimble, R. P., Snoswell, A. M., and Topping, D. L.**, Plasma and caecal volatile fatty acids in male and female rats: effects of dietary gum arabic and cellulose, *Nutr. Res.*, 4, 701, 1984.
35. **Thomsen, L. L., Roberton, A. M., Wong, J., Lee, S. P., and Tasman-Jones, C.**, Intra-caecal short chain fatty acids are altered by dietary pectin in the rat, *Digestion*, 29, 129, 1984.
36. **Demigné, C. and Rémésy, C.**, Stimulation of absorption of volatile fatty acids and minerals in the cecum of rats adapted to a very high fiber diet, *J. Nutr.*, 115, 53, 1985.
37. **Fleming, S. E., O'Donnell, A. U., and Perman, J. A.**, Influence of frequent and long-term bean consumption on colonic function and fermentation, *Am. J. Clin. Nutr.*, 41, 909, 1985.
38. **Holzgraefe, D. P., Fahey, G. C., Jr., and Jensen, A. H.**, Influence of dietary alfalfa:orchard grass hay and lasolocid on in vitro estimates of dry matter digestibility and volatile fatty acid concentrations of cecal contents and rate of digesta passage in sows, *J. Anim. Sci.*, 60, 1235, 1985.
39. **Pomare, E. W., Branch, W. J., and Cummings, J. H.**, Carbohydrate fermentation in the human colon and its relation to acetate concentrations in venous blood, *J. Clin. Invest.*, 75, 1448, 1985.
40. **Stanogias, G. and Pearce, G. R.**, The digestion of fibre by pigs. II. Volatile fatty acid concentrations in large intestine digesta, *Br. J. Nutr.*, 53, 531, 1985.
41. **Topping, D. L., Illman, R. J., and Trimble, R. P.**, Volatile fatty acid concentrations in rats fed diets containing gum arabic and cellulose separately and as a mixture, *Nutr. Rep. Int.*, 32, 809, 1985.

42. **Demigne, C., Yacoub, C., and Remesy, C.,** Effects of absorption of large amounts of volatile fatty acids on rat liver metabolism, *J. Nutr.*, 116, 77, 1986.
43. **Fleming, S. E. and Arce, D. S.,** Volatile fatty acids: their production, absorption, utilization, and roles in human health, *Clin. Gastroent.*, 15, 787, 1986.
44. **Hoverstad, T. and Midtvedt, T.,** Short-chain fatty acids in germfree mice and rats, *J. Nutr.*, 116, 1772, 1986.
45. **Walter, D. J., Eastwood, M. A., and Brydon, W. G.,** An experimental design to study colonic fibre fermentation in the rat: the duration of feeding, *Br. J. Nutr.*, 55, 465, 1986.
46. **Cheng, B. Q., Trimble, R. P., Illman, R. J., Stone, B. A., and Topping, D. L.,** Comparative effects of dietary wheat bran and its morphological components (aleurone and pericarp-seed coat) on volatile fatty acid concentrations in the rat, *Br. J. Nutr.*, 57, 69, 1987.
47. **Tulung, B., Remesy, C., and Demigne, C.,** Specific effects of guar gum or gum arabic on adaptation of cecal digestion to high fiber diets in the rat, *J. Nutr.*, 117, 1556, 1987.
48. **Walter, D. J., Eastwood, M. A., and Brydon, W. G.,** Fermentation of wheat bran and gum arabic in rats fed on an elemental diet, *Br. J. Nutr.*, 60, 225, 1988.
49. **Costa, M. A., Mehta, T., and Males, J. R.,** Effects of dietary cellulose, psyllium husk and cholesterol level on fecal and colonic microbial metabolism in monkeys, *J. Nutr.*, 119, 986, 1989.
50. **Demigné, C., Levrat, M. A., and Rémésy, C.,** Effects of feeding fermentable carbohydrates on the cecal concentrations of minerals and their fluxes between the cecum and blood plasma in the rat, *J. Nutr.*, 119, 1625, 1989.
51. **Fleming, S. E., Fitch, M. D., and Chansler, M. W.,** High-fiber diets: influence on chracteristics of cecal digesta including short-chain fatty acid concentrations and pH, *Am. J. Clin. Nutr.*, 50, 93, 1989.
52. **Guisi-Perier, A., Fiszlewicz, M., and Rerat, A.,** Influence of diet composition on intestinal volatile fatty acid and nutrient absorption in unanesthetized pigs, *J. Anim. Sci.*, 67, 386, 1989.
53. **Venter, C. S. and Vorster, H. H.,** Possible metabolic consequences of fermentation in the colon for humans, *Med. Hypotheses*, 29, 161, 1989.
54. **British Nutrition Foundation,** Energy values of complex carbohydrates, in *Complex Carbohydrates in Foods. The Report of the British Nutrition Foundation's Task Force,* Chapman and Hall, England, 1990, 56.
55. **Topping, D. L., Illman, R. J., Roach, P. D., Trimble, R. P., Kambouris, A., and Nestel, P. J.,** Modulation of the hypolipidemic effect of fish oils by dietary fiber in rats: studies with rice and wheat bran, *J. Nutr.*, 120, 325, 1990.
56. **Fleming, S. E., Choi, S. Y., and Fitch, M. D.,** Absorption of short chain fatty acids from the rat cecum in vivo, *J. Nutr.*, 121, 1787, 1991.
57. **Levrat, M. A., Behr, S. R., Remsey, C., and Demigne, C.,** Effects of soybean fiber on cecal digestion in rats previously adapted to a fiber-free diet, *J. Nutr.*, 121, 672, 1991.
58. **Ross, A. H. M., Eastwood, M. A., Brydon, W. G., Busuttil, A., and McKay, L. F.,** A study of the effects of dietary gum arabic in the rat, *Br. J. Nutr.*, 51, 47, 1984.

Chapter 6.9

EFFECTS OF DIETARY FIBER ON FECAL-LUMINAL MUTAGENIC ACTIVITIES

Hugh J. Freeman

Human feces contain mutagens and may be assessed by a variety of short-term *in vitro* methods.[1-6] Fecal mutagenic activity is postulated to influence colon cancer risk and this activity may be modulated by the diet. Generally, the methods employed have involved bacterial mutation assays; these are based on a well-established qualitative relationship between carcinogenicity and DNA damage, are sensitive, and are rapidly performed.[7] Initially, the presence of mutagenic activity was demonstrated in ether extracts of freeze-dried feces from normal healthy human male volunteers consuming a "Western diet".[1] It was subsequently claimed that stool samples contain both volatile and nonvolatile N-nitroso compounds[8] as well as nitrite and nitrates;[9] however, the precise nature of the compound or compounds in feces causing bacterial mutations still requires elucidation. Using a different approach, the genotoxic effect of human feces was demonstrated by using induction of chromosome damage in cultured Chinese hamster ovary cells as the indicator of mutagenic activity.[10] Later, fecal extracts from both carnivorous and herbivorous animals were shown[11] with high chromosome damaging potency observed in the three carnivorous species examined. It was noted that the chromosome aberrations seen were comparable to that in mammalian cells exposed to 250 to 400 rads of X-rays as well as exposure to several known carcinogens.[11]

Subsequent studies focused on changes induced in levels of mutagens by altered diets or life-styles. For example, ingestion of antioxidants such as ascorbic acid or tocopherol caused a reduction in fecal mutagenic activity followed by a gradual return to control values over a 1-month period.[12] Later, fecal mutagen levels were determined in a single stool sample from each individual in groups of South Africans (i.e., urban whites, urban blacks, and rural blacks) with differing colon cancer risks.[13] Urban whites, a high colon cancer risk population, had a significantly higher percentage of mutagen-positive stools compared to the two low-risk black populations. It was subsequently suggested that bacterial flora are involved in the formation of this mutagenic activity.[14] Others[15] examined fecal mutagens in three groups: Seventh Day Adventists living in New York and consuming an ovo-lacto vegetarian diet (milk and milk products but no fish, poultry, or meat) with a low colon cancer risk, inhabitants of Kuopio, Finland with a low risk, and omnivorous New Yorkers, a high-risk group. The Finns consumed more milk, dairy products, and fiber but less animal fat than New Yorkers. No Adventist sample was mutagenic; however, positive activity was observed in 13% of Finnish samples compared to 22% of New Yorkers. In Vancouver, Canada, fecal mutagens were determined in strict vegetarians, ovo-lacto vegetarians, and nonvegetarians[16] using the fluctuation test for weak mutagens.[17] Because this bacterial assay method is extremely sensitive compared to the method used in earlier studies,[1,12-15] virtually all samples showed mutagenic activity. Ovo-lacto vegetarians and strict vegetarians had significantly lower levels of fecal mutagens that nonvegetarians and the presence of at least two fecal mutagens was suggested. Later it was shown that formula-fed individuals with consistent nutrient levels had fecal mutagenic activities that did not vary significantly within an individual; however, there were significant differences between subjects on identical diets suggesting that long-term dietary and possibly genetic factors influence mutagen levels.[18] The effects of short-term dietary modification on fecal mutagens were also assessed.[19] In this study, two dietary regimes were used, a low colon cancer risk nonmeat diet was consumed for 2 weeks followed by 2 weeks on a high-risk beef diet. Within a 2-week period, fecal mutagen levels increased on the high meat diet. More recent studies have shown that fecal mutagen levels are lower in a rural low-risk colon cancer population (i.e., Kuopio, Finland) compared to an urban high-risk colon cancer population (i.e., Helsinki, Finland).[20] Multiple types of mutagens may be present as was shown in a population of New Yorkers consuming a high fat, low fiber "mixed" Western diet.[21] In another report of a healthy man consuming a normal "Western" diet, fecal mutagenic activities were determined after a period of supplementation with high fat and high fiber; although no significant change was seen in the high fat group, high fiber feeding caused a significant reduction in fecal mutagenic activities.[22] More recent human studies have demonstrated that only specific sources of ingested dietary fibers such as wheat bran or cellulose reduce the production and/or excretion of fecal mutagens.[23]

Studies specifically focused on the effect of dietary fibers per se are limited and have only recently been reported.[24] Extracts were obtained from fecal pellets and the luminal contents along the length of the GI tract in rats fed either a chemically defined fiber-free diet or nutritionally and calorically equivalent diets with differing amounts of purified cellulose or pectin (4.5 or 9.0%) or a mixture of cellulose and pectin (4.5% each). Mutagenicity was measured using the fluctuation test for weak mutagens[17] with *Salmonella typhimurium* TA 98 and TA 1535 as tester strains. Over a 6-week period only the high cellulose diet influenced fecal mutagen levels: a significant reduction was observed with the TA 1535 strain. Analysis of the contents of stomach, distal small bowel, cecum, and colon after 8 weeks on the fiber-free diet revealed that the distal small bowel had a severalfold higher mutagen concentration than any other site. These activities were significantly reduced by ingestion of either the cellulose or pectin single fiber diets. Previous studies using chemically induced animal models demonstrate protective effects for some dietary fibers in rats exposed to exogenously administered chemical carcinogens (see Chapter 7.10). This study further extended these observations to endogenous mutagenic activities and provided strong evidence that these mutagens are formed within the small bowel. Subsequently, they are presented to cecum and colon in high concentrations. Some recent studies have explored possible mechanisms for these dietary effects on mutagens. These have revealed that different fiber sources including corn bran, wheat bran, and alfalfa directly bind carcinogen in a pH-dependent manner, optimally in the pH range of 4 to 6 found in the human gastrointestinal tract and apparently through a mechanism of cation exchange.[25-28]

REFERENCES

1. **Bruce, W. R., Varghese, A. J., Furrer, R., and Land, P. C.**, A mutagen in feces of normal humans, in *Origins of Human Cancer,* Book C, Cold Spring Harbor Conferences on Cell Proliferation, Vol. 4, Hiatt, H. H., Watson, J. D., and Winsten, J. A., Eds., Cold Spring Harbor Laboratory, Cold Spring Harbor, NY, 1977, 1641.
2. **Stich, H. F. and Kuhnlein, U.**, Chromosome breaking activity of human feces and its enhancement by transition metals, *Int. J. Cancer,* 24, 284, 1979.
3. **de Vet, H. C. W., Sharma, C., and Reddy, B. S.**, Effect of dietary fried meat on fecal mutagenic and co-mutagenic activity in humans, *Nutr. Rep. Int.,* 23, 653, 1981.
4. **Nader, C. J., Potter, J. D., and Weller, R. A.**, Diet and DNA-modifying activity in human fecal extracts, *Nutr. Rep. Int.,* 23, 113, 1981.
5. **Venitt, S.**, Faecal mutagens in the aetiology of colonic cancer, in *Colonic Cardinogenesis, Falk Symposium 31,* Malt, R. A. and Williamson, R. C. N., Eds., MTP Press, Lancaster, England, 59, 1982.

6. **Wilkins, T. D., Lederman, R. L., van Tassell, R. L., Kingston, D. G. I., and Henion, J.**, Characterization of a mutagenic bacterial product in human feces, *Am. J. Clin. Nutr.*, 33, 2513, 1980.
7. **Ames, B. N., McCann, J., and Yamasaki, E.**, Methods for detecting carcinogens and mutagens with the Salmonella/mammalian microsome mutagenicity test, *Mutat. Res.*, 31, 347, 1975.
8. **Wang, T., Kakizoe, T., Dion, P., Furrer, R., Varghese, A. J., and Bruce, W. R.**, Volatile nitrosamines in normal human feces, *Nature (London)*, 276, 280, 1978.
9. **Tannenbaum, S. R., Fett, D., Young, V. R., Land, P. C., and Bruce, W. R.**, Nitrite and nitrate are formed by endogenous synthesis in the human intestine, *Science*, 200, 1487, 1978.
10. **Stich, H. F., Wei, L., and Lam, P.**, The need for a mammalian test system for mutagens: action of some reducing agents, *Cancer Lett.*, 5, 199, 1978.
11. **Stich, H. F., Stich, W., and Acton, A. B.**, Mutagenicity of fecal extracts from carnivorous and herbivorous animals, *Mutat. Res.*, 78, 105, 1980.
12. **Bruce, W. R., Varghese, A. J., Wang, S., and Dion, P.**, The endogenous production of nitroso compounds in the colon and cancer at that site, in *Naturally Occurring Carcinogens — Mutagens and Modulators of Carcinogenesis*, Miller, E. C., Ed., University Park Press, Baltimore, 1979, 221.
13. **Ehrich, M., Aswell, J. E., van Tassell, R. L., Walker, A. R. P., Richardson, N. J., and Wilkins, T. D.**, Mutagens in feces of 3 South African populations at different levels of risk for colon cancer, *Mutat. Res.*, 64, 231, 1979.
14. **Lederman, M., van Tassell, R., West, S. E. H., Erhrich, M. F., and Wilkins, T. D.**, In vitro production of human fecal mutagen, *Mutat. Res.*, 79, 115, 1980.
15. **Reddy, B. S., Sharma, C., Darby, L., Laakso, K., and Wynder, E. L.**, Metabolic epidemiology of large-bowel cancer. Fecal mutagens in high- and low-risk populations for colon cancer, *Mutat. Res.*, 72, 511, 1980.
16. **Kuhnlein, U., Bergstrom, D., and Kuhlein, H.**, Mutagens in feces from vegetarians and non-vegetarians, *Mutat. Res.*, 85, 1, 1981.
17. **Green, M. H. L. and Muriel, W. J.**, Mutagen testing using TRP$^+$ reversion in *Escherichia coli, Mutat. Res.*, 38, 3, 1976.
18. **Kuhnlein, H. V. and Kuhnlein, U.**, Mutagens in feces from subjects on controlled formula diets, *Nutr. Cancer*, 2, 119, 1981.
19. **Kuhnlein, H. V., Kuhnlein, U., and Bell, P. A.**, The effect of short-term dietary modification on human fecal mutagenic activity, *Mutat. Res.*, 113, 1, 1983.
20. **Reddy, B. S., Sharma, C., Mathews, L., Engle, A., Laasko, K., Choi, K., Puska, P., and Korpella, R.**, Metabolic epidemiology of colon cancer: fecal mutagens in healthy subjects from rural Kuopio and urban Helsinki, Finland, *Mutat. Res.*, 152, 97, 1985.
21. **Reddy, B. S., Sharma, C., Mathews, L., and Engle, A.**, Fecal mutagens from subjects consuming a mixed-western diet, *Mutat. Res.*, 135, 11, 1984.
22. **Venitt, S., Bosworth, D., and Aldrick, A. J.**, Pilot study of the effect of diet on the mutagenicity of human faeces, *Mutagenesis*, 1, 353, 1986.
23. **Reddy, B. S., Engle, A., Katsifis, S., Simi, B., Bartram, H. P., Perrino, P., and Mahan, C.**, Biochemical epidemiology colon cancer: effect of types of dietary fiber on fecal mutagens, acid, and neutral sterols in healthy subjects, *Cancer Res.*, 49, 4629, 1989.
24. **Kuhnlein, U., Gallagher, R., and Freeman, H. J.**, Effects of purified cellulose and pectin fiber diets on mutagenicity of feces and luminal contents of stomach, small and large bowel in rats, *Clin. Invest. Med.*, 6, 253, 1983.
25. **Barnes, W. S., Maiello, J., and Weisburger, J. H.**, In vitro binding of the food mutagen 2-amino-3-methylimidazo(4,5-f)quinoline to dietary fibers, *J. Natl. Cancer Inst.*, 70, 757, 1983.
26. **Morotomi, M. and Mutai, M.**, In vitro binding of potent mutagenic pyrolysates to intestinal bacteria, *J. Natl. Cancer Inst.*, 77, 195, 1986.
27. **Takeuchi, M., Hara, M., Inoue, T., and Kada, T.**, Adsorption of mutagens by refined wheat bran, *Mutat. Res.*, 204, 263, 1988.
28. **Roberton, A. M., Harris, P. J., Hollands, H. J., and Ferguson, L. R.**, A model system for studying the adsorption of a hydrophobic mutagen to dietary fibre, *Mutat. Res.*, 244, 173, 1990.

Section 7: Dietary Fiber in the Prevention and Treatment of Disease
---

Chapter 7.1

FIBER IN THE TREATMENT OF HYPERLIPIDEMIA

David J. A. Jenkins, Peter J. Spadafora, Alexandra L. Jenkins,
and Cynthia G. Rainey-Macdonald

INTRODUCTION

Until just over a decade ago, the dietary treatment for hyperlipidemia and hypercholesterolemia, in particular, included a reduction in saturated fat and cholesterol intakes, an increase in P:S ratio, elimination of alcohol consumption, and reduction of calories to achieve ideal body weight.

The major class of drugs used were few and remain so. These include cholestyramine, clofibrate, nicotinic acid and their analogs, and HMG-CoA reductase inhibitors. However, more recently there has been an interest in the pharmacology of natural products as hypolipidemic agents. Foremost among these is dietary fiber. In addition, other food constituents, including the phytosterols (β-sitosterol), saponins, and plant proteins have attracted attention. Of these, only dietary fibers and vegetable proteins have been tested extensively in therapeutic diets for hyperlipidemia.

DIETARY FIBER AND POSSIBLE MECHANISMS OF ACTION

A number of possible mechanisms are likely to be involved in the hypocholesterolemic effect of dietary fiber, and different mechanisms are likely to predominate depending on the fiber.

The pioneer studies of Kritchevsky and colleagues demonstrated that a number of fiber sources were capable of binding bile acids *in vitro*,[1-3] and provided a rationale for the increased bile acid losses seen *in vivo*. Together with this mechanism of action, there are possibly three other broad reasons why fiber lowers serum cholesterol levels, none of which are mutually exclusive in providing an explanation of the mechanism for an individual food. Indeed, it is likely that for a given food more than one mechanism is operative.

Increased Fecal Sterol Losses

From the beginning, it was recognized that increased fecal sterol losses provided one explanation for the lipid lowering effect of fiber.[1] There is general agreement that purified viscous fiber[8] administration increases bile acid outputs by 20 to 80%,[79,89] but the effect of fiber in foods is less clear.[90,91] Studies have been limited in number due to the unsavory nature of this line of work, and further data are therefore urgently required.

Increased Propionate Generation

Bacterial fermentation of fiber in the colon gives rise to short chain fatty acids (SCFA) which are absorbed. One of the SCFA, propionate, has been shown in pigs[92] and rats[93] to reduce serum cholesterol levels and to inhibit cholesterol synthesis in liver *in vitro*.[94] Propionate has also been demonstrated in man to inhibit, acutely, the acetate induced rise in serum cholesterol after rectal infusion.[95] However, human feeding studies of propionate[96,97] have not demonstrated a clear effect in reducing LDL cholesterol levels. On the other hand, when colonic fermentation is increased using the nonabsorbable sugar, lactulose, LDL cholesterol levels appear to rise rather than fall.[105] The nature of the fermentation and the type of fiber may therefore be important in determining the final outcome. This area also requires further studies for its definition.

Reduced Insulin Levels

Increased insulin levels have been linked with CHD.[98-101] A common effect of the viscous fibers and high fiber foods which reduce serum cholesterol levels is that they produce relatively flat post prandial glucose and insulin responses.[102,103] Early studies demonstrated that hepatic cholesterol synthesis in the rat increased during periods of maximum insulin secretion.[104] The explanation was that insulin induced an increase in activity of hepatic HMG-CoA reductase, a rate-limiting step in cholesterol synthesis.[104] The cholesterol-lowering effect associated with reduced insulin levels has been confirmed using a model of altered food frequency ("Nibbling")[110] to mimic slow absorption and so this mechanism of action also deserves further investigation.

Altered Lipid Absorption and Genetic Factors

Fiber delays the rate of nutrient absorption[103] and, in the longer term, may alter small intestinal morphology and lipid absorption.[106,107] Alteration in the rate and site of lipid absorption may alter the pattern of lipoprotein secretion[108] and catabolism. Vitamin A tolerance tests with added fiber indicate that some fibers appear to enhance chylomicronemia.[109] Added to this are the genetic differences which may make fiber more or less effective. Amongst genetic variants which influence serum lipids, differences in the apo E genotype have attracted much attention, and may influence the response to drugs such as gemfibrozil[80] and dietary change, including a prudent diet, dietary cholesterol, and vegetable protein.[81,82] In view of the association of E genotype with differences in remnant particle uptake, cholesterol absorption and bile acid excretion,[83-88] this genetic classification may be particularly useful in predicting responses to altered fat and fiber intakes. Other genetic markers have not, as yet, received this degree of scrutiny. At present, there are no data on the interaction of genetics and fiber, but these data are likely to appear in the near future. No detailed studies have been carried out at different levels of dietary fat to assess the effect on the different possible mechanisms of action of dietary fiber, i.e., whether some mechanisms are more or less effective at different levels of dietary fat intake. Hypothetically, fiber foods which induce a bile salt loss might be more effective if the bile salt pool is expanded through greater intakes of dietary fat. On the other hand, reduction in carbohydrate intake may minimize differences in glycemic response and hence mechanisms which relate to altered insulin secretion. In the absence of studies, however, these are simply speculations to be explored.

EXPERIENCE WITH SPECIFIC FIBERS

The early studies described the hypolipidemic effects of fibers in healthy volunteers before they were tested on patient groups. The literature relating to healthy volunteers has already been reviewed. The present discussion will therefore focus on the therapeutic use of fiber. In general, viscous fibers have proved useful in lowering serum lipids[5,16,21,25,53,64] while nonviscous fibers have for the most part been without effect.[10-12,52,61] There are exceptions to this generalization.[111]

Lignin and Cellulose

Early on, the suggestion that lignin may be hypocholesterolemic by virtue of its bile acid binding ability resulted in two conflicting clinical studies.[9,10] The dosages were small (Table 1), and the work has not been repeated. Similarly, the particulate fiber, cellulose,

TABLE 1
Effects of Lignin and Cellulose on Serum Lipid Concentrations in Normal and Hyperlipidemic Subjects

Fiber type	Fiber form/dose	Study protocol	Background diet/drugs	Lipid disorder	Cholesterol initial (mg/dl), change %					TG initial (mg/dl), change % total	Comments	Ref.
					Total	LDL	VLDL		HDL			
Lignin	"Celluline" (99% lignin), 4 g/day	Cholestyramine 12 g/day for 2 to 5 months, then celluline 1.2 g/day for 2 to 5 months, then celluline 4 g/day for 2 to 3 months	Usual therapeutic diet	6 Type II	(416) −21%						Celluline duplicated or maintained effect of cholestyramine	9
	Capsules, 2 g/day	Control diet for 4 weeks, then fiber for 4 weeks, then control for 4 weeks	Normal diet	7 Type II	(304) +8%					(168) 0%	Total-C ↓ to nearly basal level during second control period	10
	High MW, 16.7% methoxyl content, mixed with food 12 g/day	4 Weeks, crossover with no fiber as control	Normal diet	10 Healthy	(228)* NC	—	—		(62)* 6.3 NS	(68)* −2.6 NS	NC HDL/Total-C ratio	52
Cellulose	60 g/day		Reducing	60 Normal, some HLP	(−) NC					(−) NC	Reducing diet ↓ total-C by 22% with or without cellulose	11
	Powdered, in bread	LL diet plus cellulose bread for 3 months, partially substituted with soyhull cookies for 3 months	LL diet	14 Type IIa	(346) +8% NS					(99) +6% NS		12
	Microcrystalline cellulose, form not specified 15 g/day	12 Weeks, crossover	Normal diet, 19 of 22 on oral hypoglycemic drugs	22 Diabetics type II	(236)* 1.6 NS	—	—		NC	NC	NC fasting blood glucose or HBA1c	61
	99.9% Alpha cellulose fiber, mixed with food 15 g/day	4 Weeks, crossover with no fiber as control	Normal diet	10 Healthy	(209)* −5.6 NS	—	—		(66)* −11.8 NS	(74)* −10.7 NS	NC HDL/Total-C ratio	52

Note: TG, triglyceride; HLP, hyperlipoproteinemic; HC, hypercholesterolemic; LL, lipid-lowering; NC, no change; LDL-C, low-density lipoprotein cholesterol; Total-C, total cholesterol. Initial values are given in parentheses; values represent results for fiber treatment period or fiber-treated group (time period for fiber treatment is in italics). An asterisk indicates that values were converted from SI to traditional units, using factors C in mmol × 18.7-C in g/dl; TG in mmol × 88.5-TG in mg/dl.

was without effect on serum cholesterol or triglyceride levels.[11,12] More recent work has confirmed these findings (Table 1).[52,61]

Pectin

The early studies of Palmer and Dixon[13] in normal volunteers were followed by those of Miettinen and colleagues[14] on hyperlipidemic patients who consumed relatively large doses of pectin (40 to 50 g/d) (Table 2). The observation that the resulting falls in serum cholesterol levels were associated with only modest increases in fecal sterol loss suggested that increased sterol excretion was likely to be only one of a number of mechanisms responsible. No changes were seen in serum triglycerides. Palmer and Dixon demonstrated that little cholesterol-lowering effect could be seen in healthy individuals taking 6 g or less of pectin daily.[13] Subsequent studies in hyperlipidemic patients confirmed this observation.[15] However, a substantial lowering of serum total and LDL cholesterol levels was observed even when as little as 12 g of pectin daily was taken.[16] A clear dose-response is not evident from these studies. The interest in pectin has continued, in general, to support the earlier work (Table 2).[52-54,76]

Guar

Again following observations in healthy volunteers, studies testing the effects of guar were undertaken in hyperlipidemic patients.[5,17-23] The cholesterol-lowering results with guar were materially the same as those observed with pectin. The effect was predominantly reflected in the LDL-cholesterol fraction with much less or no change in the HDL-cholesterol fraction. Triglyceride levels were reduced, but the reduction was significant only when the guar was incorporated into very low fat, starchy carbohydrate foods, such as crisp bread or spaghetti.[5,18] The physicochemical nature of the guar and the formulation in which it is provided may be very important factors, since greatly differing effects were reported by different investigators when doses of guar of the order of 15 g/d were given.[5,17-23] Nevertheless, in a study in which the same guar was added in powder form to fruit juices and soup, baked into conventional breads, or incorporated into a dry crisp bread or melba toast-type formulation, all were equally effective.[18] These findings suggested that prehydration was not a prerequisite for the hypolipidemic action of this viscous fiber.

In 2-week studies in which the maximum acceptable dose of guar given in crisp bread form was compared with the maximum acceptable dose of cholestyramine in the same patients, the falls in total and LDL cholesterol were comparable.[18] This indicated that, in pharmacological terms, the effects of viscous fiber on lipid metabolism might have significant clinical utility.

In the majority of the guar and pectin studies, fiber was added to the patients' preexisting diet and/or drug therapy, which was then maintained constant. This included low fat, low cholesterol diets, with or without cholestyramine, clofibrate, or their analogs. It is not possible at present to say whether the mechanism or action of fiber overlap with those of the established hypolipidemic drugs and whether specific combinations might bestow an advantage. In view of the relatively small bile acid losses seen with pectin[4,14,24] and guar[4] compared with specific drugs, it is likely that the mechanisms of fiber will complement those of the bile salt binding (anion exchange) resins (e.g., cholestyramine). On the other hand, when the maximum effect has been achieved with clofibrate, it is possible that any further effect of the fiber may be reduced.[20] Recent work has contributed further support to previous evidence (Table 2).[55-61,67,78]

Locust Bean Gum

This viscous fiber has also been used successfully in a range of hyperlipidemic patients to lower serum cholesterol[25] (Table 2). Its advantage has been claimed to be its superior

TABLE 2
Effects of Soluble, Purified Fibers on Lipid Concentrations in Normal and Hyperlipidemic Subjects

Fiber type	Fiber form/dose	Study protocol	Background diet/drugs	Lipid disorder	Cholesterol initial (mg/dl), change %				TG initial (mg/dl), change % total	Comments	Ref.
					Total	LDL	VLDL	HDL			
Pectin	Powdered, in jam, 40–50 g/day	LL diet for 2 weeks, then pectin for 2 weeks	LL diet	4 Type IIa, 1 type IV, 2 secondary HLP, 2 healthy	(307)* −13%				(157) −5% NS	Fecal bile acids ↑ 57%; total fecal sterols ↑ 27%; increased plasma methyl sterols	14
	Lemon or apple, 6 g/day (10.5% methoxyl content)	LL diet for 6 weeks, then either (1) lemon pectin, (2) apple pectin, or (3) clofibrate	LL diet	18 Type IIa, 3 type IIb, 10 type III, 2 type IV, (or IIb)	(i)(301) +5% NS (ii)(321) −4% NS (iii)(306) −13% NS				(i)(142) +0.7% NS (ii)(109) +36% NS (iii)(139) −30%		15
	Apple, as granulate, 12 g/day (12% methoxyl content)	LL diet for 8 weeks then cholestyramine added for 10 weeks, then pectin added for 8 weeks	LL diet, cholestyramine, 16 g/day	6 Type IIa (male)	(377)*a −19%	(285) −22%	(−) NC	(45) −12% NS	(199) −0.4%	↓ Lipids evident at 4 weeks enhanced over 8 weeks; TG ↑ of 25% after LL diet + drug persisted with pectin	16
	Citrus pectin as gel, 15 g/day	4 Weeks, 1 week control, 3 weeks pectin	Normal Western diet	10 Healthy	(206) −18 p < 0.05	NC	—	NC	NC	Decline in anaerobe to aerobe ratio	53
	Grapefruit pectin in capsule, 15 g/day	4 Weeks, crossover	Normal diet	27 HC	(275) −7.6 p ≤ 0.008	(195) −10.7 p ≤ 0.07	(38) 2.4 NS	(42) −1.2 NS	(188) 2.7 NS	Decline LDL:HDL 9.8% (p ≤ 0.03)	54
	Breakfast cereal, 57 g/day	6 Weeks	AHA Step 1 diet	58 HC males	(220)* −2.1 NS	(152)* −3.9 NS	—	(46)* 2.5 NS	(111)* 3.7 NS	Body wt, serum glucose, and iron unchanged	76
	Citrus pectin 9.3% methoxyl content, mixed with food, 12 g/day	4 Weeks, crossover with no fiber as control	Normal diet	10 Healthy	(225)* NC	—	—	(62)* NC	(86)* 4.1 NS	NC HDL/Total-C ratio	52
	Psyllium Granule, 6–12 g/day	5 Weeks	Normal diet	9 Healthy males	(189) −14.4 NS	(LDL + VLDL 145) −25.6 p < 0.01		(44) 22.1 NS	(161) −11.7 NS	Weight loss with psyllium	62

TABLE 2 (continued)
Effects of Soluble, Purified Fibers on Lipid Concentrations in Normal and Hyperlipidemic Subjects

Fiber type	Fiber form/dose	Study protocol	Background diet/drugs	Lipid disorder	Cholesterol initial (mg/dl), change % Total	LDL	VLDL	HDL	TG initial (mg/dl), change % total	Comments	Ref.
	Metamucil, 10.6 g/day	8 Weeks, parallel design	Normal diet	14 HC males	(247) −14.8 p < 0.01	(162) −20.2 p < 0.01	—	(54) −6.5 NS	(147) −12.7 NS	LDL/HDL ratio decline 14.8% (p < 0.01)	63
	Ground husk, 21 g/day	3 Weeks	Normal Western diet	7 Healthy	(187) −16 p < 0.002	(83)+ −18 p < 0.01	—	(49)+ −8.2 p < 0.03	—	Total fecal steroid excretion NC	64
	Metamucil, 10.2 g/day	8 Weeks	LL Step 1 diet	40 HC	(228)* −4.2 p < 0.05	(156)* −7.7 p < 0.05	—	(53)* 1.9 NS	(101)* 2.6 NS	Apo B declined 8.8% with psyllium p < 0.01	65
	Breakfast cereal, 57 g/day	6 Weeks	AHA Step 1 diet	58 HC males	(218)* −5.9 p = 0.001	(148)* −5.7 p = 0.0066	—	(47)* −1.6 NS	(106)* −10.9 NS	Body wt, serum glucose, and iron unchanged	76
	Vi-Siblin, 30 g/day	11 Days	Low cholesterol, moderate fiber intake	9 HLP type IIa, IIb	(321)* −6.0 p < 0.05	(255)* −9.1 p < 0.05	—	(39)* 20.0 p < 0.05	(133)* −6.0 NS	Increase in fecal bile acids and elimination of cholesterol	67
	Flavored Metamucil, 20.4 g/day	13 Weeks, after 7 weeks AHA phase I	AHA Phase I	27 HC	(266) −7.1 p < 0.01	(190) −8.6 p < 0.01	—	(44) 6.2 p < 0.05	(177) −10.9 NS	LDL/HDL ratio declined 13.3% p < 0.05	77
Guar	Added to beverage or in soup, 15 g/day	Usual drugs for 2 years, LL diet for 3 months, then pectin for 2 weeks	LL diet, cholestyramine 12 to 16 g/day for 3 patients, clofibrate 1 g/day for 1 patient	10 Type II	(345)+ −11%				(164) +13% NS		17
	In crispbread, 13 g/day	LL for 1 year, then crispbread exchanged for bread for 2 to 8 weeks	LL diet, 2 patients on cholestyramine, 2 on clofibrate	11 Type II or IV	(259)*b −14%	(259) −16%		(46) −2.6% NS	(186) −13% NS	Maximum ↓ in C evident in 2 to 3 weeks maintained at 8 weeks; patients on cholestyramine show similar responses	18
	Granules in food or drink (73% w/w guar, 15 g/day)	Drugs discontinued for at least 1 month, then patient randomized into guar, placebo, and control groups for 4 months	LL diet	32 Type II female	(320)* −3% NS			(65) 0%	(163) −3% NS	Body weight in guar-treated group, TG ↓ 29% in placebo group, seasonal variation of lipids in control group	19

Form/Dose	Duration	Background	Subjects	Col5	Col6	Col7	Col8	Col9	Comments	Ref
Granulate, 16 g/day	Bezafibrate for 2 months, then guar added for either a second or third 2-month period	LL diet, Bezafibrate 600 g/day	12 Type IIa	(351) −7%, additional to drug effect	(273) −14%	(-) NC	(55) −13% NS	(130) +28% NS	Apo-B lipoprotein ↓ 20% with nc Apo-A, ↑ total and LDL-C pretreatment levels on withdrawal of guar	20
Preparation with gel inhibitor, 18 g/day	LL drugs discontinued for several months, LL diet for 1 year, then placebo for 4 weeks, then guar for *3 to 12 months*	LL diet	1 Type IIa, 16 type IIb	(302)* −13%	(232) −18%	(23) +17% NS	(45) −0.4% NS	(230) +8% NS	LL effects of guar evident in 3 months and sustained for 12 months; fecal acidic steroids ↑ 30%; % cholesterol absorption reduced in 4/5 normals	21
In pasta 20% w/w guar 14 to 19 g/day	(i) LL drugs discontinued, LL diet for 8 to 12 days, then guar pasta for *2 weeks*	LL diet, no LL drugs	2 Type IIa, 2 type IIb, 4 type IV	(274)[b] −32%				(510) −40%	↓ LDL-C calculated to be less than 5%	5
	(ii) LL diet for 3 months, then guar pasta for *8 weeks*	LL diet, no LL drugs	4 Type IIb, 1 type IV	(290) −6%				(358) −27%	Total-C ↓ 11% and TG 40% in 3 patients followed for 20 weeks	22
Granulate, 15 g/day	Drugs discontinued for 6 months, then placebo for 4 weeks, then guar or placebo for *12 weeks* (washout 4 weeks between periods)	Normal diet, no LL drugs	14 HC, male	(329)* −15% @ 6 weeks −8% NS @ 12 weeks	(231) −22% @ 6 weeks, −14% NS @ 12 weeks	(43) −21% NS	(46) −6% NS	(145) −4% NS	Guar effect negated between 6 and 12 weeks in 11/14 subjects	22
Powder, 16 g/day	*60 Days* guar on own diets, then 60 days control	Patients' own diets	Familial, 10 men, 2 women	(297) −10%	(226) −10%	(27) −23%	(54) 2%	(191) −22%	Very detailed study showing changes in apolipoproteins	23
Guargel in water, 16 g/day	6 Weeks	Usual diet, sulphonylurea	10 Diabetics type II	(190) −11 p < 0.05	(127) −18 p < 0.01	(17) 17.9 NS	(45) −1.8 NS	(119) −10.8 NS	Fasting BG declined 9.6% and insulin declined 23% (p < 0.05)	55
Guar bars 26.4–39.6 g/day	24 Weeks	Normal diet	8 Diabetics type II	(223) 3 NS	(141) −16 NS	—	(44) −9 NS	(186) 90 p < 0.025	NC in apo B levels	56
Baked into crispbread, 11.4 g/day	2 Weeks	Controlled mixed diet	6 Healthy males	(186) −16 p < 0.05	—	—	—	(82.8) 1.8 NS	82–95% guar metabolized in bowel	57
Guar pasta, 10 g/day	4 Days	Normal weight maintenance	10 Obese women	(194) −11.9 p < 0.05	—	—	(46) 2.2 NS	(117) −6 NS	Significant decline blood glucose and insulin	58

TABLE 2 (continued)
Effects of Soluble, Purified Fibers on Lipid Concentrations in Normal and Hyperlipidemic Subjects

Fiber type	Fiber form/dose	Study protocol	Background diet/drugs	Lipid disorder	Cholesterol initial (mg/dl), change % — Total	LDL	VLDL	HDL	TG initial (mg/dl), change % total	Comments	Ref.
	Granulated 20–30 g/day	50 Weeks	Normal diet	23 HC	(388)* −10 p < 0.001	(312)* −14.9 p < 0.01	(46)* −23.5 NS	(45)* 17.9 NS	(215)* −9.9 NS	Apo AI/Apo B ratio increase 11.8% (p < 0.05)	59
	Cracker, liquid, 15 g/day	8 Weeks	Normal diet	32 HLP	(241) −5.8 NS	(163)* −9.8 NS	—	(45) −2.2 NS	(157) 12 NS	Total- and LDL-C declined with high viscosity guar	60
	Form not specified 15 g/day	12 Weeks, crossover	Normal diet 19 of 22 on oral hypoglycemic drugs	22 Diabetics type II	(255) −10.6 p < 0.01	—	—	NC	NC	Trend towards lower glucose, HBA1c	61
	Gel, 40 g/day	11 Days	Low cholesterol, low fiber	8 Hospitalized patients with symptomatic diverticular disease	(201)* −9.6 p < 0.05	(147)* −13.2 p < 0.05	(21)* −3.7 NS	(34)* −1.1 NS	(192)* −2.1 NS	Bile acid output doubled	67
	Powder in fluid, 15 g/day	21 Days	Normal diet	13 Subjects moderately elevated lipids	(244) −10	(152) −17	(30) −3	(62) 1.6	(145) −1.4		78
Locust bean gum	18–30 g/day	LL diet, then 8 weeks of locust bean gum or 4 weeks locust, 4 weeks control, and 4 weeks locust	LL diet	18 familial HC, adults, and children, 10 normals	(260) −6 to −19%	(188) −10 to −19%	(22) −10 to −19%	(50) −0 to −17%	(95) −10%		25

Note: Abbreviations: TG, triglyceride; HLP, hyperlipoproteinemic; HC, hypercholesterolemic; LL, lipid-lowering; NC, no change; LDL-C, low-density lipoprotein cholesterol; Total-C, total cholesterol. Initial values are given in parentheses; values represent results for fiber treatment period or fiber-treated group (time period for fiber treatment is in italics). An asterisk indicates that values are converted from SI to traditional units, using factors: C in mmol × 38.7-C in g/dl; TG in mmol × 83.5, TG in mg/dl. A plus sign indicates that values are approximated from graphs.

[a] Initial values = @ 8 weeks diet + drug; % changes = @ 8 weeks diet + drug + pectin.

[b] 10 Patients also participated in earlier 2-week studies comparing effects of cholestyramine with guar in semihydrated (bread) or hydrated (soup) forms; values are for 7 patients given crispbread who were followed for 8 weeks.

[c] Values are for 14 patients who completed 12 months of treatment.

taste (or lack of taste) by comparison with guar. However, the taste of guar depends on its purity and, since both substances are galactomannans, direct comparative studies must be undertaken before any statement about their relative efficacy can be made.

Wheat Bran

Of the wheat brans, only hard red spring wheat bran has been convincingly shown to lower serum cholesterol levels in normal man.[26] This fiber source has not yet been tested in hyperlipidemic patients. As with normal volunteers, almost all studies which have used other wheat bran preparations have failed to show significant reductions in blood lipid levels of hyperlipidemic individuals[27,28] (Table 3), although there is one report of a significant rise in HDL cholesterol.[29] The lack of consistent effect of wheat bran on blood lipids is of interest from the standpoint of mechanisms, since the bile acid losses in the stool following bran consumption have been shown to be comparable to those following pectin,[4] which consistently lowers serum cholesterol.

Oat Bran

Since the early studies of DeGroot,[30] it was realized that oat constituents may have hypocholesterolemic effects. Unlike wheat bran, oat fiber contains an appreciable proportion of viscous fiber (β-glucan), and it is likely that this constituent may be one of its active hypolipidemic ingredients. More recently, studies of Anderson and co-workers have demonstrated the lipid-lowering effect of oat bran given to hyperlipidemic patients (predominantly Types IIa and IIb) for 10 days to 2 years[7,31,32] (Table 3). Although there were highly significant falls in all cholesterol fractions together with serum triglyceride during the initial 3 weeks of fiber treatment, the HDL cholesterol level increased slowly, to almost approximately the starting value by 24 weeks. The other fractions remained low throughout the maintenance treatment period and for the four patients who were followed for 2 years.[32] Again, the increase in fecal acidic steroids was small and in proportion to the increase in fecal bulk, and unlikely to provide more than a small part of the explanation of the hypocholesterolemic action of oat bran. In this respect, it has been proposed that the volatile fatty acids from oat bran and other viscous fibers, which arise from colonic fermentation of fiber and are subsequently absorbed, may produce metabolic changes which favor reduced cholesterol synthesis.[7] Despite early enthusiasm and then apparent despair, the body of evidence supports that oat bran will have a significant, although small, beneficial effect on serum lipids (Table 3).[66,68,72,78]

Dried Legumes

Cooked, dried legumes have been shown to lower serum cholesterol levels of middle-aged men,[33] although not of young student volunteers.[34] More recently, with interest in their effect of improving glucose tolerance[35] and other aspects of diabetic control,[36] high legume diets have been studied in types IIa and IV hyperlipidemic patients[7,32,37,39] (Table 3). All studies have shown falls in serum cholesterol irrespective of the class of hyperlipidemia studies. One investigator also recorded falls in serum triglyceride comparable to those seen with oat bran of equivalent soluble fiber content (20 g/day).[32] As with oat bran, the effects on blood lipids appear to be sustained for 4 months to 2 years.[32]

The reasons for the effects, however, are not clear. Increases in fecal output on 115 g of beans are small and not significant in the hyperlipidemic individuals.[7] In addition, where recorded, increases in fecal acidic steroid losses were not noted.

Nevertheless, the falls in blood lipids, especially triglycerides, may be related to the flatter postprandial glucose and insulin responses elicited by legumes.[35] These may result in a chronically reduced stimulus to hepatic triglyceride synthesis and hepatic lipid synthesis

TABLE 3
Effects of Fiber-Rich Whole Foods and Supplements on Serum Lipids

Fiber type	Fiber form/dose	Study protocol	Background diet/drugs	Lipid disorder	Cholesterol initial (md/dl), change %					TG initial (mg/dl), change % total	Comments	Ref.
					Total	LDL	VLDL	HDL				
Unprocessed wheat bran	50 g/day	Bran added to normal diet for 3 months	Normal diet	5 Type IV	(259)* + 3% NS	(178) −2% NS	(39) +20% NS	(39) +30% NS		(283) 0%		27
	50 g/day	Bran added to normal diet for 2 months	Normal diet	8 Secondary HLP, male	(252)* −2% NS					(195) +5% NS		28
Supplement wheat bran	"Fiberform" 10.5 g/day (8.2 g/day fiber)	Bran or placebo added to LL diet for 8 weeks (crossover)	LL diet	12 HC, male	(284)* +0.7% NS	(217) −2% NS	(24) −30% NS	(43) +23%		(166) −24%	↓ TG in lipoprotein fractions; NC during placebo period; seasonal variation may have masked C-lowering effect in bran-treated group	29
				14 Normal	(208)* +9%	(145) +8%		(47) −2%		(119) +9% NS		
Oat bran	In muffins, as cereal, 100 g/day (26 g total, 15 g soluble fiber) (23 g/day total fiber more than control diet)	No LL drugs for 3 months, then either/or bran-enriched diet for 10 days, sequence randomized	Normal control diet (identical except for bran content)	6 Type II, 2 normal	(269) −13%	(184) −14%		(49) −2% NS		(161) −9% NS	NC lipids during control period; fecal bile acids 54% higher and neutral sterols slightly lower on oat bran than on control diets	31
	Baked in muffins, 17 g/day	28 Days	Normal diet	19 Healthy	(179) −5 NS	(108) −9 NS	—	(55) +2 NS		(77) − 8 NS	—	69
	Flakes, Chex biscuits, 25 g/day	2 Weeks	Normal Western diet	12 HC males	(260)* −5.4 p < 0.05	(180)* −8.5 p < 0.025	—	(38)* −3.3 NS		(202)* 8.7 NS	Decline in Apo B 9.8% NS	72
	Bread, muffins, 95 g/day	4 Weeks crossover	Low dietary fiber diet	24 HC males	(245)* −4.9	(176)* −6.8	—	(41)* 2.9		(62)* −3.1	NC blood glucose, insulin, blood pressure	66
	Powder in fluid, 77 g/day	21 Days	Normal diet	13 Adults moderately elevated lipids	(244) −3.3	(152) −5.9	(30) 3.3	(62) NC		(145) 5.5	200 calories extra added/day with oat bran	78

Mixed	52 fiber/2000 kcal (30 g/day more than regular diet) as part of modified U.K. LL diet	Habitual diet for 8 weeks, then test diet (iso- or hypocaloric) for 5 to 11 months	Habitual diet	16 Type IIa, 11 type IIb, 1 type III, 3 type IV, 6 normal	(302)*,a −22%	(213) −25%	(48) −37% NS	(52) −4% NS	(235) −24%	NC HDL₁-C	50
Beans	50 g/day (100 g/ 2 days) dried	Beans added to usual diet 3 to 6 months; (18 responders continued up to 12 months)	Usual Chinese diet, no LL drugs	136 HLP	(282)ᵇ −17%				(−)ᶜ +13 to 32% NS	NC for subjects given control diets; pronounced LL effect was seen in 1 month	37
				106 Normal	(205)ᵇ −9%				(−)* +13 to 32% NS		
	Canned, 110 g/ day (dry weight)	Clofibrate withdrawn for 1 year for Type IV patients, then 50% carbohydrate exchanged for beans for 2 weeks	LL diet, usual drugs (except for clofibrate)	6 type IIa, 6 type IIb, 5 type IV	(290)* −8%				(212) −25% NS		38
	Cooked or canned, 140 g/ day (dry wt) = 15 g/day fiber	LL diet, then high legume diet for 4 months (increase of 15 g fiber per day for high legume diet)	LL diet	2 Type IIa, 1 type IIb, 4 type IV	(269) −7%	(189) −5% NS		(37) −15% NS	(238) −25%	Relatively high animal protein content (56%) of test diet could have negated effect of vegetable protein on cholesterol	39
Baked beans	450 g/day in tomato sauce	2 Weeks	Normal diet	13 Healthy males	(192)* −12 p < 0.05	—	—	(52)* −14.8 p < 0.001	(94)* 7.5 NS	3.7% Decline in HDL:Total-C ratio NS	71
	120–162 g per day as pork and beans or in tomato sauce	3 Weeks, single or double dose	Normal Western diet	24 HLP type IIa or IIb	(295)* −10.4 p < 0.001	(201)* −8.4 p < 0.005	—	(42)* −6.9 p <0.05	(256)* −10.8 p < 0.025	Decline in body weight with bean diet	73
Beans/oat bran	(i) Oat bran, or beans (dry wt) 100 g/day (48 g total, 18 g soluble fiber per day)	No LL drugs for 3 months, control diet for 7 days, then randomized into oat bran or bean diets for 3 weeks	No LL drugs, LL diet	10 Type II, male	(294) −23%	(216) −23%		(37) −20%	(203) −21%		32
	(ii) 50 g day oat bran (dry wt) or 145 g beans (wet wt)	Oat bran or bean supplement at home for 24 weeks, 4 patients were followed for 99 weeks	High carbohydrate, high fiber maintenance diet	10 Type II, male	(226) −4% fall maintained	(167) −2%, fall maintained		(30) +17% NC	(161) −6%, fall maintained	Reduced cholesterol and fat intake during maintenance study may have contributed to results	
	100 g oat bran (dry wt)	Normal diet, oat bran for 3 weeks	Normal diet	10 Type IIa and type IIb	(280) −19%	(190) −23%	(—)	(31) −6% NS	(289) −18%	Modest ↑ in fecal weight and proportionate ↑ in bile acid losses	7

TABLE 3 (continued)
Effects of Fiber-Rich Whole Foods and Supplements on Serum Lipids

Fiber type	Fiber form/dose	Study protocol	Background diet/drugs	Lipid disorder	Cholesterol initial (md/dl), change %				TG initial (mg/dl), change % total	Comments	Ref.
					Total	LDL	VLDL	HDL			
	115 g beans (dry wt)	Normal diet, beans *for 3 weeks*	Normal diet	10 Type IIa and type IIb	(300) −10%	(221) −24%	(—)	(32) −12%	(233) −3% NS	No ↑ in fecal weight or bile acid losses	
Wheat bran	Bread, muffins, 35 g/day	4 Weeks crossover	Low dietary fiber diet	24 HC males	(245)* 0.8	(176)* 0.2	—	(41)* 3.8	(62)* 3.1	NC blood glucose, insulin, blood pressure	66
Oats	Instant oats, 56.7 g/day	8 Weeks, parallel with control	Normal diet	42 HC	(254)* −6.3	(177)* −9.2	(27)* 1.4	(50)* 0.8	(135)* 1.3	NC in blood pressure	68
Oatmeal	Breakfast cereal, muffins, 56 g/day	8 Weeks	AHA phase II	113 Healthy	(193) −3 NS	— NS	—	— NS	— NS	Total-C and LDL-C declined in subgroup ≥ 198 mg/dL (4 weeks)	70

Note: Abbreviations: TG, triglyceride; HLP, hyperlipoproteinemic; HC, hypercholesterolemic; LL, lipid lowering; NC, no change; LDL-C, low-density lipoprotein cholesterol; Total-C, total cholesterol. Initial values are given in parentheses; values represent results for fiber treatment period or fiber-treated group (time period for fiber treatment is in italics). An asterisk indicates that values are converted from SI to traditional units, using factors: C in mmol × 38.7-C in g/dl; TG in mmol × 83.5, TG in mg/dl. A plus sign indicates that values are approximated from graphs.

[a] Initial values = @ 8 weeks diet + drug; % changes = @ 8 weeks diet + drug + pectin.
[b] 10 Patients also participated in earlier 2-week studies comparing effects of cholestyramine with guar in semihydrated (bread) or hydrated (soup).
[c] Values are for 14 patients who completed 12 months treatment.

in general. Evidence for this hypothesis has been drawn together in the studies of Albrink et al.[6] in healthy volunteers and is supported by the observation, also in healthy volunteers, that 24-h urinary C-peptide outputs were reduced on high legumes diets.[40]

Legume Protein

In addition to legume fibers (e.g., guar and locust bean gum), some legume proteins, notably soya protein, have been shown to reduce cholesterol levels of hyperlipidemic patients (total and LDL)[41-47] (Table 4). The effect does not appear to be related to associated fiber or saponins, since it is also found after administration of soya isolate. However, the capacity to lower blood lipids is not a universal property of all legume proteins, since fava protein isolate failed to achieve the desired effect.[46]

The mechanisms for the hypolipidemic action of soy protein remain obscure, but may relate to the amino acid profile[49] or the presence of specific pharmacologically active peptides liberated during digestion. With respect to the whole bean, although specific fiber and protein effects may be relevant to the action of some beans, other factors will have to be uncovered to explain the general hypolipidemic effect of legumes in hyperlipidemic individuals. Data continue to accumulate supporting the lipid lowering effect of legume protein (Table 4).[74,75]

Effective Fiber Dosage

In general, the effective dose of the viscous fibers required to lower serum cholesterol levels has been of the order of 12 to 30 g/d. Interestingly, the levels of fiber in the oat bran- and bean-containing diets have also been of this order of magnitude, since soluble fiber comprises approximately 20% of the dry weight of both beans and oat bran. However, the effectiveness of the supplement in hyperlipidemia may be determined by its formulation, in addition to the background diet. This fact is well illustrated by the guar-enriched spaghetti studies of Gatti and colleagues, which showed the greatest lowering of cholesterol and triglyceride levels of all the studies to date.[5] Spaghetti is already recognized as a slowly digested carbohydrate form which causes an unexpectedly low rise in blood glucose.[50] This effect is likely to have been greatly enhanced by the addition of guar, resulting in the creation of a very effective sustained release carbohydrate source. The addition of guar would likely not only have enhanced the reduction of glycemic and insulinemic responses to the pasta, but may, in effect, have resulted in a proportion of the pasta starch being converted to "fiber", i.e., carbohydrate which is unavailable for small intestinal absorption, but which acts as an additional source for synthesis of SCFAs in the colon. The choice by Gatti and co-workers of spaghetti as the vehicle for delivery of the fiber may have been in large measure the reason for the success of their trial, since it encompassed many of the mechanisms responsible for reducing blood lipids. One of the important directions for future development in this field would, therefore, appear to lie in finding the most effective food vehicles in which to incorporate fiber.

CONCLUSION

Viscous fibers such as pectin, guar, and locust bean gum, and high fiber foods such as oat bran and dried beans, all providing 12 to 30 g fiber daily, have been shown to reduce serum total and LDL cholesterol levels by 10 to 20% and with a lesser fall in HDL cholesterol levels. When the fiber was provided in a starchy food such as pasta, crisp bread, oat bran, or beans, significant falls in serum triglyceride levels have also been observed.

The mechanisms of action of fiber are likely to be complex and possibly include increased bile salt loss, altered site and rate of absorption, reduced hepatic lipogenesis secondary to

TABLE 4
Effects of Legume Protein (± Saponins) on Serum Lipid Concentrations of Hyperlipidemic Subjects

Fiber type	Fiber form/dose	Study protocol	Background diet/drugs	Lipid disorder	Total	LDL	VLDL	HDL	TG initial (mg/dl), change %, total	Comments	Ref.
Textured soybean protein	Granules	A. LL diet for 3 months, then usual diet for 1 week, then soybean or LL for 3 weeks each (crossover)	No LL drugs Soy replaced ½ animal protein	9 Type IIa, 11 type IIb	(313) −19%	(220) −18%			(217) −17%	LL diet alone was ineffective; response varied linearly with initial cholesterol levels; for patients given soy diet first, cholesterol ↑ after withdrawal soy diet	41
		B. Same preparation as A, then soy diet for 6 weeks, 500 g cholesterol added (first or second 3-week period)	ibid	8 Type II	(315) −23%				(200) NC	Cholesterol intake did not influence LL effect of soy-protein diet	
	Granules, in liquid 60 to 100 g/day "cholsoy"	Standard LL diet for 6 months (then control LL diet) for 8 weeks, then soy diet replacing all animal protein for 8 weeks, then control LL diet for 6 weeks		127 Type II	(335)+b −20%			(—) NC	(152) −11% NS	LL effect slightly greater in females than in males, familial cases less sensitive to soy diets, but show greater rise after withdrawal soy than nonfamilial cases	42
	"Cholsoy", 60 to 100 g/day	LL animal protein diet for 4 weeks, then LL soy diet for 4 weeks, then LL animal protein diet for 6 weeks, then LL soy diet, 6 meals per week for 18 months		27 Type II	(340)+b −26% @ 1st soy period, −5% NS more @ 18 months	(260) −33% during first soy diet period, −4% NS more during 18 months		(44) +15% NS @ 18 mos			51
	Cholsoy-P (texturized, lecithinated) 60 to 100 g/day	LL animal protein for 4 weeks, then LL soy diet for 4 weeks		19 Type IIa	(330)+b −21%	(255) −26%		(40) +13%		Reduced cholesterol associated with ↑ serum arginine concentrations	45
	In mixed foods	LL animal protein for 2 weeks, then test diet in which		1 Type IIa, 4 type IIb, 1 type III	(275)* −10%	(185) −9%	(70) −17% NS	(36) 0%	(230) 11% NS	LL animal protein diet reduced total-C by 25%	44

Food	Description	Subjects	Diet	TC	LDL-C	HDL-C	TG	Other	Ref
	In mixed meals	1/2 animal protein exchanged for soy for 2 weeks	12 Type II, 9 type IV, 1 normal	(241) −3% NS	(163) −0.8% NS	(29) +3% NS	(49) −12% NS	(104) +3% NS	Beef-protein LL diets ↓ total-C by 18% and LDL-C by 19%; NC lipid levels in a second study using same diets and crossover design	45
		Beef-protein LL diet for 3 weeks, then soy replacing all beef protein for 4 weeks								
	Granules, "Cholsoy" L 70–80 g/day	4 Weeks LL diet followed by 4 weeks on soy protein replaced diet followed by 4 weeks on LL diet	21 Familial HC unrelated	(392)* −20.8 p < 0.01	(313)* −25.8 p < 0.01	(19)* 32.6 NS	(43)* −7.2 NS	(143)* −69 NS	Apo B declined 14% p < 0.05 and Apo E declined 17% p < 0.05	74
	Flavored soy protein beverage, 250 mls	4 Weeks test followed by 4 weeks washout then 4 weeks test, crossover	9 Familial HC children 6–12 years	(307)* −0.5 NS	(245)* −0.2 NS	(17)* −20 p < 0.05	(45)* 4 p < 0.04	(88)* −19 p < 0.05	NC in apo A-I or apo B levels	75
Soybean flour	Defatted, in biscuits, 50 g/day (35% of protein)	Saponin-rich (22 g/kg) or saponin-depleted (4 g/kg) soyflour diets for 4 weeks each (crossover)	10 HC, free-living males	(264*)ᵃ +1% NS	(—) NC	(—) NC	(—) NC	(192) −4% NS	Neither diet affected lipid levels or distribution, or bile acid or neutral sterol excretion	47
Soybean flour	Defatted, in biscuits, 50 g/day (35% of protein)	Saponin-rich (22 g/kg) or saponin-depleted (4 g/kg) soyflour diets for 4 weeks each (crossover)	10 HC, free-living males	(264*)* +1% NS	(—) NC	(—) NC	(192) −4% NS		Neither diet affected lipid levels or distribution, or bile acid or neutral sterol excretion	47
Favabean	Fava bean protein concentrate, 11% dietary calories	2 Consecutive 18-day periods of fat reduced diet, (i) fava bean protein, (ii) egg white protein for 18 days	6 Type IIa, 1 type IIb, 1 normal	(i) (305) −13%; (ii) (320) −13% NS	(235) −17%; (240) −8% NS	(18) −5% NS; (19) −5% NS	(40) −7%; (40) −5% NS	(—) NC; (—) NC	No significant differences between fava and egg white diets apart from lower blood glucose on fava	46
	Fat reduced from 32 to 26%, carbohydrate increased from 48 to 59%									

Note: Abbreviations: TG, triglyceride; HLP, hyperlipoproteinemic; HC, hypercholesterolemic; LL, lipid-lowerings; NC, no change; LDL-C, low-density lipoprotein cholesterol; Total-C, total cholesterol. Initial values are given in brackets; values represent results for fiber treatment period or fiber-treated group (time period for fiber treatment is in italics). An asterisk indicates values are converted from SI to traditional units, using factors: C ion mmol × 38.7-C in g/dl; TG in mmol × 83.5, TG in mg/dl. A plus sign indicates that values are approximated from graphs.

ᵃ Values are means for 2, 3, and 4 weeks on diet, for saponin-rich diets; saponin-depleted diets showed similar results (final values only given for lipoprotein fractions).
ᵇ Values are averaged for men and women.

reduced postprandial glucose and insulin responses, and enhanced colonic synthesis and uptake of SCFAs.

Further developments to enhance the clinical utility of this approach should include not only a search for effective fiber types, but also the appropriate vehicles in which to deliver them.

REFERENCES

1. **Kritchevsky, D. and Story, J. A.**, Binding of bile salts in vitro by nonnutritive fiber, *J. Nutr.*, 104, 458, 1974.
2. **Kritchevsky, D. and Story, J. A.**, *Am. J. Clin. Nutr.*, 28, 305, 1975.
3. **Vahouny, G. V., Tombes, R., Cassidy, M. M., Kritchevsky, D., and Gallo, L. L.**, Dietary fibers. V. Binding of bile salts, phospholipids and cholesterol from mixed micelles by bile sequestrants and dietary fibers, *Lipids*, 15, 1012, 1980.
4. **Jenkins, D. J. A.**, Dietary fibre, diabetes and hyperlipidemia, *Lancet*, ii, 1287, 1979.
5. **Gatti, E., Catenazzo, G., Camisasca, E., Torri, A., Denegri, E., and Sirtori, C. R.**, Effects of guar-enriched pasta in the treatment of diabetes and hyperlipidemia, *Ann. Nutr. Metab.*, 28, 1, 1984.
6. **Albrink, M. J., Newman, T., and Davidson, P. C.**, Effect of high- and low-fiber diets on plasma lipids and insulin, *Am. J. Clin. Nutr.*, 32, 1486, 1979.
7. **Anderson, J. W., Story, L., Sieling, B., Chen, W.-J. L., Petro, M. S., and Story, J.**, Hypocholesterolemic effects of oat-bran or bean intake for hypercholesterolemic men, *Am. J. Clin. Nutr.*, 40(b), 1146, 1984.
8. **Jenkins, D. J. A., Wolever, T. M. S., Leeds, A. R., Gassull, M. A., Haisman, P., Dilawari, J., Goff, D. V., Metz, G. L., and Alberti, K. G. M. M.**, Dietary fibres, fibre analogues and glucose tolerance: importance of viscosity, *Br. Med. J.*, 1, 1372, 1978.
9. **Thiffault, C., Belanger, M., and Pouliot, M.**, Traitement de l'hyperlipoprotéinémie essentielle de type II par un nouvel agent pièrapeutique, la celluline, *Can. Med. Assoc. J.*, 103, 165, 1970.
10. **Lindner, P. and Moller, B.**, Lignin: a cholesterol-lowering agent?, *Lancet*, 2, 1259, 1973.
11. **Huth, K. and Fettel, M.**, Bran and blood lipids, *Lancet*, 2, 456, 1975.
12. **Palumbo, P. J., Esperanza, R., Briones, M. S., and Nelson, R. A.**, High fiber diet in hyperlipidemia. Comparison with cholestyramine treatment in Type IIa hyperlipoproteinemia, *JAMA*, 2403, 223, 1978.
13. **Palmer, G. H. and Dixon, D. G.**, Effect of pectin dose on serum-cholesterol levels, *Am. J. Clin. Nutr.*, 18, 437, 1966.
14. **Miettinen, T. A. and Tarpila, S.**, Effect of pectin on serum cholesterol, fecal bile acids and biliary lipids in normolipidemic and hyperlipidemic individuals, *Clin. Chim. Acta*, 79, 471, 1977.
15. **Delbarré, F., Rondier, J., and de Géry, A.**, Lack of effect of two pectins in ideopathic or gout-associated hyperdyslipidemia hypercholesterolemia, *Am. J. Clin. Nutr.*, 30, 463, 1977.
16. **Schwandt, P., Richter, W. O., Weisweiler, P., and Neureuther, G.**, Cholestyramine plus pectin in treatment of patients with familial hypercholesterolemia, *Atherosclerosis*, 44, 379, 1982.
17. **Jenkins, D. J. A., Leeds, A. R., Slavin, B., Mann, J., and Jepson, E. M.**, Dietary fiber and blood lipids: reduction of serum cholesterol in type II hyperlipidemia by guar gum, *Am. J. Clin. Nutr.*, 32, 16, 1979.
18. **Jenkins, D. J. A., Reynolds, D., Slavin, B., Leeds, A. R., Jenkins, A. L., and Jepson, E. M.**, Dietary fiber and blood lipids: treatment of hypercholesterolemia with guar crispbread, *Am. J. Clin. Nutr.*, 33, 575, 1980.
19. **Tuomilehto, J., Voutilainen, E., Huttunen, J., Vinni, S., and Homan, K.**, Effect of guar gum on body weight and serum lipids in hypercholesterolemic females, *Acta Med. Scand.*, 208, 45, 1980.
20. **Wirth, A., Middlehoff, G., Brauning, C. H., and Schlierf, G.**, Treatment of familial hypercholesterolemia with a combination of bezafibrate and guar, *Atherosclerosis*, 45, 291, 1982.
21. **Simons, L. A., Gayst, S., Balasubramaniam, S., and Ruys, J.**, Long-term treatment of hypercholesterolaemia with a new palatable formulation of guar gum, *Atherosclerosis*, 45, 101, 1982.
22. **Aro, A., Uusitupa, M., Voutilainen, E. V., and Korhonen, T.**, Effects of guar gum in male subjects with hypercholesterolemia, *Am. J. Clin. Nutr.*, 39, 911, 1984.
23. **Bosello, O., Cominacini, L., Zocca, I., Garbin, U., Ferrari, F., Davoli, A.**, Effects of guar gum on plasma lipoproteins and apolypoproteins C-II and C-III in patients affected by familial combined hyperlypoproteinemia, *Am. J. Clin. Nutr.*, 40(b), 1165, 1984.
24. **Kay, R. M.**, Dietary fiber, *J. Lipid Res.*, 23, 221, 1982.

25. **Zavoral, J. H., Hannan, P., Fields, D. J., Hanson, M. N., Frantz, I. D., Kuba, K., Elmer, P., and Jacobs, D. R.,** The hypocholesterolemic effect of locust bean food products in hypercholesterolemic adults and children, *Am. J. Clin. Nutr.,* 38, 285, 1983.
26. **Munoz, J. M., Sandstead, H. H., Jacob, R. A., Logan, G. M., Jr., Reck, S. J., Klevay, L. M., Dintzis, F. R., Inglett, G. E., and Shuey, W. C.,** Effects of some cereal brans and textured vegetable protein on plasma lipids, *Am. J. Clin. Nutr.,* 35, 580, 1979.
27. **Bremner, W. F., Brooks, P. M., Third, J. L. H. C., and Lawrie, T. D. V.,** Bran in hypertriglyceridaemia: a failure of response, *Br. Med. J.,* 3, 574, 1975.
28. **Brooks, P. M., Bremner, W. F., and Third, J. L. H. C.,** Bran, hypertriglyceridaemia and urate clearance, *Med. J. Aust.,* 2, 753, 1976.
29. **Lindegarde, F. and Larsson, L.,** Effects of a concentrated bran fibre preparation on HDL-cholesterol in hypercholesterolaemic men, *Hum. Nutr. Clin. Nutr.,* 38C, 39, 1984.
30. **DeGroot, A. P., Luyken, R., and Pikaar, N. A.,** Cholesterol-lowering effect of rolled oats, *Lancet,* 2, 303, 1963.
31. **Kirby, R. W., Anderson, J. W., Sieling, B., Rees, E. D., Chen, W. L., Miller, R. E., and Kay, R. M.,** Oat-bran intake selectively lowers serum low-density lipoprotein cholesterol concentrations of hypercholesterolemic men, *Am. J. Clin. Nutr.,* 34, 824, 1981.
32. **Anderson, J. W., Story, L., Sieling, B., and Chen, W. L.,** Hypocholesterolemic effects of high-fibre diets rich in water-soluble plant fibres, *J. Can. Dietet. Assoc.,* 45, 2, 140, 1984.
33. **Grande, F., Anderson, J. T., and Keys, A.,** Effect of carbohydrates and leguminal seeds, wheat and potatoes on serum cholesterol concentration in man, *J. Nutr.,* 86, 313, 1965.
34. **Grande, F., Anderson, J. T., and Keys, A.,** Sucrose and various carbohydrate containing foods and serum lipids in man, *Am. J. Clin. Nutr.,* 27, 1043, 1974.
35. **Jenkins, D. J. A., Wolever, T. M. S., Jenkins, A. L., Thorne, M. J., Lee, R., Kalmusky, J., Reichert, R., and Wong, G. S.,** The glycemic index of foods tested in diabetic patients: a new basis for carbohydrate exchange favouring the use of legumes, *Diabetologia,* 24, 257, 1983.
36. **Simpson, H. C. R., Simpson, R. W., Lonsley, S., Carter, R. D., Geekie, M., Hockaday, T. D. R., and Mann, J. I.,** A high carbohydrate leguminous fibre diet improves all aspects of diabetic control, *Lancet,* 1, 1, 1981.
37. **Bingwen Liu, Zhaofeng Wu, Wanzhen Liu, and Rongjue Zhang,** Effects of bean meal on serum cholesterol and triglycerides, *Chinese Med. J.,* 94, 7, 455, 1981.
38. **Jenkins, D. J. A. and Jepson, E. M.,** Leguminous seeds and their constituents in the treatment of hyperlipidemia and diabetes, in *Lipoproteins and Coronary Atherosclerosis,* Noseda, G., Fragiacomo, C., Fumagalli, R., and Paoletti, R., Eds., Elsevier, Amsterdam, 1982, 247.
39. **Jenkins, D. J. A., Wong, G. S., Patten, R. P., Bird, J., Hall, M., Buckley, G. C., McGuire, V., Reichert, R., and Little, J. A.,** Leguminous seeds in the dietary management of hyperlipidemia, *Am. J. Clin. Nutr.,* 38, 567, 1983.
40. **Burke, B. J., Hartog, M., Heaton, K. W., and Hooper, S.,** Assessment of the metabolic effects of dietary carbohydrate and fibre by measuring urinary excretion of C-peptide, *Hum. Nutr. Clin. Nutr.,* 36C, 373, 1982.
41. **Sirtori, C. R., Agradi, E., Conti, F., Mantero, O., and Gatti, E.,** Soybean-protein diet in the treatment of Type II hyperlipoproteinemia, *Lancet,* i, 275, 1977.
42. **Descovich, G. C., Ceredi, C., Gaddi, A., et al.,** Multicentre study of soybean protein diet for out-patient hypercholesterolemic patients, *Lancet,* ii, 709, 1980.
43. **Descovich, G. C., Benassi, M. S., Cappelli, M., Gaddi, A., Grossi, G., Piazzi, S., Songiorgi, Z., Mannino, G., and Lenzi, S.,** Metabolic effects of lecithinated and non-lecithinated textured soy protein treatment in hypercholesterolemia, in *Lipoproteins and Coronary Atherosclerosis,* Noseda, G., Fragiacomo, C., Fumagalli, R., and Paoletti, R., Eds., Elsevier, Amsterdam, 1982, 279.
44. **Vessby, B., Karlstrom, B., Lithell, H., Gustafsson, I. B., and Werner, I.,** The effects on lipid and carbohydrate metabolism of replacing some animal protein by soy-protein in a lipid-lowering diet for hypercholesterolemic patients, *Hum. Nutr. Appl. Nutr.,* 36Z, 179, 1982.
45. **Holmes, W. L., Rubel, G. B., and Hood, S. S.,** Comparison of the effect of dietary meat versus dietary soybean protein on plasma lipids of hyperlipidemic individuals, *Atherosclerosis,* 36, 379, 1980.
46. **Contaldo, F., DiBiase, G., Giacco, A., Pacioni, D., Moro, L. O., Grasso, L., Mancini, M., and Fidanza, F.,** Evaluation of the hypocholesterolemic effect of vegetable proteins, *Prevent. Med.,* 12, 138, 1983.
47. **Calvert, G. D. and Blight, L.,** A trial of the effects of soya-bean flour and soya-bean saponins on plasma lipids, fecal bile acids and neutral sterols in hypercholesterolemic men, *Br. J. Nutr.,* 45, 277, 1981.
48. **Wolfe, B. M., Giovanetti, P. M., Cheng, D. C. H., Roberts, D. C. K., and Carroll, K. K.,** Hypolipidemic effects of substituting soybean protein isolate for all meat and dairy protein in diets of hypercholesterolemic men, *Nutr. Rep. Int.,* 24, 1187, 1981.

49. **Kritchevsky, D., Tepper, S. A., and Story, J. A.,** Influences of soy protein and casein on atherosclerosis in rabbits, *Fed. Proc. Fed. Am. Soc. Exp. Biol.,* 37, 747, 1978.
50. **Jenkins, D. J. A., Wolever, T. M. S., Jenkins, A. L., Lee, R., Wong, G. S., and Josse, R.,** Glycemic response to wheat product: reduced response to pasta but no effect of fiber, *Diabetes Care,* 6, 155, 1983.
51. **Choudhury, S., Jackson, P., Katon, M. B., Marenah, C. B., Cortese, C., Miller, N. E., and Lewis, B.,** A multifactorical diet in the management of hyperlipidemia, *Atherosclerosis,* 50, 93, 1984.
52. **Hillman, L. C., Peters, S. G., Fisher, C. A., and Pomare, E. W.,** The effects of the fiber components pectin, cellulose and lignin on serum cholesterol levels, *Am. J. Clin. Nutr.,* 42, 207, 1985.
53. **Vargo, D., Doyle, R., and Floch, M. H.,** Colonic bacterial flora and serum cholesterol: alterations induced by dietary citrus pectin, *Am. J. Gastroenterol.,* 80(5), 361, 1985.
54. **Cerda, J. J., Robbins, F. L., Burgin, C. W., Baumgartner, T. G., and Rice, R. W.,** The effects of grapefruit pectin on patients at risk for coronary heart disease without altering diet or lifestyle, *Clin. Cardiol.,* 11, 589, 1988.
55. **Tagliaferro, V., Cassader, M., Bozzo, C., Pisu, E., Bruno, A., Marena, S., Cavallo-Perin, P., Cravero, L., and Pagano, G.,** Moderate guar-gum addition to usual diet improves peripheral sensitivity to insulin and lipemic profile in NIDDM, *Diab. Metabol.,* 11, 380, 1985.
56. **McIvor, M. E., Cummings, C. C., Van Duyn, M. A., Leo, T. A., Margolis, S., Behall, K. M., Michnowski, J. E., and Mendeloff, A. I.,** Long-term effects of guar gum on blood lipids, *Atherosclerosis,* 60, 7, 1986.
57. **Penagini, R., Velio, P., Bozzani, A., Castagnone, D., Ranzi, T., Bianchi, P. A., and Vigorelli, R.,** The effect of dietary guar on serum cholesterol, intestinal transit and fecal output in man, *Am. J. Gastroenterol.,* 81(2), 123, 1986.
58. **Tognarelli, M., Miccoli, R., Giampietro, O., Cerri, M., and Navalesi, R.,** Guar-pasta: a new diet for obese subjects, *Acta Diabetol.,* 23, 77, 1986.
59. **Tuomilehto, J., Silvasti, M., Aro, A., Koistinen, A., Karttunen, P., Gref, C-G., Ehnholm, C., and Uusitupa, M.,** Long term treatment of severe hypercholesterolemia with guar gum, *Atherosclerosis,* 72, 157, 1988.
60. **Superko, H. R., Haskell, W. L., Sawrey-Kubicek, L., and Farquhar, J. W.,** Effects of solid and liquid guar gum on plasma cholesterol and triglyceride concentrations in moderate hypercholesterolemia, *Am. J. Cardiol.,* 62, 51, 1988.
61. **Niemi, M. K., Keinanen-Kiukaanniemi, S. M., and Salmela, P. I.,** Long-term effects of guar gum and microcrystalline cellulose on glycemic control and serum lipids in type II diabetes, *Eur. J. Clin. Pharmacol.,* 34, 427, 1988.
62. **Nakamura, H., Ishikawa, T., Tada, N., Kagami, A., Kondo, K., Miyazima, E., and Takeyama, S.,** Effect of several kinds of dietary fibers on serum and lipoprotein lipids, *Nutr. Rep. Int.,* 26(2), 215, 1982.
63. **Anderson, J. W., Zettwoch, N., Feldman, T., Tietyen-Clark, J., Oeltgen, P., and Bishop, C. W.,** Cholesterol lowering effects of psyllium hydrophilic mucilloid for hypercholesterolemic men, *Arch. Int. Med.,* 148, 292, 1988.
64. **Abraham, Z. D. and Mehta, T.,** Three-week psyllium-husk supplementation: effect on plasma cholesterol concentrations fecal steroid excretion, and carbohydrate absorption in men, *Am. J. Clin. Nutr.,* 47, 67, 1988.
65. **Bell, L. P., Hectorne, K., Reynolds, H., Balm, T. K., and Huninghake, D. B.,** Cholesterol-lowering effects of psyllium hydrophilic mucilloid, *JAMA,* 261(23), 3419, 1989.
66. **Kestin, M., Moss, R., Clifton, P. M., and Nestel, P. J.,** Comparative effects of three cereal brans on plasma lipids, blood pressure and glucose metabolism in mildly hypercholesterolemic men, *Am. J. Clin. Nutr.,* 52, 661, 1990.
67. **Miettinen, T. A. and Tarpila, S.,** Serum lipids and cholesterol metabolism during guar gum, plantago ovata and high fiber treatments, *Clinica Chim Acta,* 183, 253, 1989.
68. **Van Horn, L., Moag-Stahlberg, A., Liu, K., Ballew, C., Ruth, K., Hughes, R., and Stamler, J.,** Effects on serum lipids of adding instant oats to usual American diets, *Am. J. Public Health,* 81(2), 183, 1991.
69. **Gold, K. V. and Davidson, D. M.,** Oat bran as a cholesterol-reducing dietary adjunct in a young, healthy population, *West J. Med.,* 148, 299, 1988.
70. **Van Horn, L., Emidy, L. A., Liu, K., Liao, Y., Ballew, C., King, J., and Stamler, J.,** Serum lipid response to a fat-modified oatmean-enhanced diet, *Prev. Med.,* 17, 377, 1988.
71. **Shutler, S. M., Bircher, G. M., Tredger, J. A., Morgan, L. M., Walker, A. F., and Low, A. G.,** The effect of daily baked bean (Phaseolus vulgaris) consumption on the plasma lipid levels of young, normo-cholesterolemic men, *Br. J. Nutr.,* 61, 257, 1988.
72. **Anderson, J. W., Spencer, D. B., Hamilton, C. C., Smith, S. F., Tietyen, J., Bryant, C. A., and Oeltgen, P.,** Oat-bran cereal lowers serum total and LDL cholesterol in hypercholesterolemic men, *Am. J. Clin. Nutr.,* 52, 495, 1990.

73. **Anderson, J. W., Gustafson, N. J., Spencer, D. B., Tietyen, J., and Bryant, C. A.**, Serum lipid response of hypercholesterolemic men to single and divided doses of canned beans, *Am. J. Clin. Nutr.*, 51, 1013, 1990.
74. **Gaddi, A., Ciarrocchi, A., Matteucci, A., Rimondi, S., Ravaglia, G., Descovich, G. C., and Sirtori, C. R.**, Dietary treatment for familial hypercholesterolemia — differential effects of dietary soy protein according to the apolipoprotein E phenotypes, *Am. J. Clin. Nutr.*, 53, 1191, 1991.
75. **Laurin, D., Jacques, H., Moorjani, S., Steinke, F. H., Gagne, C., Brun, D., and Lupien, P-J.**, Effects of a soy-protein beverage on plasma lipoproteins in children with familial hypercholesterolemia, *Am. J. Clin. Nutr.*, 54, 98, 1991.
76. **Bell, L. P., Hectorn, K. J., Reynolds, H., and Hunninghake, D. B.**, Cholesterol lowering effects of soluble fiber cereals as part of a prudent diet for patients with mild to moderate hypercholesterolemia, *Am. J. Clin. Nutr.*, 52, 1020, 1990.
77. **Neal, G. W. and Balm, T. K.**, Synergistic effects of psyllium in the dietary treatment of hypercholesterolemia, *South Med. J.*, 83(10), 1131, 1990.
78. **Spiller, G. A., Farquhar, J. W., Gates, J. E., and Nichols, S. F.**, Guar gum and plasma cholesterol. Effect of guar gum and oat fiber source on plasma lipoproteins and cholesterol in hypercholesterolemic adults, *Arteriosclerosis and Thrombosis*, 11, 1204, 1991.
79. **Kay, R. M. and Truswell, A. S.**, Effect of citrus pectin on blood lipids and fecal steroid excretion in man, *Am. J. Clin. Nutr.*, 30, 171, 1977.
80. **Manttani, M., Koskinen, P., Ehnholm, C., Hutlunen, J. K., and Manninen, V.**, Apolipoprotein E polymorphism influences the serum cholesterol response to dietary intervention, *Metabolism*, 40, 217, 1991.
81. **Kesaniemi, Y. A., Ehnholm, C., and Miettinen, T. A.**, Intestinal cholesterol absorption efficiency in man is related to Apoprotein E phenotype, *J. Clin. Invest.*, 80, 578, 1987.
82. **Gatti, A., Clanocchi, A., Matteucci, A., Rimondi, S., Ravalia, G., Descovich, G. C., and Sirtori, C. R.**, Dietary treatment of familial hypercholesterolemia — differential effects of soy protein according to the Apolipoprotein E phenotypes, *Am. J. Clin. Nutr.*, 53, 1191, 1991.
83. **Gregg, R. E., Zech, L. A., Schaefer, E. J., and Brewer, H. B.**, Apolipoprotein E metabolism in normolipoproteinemic human subject, *J. Lipid Res.*, 25, 1167, 1984.
84. **Gregg, R. E., Zech, L. A., Cabelli, C., and Brewer, H. B.**, Apo E modulates the metabolism of apo B containing lipoproteins by multiple mechanisms, in *Cholesterol Transport Systems and Their Relation to Atherosclerosis*, Steimetz, A., Kalparik, H., and Schneider, J., Eds., Springer Verlag, Berlin, 1989, 11.
85. **Breslow, J. L.**, Genetic basis of lipoprotein disorders, *J. Clin. Invest.*, 84, 373, 1989.
86. **Gotto, A. M.**, Cholesterol intake and serum cholesterol level, *New Engl. J. Med.*, 324, 912, 1991.
87. **Kern, F.**, Normal plasma cholesterol in an 88-year old man who eats 25 eggs a day. Mechanisms of adaptation, *New Engl. J. Med.*, 324, 896, 1991.
88. **Miettinen, T. A. and Kesaniemi, Y. A.**, Cholesterol absorption: regulation of cholesterol synthesis and elimination and within-population variations of serum cholesterol levels, *Am. J. Clin. Nutr.*, 49, 629, 1989.
89. **Jenkins, D. J. A., Leeds, A. R., Gassull, M. A., Houston, H., Goff, D. V., and Hill, M. J.**, The cholesterol lowering properties of guar and pectin, *Clin. Sci. Mol. Med.*, 51, 8, 1976.
90. **Raymond, T. L., Connor, W. E., Lin, D. S., Warner, S., Fry, M. M., and Connor, S. L.**, The interaction of dietary fibers and cholesterol upon the plasma lipids and lipoproteins, sterol balance and bowel function in human subjects, *J. Clin. Invest.*, 60, 1429, 1977.
91. **Anderson, J. W., Story, L., Sieling, B., Chen, W. J. L., Petro, M. S., and Story, J.**, Hypocholesterolemic effects of oat-bran or bean intake for hypercholesterolemic men, *Am. J. Clin. Nutr.*, 40(b), 1146, 1984.
92. **Thacker, P. A., Salomons, M. O., Aherne, F. X. et al.**, Influence of propionic acid on the cholesterol metabolism of pigs fed hypercholesterolemic diets, *Can. J. Anim. Sci.*, 61, 969, 1981.
93. **Chen, W. L., Anderson, J. W., and Jennings, D.**, Propionate may mediate the hypocholesterolemic effects of certain soluble plant fibers in cholesterol-fed rats (41791), *Proc. Soc. Exp. Biol. Med.*, 175, 215, 1984.
94. **Chen, W. J. L. and Anderson, J. W.**, Hypercholesterolemic effects of soluble fibers, in *Dietary Fiber: Basic and Clinical Aspects*, Kritchevsky, D. and Yahouny, G. V., Eds., Plenum Press, New York, 1986, 275.
95. **Wolever, T. M. S., Brighenti, F., and Jenkins, D. J. A.**, Serum short chain fatty acids after rectal infusion of acetate and propionate in man, *J. Clin. Nutr. Gastroenterol.*, 3, 42, 1988.
96. **Venter, C. S., Vorster, H. H., and Cummings, J. H.**, Effects of dietary propionate on carbohydrate and lipid metabolism in healthy volunteers, *Am. J. Gastroenterol.*, 85(5), 549, 1990.
97. **Todesco, T., Rao, A. V., Bosello, O., and Jenkins, D. J. A.**, Propionate lowers blood glucose and alters lipid metabolism in healthy subjects, *Am. J. Clin. Nutr.*, 54, 1991.

98. **Reaven, G. M.,** Banting Lecture 1988. Role of insulin resistance in human disease, *Diabetes,* 37, 1595, 1988.
99. **Ducimetiere, P., Eschwege, E., Papoz, L., Richard, J. L., Claude, J. R., and Rosselin, G.,** Relationship of plasma insulin levels to the incidence of myocardial infarction and coronary heart disease mortality in a middle-aged population, *Diabetologia,* 19, 205, 1980.
100. **Welborn, T. A. and Wearne, K.,** Coronary heart disease incidence and cardiovascular mortality in Busselton with reference to glucose and insulin concentrations, *Diabetes Care,* 2, 154, 1979.
101. **Pyorala, K.,** Relationship of glucose tolerance and plasma insulin to incidence of coronary heart disease: results from two population studies in Finland, *Diabetes Care,* 2, 131, 1979.
102. **Jenkins, D. J. A., Leeds, A. R., Gassull, M. A., Cochet, B., and Alberti, K. G. M. M.,** Decrease in postprandial insulin and glucose concentrations by guar and pectin, *Ann. Int. Med.,* 86, 20, 1977.
103. **Jenkins, D. J. A., Wolever, T. M. S., Leeds, A. R., Gassull, M. A., Dilawari, J. B., Goff, D. V., Metz, G. L., and Alberti, K. G. M. M.,** Dietary fibers, fiber analogues and glucose tolerance: importance of viscosity, *Br. Med. J.,* 1, 1392, 1978.
104. **Lakeshmanan, M. R., Nepokroeff, C. M., Ness, G. C., Dugan, R. E., and Porter, J. W.,** Stimulation by insulin of rat liver Beta-hydroxy-Beta-methylglutaryl coenzyme A reductase and cholesterol-synthesizing activities, *Biochem. Biophys. Res. Commun.,* 50, 704, 1973.
105. **Jenkins, D. J. A., Wolever, T. M. S., Jenkins, A. L., Brighenti, F., Vuksan, V., Rao, A. V., Cunnane, S., Ocana, A. M., Corey, P., Vezina, C., Connelly, P., Buckley, G., and Patten, R.,** Specific types of colonic fermentation may raise low-density-lipoprotein-cholesterol concentrations, *Am. J. Clin. Nutr.,* 54, 141, 1991.
106. **Vahouny, G. V. and Cassidy, M. M.,** Dietary fiber and intestinal adaptation, in *Dietary Fiber: Basic and Clinical Aspects,* Vahouny, G. V. and Kritchevsky, D., Eds., Plenum Press, New York, 1986, 181.
107. **Story, J. A.,** Modification of steroid excretion in response to dietary fiber, in *Dietary Fiber: Basic and Clinical Aspects,* Vahouny, G. V. and Kritchevsky, D., Eds., Plenum Press, New York, 1986, 253.
108. **Schneeman, B. O., Cimmarusti, J., Cohen, W., Downes, L., and Lefevre, M.,** Composition of high density lipoproteins in rats, *J. Nutr.,* 45, 564, 1976.
109. **Kasper, H., Rabast, U., Fassl, H., and Fehle, F.,** The effect of dietary fiber on the postprandial serum vitamin A concentration in man, *Am. J. Clin. Nutr.,* 32, 1847, 1979.
110. **Jenkins, D. J. A., Wolever, T. M. S., Ocana, A. M., Vuksan, V. et al.,** Metabolic effects of reducing rate of glucose ingestion by single bolus versus continuous sipping, *Diabetes,* 39, 775, 1990.
111. **Spiller, G., Gates, J., Nichols, S., Jensen, C., and Whittam, J.,** The relationship of water soluble dietary fiber (WSDF) structure to plasma cholesterol-lowering efficacy in humans. (Abstract) *FASEB J.,* 6, A1654, 1992.

Chapter 7.2

DEVELOPMENT OF THE DIETARY FIBER HYPOTHESIS OF DIABETES MELLITUS*

Hugh C. Trowell

DIABETES AND OBESITY BECAME COMMON IN EAST AFRICAN BLACKS (1930–1960)

Diabetes mellitus and obesity were extremely rare diseases in East African blacks when I started treating medical patients in Nairobi Hospital, Kenya, in 1930. After teaching medicine for nearly 30 years in East Africa, I reviewed the rising incidence of diabetes in sub-Saharan urban blacks and suggested that "their high-carbohydrate low-fat diets are protective and that low-carbohydrate high-fat diets predispose. African diets are usually high in their fiber content but in towns refined flours, sugar, and fats form a large part of the diet which may contain little fiber".[1] No earlier reference has been traced to any connection between fiber and diabetes. On returning to East Africa in 1970 I was amazed to see two new phenomena: first, many grossly obese African blacks in urban streets and second, large diabetes clinics in all towns.[2]

HIGH FIBER BRITISH NATIONAL FLOUR

In 1948 Himsworth published diabetes mortality death rates in British women during the period of the Second World War (1940 to 1945) and the postwar food rations; he attributed falling death rates to reduced fat intakes.[3] In 1966 Cleave and Campbell republished these mortality and food data but concluded that reduced sugar intakes caused the falling death rates.[4] Postwar food regulations, however, lasted until 1953. A comprehensive British government report on human food supplies from 1938 through 1958 allowed a more detailed reexamination of this problem. This reported that diabetes death rates started falling not in 1940, but in 1942, and fell until 1953, not only until 1948, 55% in men and 54% in women mainly in middle-aged and elderly groups. Diabetes death rates started to rise again in 1954. Fat and sugar supplies, however, rose in 1949 to prewar levels and continued thus thereafter, but death rates continued falling for another 5 years. High fiber high extraction national flour became mandatory for the entire British population from 1942 until 1953, then ceased and low fiber white bread was eaten. During the years of the national flour, bread consumption rose about 25%. Total energy intakes rarely decreased below 3000 kcal/day per head and were stationary during all these years.[5]

This provided the basis of the hypothesis that high fiber high *starchy* carbohydrate diets are protective against maturity-onset noninsulin-dependent Type II diabetes mellitus.[6] This protective diet, which resembles the ancient traditional diet of most peasants, is *not* the same as a high carbohydrate high fiber diet because the latter might be a diet containing much white flour and sucrose supplemented by much wheat bran. The original hypothesis carries a corollary that low fiber starchy carbohydrates, such as white wheat flour and white rice, are the main causative factors in the production of Type II diabetes mellitus. High energy diets, containing much fat and sucrose, both of which contain no fiber, encourage overweight and obesity; they are probably contributory etiological factors.

* Dr. Trowell passed away in 1989. This historical chapter is unchanged from the 1986 edition of this handbook.

GENETIC AND AUTOIMMUNE FACTORS

Genetic factors predispose strongly to Type II diabetes but are weak in Type I diabetes. Possibly viral infection or other noxious agents damage the pancreatic cells in Type I diabetes. This variety is an autoimmune disease. Many autoimmune diseases are certainly very rare in African blacks: multiple sclerosis has not yet been definitely reported; pernicious anemia and Hashimoto's thyroiditis are extremely rare; rheumatoid arthritis is certainly uncommon.[7] Unknown dietary factors or life-style protect sub-Saharan blacks from all or almost all autoimmune diseases.

NEW HIGH FIBER HIGH STARCH DIETS

In the U.S., Anderson and colleagues pioneered high fiber high starch carbohydrates in the treatment of diabetes.[8] In Britain, Mann and colleagues treated both Type I diabetes and Type II diabetes with a comparable diet; they reported improved diabetic control.[9] Jenkins studied purified fiber supplements such as pectin and guar gum; these slowed digestion and absorption, reduced GIP, and lowered enteroglucagon responses.[10]

IMPROVED DIABETIC DIETS

In 1979 the American Diabetes Association recommended that carbohydrate intakes of Type I diabetic patients be increased to 50 to 60% of total calories.[11] In 1981 the British Diabetic Association made similar recommendations.[12] These also recommended that simple sugar intakes be restricted and that carbohydrate, wherever possible, should be fiber-rich unprocessed starchy foods. One overall aim was to reduce fat consumption and hopefully in the long term to reduce the risk of cardiovascular disease.

IMPROVED DIETS FOR THE WHOLE COMMUNITY

In 1983 the (British National) Health Council recommended guidelines for nutritional changes in the whole population to decrease the incidence of modern metabolic diseases such as overweight and obesity, diabetes, coronary heart disease, and gallstones. They recommended increasing starch carbohydrates to 50% total calories by increased consumption of fiber-rich whole wheat and brown bread and potatoes, thereby increasing dietary fiber intake by 25%; they recommended that sugar intake be decreased to 50% and fat decreased by 25%.[13]

A consensus of opinion is emerging about desirable changes in modern Western diets in order to decrease the incidence of many diseases characteristic of modern affluent communities. Uncertainty about the degree of change and the desirable rate of change will continue for a decade or more.[14]

REFERENCES

1. **Trowell, H. C.**, *Non-Infective Disease in Africa,* Edward Arnold, London, 1960, 217, 218, 303.
2. **Trowell, H.**, Diabetes mellitus and dietary fiber of starchy foods, *Am. J. Clin. Nutr.,* 31, S53, 1978.
3. **Himsworth, H. P.**, Diet in the aetiology of human diabetes, *Proc. R. Soc. Med.,* 42, 323, 1949.
4. **Cleave, T. L., Campbell, G. D., and Painter, N. S.**, *Diabetes, Coronary Thrombosis, and the Saccharine Disease,* John Wright, Bristol, 1969, chap 3.

5. **Trowell, H.**, Diabetes mellitus death rates in England and Wales 1920–70 and food supplies, *Lancet*, 2, 998, 1974.
6. **Trowell, H.**, Dietary-fiber hypothesis of the etiology of diabetes mellitus, *Diabetes*, 24, 762, 1975.
7. **Trowell, H. C. and Burkitt, D. P., Eds.**, *Western Diseases, Their Emergence and Prevention*, Harvard University Press, Cambridge, MA, 1981, 439.
8. **Anderson, J. W. and Ward, K.**, Long-term effects of high carbohydrate, high fiber diets on glucose and lipid metabolism, *Diabetes Care*, 1, 77, 1982.
9. **Mann, J. L.**, Diet and diabetes, *Diabetologia*, 18, 89, 1980.
10. **Jenkins, D. J. A., Taylor, R. H., and Wolever, T. M. S.**, The diabetic diet, dietary carbohydrates and differences in digestibility, *Diabetologia*, 23, 477, 1982.
11. Committee of the American Diabetes Association on Food and Nutrition Special Report, Principles of nutrition and dietary recommendations for individuals with diabetes mellitus, *Diabetes Care*, 2, 520, 1979.
12. British Diabetic Association Medical Advisory Committee, Dietary recommendations for diabetes for the 1980s, *Hum. Nutr. Appl. Nutr.*, 36A, 378, 1982.
13. National Advisory Committee on Nutrition Education, Proposals for nutritional guidelines for health education in Britain, *Lancet*, ii, 719, 782, 835, 902, 1983.
14. **Do, R.**, Prospects for prevention, *Lancet*, i, 445, 1983.

Chapter 7.3

TREATMENT OF DIABETES WITH HIGH FIBER DIETS

James W. Anderson and Abayomi O. Akanji

INTRODUCTION

Diabetes mellitus remains more prevalent among populations with low fiber intakes than among populations with high fiber intakes.[1,2] These and other observations led Trowell[1] to postulate that diabetes was a fiber deficiency disorder. Since 1976,[3,4] many basic and clinical investigators have documented the therapeutic benefits of fiber in diabetes and its complications. There have been many recent reviews on this subject.[5-8,133,136,159-161,163]

While the clinical utility of dietary fiber in the treatment of diabetes is well established, the role of fiber in the prevention, amelioration or retardation of the development of diabetes and its complications is not established. Some studies however report that:

1. the frequency of reactive hypoglycemia is reduced in "chemical diabetics" on a high-fiber diet[12,25]
2. high fiber diets have favorable effects on blood rheology and hemostatic variables in diabetic subjects[44,63,121]
3. high fiber diets reduce the aggregate risk factors for atherosclerosis[129,163]
4. high fiber diets may ameliorate the frequency of discomfort associated with intermittent claudication in diabetic subjects[144]

The tables summarize the clinical studies of diabetic subjects using either fiber supplements or diets generous in high fiber foods (herein termed high fiber diets). The tables are an extension of our earlier report[9] and include material in the medical literature between 1976 and 1990, drawn from the following sources: (1) computer (Medline) search on diabetes and fiber, including Scientific Citation Indexes, Nutritional Abstracts, and Index Medicus, and (2) an excellent bibliographic survey of dietary fiber, up to and including the year 1986.[10]

CLINICAL STUDIES

Fiber Supplemented Meals

Table 1 summarizes the reported responses of diabetic subjects to glucose loads or meals without or with fiber supplements. The responses of normal subjects to similar test meals are described in a separate chapter. Water-soluble fibers such as guar, pectin, and psyllium extract clearly have greater effects on the glycemic response than do water-insoluble fibers such as cellulose and wheat bran. Other fiber supplements investigated in this context include cottonseed fiber,[99] soy fiber,[40,76] apple powder,[68,76] Mexican nopal leaves,[70] Indian fenugreek seeds,[88] Japanese glucomannan,[48] and xanthan gum.[83] The glucose loads or meals supplemented with these soluble fibers are followed by lower glycemic responses than are control loads without fiber. These findings could be interpreted to suggest that fiber supplements may improve long-term glycemic control.

TABLE 1
Effects of Dietary Fiber on Glycemic Responses to Single Meals for Diabetic Subjects

No. of subjects	Special group	Nature of meal	Type of fiber	Glycemic response	Comments	Ref.
11 3 IDDM 8 NIDDM	—	Breakfast	Guar and pectin	Lower	Serum insulin lower after test than after control meal	4
6 IDDM	—	Breakfast	Guar	Lower	Serum alanine, lactate, and pyruvate similar after control and test meals	11
6 IGT	"Chemical" diabetes	Breakfast	Guar and hemicellulose	Lower	Fiber decreased reactive hypoglycemia	12
6 IDDM	—	Mixed	Guar	Lower	Serum GIP lower, glucagon unchanged after test compared to control meal	13
14 NIDDM	—	Glucose solution	Wheat bran	Lower or unchanged	Metabolic clearance of radioactive glucose unaffected by bran	14
6 1 IDDM 5 NIDDM	—	Breakfast	Guar or lentils or soybeans	All lower	High fiber foods used	15
12 NIDDM	Autonomic neuropathy	Breakfast	Guar and pectin	Lower or unchanged	Fiber did not affect response of patients with autonomic neuropathy; serum insulin, glucagon, GIP unchanged	16
13 NIDDM	—	Breakfast	Guar or pectin or agar or locust bean gum	All unchanged	These fiber-supplemented meals were unpalatable	17

Subjects	Condition	Test meal	Fiber	Glucose response	Comments	Ref.
8 NIDDM	—	Breakfast	High fiber foods	Lower	Whole grain bread and apples compared to white bread and apple juice	19
12 NIDDM	—	Mixed meal	Psyllium	Lower	—	20
12 NIDDM	—	Mixed	High fiber	Unchanged	Blood glucose and insulin response similar after control and test meals	21
21 IDDM	Children	Mixed	High fiber foods	Lower	Exercise did not affect blood glucose	22
4 GDM	Gestational diabetes	Glucose solution	Guar	Lower	Glucose tolerance normalized	23
10 DM	—	Oatmeal	Guar	Lower	Gastric emptying time similar after control and test meals	24
8 IGT	"Chemical" diabetes	Glucose	Pectin or cellulose phosphate or cellulose	Lower for pectin and cellulose phosphate; unchanged for cellulose	Variable changes in serum insulin	25
4 IDDM	—	Mixed meal	Pectin	—	Insulin needs with artificial pancreas lower after test than control meals	26
9 3 IDDM 6 NIDDM	—	Glucose solution	Guar	Lower	Guar biscuit used	27
6 IDDM	—	Breakfast and lunch	Guar	Lower	HF breakfast had no effect on glucose tolerance to lunch (insulin pump treatment)	28
5 2 IDDM 3 NIDDM	—	Pasta breakfast	Guar	Lower	—	29

TABLE 1 (continued)
Effects of Dietary Fiber on Glycemic Responses to Single Meals for Diabetic Subjects

No. of subjects	Special group	Nature of meal	Type of fiber	Glycemic response	Comments	Ref.
8 NIDDM	—	Breakfast	Mixed and rye	Lower	Postprandial C-peptide, GIP response reduced	30
14 NIDDM	—	OGTT	Psyllium	Unchanged	Insulin response unchanged	31
7 IDDM	—	Lunch or supper	Wheat bran	Unchanged	Insulin requirement unchanged with artificial pancreas	32
5 NIDDM	Lean	Breakfast	Wheat bran	Lower	Xylose absorption reduced; insulin levels unchanged	33
10 NIDDM	—	Breakfast	Guar	Lower	Absorption of lactose from milk-containing foods reduced	34
9 NIDDM	—	Breakfast	Wheat flour: extrusion vs. baking	Lowest with whole grain bread	Insulin response lowest with conventional whole grain bread	35
37 16 IDDM 21 NIDDM	—	Breakfast	Rye bread	Lower	—	36
22 20 NIDDM 2 IGT	—	Breakfast or lunch	Guar	Lower	Glycemic effect persisted through late postprandial period	37
19 8 IDDM 11 NIDDM	—	Breakfast	Mixed (and beans)	Lower with beans	Postprandial insulin response lowest with beans; effect of processed food may be different in diabetic vs. nondiabetic subjects	38
4 NIDDM	Obese subjects	Breakfast	Beans vs. potato	Lower with beans	Glucose oxidation rates, insulin, and GIP responses reduced after beans despite similar fiber content as potato	39

Subjects	Population	Test	Fiber		Comments	Ref
7 NIDDM	Obese subjects	Mixed breakfast	Soy polysaccharide	Lower	Insulin unchanged, serum triglycerides, glucagon, pancreatic polypeptide, somatostatin reduced	40
5 IGT	North Indians	OGTT	Mixed high fiber	Lower	Typical North Indian diet improves glucose tolerance	41
13 NIDDM	—	Breakfast	Mixed high fiber	Lower	Post-prandial insulin responses lower	42
22 10 IDDM 12 NIDDM	—	Breakfast	Mixed high fiber	Unchanged	Insulin requirement with artificial pancreas reduced in IDDM but not in NIDDM	43
55 DM	Indian population	OGTT	Bran	Lower	Platelet adhesiveness reduced when fiber was given with glucose	44

Note: DM, diabetes mellitus (type not indicated); IDDM, insulin-dependent (type I) diabetes mellitus; NIDDM, noninsulin-dependent (type II) diabetes mellitus; GDM, gestational diabetes mellitus; IGT, impaired glucose tolerance (formerly called chemical or latent diabetes); OGTT, oral glucose tolerance test; HF, high fiber; MFLC, moderate fiber, low carbohydrate; HCHF, high fiber, high carbohydrate; LFHC, low fiber, high carbohydrate.

Fiber-Supplemented Diets

To extend the meal studies, many investigators examined the response of diabetic subjects to fiber-supplemented diets (Table 2). Most investigators used guar or another fiber source rich in soluble fiber such as glucomannan, psyllium, or apple fiber. To improve palatability, and hence acceptability, these fiber supplements, especially guar, were incorporated into everyday foods such as bread,[15,46,95] biscuits,[27] and chocolate bars.[90] Most studies suggest that fiber supplements lower average blood glucose and cholesterol (especially LDL) levels and reduce requirements for insulin or oral hypoglycemic agents. Many of the studies[78,79,89,92,100] were adequately controlled and used random allocation, random order, or crossover techniques. The controlled studies of Uusitupa et al.[102] in NIDDM and Vaaler et al.[89] in IDDM demonstrate the effects of guar supplementation on long-term (3-month) glycemic control and blood cholesterol levels. Several studies also suggest that wheat bran supplements[14,57,89] also improve glycemic control and reduce the requirements for insulin and/or oral hypoglycemic agents.

High Fiber Diets

Table 3 summarizes the responses of diabetic subjects to high fiber diets developed from high fiber foods rather than fiber supplements. Most investigators used high carbohydrate, high fiber (HCHF) diets, although some tested high fiber (HF) diets that were similar in carbohydrate content to the control diets. Our initial studies[3,105] with HCHF diets documented that these diets improved glycemic control, lowered insulin requirements, and reduced blood lipid levels. We have extended these studies[106,109,110] and they have been confirmed by many other groups (Table 3). Many of the more recent studies were well controlled using random allocation and crossover techniques, and it is now generally accepted that diabetic subjects derive distinct advantages from both HCHF and HF diets, the former probably being more beneficial. A particularly useful study is that reported by O'Dea et al.[156] which investigated the effects of varying proportions of carbohydrate, fiber, and fat on metabolic control in NIDDM and concluded that high carbohydrate diets for diabetic patients should select carbohydrates that are unrefined and high in fiber.

Use of Dietary Fiber in Distinct Diabetic Groups

The various investigators (Tables 1,2,3) confirm that fiber confers distinct advantages to both IDDM and NIDDM subjects, including patients on the insulin pump and artificial pancreas treatment,[26,28,52] improving glycemic and lipidemic control, irrespective of body weight (lean or obese), state of diabetic control, or degree of compliance to treatment. Special groups such as children,[22,63,94,118,132] pregnant women,[23,71,75,119] and geriatric subjects[64,95] also benefit from fiber supplementation. Dietary fiber confers additional benefit in the management of diabetic patients who are hypertensive,[101,130,134,143] have chronic renal failure,[139,150] or have hepatic encephalopathy from liver cirrhosis.[85]

Mechanism of Effect of Dietary Fiber on Glycemic Control

High fiber diets, especially those with a high carbohydrate content, probably exert their effect on glycemic control by improving insulin sensitivity. This is obvious from the reduced need for antidiabetic medication in subjects on these diets. However, reports on insulin clamp studies to assess insulin sensitivity in these subjects are not consistent, being variously reported as unchanged[98,117,162] or improved.[164] However, various studies[120,123,126] report increased insulin binding to monocytes and adipocytes in subjects on HF diets. It has also been reported in both normal subjects and diabetics[165-167] that fiber taken at a meal could improve glycemic response to subsequent meals. Other possible mechanisms of action of fiber may be via modulation of the secretion of gut hormones[13,25,30,40,86,101,140] or the intermediary metabolic effects of short chain fatty acids — acetate, propionate, butyrate — derived from the colonic fermentation of fiber in the diet.[174,175]

TABLE 2
Response of Diabetic Subjects to Fiber-Supplemented Diets

No. of subjects	Special group	Type of fiber	Duration of study (days)	Glycemic response	Comments	Ref.
9 DM	—	Guar	7	—	Glycosuria with guar supplements less than half of control values	45
9 7 IDDM 2 NIDDM	—	Guar	5	—	Glycosuria 38% lower with guar crispbread than with control diet	46,49
8 IDDM	—	Cellulose in bread	10	Lower	—	47
13 NIDDM	—	Glucomannan	90	Lower	Insulin requirements, cholesterol lower	48
6 DM	—	Guar	56	—	Insulin requirements lower	50
38 IGT	—	Wheat bran	30	Lower	Serum cholesterol, triglycerides lower	51
7 IDDM	—	Guar	1	Unchanged	Insulin needs with artificial pancreas lower in 5 of 7 patients	52
22 NIDDM	Poorly controlled, poorly compliant	Guar or wheat bran	91	Unchanged	No beneficial effects	53
19 IDDM	—	Guar	5	—	Glycosuria reduced more with higher than lower carbohydrate intake	54
11 5 IGT 6 NIDDM	—	Guar + pectin	3	Lower	Glucose and insulin responses lower	55

TABLE 2 (continued)
Response of Diabetic Subjects to Fiber-Supplemented Diets

No. of subjects	Special Group	Type of fiber	Duration of study (days)	Glycemic response	Comments	Ref.
11	—	Guar	183–365	Unchanged	Insulin requirements, serum cholesterol lower	56
8 IDDM 3 NIDDM	—	Wheat bran	14–28	Lower	Insulin requirements lower	57
9 NIDDM 10 IDDM	—	Guar	91	Unchanged	Serum cholesterol lower	59
6 IDDM	—	Guar	28	Lower	Serum cholesterol 9% lower	60
8 IDDM	—	Guar	91	Unchanged	Body weight, insulin requirements, cholesterol lower	61
8 NIDDM	—	Wheat bran	91	Unchanged	Oral hypoglycemic agent doses and cholesterol decreased	61
10 NIDDM	—	Guar	28	—	Glycosuria and cholesterol decreased	62
10 IDDM	Children	Guar	28	—	Insulin requirements decreased	63
14 NIDDM	Geriatric subjects	Guar	61	Lower	Serum cholesterol lower	64
17 IDDM	Stable and labile diabetic subjects	Wheat bran	10–15	Lower	Improved glycemic control	65
10 NIDDM	Subjects taken off all drugs	Guar	7	—	Urine glucose excretion 31% lower	66

40 NIDDM	Constipated patients	Psyllium	122	Lower	Glycohemoglobin and serum cholesterol lower	67
12 NIDDM	—	Apple fiber	49	Lower	Serum cholesterol lower	68
17 6 IDDM 11 NIDDM	—	Guar	7–21	Lower	Serum cholesterol lower	69
7 DM	—	Boiled nopal leaves (Mexico)	10	Lower	Body weight, total-, LDL-cholesterol, triglyceride reduced	70
12 IDDM	Pregnant	Guar	7	Unchanged	Improvements with guar persisted after guar was stopped	71
12 NIDDM	Obese, poorly controlled subjects	Guar + wheat bran	61	Lower	Plasma cholesterol lower on guar	72
28 IDDM	—	Guar or wheat bran	91	Lower	Guar lowered glycohemoglobin, cholesterol; bran increased cholesterol	73
17 IDDM	—	Pectin	91	Unchanged	Glycohemoglobin, glycated albumin unchanged	74
5 2 IDDM 3 NIDDM	—	Guar	14	Lower	Total cholesterol, triglyceride, drug requirements reduced	29
8 NIDDM	—	Soy hull	28	Lower	Glycosuria, glycohemoglobin unchanged, HDL-cholesterol increased	76
		Corn bran	28	Unchanged	VLDL-cholesterol, triglyceride glycohemoglobin lower	
		Apple powder	28	Unchanged	Total, LDL-cholesterol higher	

TABLE 2 (continued)
Response of Diabetic Subjects to Fiber-Supplemented Diets

No. of subjects	Special Group	Type of fiber	Duration of study (days)	Glycemic response	Comments	Ref.
79 38 IDDM 41 NIDDM	—	Guar	14	Lower	Serum cholesterol, glycosuria reduced, blood/urine chemistry unchanged	77
12 IDDM	—	Rye bran	28	Lower	Insulin requirements lower	78
4 IDDM	—	Cellulose	42	Lower	Total, HDL cholesterol lower, insulin need greater with cellulose	79
		Wheat bran	42	Lower	Glycohemoglobin, insulin need lower with wheat bran	
20 8 IDDM 12 NIDDM	—	Guar (low dose)	61	Unchanged	Glycohemoglobin, antidiabetic medication reduced	80
8 NIDDM	—	Guar	112	Unchanged	Hematologic parameters, blood chemistry, trace elements unaffected	81
13 8 IDDM 5 NIDDM	—	Guar	98	—	Serum cholesterol lower, triglyceride unchanged	82
9 NIDDM	—	Xanthan gum	42	Lower	Total-, VLDL-, LDL-cholesterol total-, VLDL-triglyceride, gastrin, and GIP responses lower	83
10 NIDDM	—	Guar	42	Lower	Insulin response, glycohemoglobin, total-, HDL-cholesterol lower, insulin sensitivity, and receptor binding greater, HDL-	84

Subjects	Fiber	n		Effects	Ref
8 NIDDM	Subjects with portal systemic encephalopathy (PSE) from liver cirrhosis	Vegetable protein and psyllium	15	Lower	phospholipids, triglycerides, hepatic glucose production unchanged	85
8 NIDDM	—	Guar	14	Unchanged	Tolbutamide dose reduced, bowel movement greater, PSE parameters unchanged	—
11 NIDDM	—	Guar	14	Unchanged	Serum cholesterol, GIP response lower, insulin, C-peptide responses unchanged	86
8 NIDDM	Obese	Guar	183	—	Serum triglyceride higher, LDL lower in men, effect not maintained over 6 months.	87
5 NIDDM	Asian Indians	Fenugreek seeds	21	Lower	Glycosuria, serum cholesterol, insulin response lower	88
28 IDDM	—	Guar	91	Lower	Glycohemoglobin, total-, LDL-cholesterol lower	89
	—	Wheat bran	91	Lower	HDL-chol/Total chol ratio higher	
16 NIDDM	—	Guar	183	—	Nutritional parameters unchanged	90
7 NIDDM	Poorly controlled, noncompliant subjects	Guar	30	Lower	Glycosuria, fasting insulin lower, erythrocyte insulin binding, serum calcium, cholesterol, and triglyceride, OGTT and glycohemoglobin unchanged	91

TABLE 2 (continued)
Response of Diabetic Subjects to Fiber-Supplemented Diets

No. of subjects	Special group	Type of fiber	Duration of study (days)	Glycemic response	Comments	Ref.
29 NIDDM	Subjects with near normal fasting plasma glucose levels	Guar	56	Unchanged	Glycohemoglobin, C-peptide, HDL-cholesterol, triglyceride unchanged, LDL-cholesterol lower	92
16 NIDDM	—	Guar	42	Unchanged	Glycohemoglobin, LDL-, total-cholesterol, triglyceride reduced	93
22 IDDM	Children	Guar	42	—	Glycosuria, glycohemoglobin, total cholesterol reduced	94
14 NIDDM	Geriatric	Guar	183	Lower	C-peptide lower, glycohemoglobin increased, HDL-cholesterol, triglycerides unchanged	95
17 NIDDM	Obese	Guar gum	112	Unchanged	No additional benefit	97
9 IDDM	Lean patients on insulin pump treatment	Guar	28	Lower	Glycohemoglobin, insulin sensitivity unchanged, insulin needs, LDL-cholesterol lower	98
12 NIDDM	—	Cottonseed fiber	30	Lower	Insulin response to test meal, serum lipids unchanged	99
8 NIDDM	—	Guar	183	—	Mineral (Fe, Cu, Zn, Ca, Mn, Mg) balance unchanged	100
12 NIDDM	—	Beet fiber	56	Unchanged	Systolic BP, cholesterol, triglycerides lower, HDL increased, postprandial insulin, pancreatic	101

					polypeptide and motilin lower in obese, glycohemoglobin unchanged	
33 NIDDM	Poorly controlled obese	Guar	396	Unchanged	Serum total cholesterol, vitamins A and E lower, plasma Zn higher	102
19 NIDDM	Obese	Guar	91	Lower	Total-, LDL-cholesterol lower (if serum cholesterol > 6.5 mmol/l)	103
12 NIDDM	—	Guar	14	Lower	Serum cholesterol, triglyceride lower, insulin enteroglucagon, glucagon, GIP, PYY unchanged, neurotensin higher.	104

Note: See Table 1 for definition of abbreviations.

TABLE 3
Response of Diabetic Subjects to High Fiber Diets Developed from High Fiber Foods

No. of subjects	Special group	Nature of diet	Duration of study (days)	Glycemic response	Comments	Ref.
13 8 IDDM 5 NIDDM	—	HCHF	12–28	Lower	Insulin or oral hypoglycemic agent needs, blood lipids reduced	3
14 3 IDDM 11 NIDDM	—	HCHF	1478	Lower	Insulin dose, serum cholesterol, triglycerides lower; good long-term outpatient compliance	96
10 7 IDDM 3 NIDDM	—	HCHF	182–1095	Lower	Insulin requirements, serum lipids lower	105
20 IDDM	Lean	HCHF	16	Lower	Insulin requirements, blood lipids reduced	106
14 NIDDM	—	HCHF	42	Lower	Glycohemoglobin, cholesterol lower	107
11 IDDM	—	HCHF	42	Unchanged	Insulin requirements, serum cholesterol lower	108
21 12 IDDM 9 NIDDM	Obese	HCHF	12–42	Lower	Insulin requirements, blood lipids lower	109
11 4 IDDM 7 NIDDM	—	HCHF	18–26	Lower	HCHF and LFHC diets had equivalent insulin dose-reducing effects	110
8 4 IDDM 4 NIDDM	—	HCHF	10	Lower	Serum cholesterol lower	111

Subjects	Group	Diet	Duration (days)	Blood glucose	Comments	Ref.
5 NIDDM	Geriatric nursing home residents	HF	14	Lower	Diabetic control improved	112
16 10 IDDM 6 NIDDM	—	MFLC	42	Slightly lower	With low carbohydrate, increasing fiber from 18 to 33 g/day did not change glycemic control	113
27 9 IDDM 18 NIDDM	—	HCHF	42	Lower	Serum cholesterol lower, HDL:LDL ratio higher	114
60 NIDDM	Pritikin program with exercise	HCHF	26	Lower	Insulin or oral hypoglycemic agent needs, blood lipids, body weight lower	115
8 NIDDM	Obese	HF	2	Lower	Urinary C-peptide excretion lower on high bean diet than on high bran diet	116
7 NIDDM	Very obese	HCHF	7	Unchanged	Insulin sensitivity unchanged	117
10 IDDM	Children	HF	42	Lower	Glycosuria decreased	118
20 10 IDDM 10 NIDDM	Pregnant	HCHF	28–210	Lower	Insulin requirements decreased	119
20 IDDM	—	HCHF	28	Unchanged	Insulin requirements lower; insulin binding to circulating monocytes increased	120
21 10 IDDM 11 NIDDM	—	HCHF	42	Slightly lower	Plasma clotting factors reduced	121
7 NIDDM	—	HCHF	42	—	Insulin binding to circulating monocytes increased	123
69 NIDDM	Pritikin program and exercise	HCHF	730–1095	Lower	Diet and exercise sustained lower serum lipids	124

TABLE 3 (continued)
Response of Diabetic Subjects to High Fiber Diets Developed from High Fiber Foods

No. of subjects	Special Group	Nature of diet	Duration of study (days)	Glycemic response	Comments	Ref.
35 1 IDDM 34 NIDDM	16 white, 10 black, 9 Asian, hypertensives	HCHF (low sodium)	30	—	Blood pressure lower in whites and blacks, but not in Asians	125
9 NIDDM	—	HCHF	21	Lower	Glycosuria reduced; fasting insulin unchanged; improved insulin receptor binding and sensitivity	126
10 2 IDDM 8 NIDDM	Long-term outpatient study	HF	91	Lower	Serum triglycerides lower	127
10 IDDM	—	HCHF	42	—	Serum cholesterol lower by 15%; postheparin plasma lipoprotein lipase activity unchanged	128
14 6 IDDM 8 NIDDM	—	HCHF	10	Lower	Total, LDL, VLDL-cholesterol lower	129
25 NIDDM	Mild hypertension	HF	91	—	Glyco-hemoglobin, triglyceride, mean blood pressure lower	130
14 NIDDM	—	HF	21	Lower	Insulin sensitivity improved; glycosuria, HDL, total cholesterol reduced; lipase activity in muscle or adipose tissue, i.v. fat tolerance, fecal fat, trace elements (K, Zn), hematologic variables unchanged	131

Subjects	Condition	Diet	Duration	Outcome	Comments	Ref
12 IDDM	Children	HCHF	14	Unchanged	Frequency of hypoglycemic reactions and insulin dose unchanged	132
25 5 IDDM 20 NIDDM	Mild hypertension	HCHF (low fat, low sodium)	91	—	Triglyceride, glycohemoglobin, body weight lower; same blood pressure reduction as bendrofluazide; HDL higher	134
14 6 IDDM 8 NIDDM	—	HCHF	10	Lower	LDL, HDL, total cholesterol lower, body weight higher	135
4 IDDM	—	HF	42	Lower	Glycohemoglobin, insulin requirement, total, HDL-cholesterol lower	136
6 IDDM	Self-selected foods used	HCHF	42	Unchanged	Glycosuria, insulin need, glycohemoglobin unchanged compared to MCLF (high fat) diet	137
13 IDDM	Poorly controlled	HCHF	580	Worsened	Health education is probably the best method for achieving optimal control in IDDM subjects	138
5 IDDM	Chronic renal failure (hospitalized)	HF	10	Lower	No deleterious effect on blood urea and nutritional status; plasma creatinine reduced	139
22 NIDDM	—	HCHF	42	Lower	Total, HDL cholesterol lower when diet complements intensive patient education	141
6 NIDDM	Lean	HCHF	28	Unchanged	Insulin, triglycerides, LDL, HDL, total cholesterol unchanged	142
7 NIDDM	Moderate hypertension; no drug treatment	HCHF	91	—	Glycohemoglobin, LDL-cholesterol, blood pressure, body weight lower	143

TABLE 3 (continued)
Response of Diabetic Subjects to High Fiber Diets Developed from High Fiber Foods

No. of subjects	Special Group	Nature of diet	Duration of study (days)	Glycemic response	Comments	Ref.
17 6 IDDM 11 NIDDM	Intermittent claudication	HF (low fat, low sodium)	91	—	Blood pressure, LDL-cholesterol, triglyceride, glycohemoglobin, body weight lower; symptom frequency reduced; Doppler ankle/arm ratios unchanged	144
35 15 IDDM 20 NIDDM	—	HCHF	365	Unchanged	Glycohemoglobin, cholesterol, body weight unchanged	145
15 NIDDM	Poorly controlled in metabolic ward study	HF (legumes)	21	Lower	Glycosuria lower, insulin, insulin sensitivity unchanged	146
1 GDM		Mixed HF	30	Lower	Control through pregnancy with high cereal, legumes, and fiber diet without need for insulin	147
14 NIDDM	Obese, geriatric	HF	56	Lower	Total, LDL-cholesterol, LDL/HDL ratio lower; glycohemoglobin, insulin, C-peptide, glucagon, somatostatin unchanged	149
6 IDDM	Chronic renal failure — moderate protein restriction	HCHF	10	Lower	Total cholesterol lower, triglyceride renal function, nitrogen balance, nutritional status unchanged; serum phosphate increased	150
28 NIDDM	Poorly controlled	HF	183	Elevated	Glycohemoglobin, total- and HDL-cholesterol unchanged	151

Subjects	Condition	Diet	N	Glucose	Other effects	Ref.
13 NIDDM	Poorly controlled	HCHF	21	Lower	Glycosuria, total, HDL-cholesterol, triglyceride, glucagon reduced; insulin, fatty acids, insulin receptor binding unchanged	152
10 IDDM	Patients on insulin pump treatment	HF	42	Unchanged	Body weight, insulin needs, blood lipids unchanged	153
40 19 IDDM 21 NIDDM	Retrospective evaluation of 3 studies	HCHF	700	—	Subjects complied best to fiber recommendation; least compliance was to carbohydrate recommendation	154
10 NIDDM	Outpatient study	HCHF	14	Lower	Body weight, body mass index, total, LDL cholesterol, insulin responses reduced, OGTT improved	156
16 NIDDM	To compare low glycemic index (GI) with high GI foods	About 45% carbohydrate	84	Lower on low GI diet	Glycohemoglobin, glycosuria reduced on low GI diet; lipoproteins unchanged	158

Note: See Table 1 for definition of abbreviations.

Long-term Safety of Fiber Preparations

Many investigators have reported on the long-term efficacy and safety of high fiber diets.[90,100,102,157] The consensus is that there are no significant long-term nutritional risks for patients on these diets. Vitamin, mineral, and trace element levels were generally unaffected, as was absorption of simultaneously administered drugs.[168,169] A potential problem is with acceptability and palatability of the diets especially in light of abdominal discomfort routinely experienced by many patients. This has partially been obviated by the use of low dose guar preparations,[80,93] impregnation of guar with fructose for children,[94] and incorporation of natural high fiber foods rather than fiber-enriched supplements. The major potential problems with prolonged fiber intake remain hypertriglyceridemia especially in HCHF diets[155] and small bowel obstruction,[170] although the latter appears quite rare.

CONCLUSIONS

High fiber diets provide many benefits for diabetic patients, by lowering blood glucose concentrations, reducing postprandial insulin levels and antidiabetic drugs' requirements, and decreasing blood lipid concentrations. For lean individuals with type 1 diabetes, these diets can reduce insulin requirements by 25 to 50% and improve glycemic control.[171] For lean individuals with type II diabetes these diets can lower insulin needs by 50 to 100% and often eliminate the need for insulin.[171] For obese persons with diabetes these diets associated with high satiety promote weight loss and usually provide reasonable glycemic control without specific antidiabetic medication. These diets also lower blood glycohemoglobin levels, plasma cholesterol levels (20 to 30%), triglycerides (rather variably), and blood pressure (average of 10%). However, these effects are not always consistent, and even now remain controversial.[97,151,172,173]

We routinely recommend a prudent diabetic diet containing:[7,161]
1. 55 to 60% of energy from carbohydrate (two thirds derived from the complex forms).
2. 12 to 16% of total calories from protein (or daily intake of 0.8 g/kg desirable body weight to a maximum of 45 g. This amount should be reduced in individuals with nephropathy.[176]
3. Less than 30% of total calories from fat, consistent with the American Heart Association recommendations[177] with less than 10% saturated fat and daily cholesterol intake of less than 200 mg. When increased fiber intake cannot be tolerated or is impossible, total fat intake could be increased to 30 to 40% energy, comprising mainly monounsaturated fats. While still controversial with yet unclear long-term effects,[179] a high monounsaturated fat diet has been shown to increase HDL cholesterol levels and reduce the risk of hypertriglyceridemia associated with high carbohydrate, fiber-deficient diets.[135,148,155,178]
4. Dietary fiber of about 40 g/d (or 15 to 25 g/1000 kcal), to include soluble and insoluble fibers from commonly available foods. Diets high in carbohydrate but not fiber content do not consistently improve glycemic control[122,140,155,157] and, as indicated above, may also adversely affect blood lipid levels.

Other features of the diabetes diet, especially in relation to total calorie intake, use of alternative sweeteners, intake of salt and vitamin and mineral supplements, as well as alcohol ingestion, have recently been reviewed elsewhere.[7,161]

REFERENCES

1. **Trowell, H. C.,** Dietary fiber hypothesis of the etiology of diabetes mellitus, *Diabetes,* 24, 762, 1975.
2. **Anderson, J. W.,** The role of dietary carbohydrate and fiber in the control of diabetes, *Adv. Intern. Med.,* 26, 67, 1980.
3. **Kiehm, T. G., Anderson, J. W., and Ward, K.,** Beneficial effects of a high carbohydrate, high fiber diet on hyperglycemic diabetic men, *Am. J. Clin. Nutr.,* 29, 895, 1976.
4. **Jenkins, D. J. A., Goff, D. V., Leeds, A. R., Alberti, K. G. M. M., Wolever, T. M. S., Gassull, M. A., and Hockaday, T. D. R.,** Unabsorbable carbohydrates and diabetes: decreased postprandial hyperglycaemia, *Lancet,* 2, 172, 1976.
5. **Wahlquist, M. L.,** Dietary fiber and carbohydrate metabolism, *Am. J. Clin. Nutr.,* 45, 1232, 1987.
6. **Vinik, A. I. and Jenkins, D. J. A.,** Dietary fiber in management of diabetes, *Diabetes Care,* 11, 160, 1988.
7. **Anderson, J. W. and Geil, P. B.,** New perspectives in nutrition management of diabetes mellitus, *Am. J. Med.,* 85, 159, 1988.
8. **Council on Scientific Affairs, American Medical Association,** Dietary fiber and health, *JAMA,* 262, 542, 1989.
9. **Anderson, J. W.,** Treatment of diabetes with high fiber diets, in *CRC Handbook of Dietary Fiber in Human Nutrition,* Spiller, G. A., Ed., CRC Press, Boca Raton, FL, 1984, 349.
10. **Leeds, A. R. and Burley, V. J., Eds.,** Dietary Fibre Perspectives. Reviews and Bibliography, Vol. 2. John Libbey, London, 1990.
11. **Goulder, T. J., Alberti, K. G. M. M., and Jenkins, D. A.,** Effect of added fiber on the glucose and metabolic response to a mixed meal in normal and diabetic subjects, *Diabetes Care,* 1, 351, 1978.
12. **Monnier, L., Pham, C., Aquirre, L., Orsetti, A., and Mirouze, J.,** Influence of indigestible fibers on glucose tolerance, *Diabetes Care,* 1, 83, 1978.
13. **Morgan, L. M., Goulder, T. J., Tsiolakis, D., Marks, V., and Alberti, K. G. M. M.,** The effect of unabsorbable carbohydrate on gut hormones, *Diabetologia,* 17, 85, 1979.
14. **Hall, S. E. H., Bolton, T. M., and Hetenyi, G.,** The effect of bran on glucose kinetics and plasma insulin in noninsulin-dependent diabetes mellitus, *Diabetes Care,* 3, 520, 1980.
15. **Jenkins, D. J., Wolever, T. M., Taylor, R., Barker, M., Fielden, H., and Jenkins, A. L.,** Effect of guar crispbread with cereal products and leguminous seeds on blood glucose concentrations of diabetics, *Br. Med. J.,* 281, 1248, 1980.
16. **Levitt, N. S., Vinik, A. I., Sive, A. A., Child, P. T., and Jackson, W. P. U.,** The effect of dietary fiber on glucose and hormone responses to a mixed meal in normal subjects and in diabetic subjects with and without autonomic neuropathy, *Diabetes Care,* 3, 515, 1980.
17. **Williams, D. A. R., James, W. P. T., and Evans, I. E.,** Dietary fiber supplementation of a 'normal' breakfast administered to diabetics, *Diabetologia,* 18, 379, 1980.
18. **Vaaler, S., Hanssen, K. F., and Aagenase, O.,** Effect of different kinds of fiber on postprandial blood glucose in insulin-dependent diabetics, *Acta Med. Scand.,* 208, 389, 1980.
19. **Asp, N. G., Agardh, C. D., Ahren, B., Dencker, I., Johansson, G., Lundquist, I., Nyman, M., Sartor, G., and Schersten, B.,** Dietary fiber in type II diabetes, *Acta Med. Scand.,* 656(Suppl.), 47, 1981.
20. **Sartos, G., Carlstrom, S., and Schersten, B.,** Dietary supplementation of fibre (Lunelax) as a means to reduce postprandial glucose in diabetics, *Acta Med. Scand.,* 656(Suppl.), 51, 1981.
21. **Simpson, R. W., McDonald, J., Wahlquist, M., Balasz, N., and Dunlop, M.,** Effect of naturally occurring dietary fiber in Western foods on blood glucose, *Aust. N.Z. J. Med.,* 11, 484, 1981.
22. **Baumer, J. H., Drakeford, J. A., Wadsworth, J., and Savage, D. C. L.,** Effects of dietary fiber and exercise in mid-morning diabetic control — a controlled study, *Arch Dis. Child.,* 57, 905, 1982.
23. **Gabbe, S. G., Cohen, A. W., Herman, G. O., and Schwartz, S.,** Effect of dietary fiber on the oral glucose tolerance test in pregnancy, *Am. J. Obstet. Gynecol.,* 143, 514, 1982.
24. **Leatherdale, B. A., Green, D. J., Harding, L., Griffin, D., and Bailey, C. J.,** Guar and gastric emptying in noninsulin dependent diabetes, *Acta Diabetol. Lat.,* 19, 339, 1982.
25. **Monnier, L. H., Colette, C., Aquirre, L., Orsetti, A., and Combeaue, D.,** Restored synergistic enterohormonal response after addition of dietary fiber to patients with impaired glucose tolerance and reactive hypoglycaemia, *Diabetes Metab.,* 8, 217, 1982.
26. **Poynard, T., Slama, G., and Tchobroutsky, G.,** Reduction of postprandial insulin needs by pectin as assessed by the artificial pancreas in insulin-dependent diabetics, *Diabetes Metab.,* 8, 187, 1982.
27. **Smith, J., Rosman, M. S., Levitt, N. S., and Jackson, W. P. U.,** Guar biscuits in the diabetic diet, *S. Afr. Med. J.,* 61, 196, 1982.

28. **Chenon, D., Phaka, M., Monnier, L. H., Colette, C., Orsetti, A., and Mirouze, J.**, Effects of dietary fiber on postprandial glycemic profiles in diabetic patients subjected to continuous programmed insulin infusion, *Am. J. Clin. Nutr.,* 40, 58, 1984.
29. **Gatti, E., Catenazzo, G., Camisasca, E., Torri, A., Denegri, E., and Sirtori, C. R.**, Effects of guar-enriched pasta in the treatment of diabetes and hyperlipidemia, *Ann. Nutr. Metab.,* 28, 1, 1984.
30. **Hagander, B., Schersten, B., Asp, N-G., Sartor, G., Agardh, C-D., Schrezenmeir, J., Kasper, H., Ahren, B., and Lundquist, I.**, Effect of dietary fiber on blood glucose, plasma immunoreactive insulin, C-peptide and GIP responses in non-insulin-dependent (type II) diabetics and controls, *Acta Med. Scand.,* 215, 205, 1984.
31. **Jarjis, H. A., Blackburn, N. A., Redfern, J. S., and Read, N. W.**, The effect of ispaghula (Fybogel and Metamucil) and guar gum or glucose tolerance in man, *Br. J. Nutr.,* 51, 371, 1984.
32. **McMurry, J. F. and Baumgardner, B.**, A high wheat bran diet in insulin treated diabetes mellitus: assessment with the artificial pancreas, *Diabetes Care,* 7, 211, 1984.
33. **Parsons, S. R.**, Effects of high fiber breakfasts on glucose metabolism in non-insulin-dependent diabetics, *Am. J. Clin. Nutr.,* 40, 66, 1984.
34. **Uusitupa, M., Aro, A., Korhonen, T., Tuunainen, A., Harlund, H., and Penttila, I.**, Blood glucose and serum insulin responses to breakfast including guar gum and cooked or uncooked milk in type 2 (non-insulin-dependent) diabetic patients, *Diabetologia,* 26, 453, 1984.
35. **Hagander, B., Bjorck, I., Asp, N-G., Lundquist, I., Nilsson-Ehle, P., Schrezenmeir, J., and Scherstein, B.**, Hormonal and metabolic responses to breakfast meals in NIDDM: comparison of white and whole-grain wheat bread and corresponding extruded products, *Hum. Nutr. Appl. Nutr.,* 39A, 114, 1985.
36. **Heinonen, L., Korpela, R., and Mantere, S.**, The effect of different types of Finnish bread on postprandial glucose response in diabetic patients, *Hum. Nutr. Appl. Nutr.,* 39A, 108, 1985.
37. **McIvor, M. E., Cummings, C. C., Leo, T. A., and Mendeloff, A. I.**, Flattening postprandial blood glucose responses with guar gum: acute effects, *Diabetes Care,* 8, 274, 1985.
38. **Simpson, R. W., McDonald, J., Wahlquist, M. L., Atley, L., and Outch, K.**, Food physical factors have different metabolic effects in nondiabetics and diabetics, *Am. J. Clin. Nutr.,* 42, 462, 1985.
39. **Tappy, L., Wursch, P., Randin, J. P., Felber, J. P., and Jequier, E.**, Metabolic effect of pre-cooked instant preparations of bean and potato in normal and in diabetic subjects, *Am. J. Clin. Nutr.,* 43, 30, 1986.
40. **Tsai, A. C., Vinik, A. I., Lasichak, A., and Lo, G. S.**, Effects of soy polysaccharide on postprandial plasma glucose, insulin, glucagon, pancreatic polypeptide, somatostatin, and triglyceride in obese diabetic patients, *Am. J. Clin. Nutr.,* 45, 596, 1987.
41. **Bhatnagar, D.**, Glucose tolerance in North Indians taking a high fibre diet, *Eur. J. Clin. Nutr.,* 42, 1023, 1988.
42. **Karlstrom, B., Vessby, B., Asp, N-P., and Ytterfors, A.**, Effects of four meals with different kinds of dietary fiber on glucose metabolism in healthy subjects and non-insulin-dependent diabetic subjects, *Eur. J. Clin. Nutr.,* 42, 519, 1988.
43. **Schrezenmeir, J., Tato, F., Tato, S., Kustner, E., Krause, U., Hommel, G., Asp, N. G., Kasper, M., and Beyer, J.**, Comparison of glycaemic response and insulin requirements after mixed meals of equal carbohydrate content in healthy, type 1 and type 2 diabetic man, *Klin. Wochenschr.,* 67, 985, 1989.
44. **Khan, H. S., Siddiqui, M. A., Mittal, A. K., and Ajmal, M. R.**, Role of dietary fiber on platelet adhesiveness, *J. Assoc. Phys. India,* 38, 219, 1990.
45. **Jenkins, D. J. A., Wolever, T. M. S., Hockaday, T. D. R., Leeds, A. R., Howarth, R., Bacon, S., Apling, E. C., and Dilawari, J.**, Treatment of diabetes with guar gum. Reduction of urinary glucose loss in diabetics, *Lancet,* ii, 779, 1977.
46. **Jenkins, D. J. A., Wolever, T. M. S., Nineham, R., Taylor, R., Metz, G. L., Bacon, S., and Hockaday, T. D. R.**, Guar crispbread in the diabetic diet, *Br. Med. J.,* 2, 1744, 1978.
47. **Miranda, P. M. and Horwitz, D. L.**, High fiber diets in the treatment of diabetes mellitus, *Ann. Intern. Med.,* 88, 482, 1978.
48. **Doi, K., Matsuura, M., Kawara, A., and Baba, S.**, Treatment of diabetes with glucomannan (Konjac mannan), *Lancet,* 1, 987, 1979.
49. **Jenkins, D. J. A., Hockaday, T. D. R., Wolever, T. M. S., Nineham, R., Goff, D. V., Haisman, P., Charnock, R., Taylor, R. H., and Bacon, S.**, Dietary fiber and ketone bodies: reduced urinary 3-hydroxybutyrate excretion in diabetics on guar, *Br. Med. J.,* 2, 1555, 1979.
50. **Jenkins, D. J. A., Wolever, T. M. S., Nineham, R., Bacon, S., Smith, R., and Hockaday, T. D. R.**, Dietary fiber and diabetic therapy: a progressive effect with time, *Adv. Exp. Med. Biol.,* 119, 275, 1979.
51. **Bosello, O., Ostuzzi, R., Armellini, F., Micciolo, R., and Scuro, L. A.**, Glucose tolerance and blood lipids in bran-fed patients with impaired glucose tolerance, *Diabetes Care,* 3, 46, 1980.
52. **Christiansen, J. S., Bonnevie-Neilsen, V., Svendsen, P. A., Rubin, P., Ronn, B., and Nerup, J.**, Effect of guar gum on 24-hour insulin requirements of insulin-dependent diabetic subjects as assessed by the artificial pancreas, *Diabetes Care,* 3, 659, 1980.

53. **Cohen, M., Leong, W., Salmon, E., and Martin, F. I. R.**, Role of guar and dietary fibre in the management of diabettes mellitus, *Med. J. Aust.*, 1, 59, 1980.
54. **Jenkins, D. J. A., Wolever, T. M. S., Bacon, S., Nineham, R., Leeds, R., Rowden, R., Love, M., and Hockaday, T. D. R.**, Diabetic diets: high carbohydrate combined with high fiber, *Am. J. Clin. Nutr.*, 33, 1729, 1980.
55. **Kanter, Y., Eitan, N., Brook, G., and Barzilai, D.**, Improved glucose tolerance and insulin response in obese and diabetic patients on a fiber-enriched diet, *Isr. J. Med. Sci.*, 16, 1, 1980.
56. **Jenkins, D. J. A., Wolever, T. M. S., Taylor, R. H., Reynolds, D., Nineham, R., and Hockaday, T. D. R.**, Diabetic glucose control, lipids, and trace elements on long-term guar, *Br. Med. J.*, 1, 1353, 1980.
57. **Nygren, C., Berglund, O., Hallmans, G., Lithner, F., and Taljehahl, I. B.**, The effect of a high bran diet on diabetes in mice and humans, *Acta Endocrinol.*, 94 (S 237), 66, 1980.
58. **Aro, A., Uusitupa, M., Voitilainen, E., Hersio, K., Korhonen, T., and Siitonen, O.**, Improved diabetic control and hypocholesterolaemic effect induced by long-term dietary supplementation with guar gum in type II (non-insulin-dependent) diabetes, *Diabetologia*, 21, 29, 1981.
59. **Botha, A. P. J., Steyn, A. F., Esteruysen, A. J., and Slabbert, M.**, Glycosylated hemoglobin, blood glucose and serum cholesterol levels in diabetics treated with guar gum, *S. Afr. Med. J.*, 59, 333, 1981.
60. **Carroll, D. G., Dykes, A., and Hodgson, W.**, Guar gum is not a panacea in diabetes management, *N.Z. Med. J.*, 93, 292, 1981.
61. **Dodson, P. M., Stocks, J., Holdsworth, G., and Galton, D. J.**, High fiber and low fat diets in diabetes mellitus, *Br. J. Nutr.*, 46, 289, 1981.
62. **Johansen, K.**, Decreased urinary glucose excretion and plasma cholesterol level in non-insulin-dependent diabetic patients with guar, *Diabetes Metab.*, 7, 87, 1981.
63. **Koepp, P. and Hegewisch, S.**, Effect of guar on plasma viscosity and related parameters in diabetic children, *Eur. J. Pediatr.*, 137, 31, 1981.
64. **Kyllastinen, M. and Lahikainen, T.**, Long-term dietary supplementation with a fiber product (guar gum) in elderly diabetics, *Curr. Ther. Res.*, 30, 872, 1981.
65. **Monnier, L. H., Blotman, M. J., Colette, C., Monnier, M. P., and Mirouze, J.**, Effects of dietary fiber supplementation in stable and labile insulin-dependent diabetics, *Diabetologia*, 20, 12, 1981.
66. **Stokholm, K. H., Laursten, H. B., and Larsen, H.**, Reduced glycosuria during guar gum supplementation in non-insulin-dependent diabetes, *Dan. Med. Bull.*, 28, 41, 1981.
67. **Fagerberg, S. E.**, The effects of a bulk laxative (metamucil) on fasting blood glucose, serum lipids, and other variables in constipated patients with non-insulin dependent adult diabetes, *Curr. Ther. Res.*, 31, 166, 1982.
68. **Mayne, P. D., McGill, R., Gormley, T. R., Tomkin, G. H., Julian, T. R., and O'Moore, R. R.**, The effect of apple fiber on diabetic control and blood lipids, *Ir. J. Med. Sci.*, 151, 36, 1982.
69. **Smith, U. and Holm, G.**, Effect of a modified guar gum preparation on glucose and lipid levels in diabetics and healthy volunteers, *Atherosclerosis*, 45, 1, 1982.
70. **Frati-Munari, A. C., Fernandez-Harp, J. A., De La Riva, H., Ariza-Andraca, R., and Torres, M. D. C.**, Effects of nopal (Opuntia sp) on serum lipids, glycemia and body weight, *Arch. Invest. Med. (Mex.)*, 14, 117, 1983.
71. **Kuhl, C., Molsted-Pederson, L., and Hornnes, P. J.**, Guar gum and glycemic control of pregnant insulin-dependent diabetic patients, *Diabetes Care*, 6, 152, 1983.
72. **Ray, T. K., Mansell, K. M., Knight, L. C., Malmud, L. S., Owen, O. E., and Boden, G.**, Long-term effects of dietary fiber on glucose tolerance and gastric emptying in non-insulin-dependent diabetic patients, *Am. J. Clin. Nutr.*, 37, 376, 1983.
73. **Vaaler, S., Hanssen, K. F., Dahl-Jorgensen, K., Frolich, W., Aaseth, J., Odegaard, B., and Aagenaes, O.**, Improvement in long-term diabetic control after high fibre (bran and guar) diets, *Diabetologia*, 25, 200, 1983.
74. **Gardner, D. F., Schwartz, L., Krista, M., and Merimee, T. J.**, Dietary pectin and glycemic control in diabetes, *Diabetes Care*, 7, 143, 1984.
75. **Fraser, R. B., Ford, F. A., and Milner, R. D. G.**, A controlled trial of a high dietary fiber intake in pregnancy — effects on plasma glucose and insulin levels, *Diabetologia*, 25, 238, 1983.
76. **Mahalko, J. R., Sandstead, H. H., Johnson, L. K., Inman, L. F., Milne, D. B., Warner, R. C., and Haunz, A.**, Effect of consuming fiber from corn bran, soy hulls of apple powder on glucose tolerance and plasma lipids in type II diabetes, *Am. J. Clin. Nutr.*, 39, 25, 1984.
77. **Najemnik, C., Kritz, H., Irsigler, K., Laube, H., Knick, B., Klimm, H. D., Wahl, P., Vollmar, J., and Brauning, C.**, Guar and its effects on metabolic control in type II diabetic subjects, *Diabetes Care*, 7, 215, 1984.
78. **Nygren, C., Hallmans, G., and Lithner, F.**, Effects of high bran bread on blood glucose control in insulin-dependent diabetic patients, *Diabete Metab.*, 10, 39, 1984.

79. Harold, M. R., Reeves, R. D., Bolze, M. S., Guthrie, R. A., and Guthrie, D. W., Effect of dietary fiber in insulin-dependent diabetics: insulin requirements and serum lipids, *J. Am. Diet. Assoc.*, 85, 1455, 1985.
80. Jones, D. B., Slaughter, P., Lousley, S., Carter, R. D., Jelfs, R., and Mann, J. I., Low dose guar improves diabetic control, *J. R. Soc. Med.*, 78, 546, 1985.
81. McIvor, M. E., Cummings, C. C., and Mendeloff, A. I., Long-term ingestion of guar gum is not toxic in patients with non-insulin-dependent diabetes mellitus, *Am. J. Clin. Nutr.*, 41, 891, 1985.
82. McNaughton, J. P., Morrison, D. D., Huhner, L. J., Earnest, M. M., Ellis, M. A., and Howell, G. L., Changes in total serum cholesterol levels of diabetics fed five grams guar gum daily, *Nutr. Rep. Int.*, 31, 505, 1985.
83. Osilesi, O., Trout, D. L., Glover, E. E., Harper, S. M., Koh, E. T., Behall, K. M., O'Doriso, T. M., and Tartt, J., Use of xantham gum in dietary management of diabetes mellitus, *Am. J. Clin. Nutr.*, 42, 597, 1985.
84. Tagliaferro, V., Cassader, M., Bozzo, C., Pisu, E., Bruno, A., Marena, S., Cavalla-Perin, P., Cravero, L., and Pagano, G., Moderate guar gum addition to usual diet improves peripheral sensitivity to insulin and lipaemic profile in NIDDM, *Diabete Metab.*, 11, 380, 1985.
85. Uribe, M., Dibildox, M., Malpica, S., Guillermo, E., Villallobos, A., Nieto, L., Vargas, F., and Ramos, G. G., Beneficial effect of vegetable protein diet supplemented with psyllium plantago in patients with hepatic encephalopathy and diabetes mellitus, *Gastroenterology*, 88, 901, 1985.
86. Groop, P-H., Groop, L., Totterman, K. J., and Fyhrquist, F., Relationship between changes in GIP concentrations and changes in insulin and C-peptide concentrations after guar gum therapy, *Scand. J. Clin. Lab. Invest.*, 46, 505, 1986.
87. McIvor, M. E., Cummings, C. C., Van Duyn, M. A., Leo, T. A., Margolis, S., Behall, K. M., Michnowski, J. E., and Mendeloff, A. I., Long-term effects of guar gum on blood lipids, *Atherosclerosis*, 60, 7, 1986.
88. Sharma, R. D., Effect of fenugreek seeds and leaves on blood glucose and serum insulin responses in human subjects, *Nutr. Res.*, 6, 1353, 1986.
89. Vaaler, S., Hanssen, K. F., Dahl-Jorgensen, K., Frolich, W., Aaseth, J., Odegaard, B., and Aagenaes, O., Diabetic control is improved by guar gum and wheat bran supplementation, *Diab. Med.*, 3, 230, 1986.
90. Van Duyn, M. A. S., Leo, T. A., McIvor, M. E., Behall, K. M., Michnowski, J. E., and Mendeloff, A. I., Nutritional risk of high-carbohydrate, guar gum dietary supplementation in non-insulin-dependent diabetes mellitus, *Diabetes Care*, 9, 497, 1986.
91. Atkins, T. W., Al-Hussary, N. A. J., and Taylor, K. G., The treatment of poorly controlled non-insulin-dependent diabetic subjects with granulated guar gum, *Diab. Res. Clin. Pract.*, 3, 153, 1987.
92. Holman, R. R., Steemson, J., Darling, P., and Turner, R. C., No glycemic benefit from guar administration in NIDDM, *Diabetes Care*, 10, 68, 1987.
93. Peterson, D. B., Ellis, P. R., Baylis, J. M., Fielden, P., Ajodhia, J., Leeds, A. R., and Jepson, E. M., Low dose guar in a novel food product: improved metabolic control in non-insulin-dependent diabetes, *Diab. Med.*, 4, 111, 1987.
94. Paganus, A., Maenpaa, J., Akerblom, H. K., Stenman, U-H., Knip, M., and Simell, O., Beneficial effects of palatable guar and guar plus fructose diets in diabetic children, *Acta Paediatr. Scand.*, 76, 76, 1987.
95. Sels, J. P., Flendrig, J. A., Postmes, Th. J., The influence of guar gum bread on the regulation of diabetes mellitus type II in elderly patients, *Br. J. Nutr.*, 57, 177, 1987.
96. Story, L., Anderson, J. W., Chen, W. J., Karounos, D., and Jefferson, B., Adherence to high-carbohydrate, high fiber diets: long-term studies of non-obese diabetic men, *J. Am. Diet. Assoc.*, 85, 1105, 1985.
97. Beattie, A., Edwards, C. A., Hosker, J. P., Cullen, D. R., Ward, J. D., and Read, N. W., Does adding fiber to a low energy, high carbohydrate, low fat diet confer any benefit to the management of newly diagnosed and overweight type II diabetics? *Br. Med. J.*, 296, 1147, 1988.
98. Ebeling, P., Yki-Jarvinen, H., Aro, A., Helve, E., Sinisalo, M., and Koivisto, V. A., Glucose and lipid metabolism and insulin sensitivity in type I diabetes: the effect of guar gum, *Am. J. Clin. Nutr.*, 48, 98, 1988.
99. Madar, Z., Nir, M., Troster, N., and Norenberg, C., Effects of cottonseed dietary fiber on metabolic parameters in diabetic rats and non-insulin-dependent diabetic humans, *J. Nutr.*, 118, 1143, 1988.
100. Behall, K. M., Scholfield, D. J., McIvor, M. E., Van Duyn, M. S., Leo, T. A., Michnowski, J. E., Cummings, C. C., and Mendeloff, A. I., Effect of guar gum on mineral balances in NIDDM adults, *Diabetes Care*, 12, 357, 1989.
101. Hagander, B., Asp, N-G., Ekman, R., Nilsson-Ehle, P., and Scherstein, B., Dietary fiber enrichment, blood pressure, lipoprotein profile and gut hormones in NIDDM patients, *Eur. J. Clin. Nutr.*, 43, 35, 1989.

102. **Uusitupa, M., Siitonen, O., Savolainen, K., Silvasti, M., Penttila, I., and Parvianen, M.,** Metabolic and nutritional effects of long-term use of guar gum in the treatment of non-insulin-dependent diabetes of poor metabolic control, *Am. J. Clin. Nutr.,* 49, 345, 1989.
103. **Lalor, B. C., Bhatnagar, D., Winocour, P. H., Ishola, M., Arrol, S., Brading, M., and Durrington, P. N.,** Placebo-controlled trial of the effects of guar gum and metformin on fasting blood glucose and serum lipids in obese, type 2 diabetic patients, *Diab. Med.,* 7, 242, 1990.
104. **Requejo, F., Uttenhal, L. O., and Bloom, S. R.,** Effects of alpha-glucosidase inhibition and viscous fiber on diabetic control and postprandial gut hormone responses, *Diab. Med.,* 7, 515, 1990.
105. **Anderson, J. W. and Ward, K.,** Long-term effects of high carbohydrate, high fiber diets on glucose and lipid metabolism: a preliminary report on patients with diabetes, *Diabetes Care,* 1, 77, 1978.
106. **Anderson, J. W. and Ward, K.,** High carbohydrate, high fiber diets for insulin-treated men with diabetes mellitus, *Am. J. Clin. Nutr.,* 32, 2312, 1979.
107. **Simpson, R. W., Mann, J. I., Eaton, J., Moore, R. A., Carter, R. D., and Hockaday, T. D. R.,** Improved glucose control in maturity onset diabetes treated with high carbohydrate, modified fat diet, *Br. Med. J.,* 1, 1753, 1979.
108. **Simpson, R. W., Mann, J. I., Eaton, J., Carter, D., and Hockaday, T. D. R.,** High carbohydrate diets and insulin dependent diabetes, *Br. Med. J.,* 2, 523, 1979.
109. **Anderson, J. W. and Sieling, B.,** High fiber diets for obese diabetic patients, *Obesity/Bariatric Med.,* 9, 109, 1980.
110. **Anderson, J. W., Chen, W. L., and Sieling, B.,** Hypolipidemic effects of high-carbohydrate, high fiber diets, *Metabolism,* 29, 551, 1980.
111. **Rivellese, A., Riccardi, G., Giacco, A., Pacioni, D., Genovese, S., Mattiole, P. L., and Mancini, M.,** Effect of dietary fiber on glucose control and serum lipoproteins in diabetic patients, *Lancet,* ii, 447, 1980.
112. **Kay, R. M., Grobin, W., and Track, N. S.,** Diets rich in natural fibre improve carbohydrate tolerance in maturity-onset, non-insulin dependent diabetics, *Diabetologia,* 20, 18, 1981.
113. **Manhire, A., Henry, C. L., Hartog, M., and Heaton, K. W.,** Unrefined carbohydrate and dietary fibre in the treatment of diabetes mellitus, *J. Hum. Nutr.,* 35, 99, 1981.
114. **Simpson, H. C., Simpson, R. W., Lousley, S., Carter, R. D., Geekie, M., Hockaday, T. D. R., and Mann, J. I.,** A high carbohydrate leguminous fibre diet improves all aspects of diabetic control, *Lancet,* i, 1, 1981.
115. **Barnard, R. J., Lattimore, L., Holly, R. G., Cherny, S., and Pritikin, N.,** Response of non-insulin-dependent diabetic patients to an intensive program of diet and exercising, *Diabetic Care,* 5, 170, 1982.
116. **Burke, B. J., Hartog, M., Heaton, K. W., and Hooper, S.,** Assessment of the metabolic effects of dietary carbohydrate and fiber by measuring urinary excretion of C-peptide, *Hum. Nutr. Clin. Nutr.,* 36C, 373, 1982.
117. **Hoffman, C. R., Fineberg, S. E., Howey, D. C., Clark, C. M., and Pronsky, Z.,** Short-term effects of a high fiber, high carbohydrate diet in very obese diabetic individuals, *Diabetes Care,* 5, 506, 1982.
118. **Kinmonth, A. L., Angus, R. M., Jenkins, A., Smith, M. A., and Baum, J. D.,** Whole foods and increased dietary fiber improve blood glucose control in diabetic children, *Arch. Dis. Child.,* 57, 187, 1982.
119. **Ney, D., Hollingsworth, D. R., and Cousins, L.,** Decreased insulin requirement and improved control of diabetes in pregnant women given a high carbohydrate, high fiber, low fat diet, *Diabetes Care,* 5, 529, 1982.
120. **Pedersen, O., Hjollund, E., Lindkov, H. O., Helms, P., Sorensen, N. S., and Ditzel, J.,** Increased insulin receptor binding to monocytes from insulin dependent diabetic patients after a low fat, high starch, high fiber diet, *Diabetes Care,* 5, 529, 1982.
121. **Simpson, H. C., Mann, J. I., Chakrabarti, R., Imeson, J. D., Stirling, Y., Tozer, M., Woolf, L., and Meade, T. W.,** Effect of high fiber diet on haemostatic variables in diabetes, *Br. Med. J.,* 284, 1608, 1982.
122. **Simpson, H. C. R., Carter, R. D., Lousley, S., and Mann, J. I.,** Digestible carbohydrate — an independent effect on diabetic control in type 2 (non-insulin-dependent) diabetic patients?, *Diabetologia,* 23, 235, 1982.
123. **Ward, G. M., Simpson, R. W., Simpson, H. C. R., Naylor, B. A., Mann, J. I., and Turner, R. C.,** Insulin receptor binding increased by high carbohydrate low fat diet in non-insulin-dependent diabetics, *Eur. J. Clin. Invest.,* 12, 93, 1982.
124. **Barnard, R. J., Massey, M. R., Cherny, S., O'Brien, L. T., and Pritikin, N.,** Long term use of a high complex carbohydrate, high fiber, low fat diet and exercise in the treatment of NIDDM patients, *Diabetes Care,* 6, 268, 1983.
125. **Dodson, P. M., Pacy, P. J., Beevers, M., Bal, P., Fletcher, R. F., and Taylor, K. G.,** The effects of a high fiber, low fat and low sodium dietary regime on diabetic hypertensive patients of different ethnic groups, *Postgrad Med. J.,* 59, 641, 1983.

126. **Hjollund, E., Pedersen, O., Richelsen, B., Beck-Nielsen, H., and Sorensen, N. S.,** Increased insulin binding to adipocytes and monocytes and increased insulin sensitivity off glucose transport and metabolism in adipocytes from non-insulin-dependent diabetics after a low-fat/high starch/high fiber diet, *Metabolism*, 32, 1067, 1983.
127. **Rosman, M. S., Smith, C. J., and Jackson, W. P. U.,** The effect of long-term high fiber diets in diabetic outpatients, *S. Afr. Med.J.*, 63, 310, 1983.
128. **Taskinen, M., Nikkila, E. A., and Allus, A.,** Serum lipids and lipoproteins in insulin dependent diabetic subjects during high carbohydrate, high fiber diet, *Diabetes Care*, 6, 224, 1983.
129. **Rivellese, A., Riccardi, G., Giacco, A., Postiglione, A., Mastranzo, P., and Mattioli, P. L.,** Reduction of risk factors for atherosclerosis in diabetic patients treated with a high-fiber diet, *Prev. Med.*, 12, 128, 1983.
130. **Dodson, P. M., Pacy, P. J., Bal, P., Kubicki, A. J., Fletcher, R. F., and Taylor, K. G.,** A controlled trial of a high fiber, low fat and low sodium diet for mild hypertension in type 2 (non-insulin-dependent) diabetic patients, *Diabetologia*, 27, 522, 1984.
131. **Karlstrom, B., Vessby, B., Asp, N-G., Boberg, M., Gustafsson, I-B., Lithell, H., and Werner, I.,** Effects of an increased content of cereal fiber in the diet of type II (non-insulin-dependent) diabetic patients, *Diabetologia*, 26, 272, 1984.
132. **Lindsay, A. N., Hardy, A., Jarrett, L., and Rallison, M. L.,** High carbohydrate, high fiber diet in children with type I diabetes, *Diabetes Care*, 7, 63, 1984.
133. **Anderson, J. W.,** Physiologic and metabolic effects of dietary fiber, *Fed. Proc.*, 44, 2902, 1985.
134. **Pacy, P. J., Dodson, P. M., Kubicki, A. J., Fletcher, R. F., and Taylor, K. G.,** Comparison of the hypotensive and metabolic effects of bendrofluazide therapy and a high fiber, low fat, low sodium diet in diabetic subjects with mild hypertension, *J. Hypertension*, 2, 215, 1984.
135. **Riccardi, G., Rivellese, A., Pacioni, D., Genevese, S., Mastranzo, P., and Mancini, M.,** Separate influence of dietary carbohydrate and fiber on the metabolic control of diabetes, *Diabetologia*, 26, 116, 1984.
136. **Anderson, J. W.,** Fiber and health: an overview, *Am. J. Gastroenterol.*, 81, 892, 1986.
137. **Hollenbeck, C. B., Riddle, M. C., Connor, W. E., and Leklem, J. E.,** The effects of subject-selected high carbohydrate, low fat diets on glycaemic control in insulin-dependent diabetes mellitus, *Am. J. Clin. Nutr.*, 41, 293, 1985.
138. **McCulloch, D. K., Mitchell, R. D., Ambler, J., and Tattersall, R. B.,** A prospective comparison of 'conventional' and high carbohydrate/high fiber/low fat diets in adults with established type I (insulin-dependent) diabetes, *Diabetologia*, 27, 208, 1985.
139. **Rivellese, A., Parillo, M., Giacco, A., Marco, F. D., and Riccardi, G.,** A fiber-rich diet for the treatment of diabetic patients with chronic renal failure, *Diabetes Care*, 8, 620, 1985.
140. **Sestoft, L., Krarup, T., Palmvig, B., Meinertz, H., and Faergeman, O.,** High carbohydrate, low fat diet: effect on lipid and carbohydate metabolism, GIP and insulin secretion in diabetics, *Dan. Med. Bull.*, 32, 64, 1985.
141. **Stevens, J., Burgess, M. B., Kaiser, L., and Sheppa, M.,** Outpatient management of diabetes mellitus with patient education to increase dietary carbohydrate and fiber, *Diabetes Care*, 8, 359, 1985.
142. **Hollenbeck, C. B., Coulston, A. M., and Reaven, G. M.,** To what extent does increased dietary fiber improve glucose and lipid metabolism in patients with noninsulin-dependent diabetes mellitus (NIDDM)? *Am. J. Clin. Nutr.*, 43, 16, 1986.
143. **Pacy, P. J., Dodson, P. M., and Fletcher, R. F.,** Effect of a high carbohydrate, low sodium and low fat diet in type 2 diabetics with moderate hypertension, *Int. J. Obesity*, 10, 43, 1986.
144. **Pacy, P. J., Dodson, P. M., and Taylor, K. G.,** The effect of a high fiber, low fat, low sodium diet on diabetics with intermittent claudication, *Br. J. Clin. Pract.*, 46, 313, 1986.
145. **Teuscher, A.,** Die kohlenhydrate und nahrungsfasern in der diabetesdiat, *Schweiz. Med. Wechenschr.*, 116, 282, 1986.
146. **Karlstrom, B., Vessby, B., Asp, N-G., Boberg, M., Lithell, H., and Berne, C.,** Effects of leguminous seeds in a mixed diet in NIDDM (non-insulin-dependent) diabetic patients, *Diab. Res.*, 5, 199, 1987.
147. **Paisley, R. B., Hartog, M., and Savage, P.,** A high fiber diet in gestational diabetes — wheat fiber, leguminous fiber or both?, *Hum. Nutr. Appl. Nutr.*, 41A, 146, 1987.
148. **Garg, A., Bonanome, A., Grundy, S. M., Zhang, Z., and Unger, R. H.,** Comparison of a high carbohydrate diet with a high monounsaturated fat diet in patients with non-insulin-dependent diabetes mellitus, *N. Engl. J. Med.*, 319, 829, 1988.
149. **Hagander, B., Asp, N-G., Efendic, S., Nilsson-Ehle, P., and Scherstein, B.,** Dietary fiber decreases fasting blood glucose levels and plasma LDL concentration in noninsulin-dependent diabetes mellitus patients, *Am. J. Clin. Nutr.*, 47, 852, 1988.

150. **Parillo, M., Riccardi, G., Pacioni, D., Iovine, C., Contaldo, F., Isernia, C., De Marco, F., Perrotti, N., and Rivellese, A.,** Metabolic consequences of feeding a high-carbohydrate, high-fiber diet to diabetic patients with chronic kidney failure, *Am. J. Clin. Nutr.,* 48, 255, 1988.
151. **Scott, A. R., Attenborough, Y., Peacock, I., Fletcher, E., Jeffcoate, W. J., and Tattersall, R. B.,** Comparison of high fiber diets, basal insulin supplements, and flexible insulin treatment for non-insulin-dependent (type II) diabetics poorly controlled with sulphonylureas, *Br. Med. J.,* 297, 707, 1988.
152. **Simpson, R. W., McDonald, J., Wahlquist, M. L., Balasz, N., Sissons, M., and Atley, L.,** Temporal study of metabolic change when poorly controlled noninsulin-dependent diabetics change from low to high carbohydrate and fiber diet, *Am. J. Clin. Nutr.,* 48, 104, 1988.
153. **Venhaus, A. and Chantelau, E.,** Self-selected unrefined and refined carbohydrate diets do not affect metabolic control in pump-treated diabetic patients, *Diabetologia,* 31, 153, 1988.
154. **Anderson, J. W. and Gustafson, N. J.,** Adherence to high carbohydrate, high fiber diets, *Diabetes Educator,* 15, 429, 1989.
155. **Coulston, A. M., Hollenbeck, C. B., Swislocki, A. L. M., and Reaven, G. M.,** Persistence of hypertriglyceridemic effect of low-fat high-carbohydrate diets in NIDDM patients, *Diabetes Care,* 12, 94, 1989.
156. **O'Dea, K., Traianedes, K., Ireland, P., Niall, M., Sadler, J., Hopper, J., and De Luise, M.,** The effects of diet differing in fat, carbohydrate, and fiber on carbohydrate and lipid metabolism in type II diabetes, *J. Am. Diet. Assoc.,* 89, 1076, 1989.
157. **Garg, A., Bonanome, A., Grundy, S. M., Unger, R. H., Breslau, N. A., and Pak, C. Y. C.,** Effects of dietary carbohydrates on metabolism of calcium and other minerals in normal subjects and patients with non-insulin-dependent diabetes mellitus, *J. Clin. Endocrinol. Metab.,* 70, 1007, 1990.
158. **Brand, J. C., Colagiuri, S., Crossman, S., Allen, A., Roberts, D. C. K., and Truswell, A. S.,** Low glycemic index foods improve long-term glycemic control in NIDDM, *Diabetes Care,* 14, 95, 1991.
159. **Anderson, J. W. and Bryant, C. A.,** Dietary fiber: diabetes and obesity, *Am. J. Gastroenterol.,* 81, 898, 1986.
160. **Anderson, J. W.,** Dietary fiber in nutrition management of diabetes, in *Dietary Fiber (Basic and Clinical Aspects),* Vahouny, G. V. and Kritchevsky, D., Eds., Plenum Press, New York, 1986, 343.
161. **Anderson, J. W.,** Nutrition management of diabetes mellitus, in *Modern Nutrition in Health and Disease,* 3rd ed., Shils, M. E. and Young, V. R., Eds., Lea and Febiger, Philadelphia, 1988.
162. **Nestel, P. J., Nolan, C., Bazelmans, J., and Cook, R.,** Effects of a high-starch diet with low or high fiber content on postabsorptive glucose utilization and glucose production in normal subjects, *Diabetes Care,* 7, 207, 1984.
163. **Anderson, J. W., Deakins, D. A., Floore, T. L., Smith, B. M., and Whitis, S. E.,** Dietary fiber and coronary heart disease, *CRC Crit. Rev. Food Sci. Nutr.,* 29, 95, 1990.
164. **Fukagawa, N. K., Anderson, J. W., Hageman, G., Young, V. R., and Minaker, K. L.,** High carbohydrate, high fiber diets increase peripheral insulin sensitivity in healthy young and old adults, *Am. J. Clin. Nutr.,* 52, 524, 1990.
165. **Nestler, J. E., Barlascini, C. O., Clore, J. N., and Blackard, W. G.,** Absorption characteristic of breakfast determines insulin sensitivity and carbohydrate tolerance for lunch, *Diabetes Care,* 11, 755, 1988.
166. **Trinick, T. R., Laker, M. F., Johnston, D. G., Keir, M., Buchanan, K. D., and Alberti, K. G. M. M.,** Effect of guar on second-meal glucose tolerance in normal man, *Clin. Sci.,* 71, 49, 1986.
167. **Sundell, I. B., Hallmans, G., Nilsson, T. K., and Nygren, C.,** Plasma glucose and insulin, urinary catecholamine and cortisol responses to test breakfasts with high or low fiber content: the importance of the previous diet, *Ann. Nutr. Metab.,* 33, 333, 1989.
168. **Huupponen, R., Karhuvaara, S., and Seppala, P.,** Effect of guar gum on glipizide absorption in man, *Eur. J. Clin. Pharmacol.,* 28, 717, 1985.
169. **Huupponen, R.,** The effect of guar gum on the acute metabolic response to glyburide, *Res. Commun. Chem. Pathol. Pharmacol.,* 54, 137, 1986.
170. **Miller, D. L., Miller, P. F., and Dekker, J. J.,** Small bowel obstruction from bran cereal, *JAMA,* 263, 813, 1990.
171. **Anderson, J. W.,** Nutrition Management of Metabolic Conditions. HCF Diabetes Research Foundation, Lexington, KY, 1981.
172. **Hockaday, T. D. R.,** Fibre in the management of diabetes. I. Natural fibre useful as part of total dietary prescription, *Br. Med. J.,* 300, 1334, 1990.
173. **Tattersall, R. and Mansell, P.,** Fibre in the management of diabetes. II. Benefits of fibre itself are uncertain, *Br. Med. J.,* 300, 1336, 1990.
174. **Anderson, J. W. and Bridges, S. R.,** Short-chain fatty acid fermentation products of plant fiber affect glucose metabolism of isolated rat hepatocytes, *Proc. Soc. Esp. Biol. Med.,* 177, 372, 1984.
175. **Akanji, A. O., Peterson, D. B., Humphreys, S., and Hockaday, T. D. R.,** Change in plasma acetate levels in diabetic subjects on mixed high fiber diets, *Am. J. Gastroenterol.,* 84, 1365, 1989.

176. **Ciavarella, A., Gianfranco, D. M., Stefoni, S., Borgnino, L. C., and Vannini, P.,** Reduced albuminuria after dietary protein restriction in insulin-dependent diabetic patients with clinical nephropathy, *Diabetes Care,* 10, 407, 1987.
177. American Heart Association, Position statement. Dietary guidelines for healthy American adults, *Circulation,* 77, 721A, 1988.
178. **Rivellese, A. A., Giacco, R., Genovese, S., Patti, L., Marotta, G., Pacioni, D., Annuzzi, G., and Riccardi, G.,** Effects of changing amount of carbohydrate in diet on plasma lipoproteins and apoproteins in type II diabetic patients, *Diabetes Care,* 13, 446, 1990.
179. **Anderson, J. W. and Akanji, A. O.,** Dietary fiber — an overview, *Diabetes Care,* 14, 1126, 1991.

Chapter 7.4

GALLSTONES

Kenneth W. Heaton

CURRENT DIETARY THEORIES

Theories which currently have credibility attribute gallstones to excess calories (overnutrition), to a fiber-depleted diet, and to high cholesterol intake. The arguments for and against these theories have been set out in full elsewhere.[1] If, as seems likely, fiber-depleted foods encourage overnutrition or even make it inevitable, then they may be considered as responsible, at least in part, for gallstones via overnutrition as well as by more specific mechanisms.

One speculative mechanism is via *hyperinsulinemia*. Fiber-depleted sugar generally evokes greater insulin responses than naturally sweet food;[2,3] insulin promotes hepatic cholesterol synthesis *in vitro*;[4] patients with gallstones tend to have fasting hyperinsulinemia.[5,6] More direct evidence is lacking.

The best established mechanism linking fiber-depleted diets and gallstones is via increased formation and/or absorption of deoxycholic acid from the colon (see below).

LESSONS FROM EPIDEMIOLOGY

Prevalence figures for gallstones in different communities are only just becoming available through ultrasonographic surveys and it is not yet possible to make valid statistical comparisons of dietary intake and gallstone prevalence. However, autopsy surveys and clinical experience strongly suggest that gallstones are rare in primitive, rural communities and are most common in urban, Westernized societies.[7,8]

Increasing prevalence of cholesterol-rich gallstones and decreasing prevalence of pigment-rich stones has been well documented in Japan.[9] British vegetarians have half the expected prevalence of gallstones.[10]

ASSOCIATED DISEASES AND METABOLIC DISTURBANCES (TABLE 1)

Statistically supported associations are given in Table 1. Of the seven associated disorders, six have been plausibly linked with fiber-depleted foods. Other important risk factors for gallstones are age, sex, and parity.[12]

CASE-CONTROL STUDIES

Only a few case-control studies have been methodologically sound and have included dietary fiber or fiber-rich food (Table 2). Of the six studies in which vegetable intake was measured, four showed them to have a protective effect and the two which failed to do so were the smallest. This is consistent with the finding of fewer than expected gallstones in vegetarians.[10] Case-control studies have not shown any differences in cereal fiber intake, but this may be due to lack of variation in the populations studied. Two studies showed a protective effect from beans but, paradoxically, a high intake of beans has been found to make gallbladder bile more saturated with cholesterol.[29]

TABLE 1
Diseases and Metabolic Disturbances Statistically Associated with Gallstones and Increased Cholesterol Saturation of Bile

Definite	Probable
Obesity[11]	Low plasma HDL cholesterol[16,17]
Diabetes[12] (especially type 2[13])	Hiatus hernia[18]
Hypertriglyceridemia[14]	Diverticular disease[19]
Ileal resection and disease[15]	

TABLE 2
Case-Control Studies of Dietary Fiber and Gallstones

Authors and city	Number of cases — controls	Findings with respect to fiber, fiber-rich food
Scragg et al., Adelaide[20]	267 — 241	Fiber protective only on controlling for fat or energy
Alessandrini et al., Rome[21]	160 — 160	Cases ate less fruit and vegetable fiber, no difference in cereal fiber
Attili et al., Rome[22]	60 — 917 (women)	No difference in fruit and vegetable
Attili et al., Rome[23]	64 — 1,081 (men)	No difference in fruit and vegetable
Pixley and Mann, Oxford[24]	121 — 121	No difference in fiber
Thijs and Knipschild, Limburg[25]	204 — 615	"Beans and legumes" protective
Pastides et al., Athens[26]	84 — 171	Vegetables protective
MacLure et al.,[a] Boston[27]	612 — 88,225	Vegetables, especially beans, protective after controlling for weight, energy, and alcohol
Diehl et al., San Antonio[28]	108 — 1,135	High fiber intake increased risk in men but not in women

[a] Prospective study.

Two studies have incriminated fiber-depleted sugar.[20,21] The others have failed to do so but have mostly been smaller studies.

DEOXYCHOLIC ACID AND THE CHOLESTEROL SATURATION OF BILE

There is much evidence to incriminate deoxycholic acid (DCA) as a risk factor for bile supersaturated with cholesterol and hence for gallstones.[30]

There are two ways in which DCA may increase the cholesterol content of bile. First, being the most detergent of the major bile acids, DCA leaches out large amounts of cholesterol from the liver cell as it is being secreted into bile.[31] Second, DCA displaces chenodeoxycholic acid from the bile (either by competing with it for intestinal absorption or by suppressing its synthesis).

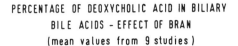

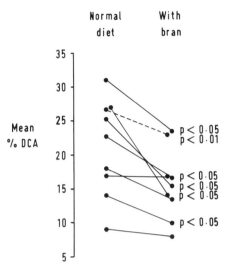

FIGURE 1. Summary of published studies on the effect of wheat bran on the percentage of deoxycholic acid in the bile acid pool. Each line represents the results from one study, and each point is a mean value for a group of subjects.[32]

EFFECTS OF WHEAT BRAN AND OF FIBER-RICH DIET ON BILE COMPOSITION

Figure 1 shows the effects of wheat bran on the DCA content and Figure 2 on the cholesterol saturation of bile.

Lactulose also reduces bile DCA and cholesterol saturation.[32] Lactulose is known to lower the pH in the cecum[33] to a point where the bacterial 7α-dehydroxylase which produces DCA from cholic acid is inhibited.[34] This suggests that bran, which is partly fermented, may act in the same way. However, there are other possibilities listed in Table 3.

The effects of a naturally fiber-rich diet, that is one low in refined sugars as well as rich in full-fiber foods, have been studied by Thornton et al.[39] The cholesterol saturation index of bile averaged 1.50 on a fiber-depleted diet and 1.20 on the full-fiber diet. There was little change in the deoxycholate content of bile, so it was not thought that full-fiber foods exerted benefit via the "bran effect". We speculated that benefit was due to the drastic reduction in the intake of refined sugars (from 106 to 6 g/d).[39] However, in a subsequent 6-week crossover study comparing two diets closely similar except for their sucrose contents (112 and 16 g/d, respectively), there was no difference in the bile saturation index.[40] Thus, the beneficial effect of the full-fiber diet is still unexplained.

ANIMAL EXPERIMENTS

No animal experiments have been reported which were designed to test the hypothesis that fiber-depleted food favors gallstone formation. However, many lithogenic dietary regimes have been reported, and while the diets vary widely, they have one feature in common — they are all semisynthetic or semipurified. In practice this means that their carbohydrate

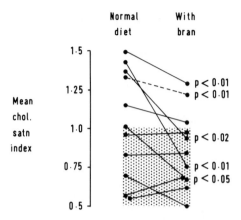

FIGURE 2. Summary of published studies on the effect of wheat bran on the cholesterol saturation index of gallbladder bile (aspirated from the duodenum). Each line represents the results from one study, and each point is a mean value for a group of subjects. If the index is over 1.0, the bile is theoretically supersaturated and liable to precipitate cholesterol crystals.[32]

TABLE 3
Possible Mechanisms Whereby Bran Reduces the DCA Content of Bile

Mechanism	By analogy with
Adsorption of DCA, preventing absorption	Lignin, other residues[35,36]
Fermentation of short-chain fatty acids leading to lower pH in colon, hence:	
Precipitation of DCA	
Reduced formation of DCA (inhibited dehydroxylation)[35]	Lactulose[33]
Rapid transit, reducing absorption	Senokot[38]

component is always in refined or fiber-depleted form, usually glucose or sucrose, but sometimes corn starch. The idea that lack of fiber explains the lithogenicity of these diets is supported by the fact that the diet loses its lithogenic effect if it is supplemented with lignin, with bulking agents such as agar and carboxymethyl cellulose, or even if the animal is allowed to eat the straw laid on the floor of its cage.

CONCLUSIONS

Experimental work suggests that a low intake of wheat bran or similar cereal fiber should promote gallstones. Epidemiological studies have provided no support for this idea but suggest that a low intake of vegetables is probably important and a high intake of sugar may be so. It is not clear how any protective effect of vegetables is mediated. If fiber-depleted foods promote obesity, then they promote gallstones through this means, and, if such foods cause hyperinsulinemia, this may be another way in which they favor gallstones.

REFERENCES

1. **Heaton, K. W.,** The role of diet in the aetiology of cholelithiasis, *Rev. Clin. Nutr.,* 54, 549, 1984.
2. **Haber, G. B., Heaton, K. W., Murphy, D., and Burroughs, L.,** Depletion and disruption of dietary fibre. Effects of satiety, plasma-glucose, and serum-insulin, *Lancet,* ii, 679, 1977.
3. **Bolton, R. P., Heaton, K. W., and Burroughs, L. F.,** The role of dietary fiber in satiety, glucose, and insulin: studies with fruit and fruit juice, *Am. J. Clin. Nutr.,* 34, 211, 1981.
4. **Neprokoeff, C. M., Lakshmanan, M. R., Ness, G. C., Dugan, R. E., and Porter, J. W.,** *Arch. Biochem. Biophys.,* 160, 387, 1974.
5. **Scragg, R. K. R., Calvert, G. D., and Oliver, J. R.,** The role of plasma lipids and insulin in gallstone disease, *Br. Med. J.,* 289, 521, 1984.
6. **Heaton, K. W., Braddon, F. E. M., Emmett, P. M., Mountford, R. A., Hughes, A. O., Bolton, C. H., and Ghosh, S.,** Why do men get gallstones? Roles of abdominal fat and hyperinsulinaemia, *Eur. J. Gastroenterol. Hepatol.,* 3, 745, 1991.
7. **Heaton, K. W.,** Gallstones, in *Western Diseases: Their Emergence and Prevention,* Trowell H. C. and Burkitt, D. P., Eds., Edward Arnold, London, 1981, 47.
8. **Acalovschi, M., Dumitrascu, D., Caluser, I., and Ban, A.,** Comparative prevalence of gallstone disease at 100-year interval in a large Romanian town, a necropsy study, *Dig. Dis. Sci.,* 32, 354, 1987.
9. **Kameda, H.,** Gallstones, compositions, structural characteristics and geographical distribution, in *Proceedings of 3rd World Congress of Gastroenterology, Tokyo 1966,* Vol. 4, S. Karger, Basel, 1967, 117.
10. **Pixley, F., Wilson, D., McPherson, K., and Mann, J.,** Effect of vegetarianism on development of gallstones in women, *Br. Med. J.,* 291, 11, 1985.
11. **Bennion, L. J. and Grundy, S. M.,** Effects of obesity and caloric intake on biliary lipid metabolism in man, *J. Clin. Invest.,* 56, 996, 1975.
12. **Bennion, L. J. and Grundy, S. M.,** Risk factors for the development of cholelithiasis in man, *New Engl. J. Med.,* 299, 1161, 1978.
13. **Haber, G. B. and Heaton, K. W.,** Lipid composition of bile in diabetics and obesity-matched controls, *Gut,* 20, 518, 1979.
14. **Ahlberg, J., Angelin, B., Einarsson, K., Hellstrom, K., and Leijd, B.,** Biliary lipid composition in normo- and hyperlipoproteinemia, *Gastroenterology,* 79, 90, 1980.
15. **Heaton, K. W. and Read, A. E.,** Gallstones in patients with disorders of the terminal ileum and disturbed bile salt metabolism, *Br. Med. J.,* 3, 494, 1969.
16. **Petitti, D. B., Friedman, G. D., and Klatsky, A. L.,** Association of a history of gallbladder disease with a reduced concentration of high-density-lipoprotein cholesterol, *N. Engl J. Med.,* 304, 1396, 1981.
17. **Thornton, J. R., Heaton, K. W., and Macfarlane, D. G.,** A relation between high-density-lipoprotein cholesterol and bile cholesterol saturation, *Br. Med. J.,* 283, 1352, 1981.
18. **Capron, J.-P., Payenneville, H., Dumont, M., Dupas, J.-L., and Lorriaux, A.,** Evidence for an association between cholelithiasis and hiatus hernia, *Lancet,* 2, 329, 1978.
19. **Capron, J.-P., Piperaud, R., Dupas, J.-L., Delamarre, J., and Lorriaux, A.,** Evidence for an association between cholelithiasis and diverticular disease of the colon: a case controlled study, *Dig. Dis. Sci.,* 26, 523, 1981.
20. **Scragg, R. K. R., McMichael, A. J., and Baghurst, P. A.,** Diet, alcohol, and relative weight in gallstone disease: a case-control study, *Br. Med. J.,* 288, 1113, 1984.
21. **Alessandrini, A., Fusco, M. A., Gatti, E., and Rossi, P. A.,** Dietary fibres and cholesterol gallstones: a case-control study, *Ital. J. Gastroenterol.,* 14, 156, 1982.
22. **Attili, A. F. and the GREPCO Group,** Dietary habits and cholelithiasis, in *Epidemiology and Prevention of Gallstone Disease,* Capocaccia, L., Ricci, G., Angelico, F., Angelico, M., and Attili, A. F., Eds., MTP Press, Lancaster, 1984, 175.
23. **Attili, A. F. and the Rome Group for the Epidemiology and Prevention of Cholelithiasis (GREPCO),** Diet and gallstones: result of an epidemiologic study performed in male civil servants, in *Nutrition in Gastrointestinal Disease,* Barbara, L., Bianchi Porro, G., Cheli, R., and Lipkin, M., Eds., Raven Press, New York, 1987, 225.
24. **Pixley, F. and Mann, J.,** Dietary factors in the aetiology of gallstones: a case-control study, *Gut,* 29, 1511, 1988.
25. **Thijs, C. and Knipschild, P.,** Legume intake and gallstone risk: results from a case-control study, *Int. J. Epidemiol.,* 19, 660, 1990.
26. **Pastides, H., Tzonou, A., Trichopoulos, D., et al.,** A case-control study of the relationship between smoking, diet, and gallbladder disease, *Arch. Intern. Med.,* 150, 1409, 1990.
27. **MacLure, K. M., Hayes, K. C., Colditz, G. A., Stampfer, M. J., and Willett, W. C.,** Dietary predictors of symptom-associated gallstones in middle-aged women, *Am. J. Clin. Nutr.,* 52, 916, 1990.

28. **Diehl, A. K., Haffner, S. M., Knapp, J. A., Hazuda, H. P., and Stern, M. P.,** Dietary intake and the prevalence of gallbladder disease in Mexican Americans, *Gastroenterology,* 97, 1527, 1989.
29. **Nervi, F., Covarrubias, C., Bravo, P., et al.,** Influence of legume intake on biliary lipids and cholesterol saturation in young Chilean men. Identification of a dietary risk factor for cholesterol gallstone formation in a highly prevalent area, *Gastroenterology,* 96, 825, 1989.
30. **Marcus, S. N. and Heaton, K. W.,** Deoxycholic acid and the pathogenesis of gallstones, *Gut,* 29, 522, 1988.
31. **Carulli, N., Loria, P., Bertolotti, M., Ponz de Leon, M., Menozzi, D., Medici, G., and Piccagli, I.,** Effects of acute changes of bile acid pool composition on biliary lipid secretion, *J. Clin. Invest.,* 74, 614, 1985.
32. **Heaton, K. W.,** Effect of dietary fiber on biliary lipids, in *Nutrition in Gastrointestinal Disease,* Barbara, L., Bianchiforro, G., Cheli, R., and Lipkin, M., Eds., Raven Press, New York, 1987, 213.
33. **Thornton, J. R. and Heaton, K. W.,** Do colonic bacteria contribute to cholesterol gallstone formation? Effects of lactulose on bile, *Br. Med. J.,* 282, 1018, 1981.
34. **Bown, R. L., Gibson, J. A., Sladen, G. E., Hicks, B., and Dawson, A. M.,** Effects of lactulose and other laxatives on ileal and colonic pH as measured by a radiotelemetry device, *Gut,* 15, 999, 1974.
35. **MacDonald, I. A., Singh, G., Mahony, D. E., and Meier, C. E.,** Effect of pH on bile salt degradation by mixed fecal cultures, *Steroids,* 32, 245, 1978.
36. **Eastwood, M. A. and Hamilton, D.,** Studies on the adsorption of bile salts to non-absorbed components of diet, *Biochem. Biophys. Acta,* 152, 165, 1968.
37. **Story, J. A. and Kritchevsky, D.,** Comparison of the binding of various bile acids and bile salts in vitro by several types of fiber, *J. Nutr.,* 106, 1292, 1976.
38. **Marcus, S. N. and Heaton, K. W.,** Intestinal transit, deoxycholic acid and the cholesterol saturation of bile — three inter-related factors, *Gut,* 27, 550, 1986.
39. **Thornton, J. R., Emmett, P. M., and Heaton, K. W.,** Diet and gall stones: effects of refined and unrefined carbohydrate diets on bile cholesterol saturation and bile acid metabolism, *Gut,* 24, 2, 1983.
40. **Werner, D., Emmett, P. M., and Heaton, K. W.,** Effects of dietary sucrose on factors influencing cholesterol gallstone formation, *Gut,* 25, 269, 1984.

Chapter 7.5

HUMAN EPIDEMIOLOGICAL STUDIES ON DIETARY FIBER AND COLON CANCER

Hugh J. Freeman

ORIGIN OF THE FIBER HYPOTHESIS IN COLON CANCER

The possible role of dietary fiber in human colon cancer pathogenesis became of particular interest following epidemiologic studies in different populations; colon cancer was observed to be uncommon in many developing countries but relatively common among age-matched inhabitants of most Western nations. In large part, the hypothesis that fiber consumption may prevent subsequent colon cancer development appears to have emerged subsequent to the report by Higginson and Oettle[1] on studies in the Bantu of rural South Africa. Malhotra[2] subsequently found a low incidence of colon cancer in northern India, where the usual diet apparently contains large amounts of cellulose fiber, and a high incidence of colon cancer in southern India, where the usual diet contains less cellulose. Later, the fiber hypothesis was widely popularized by Burkitt and colleagues,[3-5] and the possible role of fiber in the prevention of the disease was emphasized.

FIBER STUDIES IN HUMANS

Following the development of the fiber hypothesis, a number of epidemiologic reports appeared either supporting or refuting the importance of dietary fiber in colon cancer pathogenesis. A case-control study from Israel[6] described a highly significant inverse correlation between colon cancer and ingestion of certain fiber-containing foods. Interviewers were not aware of which patients had histologically confirmed malignant disease of the large bowel. Black patients from the San Francisco[7] Bay area reported less frequent consumption of foods containing 0.5% fiber, although methods used to determine fiber content were not indicated. A report by Graham and associates[8] suggested that the frequency of ingestion of certain vegetables, especially cabbage, sprouts, and broccoli, but not beef or other meats, was less in white males with an increased colon cancer incidence.

Certain groups of Inuit in the Canadian Arctic, however, are not unusually prone to colon cancer despite a diet low in plant fiber,[9] yet the Inuit eat large amounts of animal connective tissues composed of apparently nondigestible aminopolysaccharides.[10] Although this dietary characteristic is thought to be shared with certain African tribes, the role of these dietary substances, if any, in the pathogenesis of colon cancer is unknown. Seventh-Day Adventists in Loma Linda, CA are reported to eat vegetarian diets[11] and to have a low incidence of colon cancer.[12] However, other malignant diseases also occur at a low incidence in this group, and precise measurements of the content of individual fiber polymers in their diets are still needed.

Some international and in-country studies were also performed soon after this hypothesis was developed. In one, no correlation between crude dietary fiber consumption and colon cancer mortality was observed.[13] In another, cereal consumption appeared to be negatively correlated with colon cancer incidence data.[14] In a report from the U.K., differences in dietary fiber consumption within that country were correlated with its apparent protective role in colon carcinogenesis.[15]

Haenszel and colleagues[16] found a significant positive association between colon cancer and the frequency of ingestion of fiber-containing legumes in Hawaiian Japanese.* However, no other quantitative data were provided. In another study from Japan, cabbage was reported to be protective.[17] Graham and Mettlin,[18] on the other hand, drew attention to studies showing a protective role for vegetable intake, especially cruciferous vegetables rich in indoles. Similar observations supporting a possible protective role for vegetables were also previously noted.[19] While it was difficult to conduct studies on the basis of retrospective dietary histories dependent on respondent recall, discrepancies that emerged may have also reflected inadequate definition of the precise dietary fiber composition of foods ingested by the different groups.

Other earlier studies from Europe[20,21] further attempted to examine the fiber question from this perspective. Using the Southgate method, diets from population samples in an area with a low incidence of colon cancer (Kuopio, Finland) and an area with a high incidence (Copenhagen) were analyzed. Although the proportions of dietary fiber polymers were similar, the mean intakes of total dietary fiber as well as specific fiber polymers (cellulose and lignin) were significantly less in Copenhagen. Although preliminary, measured intakes of specific fiber polymers were documented for the first time and differed in human populations with different incidence rates of colon carcinoma.

RECENT STUDIES AND FUTURE DIRECTIONS

These studies served to stimulate considerable interest in the role of dietary fiber in colon cancer pathogenesis. Indeed, during the past decade, a large number of epidemiologic studies have appeared in the literature (Table 1); these now include case-control studies, international and within-country correlation studies, cohort studies, and time-trend studies concerning colon cancer and fiber, vegetables, grains, or fruit. Most have provided evidence for a protective effect while some have revealed only equivocal results or no evidence for a protective effect of fiber in colon cancer. Still, however, further investigations are needed, possibly using specific fiber polymers in long-term prospective studies. Other issues need to be addressed. These early studies have now helped to define a number of variables (Table 2) for future studies that may be very important in definition of the role of dietary fiber in colon cancer. Particular emphasis, perhaps, should be placed on prevention studies in patients with colonic disorders, such as inflammatory bowel disease and colon polyp syndromes, that predispose to colon cancer.

---

* The legumes mentioned here were mostly string beans and were associated with a high beef diet. They should not be confused with red beans, lentils, and related food products consumed as seeds. The authors mention that "beef was the only meat that yielded a significantly elevated risk". In addition, the type of starchy food consumed appeared to be from highly refined foods (macaroni, poi, white rice). A careful review of this paper seems to show a diet extremely low in cereal or red-type bean fiber.

TABLE 1
Recent Studies on Fiber in Colon Cancer

Author, year	Ref.
Evidence for Protective Effect	
Tuyns, 1986	22
Manousos et al., 1983	23
Macquart-Moulin et al., 1986	24
Kune et al., 1987	25
Slattery et al., 1988	26
Young and Wolf, 1988	27
La Vecchia et al., 1988	28
Graham et al., 1988	29
Lyon et al., 1987	30
Bristol et al., 1985	31
McKeown-Eyssen, 1984	32
Bingham et al., 1985	33
Rosen et al., 1988	34
Helms et al., 1982	35
Hirayama, 1981	36
Tuyns et al., 1988	37
Heilbrun et al., 1989	38
West et al., 1989	39
Lee et al., 1989	40
Freudenheim et al., 1990	41
Trock et al., 1990	42[a]
Equivocal or Lack of Protective Effect	
Martinez et al., 1981	43
Pickle et al., 1984	44
Rozen et al., 1981	45
Jensen, 1983	46
Boing et al., 1985	47
Phillips et al., 1985	48
Tajima et al., 1985	49
Powles et al., 1984	50
Tajima et al., 1985	51
Potter and McMichael, 1986	52
Miller et al., 1983	53
Willett et al., 1990	54

[a] Meta-analyses of other published studies.

TABLE 2
Variables for Future Fiber Studies

Dietary factors
    Individual fiber components (cellulose, pectins, etc.)
    Fiber-macronutrient interactions (fat, protein, etc.)
    Fiber-micronutrient interactions (trace elements, vitamins, etc.)
    Digestion products of fiber (short chain fatty acids, etc.)
    Source of dietary fiber components (grains, vegetables, etc.)

Patient or population factors
    Sex and age
    Geographic locale
    Genetic variables (Blood type, HLA type, etc.)
    Environmental variables (smoking, etc.)
    Medications for treatment (antibiotics, ulcer drugs)
    Medications for prophylaxis (aspirin, vitamin C)

Colonic factors
    Colonic site-specific effects (e.g., cecal vs. rectosigmoid)
    Preneoplastic disorders (ulcerative colitis, Crohn's disease)
    Other colonic neoplastic disorders (colon polyps, polyposis)
    Underlying gastrointestinal or other diseases (diabetes, etc.)

REFERENCES

1. **Higginson, J. and Oettle, A. G.**, Cancer incidence in Bantu and "Cape coloured" races of South Africa. Report of a cancer survey of the Transvaal (1953–1955), *J. Natl. Cancer Inst.*, 24, 589, 1960.
2. **Malhotra, S. L.**, Geographical distribution of gastrointestinal cancers in India with special reference to causation, *Gut*, 8, 361, 1967.
3. **Burkitt, D. P.**, Epidemiology of cancer of the colon and rectum, *Cancer*, 28, 1971.
4. **Burkitt, D. P., Walker, A. R. P., and Painter, N. S.**, Effect of dietary fiber on stools and transit-times, and its role in the causation of disease, *Lancet*, 2, 1408, 1972.
5. **Walker, A. R. P. and Burkitt, D. P.**, Colonic cancer — hypothesis of causation, dietary prophylaxis, and future research, *Am. J. Dig. Dis.*, 21, 910, 1976.
6. **Modan, B., Barell, V., Lubin, F., Modan, M., Greenberg, R. A., and Graham, S.**, Low-fiber intake as an etiologic factor in cancer of the colon, *J. Natl. Cancer Inst.*, 55, 15, 1975.
7. **Dales, L. G., Friedman, G. D., Ury, H. K., Grossman, S., and Williams, S. R.**, A case-control study of relationships of diet and other traits to colorectal cancer in American blacks, *Am. J. Epidemiol.*, 10, 132, 1979.
8. **Graham, S., Dayal, H., Swanson, M., Mittelman, A., and Wilkinson, G.**, Diet in the epidemiology of cancer of the colon and rectum, *J. Natl. Cancer Inst.*, 61, 709, 1978.
9. **Schaefer, O.**, Medical observations and problems in the Canadian Arctic. II. Nutrition and Nutritional deficiencies, *Can. Med. Assoc. J.*, 81, 396, 1959.
10. **Trowell, H., Godding, E., and Spiller, G.**, Fiber bibliographies and terminology, *Am. J. Clin. Nutr.*, 31, 1489, 1978.
11. **Goldin, B. and Gorbach, S. L.**, Colon cancer connection: beef bran, bile and bacteria, *Viewpoints Dig. Dis.*, 10, 3, 1978.
12. **Lemon, F. R., Walden, R. T., and Woods, R. W.**, Cancer of the lung and mouth in Seventh-Day Adventists. Preliminary report on a population study, *Cancer*, 17, 486, 1964.
13. **Draser, B. S. and Irving, D.**, Environmental factors in cancer of the colon and breast, *Br. J. Cancer*, 27, 167, 1973.
14. **Armstrong, B. and Doll, R.**, Environmental factors in cancer incidence and mortality in different countires, with special reference to dietary practices, *Int. J. Cancer.*, 15, 617, 1975.

15. **Bingham, S., Williams, D. R. R., Cole, T. F., and James, W. P. T.,** Dietary fibre and regional large bowel cancer mortality in Britain, *Br. J. Cancer,* 40, 456, 1979.
16. **Haenszel, W., Berg, J. W., Segi, M., Kurihara, M., and Locke, F. B.,** Large-bowel cancer in Hawaiian Japanese, *J. Natl. Cancer Inst.,* 51, 1765, 1973.
17. **Haenszel, W., Locke, F. B., and Segi, M.,** A case control study of large bowel cancer in Japan, *J. Natl. Cancer Inst.,* 64, 17, 1980.
18. **Graham, S. M. and Mettlin, C.,** Diet and colon cancer, *Am. J. Epidemiol.,* 109, 1, 1979.
19. **Stocks, P. and Karn, M. K.,** A cooperative study of the habits, home life, dietary and family histories of 450 cancer patients and an equal number of control patients, *Ann. Eugen.,* 5, 237, 1933.
20. **International Agency for Research on Cancer, Intestinal Microecology Group,** Dietary fibre, transit-time, faecal bacteria steroids, and colon cancer in two Scandinavian populations, *Lancet,* 2, 207, 1977.
21. **Jensen, O. M., MacLennan, R., Wahrendorff, J., and IARC, Large Bowel Cancer Group,** Large bowel cancer in Scandinavia in relation to diet and faecal characteristics, *Nutr. Cancer,* 4, 5, 1982.
22. **Tuyns, A. J.,** A case-control study on colorectal cancer in Belgium, *Soz. Praventivemed.,* 31, 81, 1986.
23. **Manousos, O. Day, N. E., and Trichopoulos, D.,** Diet and colorectal cancer: a case-control study in Greece, *Int. J. Cancer.,* 32, 1, 1983.
24. **Macquart-Moulin, G., Riboli, E., Cornee, J., Charnay, B., Berthezene, P., and Day, N.,** Case-control study on colorectal cancer and diet in Marseilles, *Int. J. Cancer,* 38, 183, 1986.
25. **Kune, S., Kune, G. A., and Watson, L. F.,** Case-control study of dietary etiological factors: the Melbourne colorectal cancer study, *Nutr. Cancer,* 9, 21, 1987.
26. **Slattery, M. L., Sorenson, A. W., Mahoney, A. W., French, T. K., Kritchevsky, D., and Street, J. C.,** Diet and colon cancer: assessment of risk by fiber type and food source (published erratum appears in *J. Natl. Cancer Inst.,* 81, 1042, 1989), *J. Natl. Cancer Inst.,* 80, 1474, 1988.
27. **Young, T. B. and Wolf, D. A.,** Case-control study of proximal and distal colon cancer and diet in Wisconsin, *Int. J. Cancer,* 42, 167, 1988.
28. **La Vecchia, C., Negri, E., and Decarli, A.,** A case-control study of diet and colorectal cancer in northern Italy, *Int. J. Cancer,* 41, 492, 1988.
29. **Graham, S., Marshall, J., Haughey, B., Mittelman, A., Swanson, M., Zielezny, M., Byers, T., Wilkinson, G., and West, D.,** Dietary epidemiology of cancer of the colon in western New York, *Am. J. Epidemiol.,* 128, 490, 1988.
30. **Lyon, J. L., Mahoney, A. W., West, D. W., Gardner, J. W., Smith, K. R., Sorenson, A. W., and Stanish, W.,** Energy intake: its relationship to colon cancer risk, *J. Natl. Cancer Inst.,* 78, 853, 1987.
31. **Bristol, J. B., Emmett, P. M., and Heaton, K. W.,** Sugar, fat and the risk of colorectal cancer, *Br. Med. J.,* 291, 1467, 1985.
32. **McKeown-Eyssen, G. E. and Bright-See, E.,** Dietary factors in colon cancer: international relationships. An update, *Nutr. Cancer,* 6, 160, 1984.
33. **Bingham, S. A., Williams, D. R. R., and Cummings, J. H.,** Dietary fibre consumption in Britain: new estimates and their relation to large bowel cancer mortality, *Br. J. Cancer,* 52, 399, 1985.
34. **Rosen, M., Nystrom, L., and Wall, S.,** Diet and cancer mortality in the counties of Sweden, *Am. J. Epidemiol.,* 127, 42, 1988.
35. **Helms, P., Jorgensen, I. M., and Paerregaard, A.,** Dietary patterns in Them and Copenhagen, Denmark, *Nutr. Cancer,* 4, 34, 1982.
36. **Hirayama, T.,** A large-scale cohort study on the relationship between diet and selected cancers of digestive organs, in *Gastrointestinal Cancer: Endogenous Factors,* Bruce, W. R., Correa, P., and Lipkin, M., Eds., Cold Spring Harbor Laboratory, Cold Spring Harbor, NY, 1981, 409.
37. **Tuyns, A. J., Kaaks, R., and Haelterman, M.,** Colorectal cancer and the consumption of foods: a case-control study in Belgium, *Nutr. Cancer,* 11, 189, 1988.
38. **Heilbrun, L. K., Nomura, A., Hankin, J. H., and Stemmermann, D. N.,** Diet and colorectal cancer with special reference to fiber intake, *Int. J. Cancer,* 44, 1, 1989.
39. **West, D. W., Slattery, M. L., Robison, L. M., Schuman, K. L., Ford, M. H., Mahoney, A. W., Lyon, J. L., and Sorensen, A. W.,** Dietary intake and colon cancer: sex- and anatomic site-specific associations, *Am. J. Epidemiol.,* 130, 883, 1989.
40. **Lee, H. P., Gourley, L., Duffy, S. W., Estieve, J., Lee, J., and Day, N. E.,** Colorectal cancer and diet in an Asian population — a case-control study among Singapore Chinese, *Int. J. Cancer,* 43, 1007, 1989.
41. **Freudenheim, J. L., Graham, S., Horvath, P. J., Marshall, J. R., Haughey, B. P., and Wilkinson, G.,** Risks associated with source of fiber and fiber components in cancer of the colon and rectum, *Cancer Res.,* 50, 3295, 1990.
42. **Trock, B., Lanza, E., and Greenwald, P.,** Dietary fiber, vegetables, and colon cancer: critical review and meta-analyses of the epidemiologic evidence, *J. Natl. Cancer Inst.,* 82, 650, 1990.

43. **Martinez, I., Torres, R., and Frias, Z.,** Factors asscoiated with adenocarcinomas of the large bowel in Puerto Rico, *Rev. Latinoam. Oncol. Clin.,* 13, 13, 1981.
44. **Pickle, L. W., Greene, M. H., and Ziegler, R. G.,** Colorectal cancer in rural Nebraska, *Cancer Res.,* 44, 363, 1984.
45. **Rozen, P., Hellerstein, S. M., and Horwitz, C.,** The low incidence of colorectal cancer in a "high-risk" population: its correlation with dietary habits, *Cancer,* 48, 2692, 1981.
46. **Jensen, O. M.,** Cancer risk among Danish male Seventh-Day Adventists and other temperance society members, *J. Natl. Cancer Inst.,* 70, 1011, 1983.
47. **Boing, H., Martinez, L., and Frentzel-Beyme, R.,** Regional nutritional pattern of cancer mortality in the Federal Republic of Germany, *Nutr. Cancer,* 7, 121, 1985.
48. **Phillips, R. L. and Snowdon, D. A.,** Dietary relationships with fatal colorectal cancer among Seventh-Day Adventists, *J. Natl. Cancer Inst.,* 74, 307, 1985.
49. **Tajima, K., Hirose, K., and Nakagawa, N.,** Urban-rural difference in the trend of colo-rectal cancer mortality with special reference to the subsites of colon cancer in Japan, *Jpn. J. Cancer Res.,* 76, 717, 1985.
50. **Powles, J. W. and Williams, D. R.,** Trends in bowel cancer in selected countries in relation to wartime changes in flour milling, *Nutr. Cancer,* 6, 40, 1984.
51. **Tajima, K. and Tominaga, S.,** Dietary habits and gastro-intestinal cancers: a comparative case-control study of stomach and large intestinal cancers in Nagoya, Japan, *Jpn. J. Cancer Res.,* 76, 705, 1985.
52. **Potter, J. D. and McMichael, A. J.,** Diet and cancer of the colon and rectum: a case-control study, *J. Natl. Cancer Inst.,* 76, 557, 1986.
53. **Miller, A. B., Howe, G. R., Jain, M., Craib, K. J., and Harrison, L.,** Food items and food groups as risk factors in a case-control study of diet and colo-rectal cancer, *Int. J. Cancer.,* 32, 155, 1983.
54. **Willett, W. C., Stampfer, M. J., Colditz, G. A., Rosner, B. A., and Speizer, F. E.,** Relation of meat, fat, and fiber intake to the risk of colon cancer in a prospective study among women, *N. Engl. J. Med.,* 323, 1664, 1990.

Chapter 7.6

FIBER AND COLONIC DIVERTICULAR DISEASE

Hugh J. Freeman

Colonic diverticular disease is an acquired deformity of the colon that is generally irreversible, but usually asymptomatic.[1] In developed nations, the disorder is extremely common and prevalence correlates well with increasing age.[2] Although there are different anatomical forms of colonic diverticulosis, the basic abnormality observed in most North American and European populations is the pseudodiverticulum; this is a herniation of mucosa and submucosa through the colonic muscle wall. Most often, these are multiple and involve the left side of the colon, especially the sigmoid colon. While precise figures are not available, it has been estimated that about 20% of patients with diverticulosis will develop symptoms and signs of illness, but only a small minority will endure more serious complications including diverticulitis, sepsis, obstruction, and hemorrhage.[1,3]

Dietary fiber was recommended for symptomatic diverticular disease as early as 1929 by Spriggs.[4] Subsequently, Painter and Burkitt published their hypothesis that diverticular disease was caused by a reduced intake of dietary fiber.[5] Later, this "fiber hypothesis" was examined in carefully matched population groups from Oxford; diverticulosis was observed to be significantly more frequent in nonvegetarians compared to vegetarians.[6]

A variety of epidemiologic studies on the relationship between dietary fiber consumption and diverticular disease has been done both from a historical as well as a geographical perspective. Although it has been suggested that the prevalence of diverticular disease has increased over the past century,[7] precise analyses are not available. Barium enema, for example, remains the most common current method of diagnosis, but this technique was not available to earlier clinicians; indeed, most radiographic appearances were not described in detail until 1925.[8] Interestingly, Brodribb has cited several early autopsy studies reporting very high prevalences of diverticular disease (Graser in 1899, 64%; Sudsuki in 1900, 37.5%; and Mourges in 1913, 30%).[9] To date, therefore, historical data providing strong support for an increased prevalence of colonic diverticulosis at the present time are limited and controversial.

More interesting information comes from geographical studies. Painter and Burkitt, using a variety of anecdotal sources,[7] suggested that diverticulosis is rare in many parts of Africa, except among Europeans, uncommon in the Indian subcontinent, Middle East, Far East, and South America; all are economically developing areas with cereal-based diets typically high in fiber. This contrasts with well-developed countries in Europe and North America where diets tend to be highly refined and fiber-depleted and where a high prevalence of diverticular disease is observed. This relationship between decreasing dietary fiber and increasing prevalence of diverticular disease has also been reported in urban South African blacks[10] and Hawaiian Japanese[11] but not in the Orient, including Japan.[12] Indeed, recent studies on the distributional pattern of diverticular disease contrast the increased frequency in the left colon in Western communities compared to the right colon in Oriental populations.[13] Similar observations have been reported from Europe.[14-16] Although intriguing, the true incidence of diverticular disease in these populations is not known, in part, because of variable diagnostic methods and availability of accurate postmortem studies. In those populations with available data, it is unknown how accurately these reflect the true frequency in the population as a whole. Finally, a major weakness of such correlative studies relates to the dietary component of the equation and, specifically, methods used to precisely calculate the fiber content of the diet or specific fiber components.

Although a definitive role for fiber-deficient diets in the pathogenesis of colonic diverticulosis has not been proven, a number of uncontrolled trials suggested that added fiber in the form of bran supplements may be therapeutically beneficial.[17-19] In addition, some supportive evidence for a role for deficient dietary fiber in the pathogenesis of diverticulosis comes from animal studies. As early as 1937, Lubbock et al.[20] fed low fiber diets to rats and showed the development of diverticulae. Carlson and Hoelzel[21] found that about 57% of a colony of Wistar rats more than 100 weeks old had diverticulae in the proximal colon while only 4% of rats fed a psyllium seed supplement developed diverticulae. Similar observations have been reported in rats and rabbits, but the presence of a large cecum in these animals raises doubts regarding the applicability of these results to humans; indeed, many dietary fibers are more extensively degraded in these animals than in humans. Brodribb et al.[22] chose the stub-tailed monkey with a gastrointestinal anatomy more similar to humans as a model for colonic studies. He found that colonic intraluminal pressure increased as the amount of fiber in the diet decreased gradually from 20 to 15, 10, 5, and 0 grams per day. More recent studies in adult female vervet monkeys revealed that diverticulosis frequently developed in those administered a Western-type high fat, low fiber diet compared to diets with low fat and higher fiber content.[23] Subsequently, the role of bran was examined in five controlled trials (Table 1).[24-28] In addition, ispaghula alone[29] and methylcellulose alone[30] have been studied in controlled trials; subjective improvement was reported with ispaghula but no effect was noted with methylcellulose. It appears that a high fiber diet may be effective treatment for symptoms in some patients with uncomplicated diverticular disease, especially if symptoms are severe but the data remain limited. Moreover, the most comprehensive and best conducted study,[27] largely using patients with mild symptoms, showed no major benefit in pain scores but there was improvement in constipation.

Additional studies, especially in humans, are still required to determine if high fiber diets can alter the natural history of diverticular disease over the long term or prevent its complications. In one interesting report, Hyland and Taylor[31] described 100 patients that had been retrospectively reviewed after 5 to 7 years on a high fiber diet — over 90% had remained symptom-free.

TABLE 1
Controlled Clinical Trials of Bran in Colonic Diverticular Disease

Fiber type and form	Number of patients	Study protocol	Results	Comments	Author(s) and reference
Wheat vs. bran crispbread	18 with X-ray diagnosis	Double-blind control trial × 12 weeks	Reduced symptom pain scores early placebo effect noted	Symptoms moderate to severe; pain scores subjective	Brodribb[24]
Wheat bran (coarse) vs. ispaghula vs. lactulose	31 with X-ray diagnosis	Control trial × 4 weeks	Symptoms relieved to an equivalent extent in all groups; only bran reduced colon motility and pressures		Eastwood et al.[25]
Coarse bran vs. sterculia with or without antispasmotic	20, but diagnostic method not defined	Sterculia or bran × 4 weeks	Equivalent improvement in constipation but bran or sterculia with antispasmotic better than sterculia alone for pain relief		Srivastava et al.[26]
Bran crispbread vs. ispaghula vs. placebo (either wheat crispbread or refined wheat)	58 with X-ray diagnosis	Double-blind randomized controlled trial × 16 weeks	Pain score not improved but improvement in constipation	Pain symptoms mild in degree; near normal stool weights and transit times	Ornstein et al.[27]
Coarse bran vs. hyoscyanine vs. placebo	105 with X-ray diagnosis	Control trial up to 52 weeks	Improved symptom scale for bran and hyoscyanine	Symptom scale based on ability to work	Weinreich[28]

REFERENCES

1. **Almy, T. P. and Howell, D. A.**, Diverticular disease of the colon, *N. Engl. J. Med.*, 302, 324, 1980.
2. **Parks, T. G.**, Natural history of diverticular disease of the colon, *Clin. Gastroenterol.*, 4, 53, 1975.
3. **Hughes, L. E.**, Complications of diverticular disease: inflammation, obstruction and bleeding, *Clin. Gastroenterol.*, 4, 147, 1975.
4. **Spriggs, E. I.**, Diverticulitis, *Br. Med. J.*, 2, 569, 1929.
5. **Painter, N. G. and Burkitt, D. P.**, Diverticular disease of the colon: a deficiency disease of western civilization, *Br. Med. J.*, 2, 450, 1971.
6. **Gear, J. S. S., Ware, A., Fursdon, P., Mann, J. I., Nolan, D. J., Brodribb, A. J. M., and Vessey, M. P.**, Symptomless diverticular disease and intake of dietary fiber, *Lancet*, 1, 511, 1979.

7. **Painter, N. S. and Burkitt, D. P.**, Diverticular disease of the colon, a 20th century problem, *Clin. Gastroenterol.*, 4, 3, 75.
8. **Spriggs, E. I. and Marxer, O. A.**, Intestinal diverticula,, *Q. J. Med.*, 19, 1, 1925.
9. **Brodribb, J. M.**, Dietary fiber in diverticular disease of the colon, in *Medical Aspects of Dietary Fiber*, Spiller, G. A. and Kay, R. M., Eds., Plenum Press, New York, 1980, 43.
10. **Segal, I., Solomon, A., and Hunt, J. A.**, Emergence of diverticular disease in the urban South African black, *Gastroenterology*, 72, 215, 1977.
11. **Stemmermann, G. N. and Yatani, R.**, Diverticulosis and polyps of the large intestine: a necropsy study of Hawaii Japanese, *Cancer*, 31, 1260, 1973.
12. **Narasaka, T., Watanabe, H., Yamagata, S., Munakata, A., Tajima, T., and Matatsunaga, F.**, Statistical analysis of diverticulosis of the colon, *Tohoku J. Exp. Med.*, 115, 271, 1975.
13. **Segal, I. and Leibowitz, B.**, The distributional pattern of diverticular dieseases, *Dis. Colon Rectum*, 32, 227, 1989.
14. **Kohler, R.**, The incidence of colonic diverticulosis in Finland and Sweden, *Acta. Chir. Scand.*, 126, 148, 1963.
15. **Havia, T.**, Diverticulosis of the colon, *Acta. Chir. Scand.*, 137, 167, 1971.
16. **Hughes, L. E.**, Post-mortem survey of diverticular disease of the colon, *Gut*, 10, 336, 1969.
17. **Painter, N. S., Almeida, A. Z., and Colebourne, K. W.**, Unprocessed bran in treatment of diverticular disease of the colon, *Br. Med. J.*, 2, 137, 1972.
18. **Brodribb, A. J. M. and Humphreys, D. M.**, Diverticular disease: three studies, *Br. Med. J.*, 1, 424, 1976.
19. **Plumley, P. F. and Francis, B.**, Dietary management of diverticular disease, *J. Am. Dietet. Assoc.*, 63, 527, 1973.
20. **Lubbock, D. M., Thomson, W., and Garry, R. C.**, Epithelial overgrowth and diverticula of the gut, *Br. Med. J.*, 1, 1252, 1937.
21. **Carlson, A. J. and Hoelzel, F.**, Relationship of diet to diverticulosis of the colon in rats, *Gastroenterology*, 12, 108, 1949.
22. **Brodribb, A. J. M., Condon, R. E., Cowles, V., and DeCosse, J. J.**, Effect of dietary fiber on intraluminal pressure and myoelectrical activity of the left colon in monkeys, *Gastroenterology*, 77, 70, 1979.
23. **Jaskiewicz, K., Rossouw, J. E., Kritchevsky, D., van Rensburg, S. J., Fincham, J. E., and Woodroof, C. W.**, The influence of diet and dimethylhydrazine on the small and large intestine of vervet monkeys, *Br. J. Exp. Pathol.*, 67, 361, 1986.
24. **Brodribb, A. J. M.**, Treatment of symptomatic diverticular disease with a high fiber diet, *Lancet*, 1, 664, 1977.
25. **Eastwood, M. A., Smith, A. N., Brydon, W. G., and Pritchard, J.**, Comparison of bran, ispaghula, and lactulose on colon function in diverticular disease, *Gut*, 19, 1144, 1978.
26. **Srivastava, G. S., Smith, A. N., and Painter, N. S.**, Sterculia bulk-forming agent with smooth muscle relaxant versus bran in diverticular disease, *Br. Med. J.*, 1, 315, 1976.
27. **Ornstein, M. H., Littlewood, E. R., Baird, I. M., Fowler, J., North, W. R. S., and Cox, A. G.**, Are fibre supplements really necessary in diverticular disease of the colon? A controlled clinical trial, *Br. Med. J.*, 282, 1353, 1981.
28. **Weinreich, J.**, Controlled studies with dietary fibre in the therapy of diverticular disease and irritable bowel syndrome, in *Colon and Nutrition*, Goebell, H. and Kasper, H., Eds., Falk Symposium 32, MTP Press, Lancaster, England, 1982, 239.
29. **Ewerth, S., Ahlberg, J., Holmstrom, B., Persson, U., and Uden, R.**, Influence of symptoms and transit-time of Vi-Siblin in diverticular disease, *Acta. Chir. Scand. Suppl.*, 500, 49, 1980.
30. **Hodgson, W. J. B.**, The placebo effect, is it important in diverticular disease?, *Am. J. Gastroenterol.*, 67, 157, 1977.
31. **Hyland, J. M. P. and Taylor, I.**, Does a high fibre diet prevent the complications of diverticular disease?, *Br. J. Surg.*, 67, 77, 1980.

Chapter 7.7

FIBER AND INFLAMMATORY BOWEL DISEASE

J. Scott Whittaker and Hugh J. Freeman

Inflammatory bowel disease (IBD) refers to that group of conditions in which inflammation involves the small or large intestine or both. In common usage, IBD is restricted to those conditions whose etiology is unknown and generally includes Crohn's disease (CD) and ulcerative colitis (UC). As with many other intestinal conditions of undetermined or uncertain etiology, dietary factors, including fiber, have been proposed as important factors in pathogenesis.

The low incidence of Crohn's disease in the third world and its apparently increasing incidence in the Western world have led to speculation that dietary changes in the Western world that have occurred in the past few decades may be partly responsible. For example, a consistent dietary difference between patients with CD and controls is the high refined carbohydrate intake observed in CD, a finding which was first reported in 1976,[1] and which has been subsequently confirmed.[2,3]

FIBER STUDIES IN CD

Fiber consumption in CD has also been examined in some recent studies (Table 1). Kasper and Sommer employed an experienced dietitian to perform dietary histories in CD patients and controls over 7 successive days.[4] They reported that patients with CD consumed slightly, but significantly, more fiber than control subjects (26.6 vs. 22.3 g). This increase was largely in the form of a significantly increased consumption of noncellulose polysaccharide (17.3 vs. 14.5 g). In contrast, Thornton and co-workers reported that pre-illness dietary fiber intakes of 30 patients with CD were significantly less than that of 30 controls.[5] While the median duration of symptoms in the CD patients was only 15 months, the range was wide, from 1 to 92 months; this suggests that the validity of recall in some patients with longstanding symptoms may not be precise. Of interest was the finding that the CD patients consumed only about 25% of the raw fruit and vegetable fiber as the controls (0.6 vs. 2.3 g/d). A further study by Mayberry and co-workers found no difference between the dietary fiber intakes of patients with CD compared with normal controls.[2]

The observations by Thornton et al. that the pre-illness diet of Crohn's patients may have been low in fiber, especially raw fruit and vegetable fiber, led to several further studies. Heaton et al. reported the effects of treating 32 CD patients with a fiber-rich diet for a period of 4 years and 4 months.[6] CD patients not provided dietary instruction served as retrospective controls. While the study reports higher refined carbohydrate intake in controls compared with CD patients on the diet, no figures for dietary fiber intake in controls were given. The CD patients on the modified high fiber, low sugar diet had significantly fewer hospital admissions and total days in hospital compared to the control patients. While the number of operations in those patients on the special diet was fewer (1 vs. 5), the statistical significance of this was not defined.

The apparent success of this "Bristol diet" led to a prospective study by Levenstein et al. (Table 2). Thirty patients with CD placed on a "normalized" diet were compared to 28 patients given the "usual" low residue diet prescribed in Italy.[7] The number of portions of fiber consumed by those on the "normalized" diet was significantly higher than the number taken by those on the "usual" diet, but the significance of the difference in the

TABLE 1
Fiber Intake in Crohn's Disease

Number of patients	Disease duration	Fiber intake (g/day) Preillness	Fiber intake (g/day) Current	Ref.
35 Crohn's	1 Year (av)		26.6 (17.3[a])	4
70 Control			22.3 (14.5[a])	
30 Crohn's	5 Months	17.3 (0.2[b])		5
30 Control	(range: 1–92)	19.2 (2.3[b])		
16 Crohn's	Not stated		14	2
16 Control			20	

[a] Noncellulose polysaccharides.
[b] Raw fruit and vegetable fiber.

TABLE 2
Fiber Trials in Crohn's Disease

Number of patients	Study duration	Daily fiber (g)	Daily sugar (g)	Patient admissions	Operations	Ref.
Retrospective controls						
32 Fiber	52 Months	33.4	39	11 (111 d)	1	6
32 Control		Not stated	90	18 (533 d)	5	
Prospective, randomized						
30 Normalized	29 Months	13[a]			4	7
28 Low residue		3			5	
190 High fiber	2 Years	27.9[a]	9	18	7	8
162 Low fiber		15.7	92	21	14	

[a] Low refined carbohydrate, high vegetable, and fruit fiber ("Bristol diet").

total fiber intake (13 vs. 3 g) was not stated. Over a period of 29 months, there were no differences in outcome with respect to symptoms, hospitalizations, operations, complications, nutritional status, or postoperative recurrence. A second prospective randomized controlled study was reported by Ritchie et al. in which 190 patients with CD received the high fiber "Bristol diet" while 162 received a "low fiber" diet.[8] Patients in the "high fiber" group also restricted their intake of refined carbohydrate while those in the "low fiber" group were encouraged to eat refined carbohydrate. No differences were found in clinical outcome over the 2-year study period. Significantly more patients in the high fiber group withdrew from the trial for reasons other than disease deterioration.

FIBER STUDIES IN UC

Only limited studies have examined the effects of dietary fiber in UC (Table 3). Davies and Rhoades divided 39 patients with UC in remission on sulfasalazine into 2 groups.[9] Fifteen patients continued on the sulfasalazine and their regular diet while 20 of the 24 patients who tolerated a high fiber diet were continued on that diet with sulfasalazine being stopped. The increased fiber was taken in the form of whole wheat bread, vegetables, and

TABLE 3
Fiber in Ulcerative Colitis

Number of patients	Disease duration	Daily fiber (g) Preillness	Daily fiber (g) Trial	Daily sugar (g)	Relapse no. (rate)	Ref.
Restrospective controls						
30 UC	2 Months	19.9		97		10
30 Control		18.3		96		
Prospective, randomized						
15 Sulfasalazine	8.5 Years		13[a]		3(15%)	9
20 High fiber			3		15(75%)	

[a] Fiber added as bran cereal, whole wheat bread, and vegetables.

a supplement of 25 g of bran supplied as Kellogg's All Bran or Allinson's Bran Plus. The cumulative relapse rates of the sulfasalazine group and the fiber group were 20 and 70%, respectively, over 6 months. The relapse rate on the high fiber diet was similar to that expected in UC patients treated with a placebo. A second study by Thornton et al. examined the "pre-illness" diet of 30 patients with UC diagnosed within the previous 3 months.[10] No differences were detected in refined carbohydrate or fiber intakes between these UC patients and 30 control subjects.

SHORT CHAIN FATTY ACIDS AND IBD

While only limited data are available to support a prominent role for fiber in the treatment of IBD, renewed interest has resulted from the recognition that important metabolic by-products of fiber, i.e., short chain fatty acids (SCFA), in the colon may be very relevant in disease pathogenesis and, possibly, therapy. Several studies in ileostomy subjects have shown that about 90 to 100% of orally administered fiber is recoverable in the ileostomy effluent.[11-12] When the fiber reaches the colon, anaerobic bacteria metabolize a varying amount to gases (CO_2, H_2, CH_4) and SCFA (predominantly butyrate, propionate, and acetate).[13] The SCFA which are produced have been shown to be important sources of energy for colonocytes.[14] In addition, SCFA stimulate colonic sodium and water absorption.[15,16] Diversion of the fecal stream as occurs, e.g., following colostomy, may result in an inflamed distal excluded segment, so-called "diversion colitis". Harig and co-workers have recently reported improvement in diversion colitis using rectal irrigation with SCFA.[17]

In addition to a possible role for fiber in the generation of SCFA in various colonic disorders, unabsorbed complex carbohydrates per se have been hypothesized to play a part in the diarrhea pathogenesis in IBD. Of course, totally undigested fiber probably has minimal effects, since fiber has very little osmotic activity. Metabolism of fiber entering the colon to SCFA and lactic acid, however, would increase the osmotic load and provide a mechanism for diarrhea in IBD. However, as noted above, SCFA production may not lead to diarrhea due to their rapid absorption by the colon, their use as a colonic fuel, and their stimulation of sodium and water absorption.

Vernia et al. have shown that fecal lactic acid concentrations are increased in both Crohn's colitis and UC, but that fecal weights correlate with lactic acid concentrations only in UC. Fecal SCFA concentrations were found to be much lower in patients with UC than in those with Crohn's colitis, in whom fecal concentrations were similar to those of normal controls.[18,19] Holtug and co-workers have reported that some of the changes in the SCFA pattern in UC may be due to bacterial fermentation of blood.[20] Indeed, other investigators have found higher SCFA levels in severe UC when compared with normal controls.[21] The reasons for the discrepancy in these studies is not clear, but may relate to differences in methods or severity of disease.

The abnormalities in SCFA in UC led Breuer et al. to perform rectal irrigation of SCFA in patients with distal UC.[22] Twelve patients were treated with SCFA rectal irrigation over a period of 6 weeks in a nonblinded fashion. Nine were judged to be much improved. Clearly, a blinded, randomized, controlled trial will need to be conducted. If SCFA are found to be better than placebo, the importance of these substances in UC will be confirmed.

REFERENCES

1. **Martini, G. A. and Brandes, J. W.**, Increased consumption of refined carbohydrates in patients with Crohn's disease, *Klin. Wochenschr.,* 54, 367, 1976.
2. **Mayberry, J. F., Rhodes, J., and Allan, R.**, Diet in Crohn's disease. Two studies of current and previous habits in newly diagnosed patients, *Dig. Dis. Sci.,* 26, 444, 1981.
3. **Janerot, G., Jarnmark, I., and Nilsson, K.**, Consumption of refined sugar by patients with Crohn's disease, ulcerative colitis or irritable bowel syndrome, *Scand. J. Gastroenterol.,* 18, 999, 1983.
4. **Kasper, H. and Sommer, H.**, Dietary fiber and nutrient intake in Crohn's disease, *Digestion,* 20, 323, 1979.
5. **Thornton, J. R., Emmett, P. M., and Heaton, K. W.**, Diet and Crohn's disease: characteristics of the pre-illness diet, *Br. Med. J.,* 2, 762, 1979.
6. **Heaton, K. W., Thornton, J. R., and Emmett, P. M.**, Treatment of Crohn's disease with an unrefined-carbohydrate, fibre-rich diet, *Br. Med. J.,* 2, 764, 1979.
7. **Levenstein, S., Prantera, C., Luzi, C., and D'Ubaldi, A.**, Low residue or normal diet in Crohn's disease: a prospective controlled study in Italian patients, *Gut,* 26, 989, 1985.
8. **Ritchie, J. K., Wadsworth, J., Lennard-Jones, J. E., and Rogers, E.**, Controlled multicentre therapeutic trial of an unrefined carbohydrate, fibre rich diet in Crohn's disease, *Br. Med. J.,* 295, 517, 1987.
9. **Davies, P. S. and Rhodes, J.**, Maintenance of remission in ulcerative colitis with sulphasalazine or a high-fibre diet: a clinical trial, *Br. Med. J.,* 1, 1524, 1978.
10. **Thornton, J. R., Emmett, P. M., and Heaton, K. W.**, Diet and ulcerative colitis, *Br. Med. J.,* 280, 293, 1980.
11. **Englyst, H. N. and Cummings, J. H.**, Digestion of the carbohydrates of banana (Musa paradisiaca sapientum) in the human small intestine, *Am. J. Clin. Nutr.,* 44, 42, 1986.
12. **Englyst, H. N. and Cummings, J. H.**, Digestion of polysaccharides of potato in the small intestine of man, *Am. J. Clin. Nutr.,* 45, 423, 1987.
13. **Cummings, J. H.**, Short chain fatty acids in the human colon, *Gut,* 22, 763, 1981.
14. **Roediger, W. E. W.**, Utilization of nutrients by isolated epithelial cells of the rat colon, *Gastroenterology,* 83, 424, 1982.
15. **Ruppin, H., Bar-Meir, S., Soergel, K. H., Wood, C. M., and Schmitt, M. G.**, Absorption of short-chain fatty acids by the colon, *Gastroenterology,* 78, 1500, 1980.
16. **Roediger, W. E. W. and Rae, D. A.**, Trophic effect of short chain fatty acids on mucosal handling of ions by the defunctioned colon, *Br. J. Surg.,* 69, 23, 1982.
17. **Harig, J. M., Sorgel, K. H., Komorowski, R. A., and Woods, C. M.**, Treatment of diversion colitis with short chain fatty acid irrigation, *N. Engl. J. Med.,* 320, 23, 1989.
18. **Vernia, P., Gnaedinger, A., Hauck, W., and Breuer, R. I.**, Organic anions and the diarrhea of inflammatory bowel disease, *Dig. Dis. Sci.,* 33, 1353, 1988.
19. **Vernia, P., Caprilli, R., Latella, G., Barbetti, F., Magliocca, F. M., and Cittadini, M.**, Fecal lactate and ulcerative colitis, *Gastroenterology,* 95, 1564, 1988.
20. **Holtug, K., Rasmussen, H. S., and Mortensen, P. B.**, Short chain fatty acids in inflammatory bowel disease. The effect of bacterial fermentation of blood, *Scand. J. Clin. Lab. Invest.,* 48, 667, 1988.
21. **Roediger, W. E. W., Heyworth, M., Willoughby, P., Piris, J., Moore, A., and Truelove, S. C.**, Luminal ions and short chain fatty acids as markers of functional activity of the mucosa in ulcerative colitis, *J. Clin. Pathol.,* 35, 323, 1982.
22. **Breuer, R. I., Buto, S. K., and Christ, M. L.**, Rectal irrigation with short chain fatty acids for distal ulcerative colitis, *Dig. Dis. Sci.,* 36, 185, 1991.

Chapter 7.8

DISEASE PATTERNS IN SOUTH AFRICA AS RELATED TO DIETARY FIBER INTAKE

Alexander R. P. Walker

In South Africa there are four ethnic populations: blacks (25 million), coloreds (Euro-Africa-Malay) (3 million), Indians (1 million), and whites (5 million). These populations exhibit considerable differences in patterns of diseases. Indeed, between them they afford probably greater contrasts, as juxtaposed populations, than are encountered elsewhere in the world. Thus, the Asian population exhibits high frequencies of obesity, hypertension, diabetes, and coronary heart disease (CHD).[1-3] Among rural blacks there are very low frequencies of dental caries, hypertension, CHD, noninfective bowel diseases, e.g., appendicitis and certain cancers (e.g., colon, breast).[5-9] Among urban blacks, Asians, and coloreds, rises are occurring in all these disorders and diseases. To exemplify the magnitude of changes, the teeth of urban black children are now *inferior* to those of white children.[10] Among urban black adults the frequency of hypertension (WHO criteria) now exceeds that in whites[11] (Tables 1 through 3).

Most of the differences, although not all, are related to differences in environmental factors, especially diet. In this respect there are great contrasts in the patterns consumed by the different populations and their segments. At the one extreme, the diet of rural blacks[12] (which in pattern resembles that of ancestors of Western populations[13,14]) is characterized by a relatively low intake of energy, of total protein, especially of animal protein, of total fat, especially of animal fat; yet their diet is high in fiber intake. In contrast, the diet of whites,[15] and that of the more privileged segments of the other populations, is high in energy, total protein, and fat, especially the respective moieties of animal origin; however, dietary fiber intake is low. The first pattern of diet, in contexts of indigence, is well nigh invariably associated with very low or low frequencies of degenerative disorders and diseases (although high frequencies of infections); conversely, the second is associated with very high or high frequencies of diseases of prosperity (Table 4).

As to the precise assessment of the protective role of dietary fiber intake, first it must be appreciated that patterns of health and disease are determined not only by diet, but by genetic and by nondietary factors. The latter include degree of physical activity,[16] extent of smoking practice,[17] stresses (particularly those linked with urbanization and rise in income), and the availability and utilization of medical services. Each of these components has a variable although often powerful influence in the regulation of the frequencies of the diseases mentioned. Next, it must be appreciated that the levels of a number of dietary components are powerfully correlated with level of fiber. Thus, the latter is inversely correlated with level of fat intake, especially of animal fat, of protein intake, especially animal protein, and with animal foods as a whole. So that with changes in diet, such as those which took place from the time of our ancestors to the present, and also which occurred when such changes became somewhat reversed as prevailed in certain wartime populations,[18,19] propounders of etiological hypotheses must be on their guard against overclaiming and overblaming. Account must be taken of changes and of contexts, holistically, rather than the focusing of attention and explanations almost exclusively on the changes that occurred in one or more food components. However, having said this, there is little doubt that changes in intakes of fat and of fiber are particularly influential.

TABLE 1
Frequencies of Some Diseases of Prosperity in South African Populations

	Rural blacks	Urban blacks	Coloreds	Indians	Whites
Dental caries	+	+++	+++	++++	+++
Femoral fractures	+	+	++	++	+++++
Obesity	+	+++	+++	+++	+++
Hypertension	+	++++	++++	+++	+++
Diabetes	+	+++	++++	+++++	+++
CHD	−[a]	++	+++	+++++	+++++
Stroke	+	++	+++	+++	++

[a] Implies that occurrence is rare.

TABLE 2
Cancer Patterns in South African Populations

	Rural blacks	Urban blacks	Coloreds	Indians	Whites
Lung	−[a]	++	+++	++	++++
Breast	−[a]	++	+++	+++	+++++
Colon	−	+	++	++	+++++
Stomach	−	+	+++	++	++
Pancreas	−	+	++	+	+++
Liver	++[b]	++	++	+	+
Esophagus	++++[b]	+++	++	+	+
Cervix	++	++++	+++	+	+

[a] Implies that occurrence is rare.
[b] Frequency of occurrence related to some regional but not nationwide populations.

TABLE 3
Frequencies of Noninfective Bowel Diseases in South African Populations

	Rural blacks	Urban blacks	Coloreds	Indians	Whites
Hemorrhoids	−[a]	++	++	++	+++
Appendicitis	+	++	++	++	+++++
Ulcerative colitis	−	+	+	+	+++++
Irritable bowel syndrome	−	++	++	+	++++
Diverticular disease	−	+	++	++	+++++
Colon cancer	−	+	++	++	+++++

[a] Implies that occurrence is rare.

Understandably, therefore, the *extent* of the specific involvement of dietary fiber remains a subject of uncertainty,[20-22] which does not lend itself to ready resolution. On the positive side, experimental studies on animals support the validity of a relationship,[23] as do many short-term studies on humans.[24-26] Probably the epidemiological evidence of the character already referred to provides the most persuasive support for a relationship. Briefly, there

TABLE 4
Dietary Patterns Respecting Fat, Total Carbohydrate, and Fiber Intakes

	Rural blacks	Urban blacks	Coloreds	Indians	Whites
Energy from fat (%)	10–15	20–30	30–35	30–40	35–45
Energy from carbohydrate (%)	70–75	65–75	60	60	55
Dietary fiber (g)	20–25[a]	10–20	15–20	15–20	15–20

[a] Intake depends on the season; seasonal fruits and "spinaches" are high in dietary fiber.

are similarities in the patterns of diet and disease exhibited by ancestors of Western populations and the patterns displayed by rural third world dwellers, such as South African blacks. Moreoever, in World War II, circumstances caused diets in certain countries to change, involving, *inter alia,* reductions in fat intake and increase in fiber intake.[18,19] There were associated changes in disease pattern; e.g., there were falls in dental caries, obesity, diabetes, atherosclerotic lesions of aorta and coronary vessels, constipation, and appendicitis.[18,19,27-29] Additionally, among church groups such as Seventh Day Adventists,[30,31] and among vegetarians whose diet usually contains much more dietary fiber than the diet of omnivorous eaters, there are lower frequencies of a number of diseases[32] — obesity,[33] hypertension,[34] diabetes,[35] CHD,[36] appendicitis,[37] diverticular diseases,[38] cancers of the breast[39] and colon,[30,31] and osteoporosis.[40]

In fairness, it must be stressed that although ameliorative decreases in degenerative diseases *can* be accomplished by changes in diet, the magnitude of the alterations required is too great to win widespread public acceptance. As evidence of this, prosperous Western populations are having enormous difficulties in seeking to reduce their energy intake from fat to that level recommended, of 30%. Equally great problems are latent in endeavors to, say, double intake of dietary fiber. Only a very small proportion of populations has changed their eating habits and adopted a "prudent diet".[41]

A perplexing fact in the present local situation in South Africa is that among urban blacks, while their frequencies of chronic bowel diseases have risen slightly, they are still far lower than those in the white population, despite the fact of the now relatively low fiber intake of urban dwellers.[42] Can this be explained? In his recent review, Heaton[22] noted that there are many ways in which a high fiber intake "ought to" protect against colorectal cancer;[43] yet low fiber intakes are not a consistent feature of populations prone to this cancer, nor of people who actually have it.[44,45] He suggested that fiber is only a part of the story, and that if fiber exerts its anticancer effect by being fermented into short chain fatty acids, then any carbohydrate that enters the colon and is similarly fermented could be protective, since a considerable amount of the starch consumed escapes digestion and enters the colon, where it is rapidly fermented.[46] Perhaps starch intake matters as much as fiber intake in terms of protection from cancer. How much starch reaches the colon? This varies enormously, tenfold, from person to person.[47] According to one small study, people with colonic polyps are unusually efficient at digesting starch.[48] Should this be confirmed, then possibly cancer might be prevented by people eating more starch and by eating it in a less digestible form.[49] In South Africa, evidence indicates that maize, the staple food of the black population, is malabsorbed.[50] This implies that a variable, indeed, possibly a large proportion of "resistant" starch enters the colon and is therefore available for fermentation. Conceivably, therefore, it is this phenomenon which contributes to maintaining blacks' still faster transit time,[51] and lower fecal pH value,[52] and so protects them in measure against the development of chronic bowel diseases. In this type of context, it is important to keep in mind that while different sources of fiber have different physiological actions, it must be recognized that in rural Africa, *irrespective* of the source of fiber (cereals, legumes, vegetables, fruit), chronic bowel diseases are uniformly rare or very uncommon.

REFERENCES

1. **Seedat, Y. K.,** Lifestyle and disease: hypertension and ischaemic heart disease in Indian people in South African and in India, *S. Afr. Med. J.,* 61, 965, 1982.
2. **Omar, M. A. K., Seedat, M. A., Dyer, R. B., Rajput, M. C., Motala, A. A., and Joubert, S. M.,** The prevalence of diabetes mellitus in a large group of South African Indians, *S. Afr. Med. J.,* 67, 924, 1985.
3. **Seedat, Y. K., Mayet, F. G. H., Khan, S., Somers, S. R., and Joubert, G.,** Risk factors for coronary heart disease in the Indians of Durban, *S. Afr. Med. J.,* 78, 447, 1990.
4. **Walker, A. R. P., Walker, B. F., Dison, E., and Walker, C.,** Dental caries and malnutrition in rural South African Black ten to twelve-year-olds, *J. Dent. Assoc. S. Afr.,* 43, 581, 1988.
5. **Seedat, Y. K. and Hackland, D. B. T.,** The prevalence of hypertension in 4,993 rural Zulus, *Trans. R. Soc. Trop. Med. Hyg.,* 78, 785, 1984.
6. **Walker, A. R. P. and Walker, B. F.,** Appendicectomy in South African inter-ethnic school pupils, *Am. J. Gastroenterol.,* 82, 219, 1987.
7. **Walker, A. R. P. and Segal, I.,** Colorectal cancer. Some aspects of epidemiology, risk factors, treatment, screening and survival, *S. Afr. Med. J.,* 73, 653, 1988.
8. **Walker, A. R. P., Walker, B. F., Funani, S., and Walker, A. J.,** Characteristics of black women with breast cancer in Soweto, South Africa, *The Cancer J.,* 2, 316, 1989.
9. **Walker, A. R. P. and Walker, B. F.,** Coronary heart disease in blacks in underdeveloped populations, *Am. Heart J.,* 109, 1410, 1985.
10. **Steyn, N. P. and Albertse, E. C.,** Sucrose consumption and dental caries in twelve-year-old children residing in Cape Town, *J. Dent. Assoc. S. Afr.,* 42, 43, 1987.
11. **Seedat, Y. K. and Seedat, M. A.,** An inter-racial study of the prevalence of hypertension in an urban South African population, *Trans. R. Soc. Trop. Med. Hyg.,* 76, 62, 1982.
12. **Richter, M. J. C., Langenhoven, M. L., Du Plessis, J. P., Ferreira, J. J., Swanepoel, A. S. P., and Jordaan, P. C. J.,** Nutritional value of diets of blacks in Ciskei, *S. Afr. Med. J.,* 65, 338, 1984.
13. **Steven, M.,** Food and longevity in 18th century Scotland, *Nutr. Health,* 7, 3, 1990.
14. **Hollingsworth, D.,** Changing patterns of food consumption in Britain, *Nutr. Rev.,* 32, 353, 1974.
15. **Rossouw, D. J., Fourie, J. J., van Heerden, L. E., and Engelbrecht, F. M.,** A dietary survey of free-living middle-aged white males in the Western Cape, *S. Afr. Med. J.,* 48, 2528, 1974.
16. **Blair, S. N., Kohl, H. W., Paffenbarger, R. S., Clark, D. G., Cooper, K. H., and Gibbons, L. W.,** Physical fitness and all-cause mortality: a prospective study of healthy men and women, *JAMA,* 262, 2395, 1989.
17. **Stokes, J., III and Rigotti, N. A.,** The health consequences of cigarette smoking and the internist's role in smoking cessation, *Adv. Intern. Med.,* 33, 431, 1988.
18. **Banks, A. L. and Magee, H. E.,** Effect of enemy occupation on the state of health and nutrition in the Channel Islands, *Mon. Bull. Min. Health Publ. Lab. Serv.,* 16, 184, 1945.
19. **Fleisch, A.,** Nutrition in Switzerland during the war, *Schweiz. Med. Wochenschr.,* 16, 889, 1946.
20. **Council on Scientific Affairs,** Dietary fiber and health, *JAMA,* 118, 1591, 1988.
21. **Nestel, P. J.,** Dietary fibre, *Med. J. Aust.,* 153, 123, 1990.
22. **Heaton, K. W.,** Dietary fibre: After 21 years of study the verdict remains one of fruition and frustration, *Br. Med. J.,* 300, 1479, 1990.
23. **Bianchini, F., Caderni, G., Dolara, P., Fanetti, L., and Kriebel, D.,** Effect of dietary fat, starch and cellulose on fecal bile acids in mice, *J. Nutr.,* 119, 1617, 1989.
24. **Malinow, M. R.,** Regression of atherosclerosis in humans, *Postgrad. Med.,* 73, 232, 1983.
25. **DeCosse, J. J., Miller, H. H., and Lesser, M. L.,** Effect of wheat fiber and vitamins C and E on rectal polyps in patients with familial adenomatous polyposis, *J. Nat. Cancer Inst.,* 81, 1290, 1989.

26. **Ornish, D., Brown, S. E., Scherwitz, L. W., Billings, J. H., Armstrong, W. T., Ports, T. A., McLanahan, S. M., Kirkeeide, R. L., Brand, R. J., and Gould, K. L.,** Can lifestyle changes reverse coronary heart disease?, *Lancet,* 336, 129, 1990.
27. **Pezold, F. A.,** *Arteriosclerose und Ernahrung,* Steinkopf, Darmstadt, 1959, 162.
28. **Trowell, H.,** Diabetes mellitus death-rates in England and Wales 1920–70 and food supplies, *Lancet,* ii, 998, 1974.
29. **Schettler, G.,** Cardiovascular disease during and after World War II: a comparison of the Federal Republic of Germany with other European countries, *Prev. Med.,* 8, 581, 1979.
30. **Phillips, R. I.,** Role of life-style and dietary habits in risk of cancer among Seventh-Day Adventists, *Cancer Res.,* 35, 3513, 1975.
31. **Snowdon, D. A.,** Animal product consumption and mortality because of all causes combined, coronary heart disease, stroke, diabetes, and cancer in Seventh-Day Adventists, *Am. J. Clin. Nutr.,* 48, 739, 1988.
32. **Dwyer, J. T.,** Health aspects of vegetarian diets, *Am. J. Clin. Nutr.,* 48, 712, 1988.
33. **Barbosa, J. C., Shultz, T. D., Filley, S. J., and Nieman, D. C.,** The relationship among adiposity, diet, and hormone concentrations in vegetarian and nonvegetarian postmenopausal women, *Am. J. Clin. Nutr.,* 51, 798, 1990.
34. **Beillin, L. J., Rouse, I. L., Armstrong, B. K., Margetts, B. M., and Vandongen, R.,** Vegetarian diet and blood pressure levels: incidental or causal association?, *Am. J. Clin. Nutr.,* 48, 806, 1988.
35. **Anderson, J. W.,** The role of dietary carbohydrate and fibre in the control of diabetes, *Adv. Intern. Med.,* 26, 67, 1980.
36. **Burr, M. L. and Butland, B. K.,** Heart disease in British vegetarians, *Am. J. Clin. Nutr.,* 48, 830, 1988.
37. **Westlake, C. A., St Leger, A. S., and Burr, M. L.,** Appendicectomy and dietary fibre, *J. Hum. Nutr.,* 34, 267, 1980.
38. **Gear, J. S. S., Fursdon, P., Nolan, D. J., Ware, A., Mann, J. I., Vessey, M. P., and Brodribb, A. K. M.,** Symptomless diverticular disease and intake of dietary fibre, *Lancet,* i, 511, 1979.
39. **Adlercreutz, H., Hämäläinen, E., Gorbach, S. L., Goldin, B. R., Woods, M. N., and Dwyer, J. T.,** Diet and plasma androgens in postmenopausal vegetarian and omnivorous women and postmenopausal women with breast cancer, *Am. J. Clin. Nutr.,* 49, 433, 1989.
40. **Marsh, A. G., Sanchez, T. V., Michelsen, O., Chaffee, F. L., and Fagal, S. M.,** Vegetarian lifestyle and bone mineral density, *Am. J. Clin. Nutr.,* 48, 837, 1988.
41. **Anonymous,** Nutrition and cancer, facts, fallacies, and ACS activities, *Cancer News,* Summer, 18, 1987.
42. **Segal, I. and Walker, A. R. P.,** Low-fat intake with falling fiber intake commensurate with rarity of non-infective bowel diseases in Blacks in Soweto, Johannesburg, South Africa, *Nutr. Cancer,* 8, 185, 1986.
43. **Cummings, J. H. and Bingham, S. A.,** Dietary fibre, fermentation and large bowel cancer, *Cancer Surv.,* 6, 601, 1987.
44. **Jacobs, L. R.,** Fiber and colon cancer, *Gastroenterol. Clin. North Am.,* 17, 747, 1988.
45. **Rozen, P., Horwitz, C., and Tabenkin, C.,** Dietary habits and colorectal cancer incidence in a second-defined kibbutz population, *Nutr. Cancer,* 9, 177, 1987.
46. **Cummings, J. H. and Englyst, H. N.,** Fermentation in the human large intestine and the available substrates, *Am. J. Clin. Nutr.,* 45, 1243, 1987.
47. **Stephen, A. M., Haddad, A. C., and Phillips, S. F.,** Passage of carbohydrate into the colon. Direct measurements in humans, *Gastroenterology,* 85, 589, 1983.
48. **Thornton, J. R., Dryden, A., Kelleher, J., and Losowsky, M. S.,** Super-efficient starch absorption. A risk factor for colonic neoplasia?, *Dig. Dis. Sci.,* 32, 1088, 1987.
49. **Heaton, K. W., Marcus, S. N., Emmett, P. M., and Bolton, C. H.,** Particle size of wheat, maize and oat test meals: effects on plasma glucose and insulin responses and on the rate of starch digestion in vitro, *Am. J. Clin. Nutr.,* 47, 675, 1988.
50. **Segal, I., Walker, A. R. P., Naik, I., Riedel, L., Daya, B., and De Beer, M.,** Malabsorption of carbohydrate foods by blacks in Soweto, South Africa, *S. Afr. Med. J.,* 80, 543, 1991.
51. **Walker, A. R. P., Walker, B. F., Lelake, A., Manetsi, B., Tlotetsi, G. N., Verardi, M. M., and Walker, A. J.,** Transit time and fibre intake in black and white adolescents in South Africa, *S. Afr. J. Food Science Nutr.* in press.
52. **Walker, A. R. P. and Walker, B. F.,** Intra- and inter-individual variations in serial faecal pH values in South African interethnic schoolchildren, *S. Afr. J. Food Science Nutr.,* 4(1), 10, 1992.

Chapter 7.9

DISEASE PATTERNS IN JAPAN AND CHANGES IN DIETARY FIBER (1930–1980)

Keisuke Tsuji and Bunpei Mori

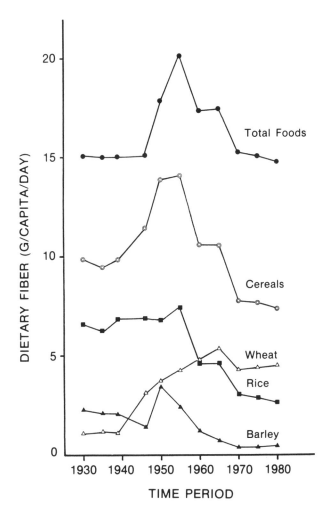

FIGURE 1. Dietary fiber (DF) intake by the Japanese people since 1930, where DF intake (grams per capita per day) = food intake × DF content. Food intake values are from Food Balance Tables of Japan.[1] DF content values are rice, 1.18 to 2.70%;[2] wheat, 1.02%;[3] barley, 4.86%.[4]

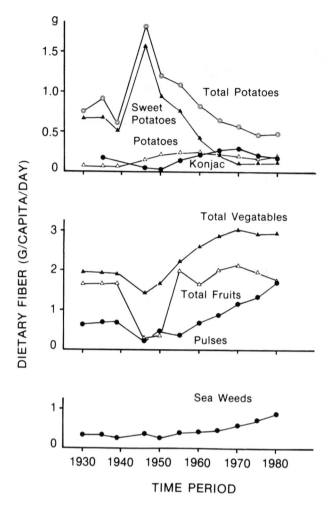

FIGURE 2. Dietary fiber (DF) intake by the Japanese people from potatoes, vegetables, fruit, pulses, and seaweeds since 1930 where: DF intake (grams per capita per day) = food intake × DF content. Food intake values are from Food Balance Tables of Japan.[1] DF content values are sweet potatoes, 1.01%;[5] potatoes, 0.54%;[5] pulses as soybeans, 7.77%;[5] total vegetables, 0.96%;[2] total fruits, 1.14%;[2] seaweeds, 23.6%;[2] konjac flour, 80%.[6]

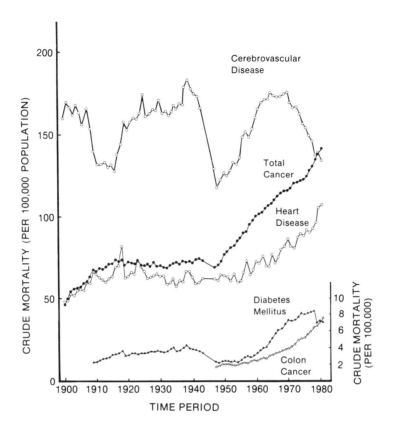

FIGURE 3. Changes of death rates from adult disease in Japan.[7]

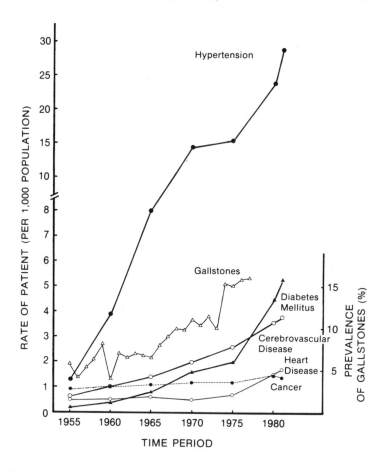

FIGURE 4. Number of patients in Japan suffering from adult diseases[8] and from gallstones.[9]

REFERENCES

1. Food Balance Tables of Japan, 1930–1980.
2. **Mori, B.,** Contents of dietary fiber in some Japanese foods and the amount ingested through Japanese meals, *Nutr. Rep. Int.*, 26, 159, 1982.
3. **Paul, A. A. and Southgate, D. A. T.,** McCance and Widdowson's, *The Composition of Foods*, 4th ed., Her Majesty's Stationery Office, London, 1978.
4. **Ayano, Y.,** *Chori Kagaku*, 15, 16, 1982.
5. **Hoshi, S. and Takehitsa, F.,** Insoluble dietary fiber contents of foodstuffs, *Eiyo to Shokuryo*, 35, 133, 1982.
6. **Tsuji, K. et al.,** unpublished data.
7. Japan Vital Statistics (1900–1980).
8. Japan Patient Survey (1955–1982).
9. **Kameta, H. et al.,** *Jpn. Med. J.*, 2924, 28, 1980.

Chapter 7.10

MODIFICATION BY DIETARY FIBER OF TOXIC OR CARCINOGENIC EFFECTS

Bandaru S. Reddy and Gene A. Spiller

The possible antitoxic effect of dietary fiber or fiber-rich foods and more specifically the possible protective role of dietary fiber in carcinogenesis has been the subject of many studies, some of them dating back to the 1950s. After the hypothesis that colon cancer may be less common in populations consuming a high fiber diet was proposed in the early 1970s (see Chapter 7.5), the number of laboratory animal model studies on chemically induced carcinogenesis in the presence of various types of dietary fiber increased rapidly. Many of the early studies were carried out by Erschoff,[1,4,9,11] a pioneer in this field in the U.S., who demonstrated that many otherwise toxic levels of various substances in foods become either less toxic or nontoxic when fed together with foods high in dietary fiber or some of the fiber polymers. This complex function of the fiber polymers, or high fiber foods, is an important one. The long-term effects of low vs. high fiber intake on the toxic effects of food components, food contaminants, and in general environmental toxic substances can have major implications on the etiology of some diseases and more specifically on the effect of carcinogens. It is interesting to note that some dietary fibers or dietary fiber-rich foods are protective for some toxic substances but not for others, and Erschoff showed that other beneficial effects such as the hypocholesterolemic effect of some fiber is often not connected with their antitoxic effect.[8] An example is locust bean gum which is hypocholesterolemic but does not prevent cyclamate toxicity in rats when cyclamate is fed at the 5% level. Other examples of the specificity of the antitoxic effect of high fiber substances are given in Tables 1 and 2. These studies point to the fact that the effect of dietary fiber depends on the composition of its fiber components.

A problem intrinsic to these animal studies is that the same toxicity experiments cannot be carried out in humans and we must limit ourself to extrapolations from animal studies. Table 1 summarizes some of the studies on protection against toxicity in general and some early carcinogenesis studies. Table 2 focuses on studies carried out in the 1970s, 1980s, and early 1990s on carcinogenesis and the possible protective effect of dietary fiber polymers or high fiber foods. Caution should be used in interpreting the results with high fiber foods as other nonfiber components of the food might be responsible for the antitoxic or cancer-preventing effect or may enhance the protective effect. Differences in research protocols, diet composition, and many other factors are certainly responsible for the differences in results obtained by various investigators. The interaction between dietary fiber polymers and other components of the diet means that the composition of the entire diet is a key factor in carcinogenesis and toxicity studies.

TABLE 1
Studies on the Antitoxic Effect of Dietary Fiber or High Fiber Foods and Early Carcinogenesis Studies in Experimental Animals[a]

Toxic substance	Dietary fiber source	Amount in diet (%)	Animal	Effect[b]	Ref.
Tween 60	Soybean meal	15	Rats	+	3
Glucoascorbic acid (4%)	Alfalfa meal	20	Rats	+	4
Tween 20	Alfalfa meal	10	Rats	+	5
Tween 60	Rye grass	10		+	
	Wheat grass	10		+	
	Fescue grass	10		+	
	Orchard grass	10		+	
	Purified cellulose	10		+	
Span 20	Alfalfa meal	20		−	
2,5-di-t-butyl-hydroquinone	Stock diet[c] vs. purified diet		Rats	+	6
Chlorazanil hydrochloride	Alfalfa		Rats	+	7
Sodium cyclamate	Locus bean gum	10	Rats	−	8
	Purified cellulose	10		−	
	Psyllium seed powder	10		+	
	Alfalfa meal	20		+	
	Carrot root powder	20		+	
	Gum karaya	10		+	
Tween 60	Sodium alginate	15	Rats	+	8
	Psyllium seed	2.5 or 5		+	
	Alfalfa meal	10		+	
	Rice straw	10		+	
	Carrot root powder	10		+	
	Purified cellulose	10		−	
FD & C Red #2	Alfalfa meal	10	Rats	+	9
	Watercress powder	10		+	
	Parsley powder	10		+	
Cadmium (CdCl$_2$)	Increased fiber[d] but different diets		Rats	+	10
Tween 60	Alfalfa meal	10	Mice	+	11
	Wheat grass meal	10		+	
	Rye grass meal	10		+	
	Sodium alginate	5		+	
	Agar	5		+	
	Alfalfa juice[c]			−	
	Locust bean gum	10		−	
	Apple powder	10		−	
2-Acetylamino-fluorene	Stock diets[d] vs. purified diets		Rats	+	12

[a] This table summarizes only selected results of the cited studies. In many of these studies, many other high fiber substances or polymers were tested.

[b] "+" Indicates a general protective effect (such as weight maintenance or survival) when compared to controls on fiber-free or lower fiber diets, without specific studies on tumorigenesis; "+ + +" indicates a specific protective effect against tumorigenesis (compared to fiber-free or lower fiber diets); "−" indicates no protective effect.

[c] Amount corresponding to the alfalfa meal fed.

[d] The term *stock diet* refers to diets based on natural foods (grains, alfalfa, etc.). These diets were usually compared to diets based on purified ingredients such as casein, starch, and glucose.

TABLE 2
Studies on the Protective Effect of Dietary Fiber or High Fiber Foods in Chemical Carcinogenesis Studies

Carcinogen	Dietary fiber source (%)	Amount in diet (%)	Animal	Effect[a]	Ref.
Colon studies					
1,2-Dimethylhydrazine	Oat bran	20	Male Sprague-Dawley rats	− −	26
1,2-Dimethylhydrazine	Guar gum	10	Male Sprague-Dawley rats	− −	26
1,2-Dimethylhydrazine	Guar gum	5	Male Sprague-Dawley rats	− −	27
Azoxymethane	Phytic acid (inositol hexaphosphate)	1	Male Fischer rats	+	28
1,2-Dimethylhydrazine	Wheat bran	20	Male Sprague-Dawley rats	+ + +	13
Azoxymethane	Wheat bran	15	Female Fischer rats	+ + +	14
Azoxymethane	Wheat bran	15	Male Fischer rats	+ + +	15
3,2-Dimethyl-4-aminobiphenyl	Wheat bran	15	Male Fischer rats	+ + +	16
Azoxymethane	Wheat bran	20	Male Sprague-Dawley rats	+ + +	17
Azoxymethane	Wheat bran	30	Male Sprague-Dawley rats	+ + +	17
1,2-Dimethylhydrazine	Wheat bran	20	Male Sprague-Dawley rats	+ + +	18
1,2-Dimethylhydrazine	Wheat bran	20	Male Fischer rats	+ + +	19
1,2-Dimethylhydrazine	Wheat bran	20	Male Sprague-Dawley rats	− −	20[b]
1,2-Dimethylhydrazine	Wheat bran	20	Male Sprague-Dawley rats	− −	18[c]
1,2-Dimethylhydrazine	Wheat bran	20	Male Balb/c mice	− −	21[d]
Methylnitrosourea	Wheat bran	15	Female Fischer rats	− −	14[e]
Azoxymethane	Citrus fiber	15	Male Fischer rats	+ + +	15
3,2-Dimethyl-4-aminobiphenyl	Citrus fiber	15	Male Fischer rats	+ + +	16
3,2-Dimethyl-4-aminobiphenyl	Corn bran	15	Male Fischer rats	− −	22
1,2-Dimethylhydrazine	Corn bran	20	Male Balb/c mice	− −	21[d]
1,2-Dimethylhydrazine	Corn bran	20	Male Fischer rats	− −	19
1,2-Dimethylhydrazine	Rice bran	20	Male Fischer rats	− −	19
1,2-Dimethylhydrazine	Soybean bran	20	Male Fischer rats	− −	19
1,2-Dimethylhydrazine	Soybean bran	20	Male Balb/c mice	− −	21[d]
Azoxymethane	Alfalfa	20	Male Sprague-Dawley rats	+ + +	17
Azoxymethane	Alfalfa	30	Male Sprague-Dawley rats	+ + +	17
Azoxymethane	Alfalfa	15	Female Fischer rats	− −	14
Methylnitrosourea	Alfalfa	15	Female Fischer rats	− −	14[e]

TABLE 2 (continued)
Studies on the Protective Effect of Dietary Fiber or High Fiber Foods in Chemical Carcinogenesis Studies

Carcinogen	Dietary fiber source (%)	Amount in diet (%)	Animal	Effect[a]	Ref.
1,2-Dimethylhydrazine	Carrot fiber	20	Male Sprague-Dawley rats	−	20[b]
Azoxymethane	Pectin	15	Female Fischer rats	+ + +	14
1,2-Dimethylhydrazine	Pectin	9	Male Wistar rats	−	23
1,2-Dimethylhydrazine	Pectin	6.5	Male Sprague-Dawley rats	−	20[b]
1,2-Dimethylhydrazine	Cellulose	4.5	Male Wistar rats	+ + +	24
1,2-Dimethylhydrazine	Cellulose	9.0	Male Wistar rats	+ + +	23
Azoxymethane	Cellulose	40	Male Fischer rats	+ + +	25
Azoxymethane	Cellulose	20	Male Sprague-Dawley rats	+ + +	17
Azoxymethane	Cellulose	30	Male Sprague-Dawley rats	+ + +	17
Azoxymethane	Cellulose	20	Male Fischer rats	−	25
3,2-Dimethyl-4-aminobiphenyl	Lignin	7.5	Male Fischer rats	+ + +	22
Mammary studies					
Methylnitrosourea	Wheat bran	10	Female Fischer rats	+ + +	26

[a] "+ + +" Indicates a protective effect against tumorigenesis in the cited study (compared to fiber-free or lower fiber diets); "−" indicates no protective effect in the cited study; "—" indicates enhancing effect in the cited study.

[b] Experimental fiber diets were fed to animals 3 days before, during, and 14 days after carcinogen treatment. The animals were then transferred to standard rat pellets and fed this diet until termination of the experiment.

[c] Effect of wheat bran on stage of initiation was studied. Wheat bran was fed to rats during the carcinogen treatment only. They were transferred to fiber-free diet which was fed until termination of the experiment.

[d] Animals fed the control diet or fiber-free diet had very low colon tumor incidence.

[e] Methylnitrosourea is a direct-acting carcinogen.

REFERENCES

1. **Ershoff, B. H.**, Antitoxic effects of plant fibers, *Am. J. Clin. Nutr.*, 27, 1395, 1974.
2. **Kritchevsky, D.**, Modification by fiber of toxic dietary effects, *Fed. Proc. Fed. Am. Soc. Exp. Biol.*, 36, 1692, 1977.
3. **Chow, B. F., Burnett, J. M., Ling, C. T., and Barrows, L.**, Effect of basal diet on the response of rats to certain dietary non-ionic surface-active agents, *J. Nutr.*, 49, 563, 1953.
4. **Ershoff, B. H.**, Beneficial effect of alfalfa and other succulent plants on glucoascorbic acid toxicity in the rat, *Proc. Soc. Exp. Biol. Med.*, 95, 656, 1957.
5. **Ershoff, B. H.**, Beneficial effect of alfalfa meal and other bulk-containing or bulk-forming materials on the toxicity of nonionic surface-active agents in the rat, *J. Nutr.*, 70, 484, 1960.
6. **Ershoff, B. H.**, Comparative effects of a purified and stock diet on DBH (2,5-di-*t*-butylhydroquinone), toxicity in the rat, *Proc. Soc. Exp. Biol. Med.*, 141, 857, 1972.
7. **Ershoff, B. H.**, Beneficial effect of alfalfa meal on chlorazanil hydrochloride toxicity in the rat, *Exp. Med. Surg.*, 17, 204, 1959.
8. **Ershoff, B. H. and Marshall, W. E.**, Protective effect of dietary fiber in rats fed toxic doses of sodium cyclamate and polyoxyethelene sorbitan monostearate (Tween 60), *J. Food Sci.*, 40, 357, 1975.
9. **Ershoff, B. H. and Thurstun, E. W.**, Effects of diet on amaranth (FD & C Red No. 2) toxicity in the rat, *J. Nutr.*, 104, 937, 1974.
10. **Wilson, R. H. and De Eds, F.**, Importance of diet in studies of chronic toxicity, *Arch. Ind. Hyg. Occup. Med.*, 1, 73, 1950.
11. **Ershoff, B. H. and Hernandez, H. J.**, Beneficial effects of alfalfa meal and other bulk-containing or bulk-forming materials on symptoms of Tween 60 toxicity in the immature mouse, *J. Nutr.*, 69, 172, 1959.
12. **Engel, B. W. and Copeland, D. H.**, Protective action of stock diets against the cancer-inducing action of 2-acetylaminofluorene in rats, *Cancer Res.*, 12, 211, 1952.
13. **Wilson, R. B., Hutcheson, D. P., and Wideman, L.**, Dimethylhydrazine-induced colon tumors in rats fed diets containing beef fat or corn oil with and without wheat bran, *Am. J. Clin. Nutr.*, 30, 176, 1977.
14. **Watanabe, K., Reddy, B. S., Weisburger, J. H., and Kritchevsky, D.**, Effect of dietary alfalfa, pectin, and wheat bran on azoxymethane- or methylnitrosourea-induced colon carcinogenesis in F344 rats, *J. Natl. Cancer Inst.*, 63, 141, 1979.
15. **Reddy, B. S., Mori, H., and Nicolais, M.**, Effect of dietary wheat bran and dehydrated citrus fiber on azoxymethane-induced intestinal carcinogenesis in Fischer 344 rats, *J. Natl. Cancer Inst.*, 66, 553, 1981.
16. **Reddy, B. S. and Mori, H.**, Effect of dietary wheat bran and dehydrated citrus fiber on 3,2'-dimethyl-4-aminobiphenyl-induced intestinal carcinogenesis in F344 rats, *Carcinogenesis*, 2, 21, 1981.
17. **Nigro, N. D., Bull, A. W., Klopfer, B. A., Pak, M. S., and Campbell, R. L.**, Effect of dietary fiber on azoxymethane-induced intestinal carcinogenesis in rats, *J. Natl. Cancer Inst.*, 62, 1097, 1979.
18. **Jacobs, L. R.**, Enhancement of rat colon carcinogenesis by wheat bran consumption during the stage of 1,2-dimethylhydrazine administration, *Cancer Res.*, 43, 4057, 1983.
19. **Barnes, D. S., Clapp, N. K., Scott, D. A., and Berry, S. G.**, Effects of wheat, rice, corn, and soybean bran or 1,2-dimethylhydrazine-induced large bowel tumorigenesis, *Nutr. Cancer*, 5, 1, 1983.
20. **Bauer, H. G., Asp, N., Oste, R., Dahlquist, A., and Fredlund, P. E.**, Effect of dietary fiber on induction of colorectal tumors and fecal β-glucuronidase activity in the rat, *Cancer Res.*, 39, 3752, 1979.
21. **Clapp, N. K., Henke, M. A., London, J. F., and Shock, T. L.**, Enhancement of 1,2-dimethylhydrazine-induced large bowel tumorigenesis in Balb/c mice by corn, soybean and wheat bran, *Nutr. Cancer*, 6, 77, 1984.
22. **Reddy, B. S., Maeura, Y., and Wayman, M.**, Effect of dietary corn bran and autohydrolyzed lignin on 3,2'-dimethyl-4-aminobiphenyl-induced intestinal carcinogenis in male F344 rats, *J. Natl. Cancer Inst.*, 71, 419, 1983.
23. **Freeman, H. J., Spiller, G. A., and Kim, Y. S.**, A double-blind study on the effects of differing purified cellulose and pectin fiber diets on 1,2-dimethylhydrazine-induced rat colonic neoplasia, *Cancer Res.*, 40, 2661, 1980.
24. **Freeman, H. J., Spiller, G. A., and Kim, Y. S.**, A double-blind study on the effects of purified cellulose dietary fiber on 1,2-dimethylhydrazine-induced rat colonic neoplasia, *Cancer Res.*, 38, 2912, 1978.
25. **Ward, J. M., Yamamoto, R. S., and Weisburger, J. H.**, Cellulose dietary bulk and azoxymethane-induced intestinal cancer, *J. Natl. Cancer Inst.*, 51, 713, 1973.
26. **Jacobs, L. R. and Lupton, J. R.**, Relationship between colonic luminal pH, cell proliferation, and colon carcinogenesis in 1,2-dimethylhydrazine treated rats fed high fiber diets, *Cancer Res.*, 46, 1727, 1986.
27. **Bauer, H. G., Asp, N. G., Dahlquist, A., Fredlund, P. E., Nyman, M., and Oste, R.**, Effect of two kinds of pectin and guar gum on 1,2-dimethylhydrazine initiation of colon tumors and on fecal β-glucuronidase activity in the rat, *Cancer Res.*, 41, 2518, 1981.

28. **Ullah, A. and Shamsuddin, A. M.,** Dose-dependent inhibition of large intestinal cancer by inositol hexaphosphate in F344 rats, *Carcinogenesis (London),* 11, 2219, 1990.
29. **Cohen, L. A., Kendall, M. E., Zang, E., Meschter, C., and Rose, D. P.,** Modulation of N-nitrosomethylurea-induced mammary tumor promotion by dietary fiber and fat, *J. Natl. Cancer Inst.,* 83, 496, 1991.
30. **Reddy, B. S.,** Dietary fiber and colon carcinogenesis: a critical review, in *Dietary Fiber in Health and Disease,* Vahouny, G. V. and Kritchevsky, D., Eds., Plenum Press, New York, 1982, 265.
31. **Freeman, H. J.,** Experimental animal studies in colon carcinogenesis and dietary fiber, in *Medical Aspects of Dietary Fiber,* Spiller, G. A. and McPherson-Kay, R., Eds., Plenum Press, New York, 1980, 83.
32. **Pilch, S. M., Ed.,** Physiological Effects and Health Consequences of Dietary Fiber, Life Sciences Research Office, Federation of American Societies for Experimental Biology, Bethesda, MD, 1987.

Section 8: Consumption Patterns of Dietary Fiber

Chapter 8.1

PATTERNS OF DIETARY FIBER CONSUMPTION IN HUMANS

Sheila Bingham

INTRODUCTION

In recent years, the majority of expert committees have recommended an increase in the fiber content of Western Diets because there is accumulating evidence that fiber is important in the prevention of a number of large bowel disorders.[1-3] However, although it is assumed that fiber intakes are greater in areas where these disorders are rare, in fact little is known of the patterns of fiber consumption worldwide. This is largely due to methodological problems in both the collection of food consumption data from representative population samples and in converting that data into grams of fiber eaten per day, using tables of food composition.

METHODS

Analytical

There are various methods in existence for the measurement of "fiber" in foods, all of which give different values for particular foods, especially cooked foods. Hence, incorporation of "fiber" values into food tables is a difficult problem and most government-sponsored food tables do not include values for it. Crude fiber analyses are not relevant to human population studies.

U.K. food tables, published in 1978,[4] included values for fiber mainly using the Southgate method, and the majority of information about fiber consumption worldwide is based on these analyses. However, recent supplements and editions now incorporate the analysis of nonstarch polysaccharides (NSP) from the analyses of Englyst.[33,36] These do not suffer from analytical problems encountered from the cooking, storage, and preservation of food, which can introduce artifactual increases in "fiber" seen in some other methods. Some information on NSP consumption is beginning to emerge, showing a reduced level using these figures compared with former estimates. In the U.S., estimates based on the table of Lanza and Butrum,[7,8] which incorporate data using four different methods, are also lower than formerly. Although the data on these new estimates is limited, they are doubtless more accurate and therefore are discussed first in this chapter.

Food consumption

In some countries, per capita data on food consumption from national statistics and household surveys are available for the reanalysis of long-term trends in dietary fiber consumption over this century, but these statistics are not available for earlier years. They are also only valid indicators of trends in countries with stable and well-documented population bases, and they give no indication of the amounts of fiber consumed by different age, sex, and occupational groups within the population. National per capita statistics also overestimate food consumption, probably by different amounts in different populations. In Britain, for example, estimates of energy consumption from national statistics are some 25% greater than the estimated energy requirement.[9] Nevertheless, published estimates of dietary fiber consumption are available for some countries using these data and are reported below.

Definitive information on food consumption is obtained from studies of individuals where the amount of food eaten is determined directly. There are many different ways in which this is done,[10] and the data from individuals can be aggregated into group estimates. It should be borne in mind, however, that the estimation of the food intake of free-living individuals is no easy undertaking since all methods rely on information supplied by the subjects themselves, which may not be correct. There are many sources of error, and average intakes estimated on the same population using one method may be up to 30% greater or less than those obtained using a different method.[10] The correct result is usually open to debate, unless actual food intakes can be observed by investigators in certain limited situations, or an independent index, such as 24-h urine N from validated urine collections, is used. Urine N should be 80 ± 5% of calculated dietary N intake in populations consuming amounts of fiber commonly found in Western-type diets.[11]

A second validity check for populations is to calculate basal metabolic rate (BMR) from body weight using published equations and to compare energy intake from the dietary survey with estimated energy expenditure which is between 1.4 to 1.6 times the BMR in sedentary populations.[12] Energy intake to BMR ratios of 1.2 or less, which have been reported in some populations, with no apparent loss of body weight is unphysiological, and hence the validity of this dietary data is questionable. The use of these markers in nutritional epidemiology is discussed elsewhere.[11,12]

NEW ESTIMATES OF NONSTARCH POLYSACCHARIDE (NSP) CONSUMPTION

Estimates of NSP and fiber using newer values are currently available for seven countries; see Table 1. All of these except one, that based on the U.S. NHANES II study, used the Englyst values for the NSP content of foods. In the NHANES II study,[7] several different methods were used to compile a table of fiber values for foods, and these included the AOAC method, neutral detergent fiber, and Englyst values.[8] The food consumption values in the table also incorporate different methods of obtaining food consumption data, ranging from 7-d weighed records in U.K. men and women,[16] 16-d weighed records in U.K. women volunteers,[17] interviews in South African urban blacks,[20] and 24-h recalls in the U.S. NHANES II[7] and Canadian students' study.[19] Recalculated data[21] from the U.S. food balance sheets, using the publication of Heller and Hackler for 1973 to 1975 to NSP, are also shown. A figure for Finnish NSP intakes, calculated from food balance sheets, is also shown.[13] In the remaining studies, in Scandinavia,[14] the U.K. National Household Food Survey,[15] Loma Linda University volunteers,[22] and in Japan,[18] duplicate diets were analyzed directly for NSP.

Overall, there is only a small range in average intakes worldwide, from 11 g in the U.S. and Japan to 18 g in men in rural Finland. Insoluble fiber is consumed in rather greater quantities than soluble, and supplies from vegetables usually predominate over cereals. The Japanese diet seems to differ from that of the West with its low content of pentose (xylose and arabinose) polysaccharides and higher intake of uronic acids. Men generally seem to consume more than women, with the exception of the small study in the U.K. South African blacks consume remarkably little compared with previous estimates using Southgate's analyses. However, starch consumption in this area is high and would have led to an overestimate in previous analyses.

There is a very large individual range in NSP intake, up to 81 g/d in Canadian students for example. However, this is probably due to the fact that single day estimates are reported in these and other estimates in U.K. volunteers and in the U.S. NHANES study. In the small U.K. study, individual intakes were averaged over 7 days, when the apparent range was reduced; see Figure 1. Nevertheless, the individual range in NSP intake, from 7 to 25 g/d, is still greater than the range in average intake worldwide.

TABLE 1
Non-Starch Polysaccharide and Fiber Intake
(grams per day)

Country	Total	SD	Range	Soluble	Insoluble	Cellulose	Hexoses	Pentoses	Uronic acids	From cereals	From vegetables	Ref.
Finland	16.0	—	—	4.8	11.2	3.8	—	—	—	9.8	3.5	13
Rural Finland	18.4	7.8	—	—	—	4.2	5.3	7.4	1.9	—	—	14
Rural Denmark	18.0	6.4	—	—	—	3.7	5.5	6.6	2.2	—	—	14
Helsinki	14.5	5.4	—	—	—	3.4	3.7	5.5	2.0	—	—	14
Copenhagen	13.2	4.8	—	—	—	3.2	3.6	4.5	1.9	—	—	14
U.K. — National Food Survey	12.4	—	—	—	—	2.6	3.4	4.5	1.8	—	—	15
U.K. — Men	11.2	3.5	5–19	5.2	6.1	3.1	2.2	4.0	1.7	4.4	5.6	16
U.K. — Women	12.5	4.1	7–25	5.4	7.2	3.3	2.2	4.8	2.0	—	—	17
U.K. — Women volunteers	15.8	5.1	1–68[a]	6.7	9.1	—	—	—	—	—	—	
Japan	10.9	—	—	4.1	6.8	3.0	2.9	1.8	3.1	—	—	18
Canada — students	12	—	1–81[a]	5	7	—	—	—	—	—	—	19
South Africa — urban black M	14	5	—	—	—	—	—	—	—	—	—	20
urban black F	13	5	—	—	—	—	—	—	—	—	—	
U.S. — National Statistics 1973–75	17	—	—	—	—	—	—	—	—	—	—	21
U.S. — NHANES II Men	13	—	1–48[a]	—	—	—	—	—	—	5.6	6.6	7
Women	9	—		—	—	—	—	—	—	—	—	
U.S. — volunteers Loma Linda Univ. Men	17	—	—	9	8	—	—	—	—	—	—	22
Women	12	—	—	6	6	—	—	—	—	—	—	22

[a] = daily range.

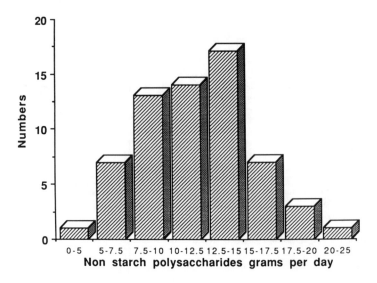

FIGURE 1. Distribution of individual nonstarch polysaccharide intakes in 63 men and women. (From Bingham et al., *J. Hum. Nutr. Dietet.*, 3, 333, 1990. With permission.)

DIETARY FIBER (SOUTHGATE ANALYSIS) CONSUMPTION

Europe

National statistics

In Table 2, data on 23 countries from Bright-See and McKeown-Eyssen[23] have been collated into 4 regions of Europe. These data, based on food analyses of Southgate, show that fiber intakes are greatest in the Mediterranean countries, with an equal contribution from vegetables and cereals. East European intakes follow a similar pattern. In Scandinavia, intakes are lowest, mainly due to the low intake of 14 g found in Iceland, and cereals contribute more than vegetables. In North and Central Europe, vegetables are the major source.

Individual surveys

Table 3 summarizes results from a number of surveys of between 30 to 2200 individuals which have been carried out in Europe. Comparisons are possible because the samples were all randomly selected from population or electoral registers, and response rates were high, usually around 80%. In all these surveys, food consumption was assessed by asking subjects to keep records of food actually consumed, and the amounts of food eaten were in most cases weighed out by the subjects themselves. Most subjects were asked to keep a record for 1 week, but in one survey in Scotland, each individual was studied for 1 month. The majority of the results were calculated using Southgate's method of analysis in the British food tables, although this was supplemented in Denmark and Finland with Englyst's values for rye flour,[26] and in the Netherlands with data from the method of Hellendoorn[37] and Katan.[38] Fiber intakes in the U.K. were measured at around the 20 g mark, with lowest intakes recorded in Scotland. The largest survey, of over 2000 individuals, recorded an intake as high as 25 g in men.[24] However, modified values for the fiber content of bread were used in these surveys.[39] Intakes in rural Finland and Denmark and in Holland and Yugoslavia were rather greater, whereas intakes in urban areas were also around 20 g/d.

TABLE 2
Per Capita Dietary Fiber Supply in Europe 1972–1974
(grams per day)[23]

Area		Total	From cereal	From vegetable	From fruit
Scandinavia[a]	(5)	21	10	7	4
North/Central[b]	(8)	25	9	11	5
Mediterranean[c]	(5)	38	16	16	6
East[d]	(5)	30	14	12	4

[a] Denmark, Finland, Iceland, Norway, Sweden.
[b] Austria, Belgium, France, Germany, Ireland, Switzerland, Netherlands, U.K.
[c] Greece, Italy, Portugal, Spain, Yugoslavia.
[d] Bulgaria, Czechoslovakia, Hungary, Poland, Romania.

Individual variation

In some of these surveys in Europe, data on the distribution of dietary fiber intakes of individuals within the overall average are published, and these are summarized in Table 3. Coefficients of variation (standard deviation/mean %) are on average 35% and the range between individuals is greater than that found between populations, for example, from 8 to 32 g/d in the Welsh and British surveys. Thus, as with NSP, even though dietary fiber intakes in Europe are comparatively low, individuals appear to vary markedly one from another within a population.

Household surveys

A commonly used method of assessing the dietary intake of populations is the household survey, whereby food entering a household over a certain period, usually 1 week, is estimated and the total food available divided by the number of people living in the household. This does not give information about the distribution of intakes between different individuals, but additional information about dietary fiber consumption in European populations is provided from a survey carried out in the EEC in 1963 to 1965 to assess levels of radioactive contamination.[40] In this survey, each family weighed all their food after preparing it, thus eliminating the need to make corrections for inedible wastage. All the areas studied were rural, and approximately 30 families were studied per month over a period of 3 years. Table 4 summarizes fiber intakes calculated from the published values on food consumption, using values for British foods, together with data from another household survey, the National Food Survey, which has been carried out every year in Britain since 1940. In this, about 6500 households are studied per year, randomly selected from each of the nine standard regions in England, Wales, and Scotland. Food entering the household is not weighed, but it is estimated from records of food purchases kept by the housewife for 1 week. Total dietary fiber intakes in Britain, a largely urban area, estimated from this survey in a comparative year, 1966, were 21 g/d. This is less than the rural areas of Europe with only 32% derived from cereals, compared with an average of 45% in the EEC, although the staple food in all of the areas was white bread.

Seasonal variations in dietary fiber estimated from these two surveys have been reported elsewhere.[34] In the rural areas, seasonal changes from month to month were substantial and in some cases greater than the variations between areas. Possible seasonal variations need therefore to be taken into account when comparing dietary fiber intake of individuals or populations, although in largely urban countries, such as Britain, quarterly seasonal variations are not as marked and are related to consumption of different types of vegetables.[34]

TABLE 3
Dietary Fiber Consumption in Europe: Individual Surveys

Country	Sample	Cooperation rate (%)	No.	Survey method	Analytical method	Total DF (g/d)	Cereal DF (g/d)	Vegetable DF (g/d)	Fruit DF (g/d)	TDF (CV%)	Range (g)	Ref.
Great Britain	Randomly selected from electoral registers, 16–64 years	70		7-d weighed record	SM							
	Men		1087			25	—	—	—	36	10–45	24
	Women		1110			19	—	—	—	36	7–33	24
England	Randomly selected from electoral registers, 20–80 years			7-d weighed record	S							
	Men	82	32			19.8	5.7	8.8	2.0	27	10–32	25
	Women	58	31			20.1	6.6	7.6	2.6	26	18–32	
Wales	Randomly selected men from prevalence study of heart disease	89	119	7-d weighed record	S	19.9	9.0	—	—	34	8–32	26
Scotland	Randomly selected men aged 40 years	78	107	7-d weighed record	S	17.5	7.6	—	—	32	6–36	27
Scotland	Randomly selected men and women aged 21–69 years	84		28-d estimated record	S							
	Men		16			16.5	—	—	—	—	—	28
	Women		27			15.0	—	—	—	—	—	
N. Ireland	Randomly selected from electoral											

	registers, 16–64 years									
	Men	74	258	7-d weighed record	S	21	—	—	—	37	—	29
	Women		334			23	—	—	—	32	—	
Netherlands	Randomly selected from electoral registers, 25–65 years										
	Men	67	44	7-d estimated record	K	27.5	7.7	9.8	3.6	28	—	30
	Women		56		S	21.3				22		
	Men, Zutphen	—	871	Diet history	H ?	30.4	—	—	—	32	—	32
Finland	Randomly selected from population registers, men aged 50–89 years										
	Rural	83	30	4-d weighed record	S	26.6	19.5	4.6	1.6	42	5–45	32, 33
	Helsinki	74	29		E	21.5	12.8	6.1	1.6	42	10–40	
Denmark	Randomly selected from population registers, men aged 50–59 years										
	Rural	63	30	4-d weighed record	S	23.4	13.5	6.5	2.7	37	10–55	32, 33
	Copenhagen	75	30		E	18.0	10.6	4.7	1.7	36	2–30	
Yugoslavia	Randomly selected men; 7 countries heart study	—	49	7-d weighed record	S	25.5	8.7	13.3	3.4	29	9–46	34, 35

Note: S[4], H[37], K[38], E[36], SM[39].

TABLE 4
Sources of Dietary Fiber in 11 Regions of the European Economic Community[a]

Area[b]	Cereal	Vegetable	Fruit, nuts	Potato	Total
Friesland (H)	8.2	5.6	2.6	6.3	22.6
Gent (B)	10.9	4.1	1.7	12.3	28.9
Liege (B)	8.0	6.0	2.3	10.5	26.8
Luxembourg	7.3	6.5	2.1	13.2	29.1
Hessen (G)	11.6	4.9	2.6	8.2	27.3
Normandy (F)	9.1	5.7	2.2	7.8	24.8
Bretagne (F)	10.2	4.9	1.8	6.9	23.8
Vendee (F)	10.1	12.7	2.8	4.0	29.6
Fruili (I)	14.7	5.1	1.3	3.8	24.9
Campania (I)	13.4	7.7	4.3	1.6	26.9
Basilicata (I)	13.5	5.7	3.9	0.7	23.8
Britain (1966)	6.7	10.3[c]	2.3	—	21.1

[a] Values are given as grams per person per day.
[b] H, Holland; B, Belgium; G, Germany; F, France; I, Italy.
[c] Includes potato.

TABLE 5
Long-Term Trends in Dietary Fiber Consumption in Europe (grams per head per day)

Year	Britain[42] Total	Britain[42] Cereal	Netherlands[30] Total	Netherlands[30] Cereal	Denmark[43] Total	Denmark[43] Cereal
1909–1913	24	11	—	—	—	—
1927	—	—	—	—	34	—
1933	—	—	—	—	32	—
1938	22	9	—	—	—	—
1944	32–40	19–25	—	—	37	—
1950–1951	—	—	27	14	31	—
1957–1960	23	9	24	10	25	—
1970–1976	23	8	25	8	23	—

Long-term trends

In Britain[42] and the Netherlands,[30] some long-term trends in dietary fiber consumption over the 20th century have been calculated from national statistics. These are summarized in Table 5, together with calculations of the dietary fiber content of diets consumed by farming households in Denmark.[42] In all three European countries, cereal dietary fiber intake has probably declined, although by only 2 to 3 g since 1909 in Britain. Cereal fiber intakes may have been greater in 1860,[34] although there are no national statistics available earlier than 1909. The decline in cereal fiber consumption has been offset somewhat by increases in vegetable sources of dietary fiber, and the most striking change in Britain was the doubling of fiber intakes during the period 1940 to 1953. This was the result of the raising of flour extraction rates, thus more than doubling the fiber content of bread and cereal fiber intakes during and after World War II. At the same time, bread and vegetable consumption was encouraged while other foods such as meat and cheese were in short supply, so that more bread was eaten.

TABLE 6
Dietary Fiber Intakes in Africa and India
(grams per head per day)

	Total	Cereal	Vegetable	Fruit, nuts	Ref.
Africa					
Kenya					
Kikuyu	86	32	54	—[a]	45
Masai					
Warriors	0	0	0	0	
Women	25	25	—	—	
Malawi (foothill village)	55	40	10	4	46
Swaziland (middle veld)	60	40	19	1	47, 48
Uganda (Buganda)	70	0	67	3	
Nigeria (urban)	63	23	40	—	49
(rural)	69	10	59	—	
India					
Andhra	23	18	—	—	50
Karnataka	42	36	—	—	
Kerala	22	10	—	—	
Tamil Nadu	32	22	—	—	

[a] Not available.

Africa

While much has been written about dietary fiber intakes in Africa, in fact, very little is known about it. No dietary surveys have been done specifically to measure fiber intake and nothing is therefore known of its main sources and composition. Dietary surveys to quantitate intakes of other nutrients have been done, and these have been used as a basis for obtaining some preliminary figures for fiber intakes. These are summarized in Table 6. Studies on dietary fiber intake, using 7-d weighed records and values for the NDF content of foods in 300 young Nigerian women, suggest intakes of 63 g in urban areas and 69 g in rural ones.[50]

Previous data[44] showing intakes of 150 g in Uganda and 130 g in the Kikuyu resulted from food analyses of 6% in plantain and 10% in maize flour.[4] These high values were almost certainly contaminated with starch, and recently published values are much lower, 2% and 4%, respectively.[5,6] The data have therefore been recalculated and result in intakes of 70 g and 90 g, respectively, in these areas (Table 6).

Intakes are still comparatively high however compared with present day estimates of 14 g in 76 urban Sowetan black males and 13 g in 113 females obtained by Segal and Walker[20] (Table 1). They state that fiber intake in the past was higher, 40 to 50 g daily in rural blacks, and that the current intake from unpublished surveys is 25 to 35 g/d. In Soweto, an urban area, refined maize meal is consumed, although there is a trend for increased consumption of brown bread. Legume consumption has decreased, and consumption of vegetables is low due to their high cost. Despite these low fiber intakes, bowel disease is rare. However, starch (including resistant starch) intakes are high and may account for the absence of Western bowel diseases.

Data from another African country, Mauritius, were obtained from food balance sheets by Bright-See and McKeown-Eyssen[23] and are shown in Table 7. The staple cereal in Mauritius is rice, so that intakes of cereal dietary fiber are similar to that of other rice-eating

TABLE 7
Per Capita Dietary Fiber Supply
1972–1974 (grams per day)

Area	Total	From cereal	From vegetables	From fruit
Australasia				
Australia and New Zealand (wheat)	24	9	10	5
Japan, Hong Kong, Singapore (rice)	28	10	14	4
America				
Chile, Cuba, Trinidad, Uruguay (wheat and rice)	25	12	10	3
Costa Rica, Mexico (maize)	33	19	9	5
North America				
United States	23	6	11	6
Canada	22	6	11	5
Other				
Israel	36	16	12	8
Mauritius	17	10	6	1

areas, such as Japan, about 10 g/d. Intakes of vegetables and fruit dietary fiber are however much lower so that total intakes are apparently one of the lowest in the world, with only Iceland having a lower value, of 14 g/d.[23]

India

Dietary fiber intakes have been calculated using data from a number of dietary surveys carried out by the National Nutritional Monitoring Bureau in 1980 in India.[49] These show a twofold range in fiber intake from 22 g/d in predominantly rice-eating states such as Kerala to 42 g/d in Karnataka where other cereals such as millet are eaten in addition. In Kerala, 9.8 g/d of dietary fiber came from cereals compared with 35.9 g/d in Karnataka (Table 6).

Australasia

A number of reports of the dietary fiber intake in New Zealand, Polynesia, and Australia are available and are summarized in Table 7. All suggest that dietary fiber intakes are low and similar to those of Europe, around 20 g/d in New Zealand women and in Australia. Intakes are three times higher in Tongan women, 65% of the dietary fiber coming from taro, cassava, and breadfruit, but surprisingly low on another Polynesian Island, Tokelau (Table 8).

Japan

With its highly urbanized society, yet disease pattern which contrasts with Western countries, Japan is of special interest to the epidemiologist, particularly since these patterns of disease change within one or two generations in Japanese who migrate.[56] Traditional Japanese diets are known to be low in fat and high in carbohydrate on which basis dietary fiber intakes might be expected to be high. However, since rice contains so little dietary fiber,[5] it might be predicted that the fiber intake of populations where rice is the staple cereal would be low. The Japanese diet is thus reported to contain only 19.4 g/d in 1979.[57]

TABLE 8
Dietary Fiber Intakes in Australasia
(grams per head per day)

	Total	Cereal	Vegetable	Fruit	Ref.
New Zealand					
Europeans[a]	18 ± 5	6	8	4	51, 52, 53
Maori[a]	16 ± 6	6	8	3	51, 52
New Zealand Tongans[a]	19 ± 6	5	10	4	51, 52
Polynesia					
Tonga[a]	72 ± 29	1	48	22	51, 52
Tokelau[a]	15	—	—	—	54
Tokelau[b]	16	—	—	—	54
Australia					
Adelaide[a]	20–22	—	—	—	55
Adelaide[b]	19–20	—	—	—	55

[a] Women.
[b] Men.

TABLE 9
Secular Changes in Major Nutrient Intakes,
1950–1979 (per capita per day) in Japan

Year	Fat (g)	Carbohydrate (g)	Dietary Fiber Total (g)	Dietary Fiber From rice (g)	Protein from animal food (g)
1950	18	418	—[a]	—	25.0
1955	20.3	411	—	—	32.0
1960	24.7	399	—	—	35.4
1965	36.0	384	21.2[b]	7.7[b]	40.0
1970	46.5	368	20.2	7.0	44.1
1975	52.0	337	20.2	5.7	48.6
1979	54.8	315	19.4	5.1	50.3

[a] Data not available.
[b] 1966.

Mori, using his own technique for analyses of Japanese foods, reported the dietary fiber content of two student meals to be 14.8 and 19.5 g/d.[58] Estimates from food balance sheet data are rather greater, 32 g/d.[23] The estimates of Far East countries are shown in Table 7. These estimates using Southgate values for fiber are less than those for NSPs, of 11 g/d (Table 1).

Long-term trends

In Japan, yearly nationwide household surveys are carried out, and this data has been used to calculate dietary fiber intakes using the British Food Tables together with neutral detergent fiber plus pectin values for some seaweed-based foods.[52,53] Total dietary fiber from rice has fallen from 7.7 g/d in 1965 to 5.1 g/d in 1979, and overall total dietary fiber intake has fallen from 21.2 g/d in 1965 to 19.4 g/d in 1979 (Table 9). These changes are small compared with a 70 g/d decline in carbohydrate intake since 1965, a threefold increase in fat intake, and a 25% increase in the amount of protein derived from animal products since 1950.

TABLE 10
Dietary Fiber Intake in North America
(grams per head per day)

	Total	Cereal	Vegetable	Fruit	Ref.
U.S.					
Men	20 ± 10	7[a]	9	5	60
Women	13 ± 6	4[a]	5	3	60
Simulated diet	19	—	—	—	61
NHANES II					
Men[b]	16	—	—	—	7
Women[b]	11	—	—	—	7
Female nurses					
Third quintile	14–17	4–5	5–7	2–3	64
American-Japanese men	12	(range 1–46 g)			65
Canada					
Men[b]	18 ± 9	9 ± 6	—	—	62
Women	19 ± 7	—	—	—	63

[a] Includes fiber from legumes.
[b] Food consumption estimated for 24-h recall.

There are no household statistics available prior to 1950, but a dietary record of an artist's family (all adults) in 1925 showed that on a typical day, rice was eaten three times a day, together with pickles, salted fish, soybean curd, radishes, spring onions, and soy sauce. Only 12 g/d of fat was eaten, but the dietary fiber content was the same as today, 18.2 g/d, although at that time rice supplied 11.3 g/d.[57]

Present day intakes

Geographical comparisons within Japan show that these changes in diet have been most marked in the urban areas.[57] In the ten largest cities in 1979, 57.5 g/d of fat were eaten, and 52% of protein was derived from animal foods. Carbohydrate and dietary fiber intakes were also lower, 296 and 17.7 g/d in these areas. This compares with less fat, 50.6 g/d less protein from animal sources, 48.2%, more carbohydrate, 332 g, and more dietary fiber, 20.2 g, in towns and villages. There is a clear trend between these extremes, depending on the size of the city.

North America

Fiber intakes calculated using Southgate analyses from the food balance sheets of Canada and the U.S. show almost identical intakes of 22 to 23 g per capita per day, 6 g from cereals and 11 g from vegetables (Table 7). Previous studies suggested an intake of about 20 g/d from individual surveys (Table 10), although the recent reanalysis of the NHANES II suggests intakes lower than this, 11 g for women and 16 g for men, 13 g on average.[7] Intakes assessed by questionnaire of the third quintile of 88,751 American female nurses ranged from 14 to 17 g/d, with 5 to 7 g obtained from vegetables and 4 to 5 g from cereals.[60] Intakes of 8000 American-Japanese men were lower, 12 g/d, range (from 24-h recall data) 1 to 46 g/d.[61]

NSP estimates (Table 1) are some 25% lower for food balance sheet estimates, 17 g/d in the U.S., of which 7 g is derived from vegetables and 6 g from cereals. NHANES estimates using the fiber table of Lanza and Butrum are 20% less, 11 g on average compared with 13 g using Southgate analyses alone.[7,8] Recalculations of data on long-term trends in food intake showed a 33% decrease in total dietary fiber and a 55% decrease in cereal dietary fiber in the U.S. from 1909 to 1975.[21,34]

South America

No individual surveys to measure dietary fiber consumption have been published in South American countries, although Bright-See and McKeown-Eyssen[23] calculated fiber intakes from food balance sheets which are summarized in Table 7. Calculated intakes were higher in the two maize eating areas, Costa Rica and Mexico. In wheat and rice areas, fiber intakes were similar to North America, although there was a wide variation; Uruguayan intakes were 20 g/d whereas those in Chile were 35 g.[23]

The Middle East

Data from food balance sheets and individual surveys are available for Israel. Food balance sheet data suggest that intakes are comparatively high, at 38 g/d (Table 7). Intakes assessed by interviews of 250 adults aged over 40 years were lower, 19 ± 6 g in Tel Aviv, and 31 ± 11 g and 23 ± 8 g in two rural Kibbutzim.[66]

CONCLUSIONS

Current evidence indicates that average dietary fiber intake is in the range of 20 to 40 g/d in the majority of populations studied throughout the world. Evidence from Japan and India suggests that in areas where rice is the staple cereal, intakes of dietary fiber are likely to be similar to those in the West.

The most accurate data using newer values for the fiber analysis of foods confirm this, with average intakes of 11 to 12 g in Japan, the U.S., and the U.K. Worldwide, newer analyses show that there is only a small range in intake to a maximum of 16 to 18 g/d in Finland.

Trends in dietary fiber intake in Holland, Denmark, and Japan are similar to those reported in the U.S. and Britain, namely a decline in cereal fiber consumption which has been offset to some extent by an increase in vegetable consumption. Relatively little data is available, however, and for some areas, such as parts of Asia, most of the Middle East, and Russia, there is no data at all due partly to continuing problems in the analysis of dietary fiber and the assessment of food consumption. More carefully standardized and well-validated studies to assess dietary fiber intake worldwide are clearly needed.

REFERENCES

1. **WHO,** *Diet, Nutrition and Chronic Diseases,* Tech. Rep. Ser. 797, World Health Organization, Geneva, 1990.
2. *COMA Report on DRV for Food Energy and Nutrients for the UK,* D. H. Rep. Health Soc. Subj. 41, Her Majesty's Stationery Office, London, 1991.
3. *Recommended Dietary Allowances 10th Edition,* Food and Nutrition Board Sub-Committee on the Tenth Edition of the RDAs, National Academic Press, 1989.
4. **Paul, A. A. and Southgate, D. A. T.,** *McCance and Widdowson's The Composition of Foods,* 4th ed., MRC Spec. Rep. 297, Her Majesty's Stationery Office, London, 1978.
5. **Holland, B., Unwin, I. D., and Buss, D. H.,** *Cereals and Cereal Products,* 3rd Suppl., Royal Society of Chemistry, Letchworth, U.K., 1988.
6. **Holland, B., Unwin, I. D., and Buss, D. H.,** *Vegetables, Herbs and Spices,* 5th Suppl., Royal Society of Chemistry, Letchworth, U.K., 1991.
7. **Lanza, E., Jones, Y., Block, G., and Kessler, L.,** Dietary fiber intakes in the US population, *Am. J. Clin. Nutr.,* 46, 790, 1987.
8. **Lanza, E. and Butrum, R.,** A critical review of fiber analysis and data, *J. Am. Diet. Assoc.,* 86, 732, 1986.

9. **Ministry of Agriculture, Fisheries and Food,** *Household Food Consumption and Expenditure 1966,* Annual Reports of National Food Survey Committee, Her Majesty's Stationery Office, London, 1968.
10. **Bingham, S.,** The dietary assessment of individuals, *Nutr. Abs. Rev.,* 57, 705, 1987.
11. **Bingham, S.,** Validations of dietary assessment through biomarkers, in *Biomarkers of Dietary Exposure,* Kok, F. J. and van't Voer, P., Eds., Smith-Gordon, London, 1991.
12. **Bingham, S. and Westerterp, K. R.,** Energy expenditure as a biomarker of energy intake: workshop report, in *Biomarkers of Dietary Exposure,* Kok, F. J. and van't Voer, P., Eds., Smith-Gordon, 1991.
13. **Varo, P., Laine, R., Veijalainen, K., Pero, K., and Koivistoinen, P.,** Dietary fibre and available carbohydrates in Finnish cereal products, vegetables and fruits, *J. Agric. Sci. Finland,* 56, 39, 1984.
14. **IARC,** Report of the Second IARC Coordinated International Study on Diet and Large Bowel Cancer in Denmark and Finland, *Nutr. Cancer,* 4, 3, 1982.
15. **Bingham, S. A., Williams, D. R. R., and Cummings, J. H.,** Dietary fibre consumption: new estimates and their relation to large bowel cancer mortality in Britain, *Br. J. Cancer,* 52, 399, 1985.
16. **Bingham, S. A., Pett, S., and Day, K. C.,** Non-starch polysaccharide intake of a representative sample of British adults, *J. Hum. Nutr. Dietet.,* 3, 333, 1990.
17. **Bingham, S. A.,** unpublished.
18. **Kuratsune, M., Honda, T., Englyst, H. N., and Cummings, J. H.,** Dietary fiber in the Japanese diet as investigated in connection with colon cancer risk, *Jpn. J. Cancer Res.,* 77, 736, 1986.
19. **Stephen, A. M.,** New perspectives on carbohydrates, *Can. Pharm. J.,* October, 443, 1990.
20. **Segal, I. and Walker, A. R. P.,** Low fat intake with falling fiber intake in Soweto, *Nutr. Cancer,* 8, 185, 1986.
21. **Heller, S. N. and Hackler, L. R.,** Changes in the crude fibre content of the American diet, *Am. J. Clin. Nutr.,* 31, 1510, 1978. (Data recalculated by S. Kingman, personal communication.)
22. **Rider, A. A., Arthur, R. S., and Calkins, B. M.,** Laboratory analysis of 3 day composite food samples, *Am. J. Clin. Nutr.,* 40, 914, 1984. Reanalysis of composites, with Englyst method (Englyst, personal communication).
23. **Bright-See, E. and McKeown-Eyssen, G. E.,** Estimates of dietary fibre supply in 38 countries, *Am. J. Clin. Nutr.,* 39, 821, 1985; 41, 824, 1985.
24. **Gregory, J., Foster, K., Tyler, H., and Wiseman, M.,** The dietary and nutritional survey of British adults, OPCS: Her Majesty's Stationery Office, London, 1990.
25. **Bingham, S., Cummings, J. H., and McNeil, N. I.,** Intakes and sources of dietary fiber in the British population, *Am. J. Clin. Nutr.,* 32, 1313, 1979.
26. **Yarnell, J. W. G., Fehilly, A. M., Milbank, J. E., Sweetnam, P. M., and Walker, C. L.,** A short dietary questionnaire for use in an epidemiological study, *Hum. Nutr. Appl. Nutr.,* 37A, 103, 1983.
27. **Thompson, M., Logan, R. L., Sharman, M., Lockerbie, L., Riemersma, R. A., and Oliver, M. F.,** Dietary survey in 40 year old Edinburgh men, *Hum. Nutr. Appl. Nutr.,* 36A, 272, 1982.
28. **Bull, N. L., Smart, G. A., and Judson, H.,** Food and nutrient intakes on Westray in the Orkney Islands, *Ecol. Food. Nutr.,* 12, 97, 1982.
29. **Barker, M. E. et al.,** Diet, lifestyle and health in Northern Ireland, University of Ulster, N. Ireland, 1989.
30. **Van Staveren, W. A., Hautvast, J. G. A., Katan, M. B., van Montfort, M. A., and van Oosten-van der Goes, H. G. C.,** Dietary fiber consumption in an adult Dutch population, *J. Am. Dietet. Assoc.,* 80, 324, 1982.
31. **Kromhout, D., Bosschieter, E. B., and Coulander, C.,** Dietary fiber and 10 year mortality in the Zutphen study, *Lancet,* ii, 518, 1982.
32. **Bingham, S., Cummings, J. H., Cole, T. J., Helms, P., and Seppanen, R.,** Individual variation in dietary fibre intake in different populations, in *Fibre in Human Nutrition,* Bulletin 20, Royal Society of New Zealand, Wellington, N.Z., 1983, 33.
33. **Englyst, H. N., Bingham, S. A., Wiggins, H. S., Southgate, D. A. T., Seppanen, R., Helms, P., Anderson, V., Day, K. C., Choolun, R., Collinson, E., and Cummings, J. H.,** Non-starch polysaccharide consumption in four Scandinavian populations, *Nutr. Cancer,* 4, 50, 1982.
34. **Bingham, S. and Cummings, J. H.,** Intakes and sources of dietary fibre in man, in *Medical Aspects of Dietary Fibre,* Spiller, G. A. and Kay, R. M., Eds., Plenum Press, New York, 1980, 261.
35. **Buzina, R., Ferber, E., Keys, A., Brodavec, A., Agneletto, B., and Horvat, A.,** Diets of rural families and heads of families in two regions of Yugoslavia, *Voeding,* 25, 629, 1964.
36. **Englyst, H.,** The determination of carbohydrate and its composition in plant material, in *The Analysis of Dietary Fibre in Food,* James, W. P. T. and Theander, O., Eds., Marcel Dekker, New York, 1981.
37. **Hellendoorn, E. W., Noordhoff, M. G., and Slagman, J.,** Enzymatic determination of the indigestible residue content of human food, *J. Sci. Food Agric.,* 26, 1461, 1975.
38. **Katan, N. and van de Bovenkamp, P.,** Determination of total dietary fiber by difference and of pectin by titration or copper titration, in *The Analysis of Dietary Fiber in Food,* James, W. P. T. and Theander, O., Eds., Marcel Dekker, New York, 1981.

39. **Wenlock, R. W., Sivell, L. M., and Agater, J. B.,** Dietary fiber fractions in cereal products in Britain, *J. Sci. Food Agric.,* 36, 113, 1985.
40. **Cresta, M., Ledermann, S., Gardiner, A., Lombardo, E., and Lacourly, G.,** A dietary survey of 11 areas of the E.E.C. in order to determine levels of radioactive contamination, *Euratom,* EUR.4218F, 1969.
41. **Ministry of Agriculture, Fisheries and Food,** *Household Food Consumption and Expenditure, 1950–1981.* Annual reports of the National Food Survey Committee, Her Majesty's Stationery Office, London, 1953–1983.
42. **Southgate, D. A. T., Bingham, S., and Robertson, J.,** Dietary fibre in the British diet, *Nature (London),* 274, 51, 1978.
43. **Helms, P., Jorgensen, I. M., Paerregaard, A., Bjerrum, L., Poulson, L., and Mosbech, J.,** Dietary patterns in Them and Copenhagen, Denmark, *Nutr. Cancer,* 4, 23, 1982.
44. **Bingham, S.,** Patterns of dietary fiber consumption in humans, in *CRC Handbook of Dietary Fiber in Human Nutrition,* Spiller, G., Ed., CRC Press, Boca Raton, FL, 1986.
45. **Orr, J. B. and Gilks, J. L.,** *Studies of Nutrition, The Physique and Health of Two African Tribes,* M.R.C. Spec. Rep. Ser. 155, Her Majesty's Stationery Office, London, 1931.
46. **Platt, B. S.,** Unpublished report on Nyasaland held at London School of Hygiene and Tropical Medicine, London, 1938/39.
47. **Jones, S.,** *A Study of Swazi Nutrition,* Report for the University of Natal for the Swaziland Government (note dated).
48. **Ruitishauser, I.,** personal communication, 1977.
49. **Mbofung, C. N., Atinmo, T., and Omolulu, A.,** Dietary fiber in the diets of urban and rural Nigerian women, *Nutr. Res.,* 4, 225, 1984.
50. **Shetty, P. S.,** Dietary fibre intakes in India, Proc. Annual Conf. Ind. Soc. Gastrol., Trivandrum, 1981.
51. **Stace, N. H., Pomare, E. W., Peters, S., Thomas, L., and Fisher, A.,** *Gastroenterology,* 89, 1291, 1981.
52. **Pomare, E. W., Stace, N. H., Peters, S. G., and Fisher, A.,** Dietary intakes, stool characteristics and biliary bile acid composition in four South Pacific populations, in *Fibre in Human and Animal Nutrition,* Bulletin 20, Royal Society of New Zealand, Wellington, N.Z., 1983, 33.
53. **Hillman, L. C., Stace, N. J., Fisher, A., and Pomare, E. W.,** Dietary intakes and stool characteristics of patients with the irritable bowel syndrome, *Am. J. Clin. Nutr.,* 36, 626, 1982.
54. **Prior, I. A., Davidson, F., Salmond, C. E., and Czochanska, Z.,** The Pukapuka and Tokelau Island studies, *Am. J. Clin. Nutr.,* 34, 1552, 1981.
55. **Potter, J. D., McMichael, A. J., and Bonnett, A. J.,** A case control study of colorectal cancer in South Australia, in *Fibre in Human and Animal Nutrition,* Bulletin 20, Royal Society of New Zealand, Wellington, N.Z. 1983, 35.
56. **Haenszel, W. and Kurihara, M.,** Studies of Japanese migrants mortality from cancer and other diseases among Japanese in the United States, *J. Natl. Cancer Inst.,* 40, 43, 1968.
57. **Minowa, M., Bingham, S., and Cummings, J. H.,** Dietary fibre intake in Japan, *Hum. Nutr.,* 37A, 113, 1983.
58. **Mori, B. and Aragane, K.,** On the determination of dietary fibre, *Nutr. Food.,* 34, 97, 1981.
59. **Nakamura, H., Tamura, A., Tanaka, H., Natsushita, C., Yamamoto, F., Yoshi, S., and Izumi, D.,** Dietary fibre content of foodstuffs for diabetes, *Nutr. Food,* 34, 71, 1981.
60. **Marlett, J. A. and Bokram, R. L.,** Relationship between calculated and crude fiber intakes of 200 college students, *Am. J. Clin. Nutr.,* 34, 335, 1981.
61. **Ahrens, E. H. and Boucher, C. A.,** The composition of a simulated American diet, *J. Am. Dietet. Assoc.,* 73, 613, 1978.
62. **Kay, R. M., Sabry, Z. I., and Csima, A.,** Multivariate analysis of diet and serum lipids in normal men, *Am. J. Clin. Nutr.,* 33, 2566, 1980.
63. **Gibson, R. S. and Scythes, C. A.,** Trace element intakes of women, *Br. J. Nutr.,* 48, 241, 1982.
64. **Willett, W. C., Stampfer, M. J., Colditz, G. A., Rosner, B. A., and Speizer, F. E.,** Relation of meat, fat and fiber intake to risk of colon cancer, *New Engl. J. Med.,* 323, 1664, 1990.
65. **Heilbrun, L. K., Nomura, A., Hankin, J., and Stemmerman, G. N.,** Diet and colorectal cancer with special reference to fiber intake, *Int. J. Cancer,* 44, 1, 1989.
66. **Rozen, P., Horwitz, C., Takenkin, C., Ron, E., and Katz, L.,** Dietary habits and colorectal cancer incidence in a second-defined Kibbutz population, *Nutr. Cancer,* 9, 177, 1987.

Chapter 8.2

THE CONSUMPTION OF FIBER IN VEGETARIANS AND NONVEGETARIANS

Beverly M. Calkins

For many years, the undigested fiber portion of foods was believed to contribute nothing to nutrition. Accordingly, information about the chemical constituents of fiber, the fiber content of foods, the requirement for or the usual intake of fiber, and the effects of fiber in nutrition and disease were largely overlooked.[1,2] However, over the past three decades an association between low fiber intake and a variety of chronic diseases has been suggested, among them being ischemic heart disease, varicose veins, obesity, bowel cancer, and diverticular disease.[3-9] For the hypothesized association to be supported by epidemiological data, vegetarians, whose diets are composed largely of plant foods, should be found to have lower mortality rates for such diseases. For ischemic heart disease and bowel cancer, reports on Seventh-Day Adventists (SDAs)* have shown this to be the case. The occurrence of ischemic heart disease among nonvegetarian SDA males is three times that of vegetarian SDA males, 35 to 64 years of age, a significant excess which persists even after accounting for a number of risk factors.[10] For bowel cancer, reports of comparisons between SDAs and non-SDAs have shown that the age-sex adjusted mortality ratio among male SDAs is 58% of U.S. white males. The mortality ratio for female SDAs is 52% of the U.S. white females.[11]

The *a priori* assumption that vegetarians have a higher intake of fiber may not necessarily be true, since the foods from meat sources could be simply replaced with dairy and egg products which also have little or no fiber to contribute to the diet. To further support the hypothesis that fiber is protective against certain diseases, vegetarians should be shown to have higher intakes of fiber. If this is demonstrated, then estimation of the quantity of fiber intake among vegetarians would provide some idea of the amounts in the diet which could be considered protective. Total dietary fiber is now regarded to be composed of a number of biochemically separate fractions.[2] The difference in intake between vegetarians and nonvegetarians of each of these fractions must also be explored. This chapter summarizes the available literature on the intake of dietary fiber and fractions of fiber in vegetarian and nonvegetarian populations.

All available reports in the literature comparing fiber intake between vegetarian and comparable nonvegetarian groups are summarized in Table 1.[12-58] The intake of fiber in vegetarians is consistently higher in every report except for King et al.[26] and Kurup et al.[29] However, in both of these studies the groups which are culturally similar show consistently higher intakes of fiber than the general population comparison group.

The studies do not agree with respect to estimation of the amount of fiber consumed. This is not unexpected since these reports are drawn from populations which differ culturally, ethnically, and socioeconomically. In addition, the studies represent data taken over a span of time during which a variety of sources for determining fiber have been used, some

---

* The Seventh-Day Adventist church is a small, conservative denomination with about 600,000 members in North America who have, for over 100 years, abstained from drinking alcoholic beverages and smoking. About 50% of SDAs also follow a lacto-ovo-vegetarian diet and also tend to avoid caffeine-containing beverages, rich, highly refined foods, and hot condiments and spices. About 60% of the SDA population are adult converts; the remainder were raised in the church recommended life-style as children of SDA parents. SDAs represent in Western cultures one of the largest single groups of individuals who follow a vegetarian dietary pattern, making study of this group logistically quite feasible.

TABLE 1
Fiber Intake of Vegetarians and Nonvegetarians

Investigator (Ref.) (Population) Characteristics	Vegetarians g/day (N) {g/1000 kcal/day}	Nonvegetarians g/day (N) {g/1000 kcal/day}	Fiber content Ref.	Diet[a] intake method
Hardinge (12) (S. California)				
Adult Males				
LOV[b]	16.3(15) {53.7}	10.7(15) {28.8}	31–33	DH
PV[b]	23.9(14) {78.7}			
Adult females				
LOV[b]	12.6(15) {51.5}	8.4(15) {31.3}		
PV[b]	20.7(11) {85.7}			
Pregnant	12.8(26) {46.7}	8.4(28) {28.2}		
Adolescent				
Males	17.8(15) {39.9}	12.2(15) {22.8}		
Females	12.9(15) {41.7}	10.6(15) {25.7}		
Holm(13) (Denmark)				
Males	11.0(29)	4.6(31)	35	DD
GP[c] — 1972 survey		5.6(?)		
Gear(14–15) (England)				
Both sexes	31.0(46)	19.0(235)	34,36	DH
With diverticular disease	33.7(7)	21.8(84)		
Without diverticular dis.	42.8(48)	22.1(105)		
Reddy(16) (New York City)				
Males	20.0(11)	12.0(18)	?	DH, 24R?
(Finland, Kupoio)				
Males		32.2(15)		
Trueherz(17) (London, both sexes)				
Adolescents	29.0(17)	4.8(17)	?	DD
Goldin(18) (Boston)				
Both sexes	8.0(13)	4.8(15)	36	DD
Freeland-Graves(19) (Texas, both sexes)				
LOV[b]	8.9(57)	4.5(41)	31	24R
LV[b]	10.8(14)			
PV[b]	16.1(8)			
Aldercruetz(20–22) (Boston, females)				
Younger	31.1(6)	9.8(7)	36	DD
Older	28.4(8)	15.2(5)		
Postmenopausal	24.2(10)	16.8(10)		
Breast cancer patients		13.8(7)		

TABLE 1 (continued)
Fiber Intake of Vegetarians and Nonvegetarians

Investigator (Ref.) (Population) Characteristics	Vegetarians g/day (N) {g/1000 kcal/day}	Nonvegetarians g/day (N) {g/1000 kcal/day}	Fiber content Ref.	Diet intake method
Abdulia(23)				
(Sweden)				
Both sexes — PV[b]	{29.0}(6)	{6.3}(35)	37	24R?
Burr(24)				
(England)				
Males	36.7(11)	24.5(18)	?	DD
Females	30.1(14)	19.5(28)		
Anderson(25)				
(Canada)				
Females	30.9(49)		36,41	FF,DD
King(25)				
(N. California, females)				
Pregnant	8.9(9) {3.6}	4.8(6) {2.0}	?	DH,DD
Nonpregnant	6.2(5) 4.7			
Abraham(26)				
(England)				
Pregnant females				
Indian	23.0(20)	22.6(20)	34,36	DD
English		16.4(20)		
Gibson(27)				
(Canada, females)				
Postmenopausal	33.2(36)	20.2(30)	34	DD
Kurup(28)				
(S. California)				
SDA Males[b,c]	PVs 71.6(9) {23.6} LOVs 67.0(15) {23.3}	67.1(14) {20.4}		Food samples
GP Males[c]		62.3(9) {16.9}		
SDA Females[b,c]	PVs 52.0(7) {27.2} LOVs 46.5(18) {25.7}	49.5(18) {20.7}		
GP Females[c]		45.7(13) {15.9}		
Ross(43)				
(California)				
Both sexes			58–59	DD
Neutral detergent fiber		51(18)		
LOV	72(20)			
PV	107(15)			
Hemicellulose		38(18)		
LOV	56(20)			
PV	72(15)			
Cellulose		22(18)		

TABLE 1 (continued)
Fiber Intake of Vegetarians and Nonvegetarians

Investigator (Ref.) (Population) Characteristics	Vegetarians g/day (N) {g/1000 kcal/day}	Nonvegetarians g/day (N) {g/1000 kcal/day}	Fiber content Ref.	Diet intake method
LOV	28(20)			
PV	48(15)			
Lignin				
		10(18)		
LOV	16(20)			
PV	24(15)			
Pectin				
		6(18)		
LOV	10(20)			
PV	11(15)			
Davis(44)				
(England)				
Both sexes				
		23(35)	36	DD
LOV	37(34)			
PV	47(31)			
Lowik(45)				
(Dutch)				
Elders				
Male	33(15)	27(225)	46	DD
	{3.9}	{2.7}		
Female	28(17)	23(216)		
	{3.9}	{3.0}		
Aldercreutz(47)				
(Finland)				
Young women				
Summer	23(11)	20(12)	36	
Winter	22	17		
Barbosa(48)				
(S. California)				
Postmenopausal women	24(12)	13(12)	49	DD
Allinger(50)				
(Sweden)				
Both sexes	30(25)	20(26)	51	24-R
Brune(52)				
(Sweden)				
Both sexes	44(13)	18(6)	51	DD
Kelsay(53)				
(United States)			38,54–55	DD
Males				
Asian Indian	12(14)			
Americans	15(14)	9(13)		
Females				
Asian Indian	9(13)			
Americans	13(15)	6(16)		

TABLE 1 (continued)
Fiber Intake of Vegetarians and Nonvegetarians

Investigator (Ref.) (Population) Characteristics	Vegetarians g/day (N) {g/1000 kcal/day}	Nonvegetarians g/day (N) {g/1000 kcal/day}	Fiber content Ref.	Diet[a] intake method
Shultz(56) (Oregon) Postmenopausal women	7(13)	5(16)	57	DD

Note: A question mark indicates that the method or source of determination is uncertain.

[a] FF = Food frequency questionnaire; 24-R = 24-h recall questionnaire; DD = diet diary; DH = diet history.

[b] LOV = Lacto-ovo-vegetarians (exclude meat, fish, and fowl only), LV = lacto-vegetarians (exclude meat, fish, fowl, and eggs only), PV = pure vegetarians (exclude meat, fish, fowl, eggs, and dairy products).

[c] SDA = Seventh-Day Adventists, GP = general population.

estimating crude fiber only and some total dietary fiber. The method of gathering dietary information also varies between these reported studies. The food frequency questionnaire, diet diary, diet history, or 24-h recall are used alone in some reports and in combination in dietary information and determining fiber intake is consistently used for all groups within each study. Thus, these considerations must necessarily limit the conclusions which can be drawn about the amount of fiber consumption which might be considered desirable. The percentage of difference between vegetarian's and nonvegetarian's fiber consumption can be evaluated by these data and is large. The mean difference is 86% (SEM = 15%) greater intake of fiber among vegetarians.

These reports are based on the estimation of fiber intake which is generally considered to be "crude fiber", cellulose, and lignin fractions only. "Total dietary fiber" as calculated from tables of fiber in foods or chemically from samples is composed of many fractions. Of those estimating total dietary fiber, two studies have measured some fractions of dietary fiber chemically. The detailed information on fractions of total dietary fiber from Kurup is summarized in Table 2, separate from the information for the Ross et al. report[43] in Table 1. It is important to note, however, that both of these reports[29,43] represent data developed on vegetarians who are also SDAs.

The intake of each of the fractions of total dietary fiber are reported in grams per day and, for the Kurup report only,[29] grams per 1000 calorie per day intake. The intake in grams per day is greater for lacto-ovo vegetarians and pure vegetarians* (sometimes called vegans), both vegetarian subgroups, in both reports for lignin, cellulose, cutin and silica, and pectin. Intake is greater for men than for women for each fraction, but when the intake is adjusted for calorie intake, the difference between men and women diminishes or disappears for all fractions.[29] After adjusting for sex, the intake of most fractions remains greater for pure vegetarians.

---

* Pure vegetarians exclude all food of animal origin, including meat, fish, fowl, dairy, eggs, and honey. Lacto-ovo vegetarians exclude meat, fish, and fowl.

TABLE 2
Intake of Total Fiber and Fiber Components of Seventh-Day Adventist Vegetarians and Nonvegetarians and the Nonvegetarian General Population

	Intake (g/day)		Intake/1000 kcal (g/day)		
	Mean	SD	Mean	SD	(N)
Total Fiber					
SDA Pure-vege	63.00	31.70	25.18	12.93	(16)
Male	71.58	35.43	23.65	13.60	(9)
Female	51.96	24.21	27.15	12.79	(7)
SDA Lacto-ovo vege	55.80	19.86	24.04	11.74	(33)
Male	66.99	18.24	23.29	12.51	(15)
Female	46.47	16.31	24.67	11.39	(18)
SDA Nonvege	57.16	19.89	20.55	7.49	(32)
Male	67.06	21.36	20.36	7.77	(14)
Female	49.46	15.12	20.70	7.48	(18)
GP Nonvege	52.53	22.95	16.31	8.54	(22)
Male	62.34	19.53	16.92	6.15	(9)
Female	45.73	23.35	15.89	10.10	(13)
Hemicellulose					
SDA Pure-vege	45.37	29.77	18.45	12.43	(16)
Male	48.86	34.58	16.24	12.57	(9)
Female	40.89	24.08	21.28	12.60	(7)
SDA Lacto-ovo vege	43.77	18.18	19.09	10.63	(33)
Male	52.25	18.79	18.43	11.61	(15)
Female	36.69	14.66	19.64	10.05	(18)
SDA Nonvege	47.62	18.45	17.08	6.69	(32)
Male	56.64	19.81	17.25	7.16	(14)
Female	40.60	14.19	16.94	6.51	(18)
GP Nonvege	43.27	22.02	13.59	8.12	(22)
Male	51.73	20.70	14.18	6.36	(9)
Female	37.42	21.73	13.18	9.38	(13)
Lignin					
SDA Pure-vege	3.46	2.29	1.37[c]	0.85	(16)
Male	4.31	2.48	1.43[c]	0.80	(9)
Female	2.36	1.55	1.31	0.96	(7)
SDA Lacto-ovo vege	2.47	1.89	1.08[e]	1.17	(33)
Male	2.75	1.39	0.89[e]	0.59	(15)
Female	2.23	2.24	1.25	1.50	(18)
SDA Nonvege	2.02	1.27	0.74[f]	0.58	(32)
Male	2.15	1.19	0.66	0.49	(14)
Female	1.93	1.35	0.80	0.64	(18)
GP Nonvege	1.52	0.83	0.44	0.21	(22)
Male	1.44	0.73	0.36	0.14	(9)
Female	1.58	0.92	0.49	0.23	(13)

TABLE 2 (continued)
Intake of Total Fiber and Fiber Components of Seventh-Day Adventist Vegetarians and Nonvegetarians and the Nonvegetarian General Population

	Intake (g/day)		Intake/1000 kcal (g/day)		
	Mean	SD	Mean	SD	(N)
Cellulose					
SDA Pure-vege	12.51	5.86	4.69[c]	1.29	(16)
Male	16.31	5.18	5.23[b,c]	1.41	(9)
Female	7.63	0.91	4.00	0.72	(7)
SDA Lacto-ovo vege	7.96	3.46	3.20[d,e]	1.38	(33)
Male	9.69	3.82	3.05[d,e]	1.53	(15)
Female	6.52	2.39	3.33	1.28	(18)
SDA Nonvege	6.44	2.10	2.30	0.87	(32)
Male	7.21	1.86	2.12	0.54	(14)
Female	5.84	2.13	2.44	1.05	(18)
GP Nonvege	6.27	2.60	1.84	0.74	(22)
Male	7.13	2.16	1.83	0.39	(9)
Female	5.68	2.80	1.85	0.93	(13)
Cutin and Silica					
SDA Pure-vege	1.74	1.29	0.68	0.62	(16)
Male	2.26	1.44	0.79	0.77	(9)
Female	1.06	0.69	0.54	0.38	(7)
SDA Lacto-ovo vege	1.51	1.79	0.57	0.90	(33)
Male	2.13	2.25	0.73	1.28	(15)
Female	1.00	1.13	0.44	0.40	(18)
SDA Nonvege	1.12	1.09	0.45	0.55	(32)
Male	1.19	1.18	0.38	0.45	(14)
Female	1.07	1.05	0.50	0.63	(18)
GP Nonvege	1.37	1.69	0.41	0.47	(22)
Male	1.84	2.43	0.48	0.66	(9)
Female	1.04	0.87	0.36	0.30	(13)
Pectin					
SDA Pure-vege	33.53	16.99	12.59[b,c]	4.32	(16)
Male	43.42	16.27	13.74[b,c]	4.56	(9)
Female	20.80	5.75	11.11	3.81	(7)
SDA Lacto-ovo vege	23.51	36.81	10.99	21.06	(33)
Male	32.95	53.71	13.90	31.08	(15)
Female	15.65	5.55	8.57[e]	5.08	(18)
SDA Nonvege	17.67	5.90	6.34	2.68	(32)
Male	20.74	5.15	6.20	2.17	(14)
Female	15.29	5.42	6.44	3.07	(18)
GP Nonvege	14.78	6.24	4.46	1.86	(22)
Male	18.16	6.18	4.74	1.52	(9)
Female	12.44	5.30	4.26	2.09	(13)

TABLE 2 (continued)
Intake of Total Fiber and Fiber Components of Seventh-Day Adventist Vegetarians and Nonvegetarians and the Nonvegetarian General Population

Note: SDA Lacto-ovo = Seventh-Day Adventist lacto-ovo vegetarian; SDA Nonvege = Seventh-Day Adventist nonvegetarian; GP Nonvege = general population nonvegetarian. (N) represents the number of subjects in each group.

[a] $p \leq$ = 0.05 for t-test difference between PVs and LOVs.
[b] $p \leq$ = 0.05 for t-test difference between PVs and NVs.
[c] $p \leq$ = 0.05 for t-test difference between PVs and GPs.
[d] $p \leq$ = 0.05 for t-test difference between LOVs and NVs.
[e] $p \leq$ = 0.05 for t-test difference between LOVs and GPs.
[f] $p \leq$ = 0.05 for t-test difference between NVs and GPs.

SUMMARY

Fiber intake among vegetarian and nonvegetarian populations has been examined from a wide variety of populations. The number of studies on populations whose vegetarian habits are unrelated to a religious affiliation has grown impressively. Collectively, these reports measure the intake of fiber among vegetarians to be about 86% higher than that of nonvegetarians. All fractions of fiber show differences between vegetarians and nonvegetarians and remain so even after adjusting for calorie intake. The more strictly a vegetarian diet is observed, as shown by data from pure vegetarians, the higher the intake of fiber and fiber fractions.

The amount of fiber intake which could be considered optimal cannot be determined from this review due to wide variation in the populations examined and the methods employed to determine dietary intake and the fiber content of the diet. This review does suggest that fiber intake could be safely doubled in nonvegetarian populations. The health or longevity benefit attributable to higher fiber intake or the specific function of particular fractions of fiber physiologically as pertains to disease prevention will require further study. These findings are consistent with the hypothesized associations of greater fiber intake with lower mortality rates for some disease, but many other factors of diet, lifestyle, medical history, etc. have not been taken into account in this analysis.

REFERENCES

1. **Trowell, H.,** The development of the concept of dietary fiber in human nutrition, *Am. J. Clin. Nutr.,* 31, S3, 1978.
2. **Huang, C. T. L., Gopalakrishna, G. S., and Nichols, B. L.,** Fiber, intestinal sterols and colon cancer, *Am. J. Clin. Nutr.,* 31, 516, 1978.
3. **Armstrong, B. and Doll, R.,** Environmental factors and cancer incidence and mortality in different countries, with special reference to dietary practices, *Int. J. Cancer,* 15, 617, 1975.
4. **Wynder, E. L., Kajitani, T., Ishikawa, S., Dodo, H., and Takano, A.,** Environmental factors of cancer of the colon and rectum. II. Japanese epidemiological data, *Cancer,* 23, 1210, 1969.
5. **Irving, D. and Drasar, B. S.,** Fiber and cancer of the colon, *Br. J. Cancer,* 28, 462, 1973.
6. **Trowell, H., Painter, N., and Burkitt, D.,** Aspects of the epidemiology of diverticular disease and ischemic heart disease, *Dig. Dis.,* 19, 864, 1974.

7. **Burkitt, D. P.,** Large-bowel cancer: an epidemiologic jigsaw puzzle, *J. Natl. Cancer Inst.,* 54, 3, 1975.
8. **Haenszel, W., Berg, J. W., Segi, M., Kurihara, M., and Locke, F. B.,** Large-bowel cancer in Hawaiian Japanese, *J. Natl. Cancer Inst.,* 51, 1765, 1973.
9. **Graham, S., Dayal, H., Swanson, M., Mittelman, A., and Wilkinson, G.,** Diet in the epidemiology of cancer of the colon and rectum, *J. Natl. Cancer Inst.,* 61, 709, 1978.
10. **Phillips, R. L., Lemon, F. R., Beeson, L., and Kuzma, J. W.,** Coronary heart disease mortality among Seventh-day Adventists with differing dietary habits: a preliminary report, *Am. J. Clin. Nutr.,* 31, S191, 1978.
11. **Phillip, R. L., Kuzma, J. W., and Lotz, T.,** Cancer mortality among comparable members of the Seven-day Adventist church, *Banbury Report 4: Cancer Incidence in Defined Populations,* Cold Spring Harbor Laboratory, Cold Spring Harbor, New York, 1980, 93.
12. **Hardinge, M. G., Chambers, A. C., Crooks, H., and Stare, F. J.,** Nutritional studies of vegetarians. III. Dietary levels of fiber, *Am. J. Clin. Nutr.,* 6, 523, 1958.
13. **Holm, C. N. and Hansen, L. P.,** Plantefibre og gastrointestinal passagetid, *Ugeskr. Laeg.,* 137, 561, 1975.
14. **Gear, J. S. S., Ware, A. C., Nolan, D. J., Fursdon, P. S., Brodribb, A. J. M., and Mann, J. I.,** Dietary fibre and asymptomatic diverticular disease of the colon, *Proc. Nutr. Soc.,* 37, 13A, 1977.
15. **Gear, J. S. S., Fursdon, P., Nolan, D. J., Ware, A., Mann, J. I., Brodribb, A. J. M., and Vessey, M. P.,** Symptomless diverticular disease and intake of dietary fibre, *Lancet,* 2, 511, 1979.
16. **Reddy, B. S., Sharma, C., Darby, L., Laadso, K., and Wynder, E. L.,** Metabolic epidemiology of large bowel cancer, fecal mutagens in high- and low-risk population for colon cancer: a preliminary report, *Metab. Res.,* 72, 511, 1980.
17. **Treuherz, J.,** Zinc and dietary fibre: observations on a group of vegetarian adolescents, *Proc. Nutr. Soc.,* 39, 10A, 1980.
18. **Goldin, B. R., Swenson, L., Dwyer, J., Sexton, M., and Gorbach, S. L.,** Effect of diet and *Lactobacillus acidophilus* supplements on human fecal bacterial enzymes, *J. Natl. Cancer Inst.,* 64, 255, 1980.
19. **Freeland-Graves, J. H., Brodzy, P. W., and Eppright, M. A.,** Zinc status of vegetarians, *J. Am. Dietet. Assoc.,* 77, 655, 1980.
20. **Adlercreutz, H., Fotsis, T., Heikkinen, R., Dwyer, J. T., Goldin, B. R., Gorbach, S. L., Lawson, A. M., and Setchell, K. D. R.,** Diet and urinary excretion of lignins in female subjects, *Med. Biol.,* 59, 259, 1981.
21. **Goldin, B. R., Adlercreutz, H., Gorbach, S., Warram, J. H., Dwyer, J. T., Swenson, L., and Woods, M. N.,** Estrogen excretion patterns and plasma levels in vegetarian and omnivorous women, *N. Engl. J. Med.,* 307, 1542, 1982.
22. **Adlercreutz, H., Heikkinen, R., Woods, M., Rotsis, T., Dwyer, J. T., Goldin, B. R., and Gorbach, S. L.,** Excretion of the lignans enterolactone and enterodiol and of equol in omnivorous and vegetarian postmenopausal women and in women with breast cancer, *Lancet,* 2, 1295, 1982.
23. **Abdulia, M., Andersson, I., Asp, N., Berthelsen, K., Birkhed, D., Dencker, I., Johansson, C., Jägerstad, M., Kolar, K., Nair, B. M., Nilsson-Ehle, P., Nord'en, A., Rassner, S., Akesson, B., and O"ckerman, P.,** Nutrient intake and health status of vegans. Chemical analysis of diets using the duplicate portion sampling technique, *Am. J. Clin. Nutr.,* 34, 2464, 1981.
24. **Burr, M. L., Bates, C. J., Fehily, A. M., and St. Leger, A. S.,** Plasma cholesterol and blood pressure in vegetarians, *J. Hum. Nutr.,* 35, 437, 1981.
25. **Anderson, B. M., Gibson, R. S., and Sabry, J. H.,** The iron and zinc status of long-term vegetarian women, *Am. J. Clin. Nutr.,* 34, 1042, 1981.
26. **King, J. C., Stein, T., and Doyle, M.,** Effect of vegetarianism on the zinc status of pregnant women, *Am. J. Clin. Nutr.,* 34, 1049, 1981.
27. **Abraham, R.,** Trace element intake in Asians during pregnancy, *Proc. Nutr. Soc.,* 41, 261, 1982.
28. **Gibson, R. S., Anderson, B. M., and Sabry, J. H.,** The trace metal status of a group of post-menopausal vegetarians, *J. Am. Dietet. Assoc.,* 82, 246, 1983.
29. **Kurup, P. A., Jayakumari, N., Indira, M., Kurup, G. M., Vargheese, T., Mathew, A., Goodman, G. T., Calkins, B. M., Kessie, G., Turjman, N., and Nair, P. P.,** Composition, intake and excretion of fiber constituents, *Am. J. Clin. Nutr.,* Suppl. 40(4), 942, 1984.
30. **Sorenson, A. W., Calkins, B. M., Connolly, M., and Diamond, E.,** Comparison of nutrient intake as determined by four dietary intake instruments, *J. Nutr. Educ.,* 17, 92, 1985.
31. **Watt, B. K. and Merrill, A. L.,** *Composition of Foods, Raw, Processed, Prepared,* U.S. Department of Agriculture Handbook No. 8, Washington, D.C., 1950.
32. **Bowes, A. deP. and Church, C. F.,** *Food Values of Portions Commonly Used,* Lippincott, New York, 1951.
33. **Chatfield, C.,** *Food Composition Tables for International Use,* FAO Nutrition Study No. 3, FAO, Rome, 1949.

34. **Southgate, D. A. T., Bailey, B., Collinow, E., and Walker, A. F.,** *J. Hum. Nutr.,* 30, 303, 1976.
35. **Hansen, L. P. and Holm, C. N.,** *Manedsskr prakt Laegegern,* 52, 630, 1974.
36. **Paul, A. A. and Southgate, D. A. T., Eds.,** *McCance and Widdowson's The Composition of Foods,* 4th ed., Her Majesty's Stationary Office, London, 1978.
37. **Asp, N.-G. and Johnson, C.-G.,** Techniques for measuring dietary fiber, principle aims of methods and a comparison of results obtained by different techniques, *The Analysis of Dietary Fibre in Food,* James, W. P. T. and Theander, O., Eds., Marcel Dekker, New York, 1980, 173.
38. **Leung, W. T. W., Burtrum, R. R., Chang, F. H., Rao, M. N., and Polacchi, W.,** *Food Composition Table for Use in E. Asia,* U.S. Department of Health, Education and Welfare Publication, No. 73-465, Washington, D.C., 1972.
39. **Leung, W. T. W.,** *Food Composition Table for Use in Africa,* U.S. Department of Health, Education and Welfare, Washington, D.C., 1968.
40. **Peckham, C. G. and Freeland-Graves, J. H.,** Nutrition in household quantities of foods, Tables A-12, *Foundations of Food Preparation,* MacMillan, New York, 1979.
41. **Anon.,** *Nutrient Value of Some Common Foods,* Health and Welfare, Ottawa, Canada, 1971.
42. **Kurup, P. A., Jayakumari, N., Indira, M., Kurup, F. M., Vargheese, T., and Menon, P. V. G.,** Determination of fiber and fiber constituents in food and stools, *Am. J. Clin. Nutr.,* Suppl. 40(4), 961, 1984.
43. **Ross, J. K., Pusateri, D. J., and Shultz, T. D.,** Dietary and hormonal evaluation of men at different risks for prostate cancer: fiber intake, excretion, and composition, with in vitro evidence for an association between steroid hormones and specific fiber components, *Am. J. Clin. Nutr.,* 51, 365, 1990.
44. **Davies, G. J., Crowder, M., and Dickerson, J. W. I.,** Dietary fibre intakes of individuals with different eating patterns, *Hum. Nutr. Appl. Nutr.,* 39A, 139, 1985.
45. **Lowik, M. R. H., Schrijver, J., van den Berg, H., Hulshof, F. A. M., Wedel, M., and Ockhuizen, T.,** Effect of dietary fiber on the vitamin B_6 status among vegetarian and nonvegetarian elderly (Dutch Nutrition Surveillance System), *J. Am. Coll. Nutr.,* 9(3), 241, 1990.
46. **Hautvast, J. G. A. J.,** Ontwikkeling van een systeem om gegevens van voedingsequetes met behulp van een computer te verwerken, *Voeding,* 36, 356, 1975.
47. **Adlercreutz, H., Fotsis, T., Bannwart, C., Hamalainen, E., Bloigu, S., and Ollus, A.,** Urinary estrogen profile determination in young Finnish vegetarian and omnivorous women, *J. Steroid Biochem.,* 24(1), 289, 1986.
48. **Barbosa, J. C., Shultz, T. D., Filley, S. J., and Nieman, D. C.,** The relationship among adiposity, diet, and hormone concentrations in vegetarian and nonvegetarian postmenopausal women, *Am. J. Clin. Nutr.,* 51, 798, 1990.
49. N-squared computing, Analytical software, Nutritionist III. N-squared Computing, Salem, OR, 1987.
50. **Allinger, U. G., Johansson, G. K., Gustafsson, J. A. and Rafter, J. J.,** Shift from a mixed to a lactovegetarian diet: influence on acidic lipids in fecal water — a potential risk factor for colon cancer, *Am. J. Clin. Nutr.,* 50, 992, 1989.
51. National Food Administration, Food composition tables, LIber Tryck AB, Stockholm, Sweden, 1986.
52. **Brune, M., Rossander, L., and Hallberg, Lief,** Iron absorption: no intestinal adaptation to a high-phytate diet, *Am. J. Clin. Nutr.,* 49, 542, 1989.
53. **Kelsay, J. L., Frazier, C. W., Prather, E. S., Canary, J. J., Clark, W. M., and Powell, A. S.,** Impact of variation in carbohydrate intake on mineral utilization by vegetarians, *Am. J. Clin. Nutr.,* 48, 875, 1988.
54. U.S. Department of Agriculture, Human Nutrition Information Service, Nutrition Monitoring Division, Nutrient Data Research Branch, USDA nutrient data base for standard reference, Release 3, Hyattsville, MD, 1982.
55. Food and Agriculture Organization of the United Nations, U.S. Department of Agriculture Human Nutrition Information Division, Food composition tables for the Near East p-85, Food and Agriculture Organization, Rome, 1982.
56. **Shultz, T. D. and Leklem, J. E.,** Vitamin B-6 status and bioavailability in vegetarian women, *Am. J. Clin. Nutr.,* 46, 647, 1987.
57. **Schaum, K. D., Mason, M., and Sharp, J. L.,** Patient-oriented dietetic information system, *J. Am. Diet. Assoc.,* 63, 39, 1973.
58. **Robertson, J. B. and Van Soest, P. J.,** The detergent system of analysis and its application to human food, in *The Analysis of Dietary Fiber in Food,* James, W. P. T. and Theander, O., Eds., Marcel Dekker, New York, 1981, 123.
59. **Katan, M. B. and van de Bovenkamp, P.,** Determination of total fiber by difference and of pectin by calorimetry of copper titration, in *The Analysis of Dietary Fiber in Food,* James, W. P. T. and Theander, O., Eds., Marcel Dekker, New York, 1981, 217.

Chapter 8.3

FIBER CONSUMPTION IN AUSTRALIAN POPULATIONS

Katrine I. Baghurst, Sally J. Record, and John D. Potter

INTRODUCTION

Until the early to mid-1980s, the only nationally based information about dietary fiber intake in the Australian population came from the apparent consumption or food disappearance data collected by the Australian Bureau of Statistics. The only data available from direct survey of individuals was on selected, and usually small, samples of subpopulations. Since 1983, several national or statewide, randomized surveys of the population have been undertaken. These have indicated that dietary fiber intake has increased substantially over the past decade in Australia, from an average intake of 17 to 18 g per day in the late 1970s, to 24 to 25 g in the late 1980s. This chapter summarizes some of the earlier data and details the results of the more recent random surveys. A variety of dietary methodologies were used in these surveys, but they appear to have produced consistent results.

SUBJECTS AND METHODS

The subjects and methodologies employed in the surveys described here varied widely and are shown in Table 1, along with the mean fiber intakes obtained. Many of the studies used traditional techniques such as 24-h recall or record, 3-day records or diet history which will not be detailed here, but a large number of the surveys employed a variation of the quantitative food frequency technique developed by the CSIRO Division of Human Nutrition.[1] In this technique, the respondent is asked to complete a questionnaire concerning the usual frequency and volume of intake of 180 food and drink items. In addition, there are quantitative and qualitative questions concerned with specific brand usage, cooking, and food preparation practices, particularly as they relate to the effect on salt, sugar, fiber, vitamins, and fat intake. Data on supplementation is also collected. Answers to these questions are used to modify the nutrient intake figures attained from the food frequency section. Average daily consumption of particular foods is calculated using information supplied by the respondents regarding their usual portion size (open-ended) and how often they usually eat each food. Using this information and the nutrient content of the food item per unit weight taken from food tables, an individual's nutrient intake per day can be calculated using the FREQUAN dietary analysis program. The British McCance and Widdowson's Food Tables[2] were used as the nutrient data base with additional Australian data where this was available. Recent analytical data produced by Englyst[3] for the various types of insoluble and soluble fiber components were added to the data base and used in the later random surveys of CSIRO.

As with the methodologies used, the techniques for sampling varied widely and are detailed in Table 1. Many of the random surveys, in particular those conducted by the CSIRO, used a random selection procedure based on the Electoral Rolls of the States or the Commonwealth (national government). As voting at State and Commonwealth Elections is compulsory in Australia, all citizens or permanent residents over the age of 18 years are required to register on these rolls.

RESULTS AND DISCUSSION

Tables 1 and 2 show the dietary fiber intakes and the group mean fiber to energy ratios from nonrandomized surveys from the late 1970s and early 1980s and from randomized population surveys carried out by the Commonwealth Government and the CSIRO Division of Human Nutrition since 1983. Assessment of trends over time is difficult because of the nonrandom nature of earlier surveys and the variety of measurement techniques employed. However, if the more generally representative data from the earlier period are used for comparative purposes, it does appear that dietary fiber intake has increased over the past decade by some 3 to 4 g/day (about a 15% increase). In general, women, those in the older age bands and those of higher occupational status, have higher fiber densities. The intakes of Adventists, whether vegetarian or omnivore, were particularly high and that of the elderly institutionalized was low, even when adjusting for total energy intake.

The more recent random surveys of adults indicate that approximately 40% of dietary fiber is currently provided by cereals, 30% by vegetables and 20% by fruit. The National Schoolchildren's survey showed a similar contribution from cereals, less from vegetables and fruit but more from the "other" category which included composite dishes such as pies, pastries, and pizzas as well as snack foods, beverages, nuts, and seeds. The figures for adults indicate an increasing relative contribution from the cereal group over the last decade and a lessening of the relative contribution of vegetables and, to a lesser extent, fruit to total fiber intake.

ACKNOWLEDGMENTS

Unpublished data from some of the nonrandom surveys were supplied by Delia Flint-Richter, Drs. S. Ash, B. K. Armstrong, B. Margetts, and I. Rouse, and Professors Truswell and Wahlquist, to whom we extend our thanks.

TABLE 1
Mean Daily Fiber and Energy Consumption in Nonrandom Australian Population Samples From 1977–85

Survey	Sex	No.	Method	Energy MJ/day	Fiber g/day	Fiber/energy ratio[a]
Urban community (4)	M	481	FFQ	9.9	20.2	2.04
(random within age bands)	F	441		7.5	19.5	2.60
Fitness intervention	M	581	FFQ	9.0	21.8	2.42
group (5)	F	454		7.2	22.7	3.15
Public servants (6)	M	142	FFQ	8.8	22.4	2.54
	F	60		7.3	22.8	3.12
Parents of 10-year-olds	M	300	FFQ	10.1	24.2	2.42
(7)	F	300		7.83	23.5	3.00
10-year-old children (7)	M & F	300	FFQ	7.76	21.5	2.77
Adolescents 14–15	M	72	FFQ	12.0	19.5	1.63
years (4)	F	69		9.4	18.9	2.01
Pregnant women (8)	F	91	3 day record	9.1	22.0	2.42
Elderly						
Community (9)	M & F	27	Hist.	8.0	20.9	2.6
Institutionalized (9)	M & F	87	3-day records	7.4	11.8	1.6
Nursing home (10)	M & F	30		6.5	13.7	2.1
Religious groups (11)						
Adventist (vegetarian)	M	98	24-h Record	11.0	44.3	4.03
	F			8.6	32.6	3.79
Adventist (omnivore)	M	82	24-h Record	10.5	41.4	3.94
	F			8.0	27.1	3.39
Mormon (omnivore)	M	113	24-h Record	11.6	24.3	2.09
	F			8.4	19.7	2.34
Vietnamese migrants (12)	F	200	24-h Record	7.53	15.5	2.06

[a] Group mean ratio.

TABLE 2
Random Surveys of Australian Population Samples from 1983–90

Survey	Sex	No.	Method	Energy MJ/day	Fiber g/day	Fiber/energy ratio[a]
Commonwealth government						
National Adults survey 1983[b] (13)	M	3021	24-h Recall	11.0	23.2	2.11
	F	3234		7.4	18.7	2.53
National Schoolchildren's survey 1985[b] (14)	M (10–11 years)	912	24-h Record	8.3	18.0	2.17
	M (12–15 years)	1719		10.3	21.5	2.09
	F (10–11 years)	925		7.21	5.4	2.14
	F (12–15 years)	1668		7.72	17.0	2.20
CSIRO surveys						
Victorian State survey 1985 (15)	M	1321	FFQ	9.65	21.0	2.18
	F	1595		7.77	21.1	2.72
South Australian State survey 1988 (16)	M	445	FFQ	9.64	22.4	2.32
	F	456		7.66	23.2	3.03
National Adults survey 1988 (17)	M	716	FFQ	9.54	23.2	2.43
	F	763		7.72	23.0	2.98
National Elderly survey (55–75 years) 1989/90 (18)	M	606	FFQ	9.08	28.2	3.11
	F	707		7.85	29.7	3.78

[a] Group mean ratio.
[b] Metropolitan sample only.

TABLE 3
Intakes of Total Dietary Fiber, Insoluble, and Soluble Non-starch Polysaccharides in the Australian Population[17]

Fiber fraction	Daily intake (g/day)					
	Men			Women		
	Mean	10th percentiles	90th percentiles	Mean	10th percentiles	90th percentiles
Total dietary fiber	21.0	11.2	32.9	21.1	11.3	33.2
Total non-starch polysaccharides	15.8	8.8	24.4	16.1	8.8	24.2
Soluble NSP						
Total	6.8	4.0	10.0	6.7	3.9	10.0
Rhamnose	0.16	0.07	0.25	0.18	0.09	0.28
Fucose	0.007	0.001	0.015	0.008	0.002	0.016
Arabinose	1.5	0.9	2.3	1.4	0.8	2.1
Xylose	1.1	0.6	1.7	0.9	0.4	1.4
Mannose	0.057	0.019	0.105	0.066	0.026	0.115
Galactose	1.1	0.65	1.64	1.1	0.66	1.63
Glucose	0.7	0.3	1.2	0.6	0.3	1.1
Uronic acid	2.1	1.0	3.4	2.5	1.2	4.0
Insoluble NSP						
Total	9.0	4.5	14.7	9.3	4.7	14.7
Cellulose	4.0	2.1	6.3	4.3	2.4	6.6
Rhamnose	0.037	0.013	0.067	0.042	0.015	0.073
Fucose	0.008	0.002	0.018	0.011	0.003	0.020
Arabinose	1.4	0.5	2.7	1.4	0.5	2.5
Xylose	2.2	0.8	4.1	2.2	0.8	3.8
Mannose	0.2	0.15	0.41	0.27	0.14	0.42
Galactose	0.29	0.15	0.44	0.31	0.17	0.48
Glucose	0.45	0.18	0.82	0.44	0.18	0.76
Uronic acid	0.31	0.14	0.52	0.35	0.17	0.56

TABLE 4
Density of Total Dietary Fiber, Insoluble, and Soluble Non-starch Polysaccharides in the Australian Population[17] by Gender, Age, and Occupation

Density of fiber fractions (g/MJ)

Fiber fraction	All ages	Age group (years)				
		18–29	30–39	40–49	50–59	60+
Total dietary fiber						
M	2.3	2.0	2.3	2.2	2.4	2.6
F	2.9	2.6	2.8	2.7	3.1	3.3
Non-starch polysaccharides						
Total NSP						
M	1.7	1.5	1.7	1.7	1.8	2.0
F	2.2	2.0	2.1	2.0	2.3	2.5
Soluble NSP						
M	0.7	0.7	0.7	0.7	0.8	0.8
F	0.9	0.8	0.9	0.9	1.0	1.0
Insoluble NSP						
M	1.0	0.8	1.0	1.0	1.0	1.2
F	1.3	1.1	1.2	1.2	1.4	1.5

Fiber fraction	Occupational categories				
	Upper	Upper middle	Middle	Lower middle	Lower
Total dietary fiber					
M	2.5	2.3	2.2	2.1	1.9
F	3.0	2.8	2.7	2.7	2.5
Non-starch polysaccharides					
Total NSP					
M	1.9	1.7	1.6	1.6	1.5
F	2.3	2.1	2.0	2.0	1.9
Soluble NSP					
M	0.8	0.7	0.7	0.7	0.7
F	0.9	0.9	0.9	0.9	0.8
Insoluble NSP					
M	1.1	1.0	0.9	0.9	0.8
F	1.3	1.2	1.2	1.2	1.1

TABLE 5
Sources of Dietary Fiber in the Australian Population

	Percentage of total dietary fiber derived from food groups					
		Vegetables				
Survey	Cereals	Brassica and green-leafy	Legumes, peas, and beans	Total	Fruit	Other[a]
Urban community samples, 1978–83	32.8	4.7	13.2	37.2	23.3	6.7
Victorian State, 1983	41.7	4.6	8.0	31.0	20.2	7.1
National Adults, 1983	37.2	6.9	8.6	32.9	20.0	9.9
National Schoolchildren's, 1985	39.0	2.3	8.5	26.3	17.4	17.3

[a] Includes composite dishes such as pies, pizzas, etc.; snack foods, beverages, nuts, and seeds.

REFERENCES

1. **Baghurst, K. I. and Record, S. J.**, A computerized dietary analysis system for use with diet diaries or food frequency questionnaires, *Community Health Stud.*, 8, 11, 1984.
2. **Paul, A. A. and Southgate, D. A. T.**, *McCance and Widdowson's The Composition of Foods*, 4th ed., Her Majesty's Stationery Office, London, 1978.
3. **Englyst, H. N., Bingham, S. A., Runswick, S. A., Collinson, E., and Cummings, J. H.**, (a) Dietary fibre (non-starch polysaccharides) in fruit, vegetables and nuts, *J. Hum. Nutr. Dietet.*, 2, 247, 1988; (b) Dietary fibre (non-starch polysaccharides) in cereal products, *J. Hum. Nutr. Dietet.*, 2, 253, 1989.
4. **Baghurst, K. I. and Record, S. J.**, Intake and sources, in selected Australian subpopulations, of dietary constituents implicated in the aetiology of chronic disease, *J. Food Nutr.*, 40, 1, 1983.
5. **Baghurst, K. I., Sedgwick, A. W., and Strohm, K.**, Nutritional profile of recruits to a fitness program, *Med. J. Aust.*, 143, 188, 1985.
6. **Baghurst, K. I. and Record, K. I.**, Unpublished data.
7. **Syrette, J. and Baghurst, K. I.**, Dietary intake of ten-year old children and their parents with respect to occupational status, *Proc. Nutr. Soc. Aust.*, 12, 160, 1987.
8. **Ash, S.**, Unpublished data.
9. **Flint-Richter, D.**, Unpublished data.
10. **Baghurst, K. I., Hope, A., and Down, E.**, Dietary fibre intake in a group of institutionalised elderly and the effect of a fibre supplementation program on nutrient intake and weight gain, *Community Health Stud.*, IX, 99, 1985.
11. **Rouse, I. L., Armstrong, B. K., and Beilin, L. J.**, The relationship of blood pressure to diet and lifestyle in two religious populations, *J. Hypertension*, 1, 65, 1983.
12. **Baghurst, K. I., Syrette, J. A., and Tran, M. M.**, Dietary profile of Vietnamese women in South Australia, *Nutr. Res.*, 11, 715, 1991.
13. **English, R., Cashel, K., Bennett, S., Berzins, J., Waters, A.-M., and Magnus, P.**, National dietary survey of adults: 1983. No. 2. Nutrient intakes, Australian Government Publishing Service, Canberra, 1987.
14. **English, R., Cashel, K., Lewis, J., Waters, A.-M., and Bennett, S.**, National dietary survey of schoolchildren (aged 10–15 years): 1985. No. 2. Nutrient intakes. Australian Government Publishing Service, Canberra, 1989.
15. **Baghurst, K. I., Crawford, D. A., Worsley, A., Syrette, J., and Baghurst, P. A.**, The Victorian Nutrition Survey. Part 2. Nutrient intakes by age, sex, area of residence and occupational status, Commonwealth Scientific and Industrial Research Organization, Adelaide, 1987.
16. **Baghurst, K. I., Record, S. J., Syrette, J. A., and Baghurst, P. A.**, The South Australian Nutrition Survey, Commonwealth Scientific and Industrial Research Organization, Adelaide, 1989.

17. **Baghurst, K. I., Dreosti, I. E., Syrette, J. A., Record, S. J., Baghurst, P. A., and Buckley, R. A.,** Zinc and magnesium status of Australian adults, *Nutr. Res.*, 11, 23, 1991.
18. **Baghurst, K. I., Record, K. I., and Baghurst, P. A.,** National dietary survey of the elderly, Commonwealth Scientific and Industrial Research Organization, Adelaide, 1991.

Chapter 8.4

CONSUMPTION OF DIETARY FIBER-RICH FOODS IN CHINA

Zhi-Ping Shen and Su-Fang Zheng

China is a big country with great varieties of foodstuffs. However, the most important components of the daily diets are grains and cereals which provide about 80% of the daily caloric intake. In south China, the predominant grain is rice and in the north, the main staple foods are wheat and coarse grains including corn, millet, sorghum, etc. The amount and varieties of plant subsidiary foods are dependent on the climate. In general, Chinese diets are rich in vegetables. The supply of staple and nonstaple food varies in amount and varieties with season. National nutrition surveys carried out in China in 1959 and 1982 indicate that the consumption pattern of plant foods and crude fiber intake differ in different parts of China as shown in Table 1. Crude fiber are mainly from cereal grains and vegetables. The data in Table 2 indicate the contribution of crude fiber from various foods in north China peasant diets[1] as calculated by Zheng from the annual dietary surveys in 1979. The crude fiber content of the Chinese daily diet is much higher than the daily crude fiber intake in England, which was estimated to be about 4 g per capita.[2] The age-adjusted death rate for colorectal cancer in China was 5.49 per 100,000 in 1979, the second lowest in the world.[3]

The Chinese government has stipulated the standard of rice milling and wheat flour extraction in order to retain more nutrients. Table 3 lists the crude fiber contents of processed rice and wheat.[4]

The comparison between crude fiber and neutral detergent fiber contents in selected Chinese foods is listed in Table 4.[5]

TABLE 1
Consumption Pattern of Fiber-Containing Foods and Crude Fiber Intake in Different Parts of China (Grams/Day/Capita)

	Beijing North	Shanghai South	Jiangxi South	Hebei North	Shanxi North	Gansu Northwest
Food						
Rice	90	463	558	13	11	3
Wheat flour	314	44	13	350	173	610
Coarse grains	125	—	—	252	344	49
Starchy tubers	35	43	110	97	352	149
Legumes, dried	8	4	9	3	21	5
Vegetables	440	326	383	280	305	147
Fruits	82	9	1	30	13	34
Nuts	4	1	1	2	1	—
Crude fiber	8.5	6.9	7.7	9.3	11.3	6.6

TABLE 2
Contribution of Crude Fiber from Various Foods in North China Peasant Daily Diets

	Linxian County, Henan			Xianxiang County, Henan		
Food	Consumption (g)	Crude fiber (g)	Contribution (%)	Consumption (g)	Crude fiber (g)	Contribution (%)
Rice	13	0.06	0.5	66	0.29	2.7
Wheat flour	250	1.46	11.2	456	2.66	24.4
Coarse grains	300	4.47	34.2	225	0.02	26.3
Starchy tubers	646	2.76	21.1	11	0.42	0.2
Legumes	21	0.81	6.2	20	4.06	3.8
Vegetables	583	3.44	26.2	830	0.52	37.2
Fruits	3	0.03	0.2	85	—	4.8
Nuts	1	0.02	0.2	—	0.07	—
Seaweeds	—	—	—	1	—	0.6

TABLE 3
Crude Fiber Contents of Processed Cereal Grains in China

Rice, long grains		Wheat flour	
Grade	Crude fiber (g/100 g)	Extraction	Crude fiber (g/100 g)
Husked	0.7	Whole	2.4
Fine	0.3	75% extraction	0.2
Standard, 1st	0.4	81% extraction	0.4
Standard, 2nd	0.5	85% extraction	0.6

TABLE 4
Comparison between Crude Fiber and Neutral Detergent Fiber Contents in Selected Chinese Foods

Food	CF	NDF
	(g/100 g dried edible portion)	
Cereals		
Corn	1.70	8.42
Corn meal	0.88	4.50
Millet	0.24	1.54
Sorghum	0.28	3.19
Rice, glutinous	0.13	0.49
Rice, long grain	0.17	0.70
Rice, round grain	0.11	0.24
Whole wheat flour	2.12	9.70
Legumes, dried		
Adsuki bean	3.90	8.41
Kidney bean	4.04	7.81
Mung bean	3.74	7.16
Soybean, green	3.74	10.43
Soybean, yellow	3.50	10.03
Vegetables		
Cabbage, celery	8.37	14.53
Cabbage, Chinese	10.94	18.21
Cabbage, common	7.90	18.55
Celery stem	11.79	18.20
Chive	8.99	14.30
Garlic green	11.42	17.40
Garlic shoot	8.89	10.38
Onion shallot	6.57	11.66
Spinach	8.04	21.38
Roots		
Carrot	6.57	11.66
Lotus root	2.36	7.03
Potato	1.59	3.48
Yam	1.23	4.09

REFERENCES

1. **Zheng, S.,** The crude fiber intake of peasants in north China, unpublished.
2. **Trowell, H.,** Definition of dietary fiber and hypothesis that it is a protective factor in certain diseases, *Am. J. Clin. Nutr.,* 29, 417, 1976.
3. **Dai, X.,** Colorectal cancer, in *The Investigation of The Cancer Mortality in China* (in Chinese), The National Cancer Control Office of the Ministry of Health, Ed., People's Medical Publishing House, Beijing, 1979.
4. Institute of Health, Chinese Academy of Medical Sciences *Food Composition Table* (in Chinese), 3rd ed., People's Medical Publishing House, Beijing, 1981.
5. **Zao, Z.,** Comparison between crude fiber and dietary fiber contents in foods, *Acta Nutrimenta Simica,* 9, 333, 1989.

Chapter 8.5

CONSUMPTION OF DIETARY FIBER IN FRANCE (1850–1981)

Yves Le Quintrec

INTRODUCTION

Little has been published about the consumption of dietary fiber in France and, more generally, about food consumption. In this chapter we will make a distinction between direct and indirect methods for evaluating this consumption.

DIRECT METHOD OF EVALUATION

This method is based on dietary recall in a sample of people as representative as possible of the general population. The dietary fiber consumption can then be calculated by tables using the Paul-Southgate method[1] to obtain the total fiber consumption and not just the crude fiber consumption.

Three studies of this type have been published in France (Table 1). The results are identical in two studies but, in the third[4] the consumption of dietary fibers is far more important. This difference can be partly explained: in the first and second studies, the calculation of the dietary fiber content was made with Southgate's table[1] which is based on English alimentation, and in particular, English bread; in the third study, the content of dietary fiber was calculated with a new analysis of fiber content carried out by Southgate himself on French bread and flour which showed a higher proportion of fiber in French products (Table 2). Therefore, while the consumption of cereal fiber is virtually the same in the three studies, the total consumption of fiber is higher in the study by Macquart-Moulin et al.[4]

INDIRECT METHODS OF EVALUATION

These methods consist of measuring the total consumption of a given food in a given population and then dividing it by the number of individuals to obtain an evaluation of the average per capita consumption. We have, therefore, two major sources of information in France:

1. Inquiries by INSEE (National Institute of Statistic and Economic studies[5]); 10,000 households, statistically representative of the total French population, are each examined for 1 week, the study being completed in the course of 1 year. Unfortunately, only the "at-home" consumption is estimated and not the away-from-home consumption (including restaurants, canteens, etc.). Therefore, food consumption is always underestimated; still, interesting comparisons between different population subgroups can be made.

2. Agricultural Statistics of the CEE (European Economic Community) or Eurostat.[6] Here, consumption means the gross amount of foodstuffs made available at the wholesale stage, in all forms: direct, preserved, and processed products. Consequently the consumption is overestimated, because no account is taken of losses at the retail trade stage, nor at the household level.

TABLE 1
Average Daily Consumption of Dietary Fiber in France Calculated from Dietary Recall

	Total dietary fiber (g/day)	Cereal fiber (g/day)	Ref.
Females	12.7 ± 5.8	3.6 ± 0.8	2
Females			
May	11.81 ± 1.88		
October	8.64 ± 0.70		3
Males			
May	10.61 ± 0.70		
October	8.34 ± 1.08		
Females	28.0 ± 7.0	6.6 ± 4.0	4
Males	28.0 ± 8.3	11.6 ± 6.4	

TABLE 2
Dietary Fiber Content (g/%) of Bread and Flour from Southgate

French bread[4]	English bread[1]	French flour[4]	English flour[1]
5.67–5.96	2.7	3.71–3.93	3.0

CEREAL CONSUMPTION (TABLES 3 TO 7)

The total cereal consumption has been quite stable for the last 10 years. The major cereal in France is wheat (soft wheat). The consumption of rice is increasing but is still very low.

The consumption of bread has been decreasing for many years, but this tendency seems to have now stopped. Still, bread remains the chief source of cereal fiber in the French diet. Bread consumption appears to be higher in the agricultural population than in the urban (Table 6), but this result may be due to the lack of information about away-from-home consumption (lunch is frequently taken in a restaurant or a canteen by the urban population).

CONSUMPTION OF FRUITS AND VEGETABLES (TABLES 8 TO 12)

The consumption of potatoes has been steadily decreasing for many years. Nevertheless, it remains high in the agricultural population and constitutes a large percentage of the total away-from-home consumption of vegetables. The consumption of dried pulses is very small.

The consumption of other vegetables and fresh fruits, except for citrus fruits, is no longer on the rise. There is a great discrepancy between the data on this consumption collected by Eurostat (Table 9) and INSEE (Table 11). The estimation by Eurostat probably is more realistic because it reflects all forms of consumption including preserves, jam, etc. It also includes the away-from-home consumption, which represents at least 10% of the total consumption of vegetables and about 15% of the fruit consumption.[7]

According to the data of INSEE, the consumption of fruits (including bananas and citrus fruits) is certainly higher in the urban population than in the highest classes of society (Table 11).

TABLE 3
Total Human Consumption of Cereals in France
(1000 t/year) (Eurostat's Data)[6]

Year	Total cereals (excluding rice)	Total wheat	Soft wheat	Other cereals (excluding wheat and rice)	Rice
1970–1971	5089	4978	4444	111	160
1975–1976	5016	4898	4426	118	211
1980–1981	5344	5180	4650	164	278

TABLE 4
Average Annual Consumption of Cereal (Kilograms per Capita) in Flour Equivalent (= Grain × 0.77) (Eurostat's Data[6])

Year	Total cereals (excluding rice)	Total wheat	Soft wheat	Other cereals (excluding wheat and rice)	Rice
Before 1970	80	78	70	2	2
1975–1976	73	79	64	2	4
1980–1981	76	75	67	1	4

TABLE 5
Average Daily Consumption of Wheat and Rice (Grams per Capita) Calculated from Annual Consumption

Year	Total wheat	Wheat in flour equivalent	Bread	Rice
1970–1971	268	206	199	5.5
1975–1976	257	198	182	11
1980–1981	261	201	148	12.5

TABLE 6
Average Annual at Home Consumption of Cereal Foods (Kilograms per Capita) (INSEE's Data 1980[5])

	Bread (total)	Noodles	Wheat flour	Rice
Total population	48.57	5.49	4.16	3.86
Agricultural population	78.57	7.41	5.78	2.58
Nonagricultural population	45.32	5.28	3.98	4.00
Population of the greater Paris area	37.72	4.65	3.37	5.93

INTAKE OF DIETARY FIBER

An estimate of average daily fiber consumption can be made from these data, with a large margin of error. From Eurostat (Table 13) the "average Frenchman's" total dietary fiber intake ranges from 17.85 to 24.60 g/day, including 11.6 g of cereal fiber. From INSEE, the at-home consumption is surprisingly not much lower: 16 to 20 g/day. If one calculates the quantity of dietary fiber in the diets of farm owners and the unemployed (Table 14),

TABLE 7
Average Annual Consumption of Cereal Foods by Occupation Group (Kilograms per Capita) INSEE's Data 1980[5]

	Farm owners	Farm laborers	Self-employed professionals	Upper-level executives	Medium-level executives	White collar workers	Blue collar workers	Unemployed
Bread	81.11	64.03	42.43	32.38	38.53	39.17	51.22	48.75
Noodles	6.96	6.50	4.39	3.92	4.53	4.87	5.63	5.41
Wheat flour	4.65	5.27	3.32	2.58	3.49	2.99	4.52	4.12
Rice	2.12	2.55	2.97	3.85	3.00	3.86	4.75	5.13

TABLE 8
Total Human Consumption of Fruits and Vegetables
(100 t/Year) (Eurostat's Data[6])

Year	Potatoes	Dried pulse	Other vegetables	Total fresh fruits	Citrus fruits
1970–1971	4897	—	6632	2819	856
1975–1976	4790	113	6257	2890	998
1980–1981	3970	73	6168	2779	1015

TABLE 9
Average Annual Consumption of Fruits and Vegetables
(Kilograms per Capita) (Eurostat's Data[6])

Year	Potatoes	Dried pulse	Other vegetables	Total fresh fruits	Citrus fruits
Before 1970	97	—	129	56	17
1975–1976	81	2.1	118	55	19
1980–1981	74	1.4	115	52	19

TABLE 10
Average Daily Consumption of Fruits and Vegetables (Grams per Capita)
Calculated from Annual Consumption

Year	Potatoes	Dried pulse	Other vegetables	Total fresh fruits	Citrus fruits
1970–1971	266	—	353	153	47
1975–1976	222	5.7	323	151	52
1980–1981	202	3.8	315	142	52

TABLE 11
Average Annual at Home Consumption of Fruits and Vegetables
(Kilograms per Capita) (INSEE's Data 1980[5])

	Potatoes	Dried pulse	Other vegetables	Metropolitan fresh fruits	Bananas and citrus fruits
Total population	55.5	1.47	64.64	40.55	22.50
Agricultural population	62.79	2.45	77.46	37.44	14.54
Nonagricultural population	54.69	1.38	63.29	40.87	22.39
Population of the greater Paris area	40.93	1.69	63.81	45.82	29.38

who probably take the greatest number of meals at home, the values are a little higher: 22 to 26 g/day and 19 to 24 g/day.

For the last century (Figure 1) the consumption of bread and potatoes has been decreasing to a considerable extent. Conversely, the consumption of fruits and vegetables has been increasing, but this increase cannot compensate for the lack of cereal fiber. Therefore, the intake of dietary fiber currently is a great deal lower than in the years 1900 to 1930.[9]

TABLE 12
Average Consumption of Fruits and Vegetables by Occupation Group (Kilograms per Capita) (INSEE's Data 1980[5])

	Farm owners	Farm laborers	Self-employed professionals	Upper-level executives	Medium-level executives	White collar workers	Blue collar workers	Unemployed
Potatoes	57.83	50.42	48.12	29.24	44.34	42.68	64.74	69.03
Dried pulse	2.24	2.35	1.24	0.88	1.01	1.45	1.54	1.77
Vegetables	73.70	58.41	58.20	60.12	60.68	57.29	54.97	83.70
Fresh fruits	35.55	28.50	33.71	42.42	40.42	34.24	36.13	52.18
Bananas and citrus fruits	13.13	17.12	20.77	27.85	21.71	23.78	21.63	24.85

TABLE 13
Average Daily Fiber Intake (Eurostat's Data[6])

	Cereals in flour equivalent	Potatoes	Vegetables	Fruits	Citrus fruits	Total
% of total that is dietary fiber	3.8	2	1.5–3	0.5–2	2	
g/day	200	200	300	145	52	
Dietary fiber (g/day)	7.6	4	4.5–9	0.75–3	1	17.85–24.6

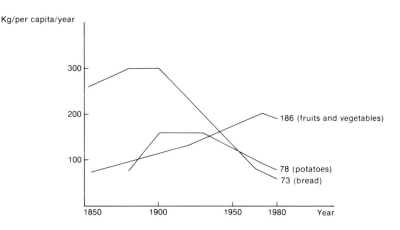

FIGURE 1. Evolution of dietary fiber in France.[9]

DIETARY FIBER INTAKE AND MORBIDITY

Statistics on this problem are very rare in France. We did not find any difference in the dietary fiber intake between two groups of women, one of which consisted of women suffering from constipation and the others of controls. In both groups the total dietary fiber intake (12.4 and 12.7 g/day) and the cereal fiber intake (3.3 and 3.6 g/day) were virtually the same.[10] Therefore, the lack of dietary fiber in alimentation cannot be considered as the only cause of constipation.

Meyer found a negative correlation between consumption of fruits and mortality due to colonic cancer,[8] but did not calculate the total dietary fiber intake, nor even the crude fiber intake. Recently, Macquart-Moulin et al.[4] found that, among other dietary factors, an increased intake of dietary fiber was correlated with a diminished relative risk of colorectal cancer.

TABLE 14
Average Daily Fiber Intake by Occupation Groups (INSEE's Data) Calculated from Southgate's Analyses

	Bread	Noodles	Wheat flour	Rice	Potatoes	Dried pulse	Vegetables	Fruits	Bananas	Total
% of total that is dietary fiber	5.8	?	3.8	2	2	15	1.5–3	0.5–2	2	
Farm owners (g/day)	222	19	13	5.8	160	6	200	97	35	
Dietary fiber	12.8	?	0.5	0.1	3.2	0.9	4–6	0.5–2	0.7	22.7–26.1
Unemployed (g/day)	133	15	11	14	190	5	230	140	68	
Dietary fiber	7.8	?	0.4	0.3	3.8	0.75	4.6–6.9	0.7–2.8	1.3	19.65–24.0
General average (g/day)	133	15	11	9.5	150	4	175	110	60	
Dietary fiber	7.8	?	0.4	0.2	3	0.6	2.6–5.2	0.55–2.2	1.2	16.35–20.6

REFERENCES

1. **Paul, A. A. and Southgate, D. A. T.**, *McCance and Widdowson's: The Composition of Foods,* Vol. 1, Her Majesty's Stationery Office, London, 1978.
2. **Meyer, F. and Le Quintrec, Y.**, Rapports entre fibres alimentaires et constipation, *Nouv. Presse Med.,* 10, 2479, 1981.
3. **Frexinos, J. and Allegret, M.**, Evaluation de la ration en fibres alimentaires dans la région Midi-Pyréneés et en Nouvelle Calédonie, *Gastroenterol. Clin. Biol.,* 4, 739, 1980.
4. **Macquart-Moulin, G., Durbec, J. P., Corvee, J., Berthezene, P., and Southgate, D. A. T.**, Alimentation et cancer recto-colique, *Gastroenterol. Clin. Biol.,* 7, 277, 1983.
5. **Mercier, M. A.**, Consommation et lieux d'achat des produits alimentaires en 1980, Vol. 1, INSEE (Ser. M, No. 99), 1983.
6. **EUROSTAT,** Statistiques de production agricole de la Communauté Européenne, Publiees par O.F.C.E., 1970 a 1980.
7. **Vlandas, S.**, Les fruits et légumes frais dans la restauration collective et communale. Centre technique interprofessionel des fruits et légumes, *Documents,* 27, 9, 1982.
8. **Meyer, F.**, Relations alimentation — cancer en France, *Gastroenterol. Clin. Biol.,* 1, 971, 1977.
9. **Meyer, F.**, Evolution de l'alimentation des Français 1781–1972. *Gastroenterol. Clin. Biol.,* 1, 1043, 1977.
10. **Le Quintrec, Y. and Meyer, F.**, Fibres alimentaires et constipation, *Gastroenterol. Clin. Biol.,* 4, 174A (summary), 1980.

Chapter 8.6

FIBER CONSUMPTION IN ITALY

Ottavio Bosello, Fabio Armellini, and Mauro Zamboni

INTRODUCTION

Epidemiological and alimentary studies on the population of Italy, from 1954 to 1978,[1] have shown a substantial increase in daily energy intake, a doubling of animal-origin proteins and animal and plant fats and a clear drop in carbohydrate consumption (Table 1). Research by the Istituto Nazionale della Nutrizione (National Institute of Nutrition: INN) for the period 1980 to 1984 (Table 4) has shown a further increase in consumption of animal-origin products and a reduction in those of plant origin. Caloric intake, on the other hand, has dropped back to 1964-1966 values.

This gradual change in Italy's traditional eating habits, going from the Mediterranean model[2] to a Western diet, has also involved a decrease in dietary fiber consumption and is more accentuated in northern Italy and less so in the south.[8]

SUBJECTS AND METHODS

The Trento Study (Table 2)

This research,* carried out in 1989, considered a representative sample of the city of Trento in northern Italy: 1697 people, 809 males and 888 females, between 25 and 69 years of age. Systematic sampling was performed on the resident population in the city and each of its suburbs. Food consumption was monitored by simultaneous recording of the food consumed during meals with total quantity evaluation for a 7-day period.[3] The diary, previously sent to the subject's residence, was then checked and discussed with the subject by a dietitian when the diary was picked up. Nutritional and fiber values were calculated using the food composition tables published by the INN.[4]

Italian INN Study (Table 4)

The INN, in the period from 1980 to 1984, carried out sample monitoring and registration[5] of family food consumption in many zones of Italy (180 towns and cities, distributed over 9 regions). Research involved about 10,000 families selected by random sampling of the civic lists of voters. Data were collected by a mixed weight and inventory method, employing specifically trained dietitians. Nutritional and dietary fiber values were calculated using the INN tables.[4]

European Economic Community Survey (Table 3)

For the European Economic Community (EEC) Dietary Survey, research was performed in Europe between 1963 and 1965, as part of studies to determine environmental radioactive contamination levels.[6] The weekly eating habits of 30 family units were studied each month for 3 years. Research in Italy involved three regions: Friuli Venezia Giulia in northeastern Italy, Campania in south-central Italy, and Basilicata in southern Italy. Each family weighed

---

* Unpublished information from an epidemiological cross-sectional study by M. Miori (Department of Internal Medicine, Trento Hospital) on a randomly selected sample of the population of Trento (northeast Italy) in 1989.

TABLE 1
Changes in Food Consumption from 1954–1978 in Italy[1]

		1954–1956	1964–1966	1976–1978
Proteins g/day	Plant	45.8	54.9	48.0
	Animal	24.8	33.6	49.4
	Total	70.6	88.5	97.4
Lipids g/day	Plant	32.6	52.1	65.8
	Animal	26.1	37.2	48.4
	Total	58.7	89.3	114.2
Carbohydrates g/day	Total	389.9	451.5	428.1
Energy MJ/day	Total	9.4	11.9	13.3

the food after preparation but before cooking, thus avoiding the need to make corrections for waste. Fiber intake was calculated, using British food composition tables,[7] on the food intakes as measured.

Verona Vegetarian Study (Table 7)

This study* was performed in 1989 on 11 members of the vegetarian community in Verona (northeastern Italy). Comparisons were made on a one-to-one basis with a group of subjects of equal age, weight, body mass index, degree of physical activity, and sociocultural level. Nutritional parameters were obtained using a diary with simultaneous registration of foods consumed during meals, measured by quantity, for 7 days.[3] Data were subsequently checked by a dietitian. Nutritional and dietary fiber values were calculated using the INN tables.[4]

CONSUMPTION PATTERNS

Table 2 gives a few results from the Trento study, separately for males and females and for three age groups. Fiber intake is indicated. The table also includes both total and percentage values for daily energy intake from each of the three main nutrients. There is a tendency for greater fiber consumption in older age groups, both for males (21 ± 9 g/day in the oldest age group, 17 ± 8 g/day in the youngest) and for females (20 ± 9 g/day in the oldest, 17 ± 8 g/day in the youngest).

Table 3 gives total and food-group fiber consumption, measured during the EEC study. These results show that Italian fiber intake from potatoes is low (0.7 to 3.8 g per person per day) and that from grains high (13.4 to 14.7 g per person per day). Other European countries show a totally opposite picture.[8]

Table 4 gives mean values for fiber consumption and total and percentage energy intake per nutrient for Italians as indicated by the Italian INN study. A look at four geographical areas shows moderate variations (Table 5) from one area to another of Italy.[9] Table 5 gives interesting data regarding energy and nutrients. Whereas, in fact, average total protein and lipid consumption values show only small percentage differences with respect to totals between geographical areas, these same consumption values vary much more strongly when they are subdivided into plant and animal protein and lipid values. Percentage differences

---

* Unpublished information from a case-control study by M. Zamboni about dietary fiber consumption in lacto-ovo vegetarians and omnivores living in Verona (northeast Italy) in 1989.

TABLE 2
Mean (±SD) Daily Energy, Nutrient (as % Daily Energy) and Dietary Fiber Consumption in an Urban Northern Italian Population by Sex and Age, in 1989[a]

Sex	Age (years)	Number of subjects	Energy MJ/day	Carbohydrates (% daily energy)	Lipids (% daily energy)	Proteins (% daily energy)	Dietary fiber (g/day)
Males	25–39	227	9.7 ± 2.8	48 ± 10	35 ± 9	16 ± 4	17 ± 8
	40–54	204	9.3 ± 3.1	45 ± 10	34 ± 9	16 ± 3	20 ± 9
	55–69	177	9.5 ± 2.6	44 ± 11	35 ± 10	16 ± 3	21 ± 9
Females	25–39	256	8.2 ± 2.8	45 ± 10	39 ± 9	15 ± 4	17 ± 8
	40–54	172	8.0 ± 2.6	44 ± 10	38 ± 10	16 ± 4	17 ± 8
	55–69	222	7.9 ± 2.3	45 ± 10	38 ± 9	16 ± 3	20 ± 9

[a] Unpublished information from an epidemiological cross-sectional study by M. Miori (Department of Internal Medicine, Trento Hospital) on a randomly selected sample of the population of Trento (northeast Italy) in 1989.

TABLE 3
Dietary Fiber Intake from Food (g per person per day),
in Three Italian Regions, 1963–1965[6]

Region	Cereals	Vegetables	Fruit and nuts	Potatoes	Total
Friuli Venezia Giulia (Northeast)	14.7	5.1	1.3	3.8	24.9
Campania (central)	13.4	7.7	4.3	1.6	26.9
Basilicata (south)	13.5	5.7	3.9	0.7	23.8

TABLE 4
Mean (±SE) Fiber, Nutrients, and
Energy Intake in Italy, 1980–1984[5]

Fiber g/day	20.9 ± 0.04
Protein g/day	
Animal	59.7 ± 0.12
Plant	38.1 ± 0.07
Total	97.8 ± 0.15
Lipids g/day	
Animal	53.6 ± 0.13
Plant	54.5 ± 0.16
Total	108.1 ± 0.22
Carbohydrates g/day	
Available	325.6 ± 0.54
Soluble	89.1 ± 0.21
Alcohol g/day	17.8 ± 0.09
Energy MJ/day	11.3 ± 0.02

in animal protein consumption, compared to the national average (59.7 g/day) given in Table 4, range from +9% in northeastern Italy to −8% in southern Italy. Plant protein consumption compared with the national average (38.1 g/day) ranges from +8% in southern Italy to −13% in northwestern Italy. For animal fats, when compared with the national average (53.6 g/day), consumption varies from +21% in northeastern Italy to −16% in southern Italy, whereas plant fat consumption compared with the national average (54.5 g/day) ranges from +7% in southern Italy to −17% in northwestern Italy. Data on fiber consumption compared with the national average (20.9 g/day), show greater consumption in central (+4%) and southern (+6%) Italy than in the north (−12 and −13%). Table 6 illustrates this same territorial variability phenomenon in terms of consumptions expressed as food preferences.

Table 7 gives results from a study on vegetarians (lacto-ovo-vegetarians) and non-vegetarians (omnivores) living in a northern Italian town. The latter demonstrate eating habits practically identical to the population at large, and this is true for fiber intake as well. The vegetarians, on the other hand, showed about twice the fiber intake (31.9 ± 4.4 g/day) compared with the nonvegetarians (17.3 ± 2.3 g/day). The fiber intake of these north Italian vegetarians is greater even than that measured in 1980 to 1984 in the southern regions of Italy (22.2 g/day); see Table 5.

TABLE 5
Percentage Intake of Fiber, Nutrients, and Energy in Four Geographical Areas, Compared with the Whole of Italy (intake = 100), 1980–1984. Actual Fiber Intake, g/day, is Given in Parentheses[9]

Fiber	Northwest 88 (18.4)	Northeast 87 (18.2)	Center 104 (21.7)	South 106 (22.2)
Protein				
Animal	106	109	104	92
Plant	87	89	100	108
Total	99	101	102	98
Lipids				
Animal	120	121	103	84
Plant	83	95	100	107
Total	102	108	102	95
Carbohydrates				
Available	95	99	99	103
Soluble	98	109	100	97
Alcohol	97	121	105	88
Energy	98	103	101	99

FIBER CONSUMPTION AND CARDIOVASCULAR DISEASE IN ITALY

In Italy, it is practically impossible to evaluate mortality trends for cardiovascular diseases and ischemic heart diseases, in particular. This is because many risk factors have undergone simultaneous changes. Starting in 1970, for example, a continuous increase in fat consumption and cigarette smoking has been counterbalanced by better control of high blood pressure, increased physical activity, and improved health care for patients with coronary disease.[10] On the other hand there have been studies in Italy that show the beneficial effects that fiber has on the main coronary risk factors.[11,12]

FIBER CONSUMPTION AND CANCER IN ITALY

One study,[13] performed on 206 women with endometrial cancer and on 206 controls, showed that the risk for contracting this disease is higher for subjects consuming the more fat-rich diets that are also poor in green vegetables, fruit, and whole foods. The risk for contracting endometrial cancer appears inversely correlated to beta-carotene and fiber intake. The same authors[14] have performed a similar case-control study on stomach cancer; foods that are especially rich in fiber and complex carbohydrates, such as whole wheat bread and whole wheat pasta, have a protective effect with regard to stomach cancer.

CONCLUSIONS

Fiber consumption in Italy is higher in central than in northern regions of Italy and is even greater in the south. These southern and central areas seem to still be fairly well tied to the Mediterranean alimentary model, where the source of proteins and lipids is predom-

TABLE 6
Food Preferences in Four Italian Geographical Areas, 1980–1984[9]

Northwest	Northeast	Center	South
More Frequently Consumed Food			
Rice	Cereals[a]	Tomatoes	Pizza
Fresh fruit	Potatoes	Vegetables	Pasta
Salted meats	Dry fruit	Citrus fruit	Dry legumes
Giblets	Fresh pork	Beef	Meat
Yogurt	Poultry	Preserved fish	Fresh fish
Medium fat cheese	Milk	Animal fats	Low fat cheese
High fat cheese	Plant fats and oils	Soup preparations	
Biscuits and cakes	Pasta sauces		
Artificial sweeteners	Sugar		
Dietetic products	Soft drinks		
Soft drinks	Wine		
	Beer		
	Spirits		
Less Frequently Consumed Food			
Pasta	Bread and pizza	Rice	Cereals[a]
Dry legumes	Tomatoes for	Potatoes	Citrus fruit
Vegetables	sauces	Giblets	Dry fruit and nuts
Fresh fish	Fresh fruit	Low fat cheese	Beef
Preserved fish	Meat	Plant fats and oils	Pork
Whole milk	Low fat cheese	Sugar and honey	Salted meats
	Eggs	Soft drinks	Poultry
	Olive oil	Beer	Nonfat milk
	Snacks		Lowfat milk
			Yogurt
			Medium fat cheese
			Animal fats
			Pasta sauces
			Soup preparations
			Biscuits and cakes
			Wine
			Spirits

[a] Excluding bread, pizza, and pasta.

inantly from plants and where there is an evident preference for the consumption of vegetables, bread, pasta, and pizza, in comparison with other Italian regions. In northern Italy, on the other hand, the influence of the Western diet is much stronger and fiber intake is low. A recent study that shows that, in the same northern Italian urban environment, there is lower fiber consumption in the younger age groups compared to the elderly, who are presumably still tied to older, but healthier, eating habits gives further confirmation of this change towards the so-called Western diet which is relatively low in fiber.

TABLE 7
Mean (±SE) Fiber, Nutrients, and Energy Intake by Lacto-ovo-vegetarians and Omnivores, Living in a Northern Italian Town, 1989[a]

	Lacto-ovo-vegetarians	Omnivores
Protein g/day		
Animal	17.9 ± 3.8	48.6 ± 6.0
Plant	42.2 ± 4.8	29.1 ± 9.3
Total	60.1 ± 5.7	77.7 ± 7.8
Lipids g/day		
Mono-unsaturated	32.8 ± 5.3	32.6 ± 4.7
Poly-unsaturated	13.3 ± 4.3	7.6 ± 1.1
Saturated	23.2 ± 3.5	28.5 ± 4.3
Total	69.0 ± 9.5	75.7 ± 10.6
Carbohydrates g/day		
Total	378.0 ± 37.4	320.1 ± 42.4
Fiber	31.9 ± 4.4	17.3 ± 2.3
Energy MJ/day	9.8 ± 0.9	9.6 ± 1.2

[a] Unpublished information from a case-control study by M. Zamboni about dietary fiber consumption in lacto-ovo vegetarians and omnivores living in Verona (Northeast Italy) in 1989.

REFERENCES

1. **Cialfa, E. and Mariani Costantini, A.**, Situazione ed evoluzione dei consumi alimentari in Italia, in *Nutrizione Umana,* Fidanza, F. and Liguori, G. Eds., Idelson, Napoli, 1981.
2. **Spiller, A. G.**, *The Mediterranean Diet in Health and Disease,* Van Nostrand Reinhold, New York, 1991.
3. **Fidanza, F.**, Tecniche di rilevamento delle abitudini e dei consumi alimentari, in *Nutrizione Umana,* Fidanza, F. and Liguori, G., Eds., Idelson, Napoli, 1981.
4. Istituto Nazionale della Nutrizione, *Tabelle di composizione degli alimenti,* edizione 1988, Litho Delta, Milano, 1989.
5. **Saba, A., Turrini, A., Mistura, G., and Cialfa, E.**, Indagine nazionale sui consumi alimentari delle famiglie 1980–84. Alcuni importanti risultati, La Rivista della Societa Italiana di Scienza dell'Alimentazione, 19(4), 53, 1990.
6. **Cresta, M., Ledermann, S., Gardiner, A., Lombardo, E., and Lacoury, G.**, A dietary survey of 11 areas of the E.E.C. in order to determine levels of radioactive contamination, *Euratom,* EUR.4218F, 1969.
7. Ministry of Agriculture, Fisheries and Food, Household Food Consumption and Expenditure, 1950–1981, Annual reports of the National Food Survey Committee, Her Majesty's Stationery Office, London, 1953–1983.
8. **Bingham, S.**, Patterns of Dietary Fiber Consumption in Humans, in *Handbook of Dietary Fiber in Human Nutrition,* Spiller, G. A., Ed., CRC Press, Boca Raton, FL, 1986.
9. **Cialfa, E., Turrini, A., and Lintas, C.**, A National food survey. Food Balance Sheets and other methodologies: a critical overview, *Human Nutrition Reviews* (ILSI), MacDonald, I., Ed., 1991, 24.
10. **Menotti, A., Capocaccia, R., Farchi, F., and Pasquali, M.**, Recent trends in coronary heart disease and other cardiovascular diseases in Italy, *Cardiology,* 72, 88, 1985.
11. **Bosello, O., Ostuzzi, R., Armellini, F., Micciolo, R., and Scuro, L. A.**, Glucose tolerance and blood lipids in bran fed patients with impaired glucose tolerance, *Diabetes Care,* 3, 46, 1980.
12. **Rivellese, A., Riccardi, G., Giacco, A., et al.**, Reduction of risk factors for atherosclerosis in diabetic patients treated with high-fiber diet, *Prev. Med.,* 12(1), 128, 1983.

13. **La Vecchia, C., De Carli, A., Fasoli, M., and Gentile, A.,** Nutrition and diet in the etiology of endometrial cancer, *Cancer,* 57, 1248, 1986.
14. **La Vecchia, C., Negri, E., De Carli, A., D'Avanzo, B., and Franceschi, S.,** A case-control study of diet and gastric cancer in northern Italy, *Int. J. Cancer,* 40, 484, 1987.

Appendix I: Tables of Dietary Fiber and Associated Substances Content in Food

APPENDIX I

Table 1

DIETARY FIBER VALUES FOR COMMON FOODS*

Sally F. Schakel, Yvonne A. Sievert, and I. Marilyn Buzzard

The dietary fiber table developed by the Nutrition Coordinating Center (NCC) contains values compiled from scientific literature: the USDA Composition of Foods Handbook No. 8 revisions,[27,28] supplement,[29] and provisional table;[73] manufacturers' information; and estimated data. Estimated values were derived from (1) a different form of the same food (e.g., raw to cooked), (2) from a similar food, or (3) from calculation of recipes or formulations. Where only two of the three fiber values were known for a food, the third was calculated using the formula: Total Dietary Fiber = Insoluble Fiber + Soluble Fiber. For some foods, the three fiber values were obtained from different references, and, therefore, the sum of the insoluble and soluble fractions may not equal the value for total dietary fiber.

Food	Amount	g	Total dietary fiber (g)	Insoluble fiber (g)	Soluble fiber (g)
NUTS AND SEEDS					
Almond butter	1 TS	5.33	0.60	0.54	0.06
Almond paste	1 TB	14.19	0.76	0.69	0.08
Almonds	1 CP	142.00	15.90	14.34	1.56
Brazil nuts	1 CP	140.00	7.56	5.74	1.82
Cashew butter	1 TS	5.33	0.32	0.30	0.02
Cashews	1 CP	130.00	7.79	7.34	0.44
Chestnuts	1 CP	143.00	28.07	25.04	3.03
Coconut, fresh	1 Piece	45.00	4.05	3.87	0.18
Coconut, shredded, sweetened	1 TS	1.94	0.17	0.16	0.01
Coconut, shredded, unsweetened	1 TS	1.67	0.24	0.23	0.01
Filberts, hazelnuts	1 CP	135.00	8.64	5.26	3.37

* Includes both analytic and estimated values. For further information regarding specific values, contact The Nutrition Coordinating Center, 2221 University Avenue S.E., Minneapolis, MN 55414

Table 1 (continued)
DIETARY FIBER VALUES FOR COMMON FOODS

Food	Amount	g	Total dietary fiber (g)	Insoluble fiber (g)	Soluble fiber (g)
Hickory nuts	1 CP	100.00	6.10	3.13	2.97
Macadamia nuts	1 CP	134.00	6.97	4.34	2.63
Mixed nuts w peanuts	1 CP	142.00	11.64	7.14	2.94
Mixed nuts w/o peanuts	1 CP	144.00	11.33	7.65	1.17
Peanut butter	1 TS	5.33	0.32	0.29	0.03
Peanuts, honey roasted	1 CP	166.00	12.67	7.92	4.75
Peanuts	1 CP	144.00	12.67	7.92	4.75
Pecans	1 CP	110.00	7.15		
Pistachio nuts	1 CP	128.00	13.82	10.42	3.40
Pumpkin seeds	1 CP	138.00	9.34	6.76	2.58
Sesame nut mix (peanuts, sesame sticks, cashews)	1 CP	93.47	6.55	4.55	2.00
Sesame seeds	1 TB	8.00	0.73	0.58	0.15
Sunflower seed butter	1 TS	5.33	0.43	0.26	0.17
Sunflower seeds, hulled	1 CP	144.00	9.79	5.23	4.56
Tahini (sesame butter)	1 TS	5.00	0.46		
Walnuts	1 CP	100.00	4.80	2.84	1.96
FRUIT JUICES					
Apple juice	1 CP	248.00	0.25	0.17	0.07
Black currant juice	1 CP	240.00	1.44	0.50	0.94
Cranapple juice	1 CP	245.00	0.56	0.51	0.05
Grape juice	1 CP	253.00	1.26	0.76	0.51
Grapefruit juice	1 CP	247.00	0.25	0.05	0.20
Lemon juice	1 CP	244.00	0.73	0.24	0.49
Nectars, apricot	1 CP	251.00	1.51	0.75	0.75
Orange juice	1 CP	249.00	0.75	0.50	0.25
Papaya juice	1 CP	250.00	1.50	0.80	0.70
Pineapple juice	1 CP	250.00	0.75	0.67	0.07
Prune juice	1 CP	256.00	1.28	0.77	0.51

FRUITS, FRESH OR UNSWEETENED

Food	Serving	Weight (g)			
Apple, fresh w/o skin	1 Medium	128.00	2.43	1.92	0.51
Apple, fresh w skin	1 Medium	138.00	2.76	1.79	0.97
Apricots, fresh	1 Medium	35.33	0.67	0.47	0.27
Banana, fresh	1 Medium	114.00	2.19	1.55	0.64
Blackberries, fresh	1 CP	144.00	4.90	3.46	1.44
Blueberries, fresh	1 CP	145.00	1.88	1.45	0.43
Cantaloupe, fresh	1 Medium	922.75	7.38	2.95	4.43
Cherries, fresh, sweet	1 CP	145.00	1.88	1.16	0.72
Cranberries, fresh	1 CP	95.00	3.99	2.04	1.95
Figs, fresh	1 Medium	50.00	1.65	1.20	0.44
Gooseberries, fresh	1 CP	150.00	3.90	2.55	1.35
Grapefruit, fresh	1 Medium	291.20	3.61	1.40	2.21
Grapes, fresh	1 CP	160.00	1.12	0.78	0.34
Honeydew melon, fresh	1 Medium	1290.00	6.45	3.87	2.58
Kiwi fruit, fresh	1 Medium	76.00	2.58	1.88	0.71
Kumquats, fresh	1 Medium	19.00	0.17	0.08	0.08
Lemon, fresh	1 Medium	58.00	1.19	0.61	0.58
Loganberries, fresh	1 CP	147.00	4.70	3.97	0.73
Mandarin orange, fresh	1 Medium	84.00	0.73	0.37	0.36
Mango, fresh	1 Medium	207.00	4.14	2.24	1.90
Nectarine, fresh	1 Medium	136.00	2.18	1.10	1.07
Orange, fresh	1 Medium	131.00	3.14	1.19	1.90
Papaya, fresh	1 Medium	140.00	3.50	1.27	2.23
Peach, fresh	1 Medium	87.00	1.39	0.54	0.85
Pear, fresh	1 Medium	166.00	4.32	3.32	1.00
Persimmons, Japanese, raw	1 Medium	168.00	2.92	2.13	0.79
Pineapple, unsweetened or juice pack, cnd	1 CP	250.00	4.12	3.60	0.52
Pineapple, fresh	1 Slice	84.00	1.01	0.75	0.26
Plantains, ckd, fresh	1 CP	154.00	2.91	1.51	1.39
Plum, fresh	1 Medium	66.00	0.99	0.33	0.66
Pomegranate, fresh	1 Medium	154.00	5.70	4.62	1.08
Raspberries, fresh	1 CP	123.00	3.32	2.46	0.86
Strawberries, fresh	1 CP	149.00	3.87	2.83	1.04
Watermelon, fresh	1 Slice	482.00	1.93	0.96	0.96

Table 1 (continued)
DIETARY FIBER VALUES FOR COMMON FOODS

Food	Amount	g	Total dietary fiber (g)	Insoluble fiber (g)	Soluble fiber (g)
FRUITS, SWEETENED					
Apple, baked w sugar, unpared	1 CP	190.00	4.75	4.56	0.95
Apples, spiced	1 Ring	24.05	0.80	0.77	0.16
Applesauce, sweetened, cnd	1 CP	255.00	4.11	2.52	1.58
Apricots, sweetened, cnd	1 CP	258.00	3.35	1.21	2.14
Cherries, sweetened, cnd	1 CP	200.00	2.80	0.50	2.30
Cranberry sauce, whole berries	1 TB	17.00	0.25	0.13	0.12
Cranberry-orange relish	1 TB	17.00	0.38	0.23	0.15
Figs, heavy syrup, cnd	1 CP	259.00	4.27	3.11	1.14
Fruit cocktail, sweetened, cnd	1 CP	256.00	3.84	1.56	2.28
Grapefruit sections, sweetened, cnd	1 CP	254.00	1.12	0.56	0.56
Mandarin orange sections, sweetened, cnd	1 CP	254.00	0.74	0.38	0.36
Peaches, sweetened, cnd	1 CP	256.00	4.04	2.41	1.64
Pear, sweetened, cnd	1 CP	255.00	7.70	6.07	1.66
Pineapple, sweetened, cnd	1 Slice	58.00	0.64	0.43	0.20
Plums, sweetened, cnd	1 CP	258.00	5.65	3.20	2.45
Rhubarb, sweetened, ckd	1 CP	240.00	4.80	2.33	2.40
Strawberries, sweetened, cnd or frozen	1 CP	255.00	4.33	3.31	1.02
FRUITS, DRIED					
Apples, dried, unckd	1 CP	86.00	8.26	5.99	2.27
Apricots, dried, unckd	1 CP	130.00	10.14	6.79	3.35
Apricots, dried, unsweetened, ckd	1 CP	250.00	6.82	4.57	2.25
Banana chips	1 CP	92.00	6.09	4.28	1.84
Dates, dried	1 CP	178.00	7.83	5.70	2.14
Figs, dried	1 CP	199.00	16.32	8.36	7.96
Peaches, dried, unsweetened, ckd	1 CP	258.00	6.76	2.63	4.13
Peaches, dried, unckd	1 CP	160.00	13.12	5.09	8.03
Pears, dried, unckd	1 CP	180.00	21.20	12.47	8.73

Pears, dried, unsweetened, ckd	1 CP	255.00	14.56	8.57	5.99
Prunes, dried, unsweetened, ckd	1 CP	212.00	6.36	2.76	3.60
Prunes, dried, unckd	1 CP	161.00	10.63	4.51	6.12
Raisins	1 TB	9.69	0.51	0.16	0.35

VEGETABLES, RAW

Broccoli, raw	1 CP	88.00	2.20	1.41	0.79
Cabbage, Chinese, (Pak-choi), raw	1 CP	70.00	1.13		
Cabbage, Chinese, (Pe-tsai), raw	1 CP	76.00	0.84		
Cabbage, raw	1 CP	70.00	1.46	0.92	0.55
Carrot, raw	1 CP	110.00	3.53	1.85	1.68
Cauliflower, raw	1 CP	100.00	2.40	1.38	1.20
Celery, raw	1 CP	120.00	1.92	1.08	0.84
Chives, fresh	1 TB	3.00	0.06	0.04	0.02
Cucumber, raw	1 CP	104.00	1.04	0.83	0.21
Endive, raw	1 CP	50.00	1.40	1.00	0.39
Garlic, fresh	1 TS	3.12	0.02		
Jicama, raw	1 CP	120.00	2.26	1.28	0.97
Kohlrabi, raw	1 CP	140.00	4.62	1.54	3.08
Lettuce, fresh	1 CP	55.00	0.48	0.38	0.11
Mushrooms, raw	1 CP	70.00	1.35	1.17	0.18
Onion, dehydrated flakes	1 TB	4.00	0.40	0.20	0.20
Onions, raw	1 CP	160.00	2.56	1.28	1.28
Parsley, fresh	1 TB	3.75	0.16	0.14	0.02
Pepper, green, raw	1 CP	100.00	1.60	1.10	0.50
Radish, raw	1 CP	116.00	2.55	1.52	1.03
Romaine, raw	1 CP	56.00	0.58		
Scallion, raw	1 CP	100.00	2.40	1.20	1.20
Seaweed, dried; Laver or "Nori"	1 Piece	2.00	0.29		
Spinach, raw	1 CP	56.00	1.46	1.01	0.45
Sprouts, alfalfa, raw	1 CP	33.00		0.73	
Sprouts, soybean, raw	1 CP	70.00	2.59	2.32	0.27
Tomatoes, raw	1 CP	180.00	2.34	1.44	0.90
Watercress, raw	1 CP	34.00	0.78	0.64	0.14
Zucchini, raw	1 CP	130.00	1.95	0.65	1.30

Table 1 (continued)
DIETARY FIBER VALUES FOR COMMON FOODS

Food	Amount	g	Total dietary fiber (g)	Insoluble fiber (g)	Soluble fiber (g)
VEGETABLES, COOKED OR CANNED					
Artichokes, ckd	1 CP	168.00	5.54	2.47	3.07
Asparagus, ckd, fresh or frozen	1 CP	180.00	2.95	2.34	0.61
Asparagus, cnd, drained solids	1 CP	242.00	5.69	4.67	1.02
Bamboo shoots, cnd	1 CP	131.00	2.88		
Beans, lima, ckd, fresh or frozen	1 CP	170.00	8.50	7.14	1.70
Beans, yellow, ckd, fresh or frozen	1 CP	135.00	4.08	3.08	1.00
Beans, yellow, cnd, drained solids	1 CP	136.00	4.07	3.09	0.98
Beets, red, ckd, fresh or frozen	1 CP	170.00	4.25	3.48	0.76
Beets, red, cnd, drained solids	1 CP	170.00	4.42	3.04	1.36
Broccoli, ckd, fresh or frozen	1 CP	184.00	5.15	2.83	2.30
Brussels sprouts, ckd, fresh or frozen	1 CP	155.00	7.02	4.18	2.82
Cabbage, Chinese, (Pak-choi), ckd	1 CP	170.00	2.72		
Cabbage, Chinese, (Pe-tsai), ckd	1 CP	119.00	1.90		
Cabbage, ckd	1 CP	150.00	3.00	1.90	1.13
Carrot juice	1 CP	246.00	1.97	1.43	0.54
Carrots, ckd, fresh or frozen	1 CP	156.00	4.84	2.96	1.87
Carrots, cnd, drained solids	1 CP	146.00	2.19	1.75	0.44
Cauliflower, ckd, fresh or frozen	1 CP	180.00	4.61	3.08	1.55
Celery, ckd, fresh or frozen	1 CP	150.00	3.30	1.86	1.44
Chard, swiss, ckd, fresh or frozen	1 CP	175.00	4.27	3.66	0.61
Chinese or chow mein vegetables, cnd (bean sprouts, bamboo shoots, water chestnuts red pepper)	1 CP	113.00	3.28	1.88	0.21
Chop suey vegetables, cnd (bean sprouts, celery, water chestnuts, onions, bamboo shoots, etc.)	1 CP	127.40	1.86	0.98	0.79
Corn, ear, ckd	1 Medium	77.00	4.39	1.62	2.77
Corn, whole kernel, fresh or frozen	1 CP	164.00	6.07	3.44	2.62
Corn, whole kernel, cnd, drained solids	1 CP	164.00	3.05	2.64	0.39

Food	Amount	Weight (g)		
Eggplant, ckd	1 CP	96.00	1.91	1.86	0.05
Green beans, ckd, fresh or frozen	1 CP	135.00	4.08	3.08	1.00
Green beans, cnd, drained solids	1 CP	136.00	4.07	3.09	0.98
Greens, collards, ckd, fresh or frozen	1 CP	128.00	2.70	2.76	1.70
Greens, turnip, ckd, fresh or frozen	1 CP	144.00	4.46	1.42	2.95
Kohlrabi, ckd, fresh or frozen	1 CP	165.00	4.37	4.19	2.73
Mixed vegetables (corn, lima beans, snap beans, peas, carrots), ckd, fresh or frozen	1 CP	182.00	6.92		
Mixed vegetables (corn, lima beans, snap beans, peas, carrots), cnd, drained solids	1 CP	163.00	6.19	3.91	2.28
Mixed vegetables, ckd, fresh or frozen (broccoli, cauliflower, carrots)	1 CP	151.20	4.22	2.56	1.65
Mushrooms, ckd or cnd	1 CP	156.00	3.43	2.96	0.47
Okra, ckd, fresh or frozen	1 CP	184.00	5.89	2.39	3.50
Onions, ckd, fresh or frozen	1 CP	210.00	2.73	1.30	1.43
Parsnips, ckd, fresh or frozen	1 CP	156.00	6.24	4.21	2.03
Peas & carrots, ckd, fresh or frozen	1 CP	160.00	5.84	4.56	1.44
Peas & carrots, cnd, drained solids	1 CP	158.00	4.17	3.52	0.65
Peas, blackeye, fresh, ckd	1 CP	165.00	6.39	5.69	0.69
Peas, edible-podded, ckd, fresh or frozen	1 CP	160.00	4.48	2.56	1.92
Peas, green, ckd, fresh or frozen	1 CP	160.00	6.72	6.08	0.96
Peas, green, cnd, drained solids	1 CP	170.00	6.44	5.54	0.90
Pepper, chili, ckd, fresh	1 CP	136.00	2.04		
Pepper, green, ckd, fresh or frozen	1 CP	136.00	1.26	0.87	0.39
Potatoes, baked or boiled, w skin	1 CP	156.00	3.90	1.56	1.40
Potatoes, baked or boiled, w/o skin	1 CP	156.00	2.34	1.81	0.53
Potatoes, cnd, drained solids	1 CP	180.00	4.52	0.99	3.53
Pumpkin, ckd or cnd	1 CP	245.00	2.69	1.71	0.98
Rutabaga, ckd, fresh or frozen	1 CP	170.00	2.43	1.27	1.16
Sauerkraut, ckd, cnd, solids and liquid	1 CP	236.00	8.26	6.21	2.05
Scallion, ckd	1 CP	219.00	5.50	2.63	2.87
Spinach, ckd, fresh or frozen	1 CP	190.00	4.14	3.21	0.95
Spinach, cnd, drained solids	1 CP	214.00	2.46	1.63	0.81
Sprouts, mung bean, ckd or cnd	1 CP	125.00	1.00	0.52	0.47
Squash, summer, all varieties, ckd, fresh or frozen	1 CP	180.00	2.52	1.98	0.54
Squash, winter, all varieties, ckd, fresh or frozen	1 CP	245.00	6.86	2.94	3.92
Sweet potato, cnd, syrup pack, drained solids	1 CP	196.00	2.39	1.49	0.92
Sweet potatoes, ckd, fresh or frozen	1 CP	255.00	7.65	4.59	3.06

Table 1 (continued)
DIETARY FIBER VALUES FOR COMMON FOODS

Food	Amount	g	Total dietary fiber (g)	Insoluble fiber (g)	Soluble fiber (g)
Sweet potatoes, cnd, vacuum pack, drained solids	1 CP	200.00	2.44	1.52	0.94
Tomato juice	1 CP	242.64	1.94	1.41	0.53
Tomato paste, cnd	1 CP	262.00	11.27	9.12	2.15
Tomato sauce, cnd w/o fat	1 CP	245.00	3.67	2.67	1.00
Tomatoes, ckd, fresh	1 CP	240.00	4.06	2.50	1.56
Tomatoes, cnd	1 CP	240.00	2.04	1.68	0.79
Turnips, ckd, fresh or frozen	1 CP	156.00	3.12	2.00	1.12
Vegetable juice, cocktail	1 CP	242.00	1.94	1.40	0.53
Waterchestnuts, cnd	1 CP	140.00	3.08	1.83	1.25
Wild spinach, ckd, fresh	1 CP	124.00	3.78		
Zucchini, ckd, fresh or frozen	1 CP	180.00	2.52	1.98	0.54
LEGUMES AND MEAT SUBSTITUTES					
Baked beans, w franks, cnd	1 CP	257.00	9.15	4.81	4.37
Baked beans, w pork & tomato sauce	1 CP	253.00	10.63	5.57	5.06
Baked beans, w pork & brown sugar	1 CP	253.00	10.63	5.57	5.06
Beans, kidney, dry, ckd or cnd	1 CP	177.00	11.04	8.27	2.78
Beans, lima, dry, ckd or cnd	1 CP	188.00	13.59	6.22	7.35
Beans, navy, dry, ckd or cnd	1 CP	182.00	15.42	6.55	5.21
Beans, northern, dry, ckd or cnd	1 CP	179.00	9.67	7.50	2.17
Beans, pinto, dry, ckd or cnd	1 CP	171.00	11.97	8.24	3.74
Beans, tepary, dry, ckd or cnd	1 CP	262.00	13.36		
Chickpeas, dry, ckd or cnd	1 CP	164.00	9.51	5.74	3.77
Lentils, dry, ckd or cnd	1 CP	198.00	10.34	9.21	1.11
Peas, blackeye, dry, ckd or cnd	1 CP	171.00	16.42	14.65	1.76
Peas, split, dry, ckd or cnd	1 CP	196.00	6.27	4.12	2.16
Breakfast strips, vegetable protein	1 Slice	8.00	0.05	0.00	0.05
Frankfurter substitute, soybean	1 OZ	28.35	0.39	0.28	0.11

Ham or canadian bacon substitute, soybean	1 Slice	22.67	0.00	0.00
Meat loaf substitute, soybean	1 OZ	28.35	0.00	0.00
Sausage substitute, soybean, link	1 OZ	28.35	0.05	0.01
Sausage substitute, soybean, patty	1 Medium	64.00	0.32	0.00
Soy flour	1 CP	85.00	9.15	2.57
Soybean curd, tofu	1 OZ	28.35	0.34	0.20
Textured vegetable protein, bacon-like bits	1 TB	7.68	0.70	0.20
Textured vegetable protein, dehydrated	1 CP	94.05	10.64	2.98
Textured vegetable protein, frozen	1 OZ	28.35	0.12	0.03

BREADS

Bagel, egg	1 Medium	55.00	0.88	0.35
Bagel, oat bran	1 Medium	55.00	2.21	0.69
Bagel, plain	1 Medium	55.00	1.15	0.48
Bagel, rye	1 Medium	66.00	3.10	0.73
Bagel, whole wheat	1 Medium	55.00	4.29	0.68
Biscuit, baking powder	1 Medium	38.00	0.97	0.25
Bread crumbs, dry grated	1 TB	6.25	0.26	0.13
Bread stick, plain, soft type	1 Medium	10.00	0.38	0.06
Bread, Boston brown	1 Slice	48.00	2.26	0.53
Bread, cheese	1 Slice	28.65	0.64	0.14
Bread, cinnamon swirl	1 Slice	21.50	0.23	0.09
Bread, diet w fiber added	1 Slice	23.00	2.60	0.14
Bread, egg	1 Slice	32.51	0.86	0.27
Bread, English muffin	1 Slice	28.35	0.45	0.19
Bread, fruit w/o nuts	1 Slice	44.80	1.45	0.33
Bread, high fiber	1 Slice	28.35	3.20	0.49
Bread, Hovis	1 Slice	28.57	1.29	0.15
Bread, Italian	1 Slice	30.00	0.81	0.51
Bread, Italian Focaccia	1 Slice	70.50	1.78	0.39
Bread, nut	1 Slice	58.05	0.93	0.28
Bread, oatmeal	1 Slice	29.96	0.94	0.26
Bread, pumpkin w/o nuts	1 Slice	44.80	0.94	0.34
Bread, raisin	1 Slice	22.50	0.85	0.36
Bread, rye	1 Slice	28.69	1.89	0.40
Bread, rye, thin sliced	1 Slice	20.00	1.32	0.28
Bread, Syrian or pita, white	1 Large	85.00	2.29	1.02

Table 1 (continued)
DIETARY FIBER VALUES FOR COMMON FOODS

Food	Amount	g	Total dietary fiber (g)	Insoluble fiber (g)	Soluble fiber (g)
Bread, Syrian or pita, whole wheat	1 Large	85.00	6.29	5.23	1.05
Bread, white	1 Slice	25.00	0.50	0.25	0.24
Bread, white, thin sliced	1 Slice	17.00	0.34	0.17	0.17
Bread, whole wheat, mixed grain, wheat germ, granola type, etc.	1 Slice	28.57	2.11	1.65	0.46
Bread, whole wheat, thin sliced	1 Slice	17.00	1.26	0.98	0.28
Bread, zucchini w/o nuts	1 Slice	44.80	0.69	0.44	0.15
Cornbread	1 Piece	58.50	1.28	1.15	0.13
Croutons, commercial	CP	35.50	1.67	0.85	0.82
Lefse	1 Piece	38.24	0.71	0.54	0.17
Muffin, bran	1 Medium	50.00	2.14	1.93	0.21
Muffin, carrot	1 Medium	58.00	1.20	0.76	0.41
Muffin, corn	1 Medium	40.00	0.82	0.76	0.06
Muffin, English, White	1 Medium	56.70	0.91	0.25	0.66
Muffin, English, whole wheat	1 Medium	56.70	2.48	1.89	0.44
Muffin, oat bran or oatmeal	1 Medium	47.00	1.01	0.65	0.35
Muffin, plain varieties	1 Medium	47.00	0.73	0.54	0.19
Muffin, pumpkin	1 Medium	58.00	1.24	0.66	0.52
Popover	1 Medium	40.00	0.48	0.36	0.12
Roll, cheese bread	1 Medium	28.00	0.62	0.40	0.14
Roll, egg bread	1 Medium	39.00	1.03	0.64	0.22
Roll, hamburger	1 Medium	43.00	0.58	0.23	0.35
Roll, hard	1 Medium	37.00	1.61	0.72	0.25
Roll, hot dog	1 Medium	43.00	0.58	0.23	0.35
Roll, kaiser	1 Medium	50.00	2.18	0.97	0.33
Roll, rich, brioche	1 Medium	77.00	1.82	1.09	0.38
Roll, rich, crescent, refrigerated dough	1 Medium	28.35	0.79	0.31	0.48
Roll, rich, croissant	1 Medium	55.00	0.73	0.45	0.15
Roll, rye	1 Medium	36.00	2.38	1.87	0.50

Roll, sourdough	1 Medium	45.00	1.21	0.45	0.76
Roll, submarine	1 Medium	100.00	2.60	1.70	0.90
Roll, white, dinner	1 Medium	36.00	1.01	0.39	0.62
Roll, whole wheat	1 Medium	36.00	2.59	2.02	0.57
Scone	1 Medium	28.00	0.64	0.47	0.17
Tortilla, corn	5 1/2" diam	21.30	1.11	0.72	0.39
Tortilla, flour	7" diam	24.00	0.70	0.52	0.18
Tortilla, flour, whole wheat	7" diam	42.50	2.46	2.05	0.41
Tortilla, taco shell	1 Medium	13.00	1.04	0.68	0.36
Coffee cake, quick bread w/o nuts	1 Piece	70.20	0.73	0.54	0.19

PASTRIES, PANCAKES, AND WAFFLES

Coffee cake, yeast w/o nuts	1 Piece	41.22	0.97	0.63	0.22
Crepes	1 Small	33.21	0.27	0.20	0.07
Doughnut, cake	1 Medium	42.00	0.79	0.57	0.20
Doughnut, yeast	1 Medium	60.00	1.00	0.65	0.23
Pancake, homemade, all varieties except whole wheat and buckwheat	1 Medium	21.00	0.30	0.22	0.08
Pancake, homemade, whole wheat	1 Medium	21.00	0.89	0.74	0.15
Pancake, prepared from a complete mix w water, all varieties	1 Medium	21.00	0.55	0.45	0.10
Pancake, prepared from a mix w whole milk, oil, & egg, all varieties	1 Medium	21.00	0.44	0.31	0.12
Panetonne, Italian coffee cake	1 Piece	45.97	1.36	0.59	0.35
Pastry, Danish	1 Medium	82.00	1.46	0.96	0.34
Pastry, toaster; Poptarts, all varieties	1 Each	52.00	0.52	0.37	0.16
Roll, sweet, yeast	1 Medium	50.00	1.14	0.70	0.24
Waffle, frozen all varieties	1 Each	34.00	0.46	0.34	0.12
Waffle, homemade, all varieties	1 Each	75.00	1.09	0.81	0.28

CEREAL AND GRAINS

Barley, pearled, ckd	1 CP	157.00	6.45	4.60	1.85
Barley, pearled, dry	1 CP	200.00	23.60	16.80	6.80
Bran, unprocessed	1 TB	3.75	1.60	1.50	0.10
Buckwheat groats, cooked	1 CP	198.00	3.29	2.85	0.46
Buckwheat groats, dry	1 CP	164.00	10.51	9.05	1.44
Bulgur, ckd	1 CP	182.00	7.94	6.59	1.33
Bulgur, dry	1 CP	140.00	25.62	21.31	4.28
Cereals, dry, All Bran	1 CP	85.05	26.15	21.82	4.34

Table 1 (continued)
DIETARY FIBER VALUES FOR COMMON FOODS

Food	Amount	g	Total dietary fiber (g)	Insoluble fiber (g)	Soluble fiber (g)
Cereals, dry, All Bran fruit & almonds	1 CP	55.28	16.22	14.79	1.43
Cereals, dry, All Bran with extra fiber	1 CP	56.70	24.26	22.67	1.59
Cereals, dry, Almond Delight	1 CP	37.80	2.00	1.33	0.67
Cereals, dry, Amaranth	1 CP	113.40	10.04	8.31	1.72
Cereals, dry, Apple Cinnamon Oh's	1 CP	28.35	0.65	0.50	0.15
Cereals, dry, Apple Jacks	1 CP	28.35	0.76	0.70	0.01
Cereals, dry, Apple Raisin Crisp	1 CP	55.28	3.08	2.13	0.95
Cereals, dry, Body Buddies (all flavors)	1 CP	28.35	0.76	0.70	0.01
Cereals, dry, Boo Berry	1 CP	28.35	0.76	0.70	0.01
Cereals, dry, Bran Buds	1 CP	84.00	29.63	23.27	6.36
Cereals, dry, Bran Chex	1 CP	42.50	9.15	7.50	1.65
Cereals, dry, Bran Flakes	1 CP	39.00	5.97	4.93	1.05
Cereals, dry, Bran News (all flavors)	1 CP	37.80	3.52	2.91	0.60
Cereals, dry, C.W. Post Hearty Granola	1 CP	113.40	6.02	4.21	1.81
Cereals, dry, Cap'n Crunch's Peanut Butter Crunch	1 CP	35.00	1.09	0.57	0.52
Cereals, dry, Captain Crunch	1 CP	37.00	1.04	0.44	0.59
Cereals, dry, Cheerios	1 CP	22.68	2.05	0.99	1.05
Cereals, dry, Chex, corn or rice	1 CP	28.35	0.51	0.51	0.00
Cereals, dry, Chex, wheat	1 CP	46.00	6.00	3.40	2.60
Cereals, dry, Cinnamon Toast Crunch	1 CP	42.50	1.26	1.02	0.21
Cereals, dry, Circus Fun	1 CP	28.35	0.48	0.40	0.09
Cereals, dry, Clusters	1 CP	56.70	5.31	4.03	1.28
Cereals, dry, Cocoa Krispies	1 CP	37.80	1.01	0.93	0.01
Cereals, dry, Cocoa Puffs	1 CP	28.35	0.66	0.65	0.01
Cereals, dry, Common Sense Oat Bran	1 CP	56.00	6.00	3.89	2.18
Cereals, dry, Common Sense Oat Bran w Raisins	1 CP	73.71	7.00	4.25	2.82
Cereals, dry, Cookie-Crisp (chocolate chip & vanilla flavor)	1 CP	28.35	0.90	0.72	0.15
Cereals, dry, Corn Bran	1 CP	42.50	5.38	4.65	0.73

Cereals, dry, Corn Flakes low sodium	1 CP	25.00	0.50	0.40	0.10
Cereals, dry, Corn Flakes (Kellogg's)	1 CP	28.35	0.45	0.35	0.10
Cereals, dry, Corn Flakes (Ralston)	1 CP	28.35	0.46	0.36	0.10
Cereals, dry, Corn Pops	1 CP	28.35	0.48	0.40	0.09
Cereals, dry, Country Corn Flakes	1 CP	28.35	0.45	0.35	0.10
Cereals, dry, Cracklin' Oat Bran	1 CP	56.70	9.37	7.61	1.76
Cereals, dry, Crispix	1 CP	28.35	0.45	0.35	0.10
Cereals, dry, Crispy Critters	1 CP	28.35	0.94	0.34	0.60
Cereals, dry, Crispy Wheats 'n Raisins	1 CP	37.80	3.51	2.91	0.60
Cereals, dry, Croonchy Stars	1 CP	28.35	0.65	0.50	0.15
Cereals, dry, Crunchy Bran	1 CP	28.35	5.24	4.82	0.43
Cereals, dry, Crunchy Nut Oh's	1 CP	28.35	1.50	1.05	0.45
Cereals, dry, Dinersaurs	1 CP	28.35	0.65	0.50	0.15
Cereals, dry, Fiber One	1 CP	56.70	21.69	19.91	1.77
Cereals, dry, Fiber 7 Flakes	1 CP	56.70	10.34	9.23	1.11
Cereals, dry, Fibre Crunch	1 CP	90.00	13.18	11.47	1.71
Cereals, dry, Food Club 100% Natural Cereal	1 CP	113.40	8.30	6.44	1.84
Cereals, dry, Fortified Oat Flakes	1 CP	42.50	3.19	1.66	1.53
Cereals, dry, Froot Loops	1 CP	28.35	0.76	0.70	0.01
Cereals, dry, Frosted Flakes	1 CP	37.80	1.01	0.93	0.01
Cereals, dry, Frosted Krispies	1 CP	37.80	1.01	0.93	0.01
Cereals, dry, Fruit Lites, rice	1 CP	24.00	0.31	0.22	0.09
Cereals, dry, Fruit Wheats (all flavors)	1 CP	56.70	7.10	6.19	0.91
Cereals, dry, Fruity Marshmallow Krispies	1 CP	29.48	0.61	0.56	0.01
Cereals, dry, Fruity Yummy Mummy	1 CP	28.35	0.99	0.87	0.10
Cereals, dry, Ghost Busters	1 CP	28.35	0.65	0.50	0.15
Cereals, dry, Golden Grahams	1 CP	37.80	0.66	0.66	0.00
Cereals, dry, Golden Wheat Lites	1 CP	28.35	2.63	2.18	0.45
Cereals, dry, Granola, commercial	1 CP	113.00	5.99	4.18	1.81
Cereals, dry, Granola, homemade w/o coconut, w/o nuts	1 CP	146.17	7.13	5.12	1.94
Cereals, dry, Grape-Nuts	1 CP	113.40	11.45	8.05	3.40
Cereals, dry, Grapenuts Flakes	1 CP	39.00	2.65	2.50	0.16
Cereals, dry, Healthy Crunch (all flavors)	1 CP	113.40	12.04	6.72	5.50
Cereals, dry, Heartwise	1 CP	42.50	7.67	3.08	4.62
Cereals, dry, Honey Bran Crunchies	1 CP	50.00	6.32	5.46	0.86
Cereals, dry, Honey Buc Wheat Crisp	1 CP	37.80	3.51	2.91	0.60
Cereals, dry, Honey Graham Oh's	1 CP	28.35	0.75	0.32	0.43

Table 1 (continued)
DIETARY FIBER VALUES FOR COMMON FOODS

Food	Amount	g	Total dietary fiber (g)	Insoluble fiber (g)	Soluble fiber (g)
Cereals, dry, Honey Nut Cheerios	1 CP	37.80	1.24	0.45	0.79
Cereals, dry, Honeycomb	1 CP	21.26	0.34	0.28	0.06
Cereals, dry, Just Right Nugget & Flake	1 CP	42.50	3.96	3.28	0.68
Cereals, dry, Kaboom	1 CP	28.35	1.28	0.92	0.33
Cereals, dry, Kenmei Rice Bran	1 CP	37.80	1.22	0.94	0.28
Cereals, dry, Kenmei Rice Bran Almond and Raisin	1 CP	52.92	2.51	1.90	0.61
Cereals, dry, King Vitamin	1 CP	21.00	0.96	0.88	0.09
Cereals, dry, Kix	1 CP	18.90	0.30	0.23	0.06
Cereals, dry, Life	1 CP	44.00	3.92	2.42	1.50
Cereals, dry, Mountain House Granola	1 CP	113.40	2.80	2.02	0.77
Cereals, dry, Mueslix Crispy Blend	1 CP	63.80	3.86	2.72	1.15
Cereals, dry, Mueslix, Golden Crunch	1 CP	68.00	4.11	2.90	1.22
Cereals, dry, Natural Bran Flakes (Post)	1 CP	42.50	6.95	5.72	1.23
Cereals, dry, Natural Bran w Raisins or w Apples & Cinnamon (Health Valley)	1 CP	113.40	18.16	16.07	2.09
Cereals, dry, Nature Valley Granola Coconut & Honey	1 CP	85.05	5.60	4.33	1.26
Cereals, dry, Nut & Honey Crunch Biscuits	1 CP	56.70	5.28	4.38	0.91
Cereals, dry, Nut & Honey Crunch Flakes	1 CP	42.50	1.32	1.14	0.11
Cereals, dry, Nutri-Grain Almond Raisin	1 CP	59.54	5.51	4.58	0.92
Cereals, dry, Nutri-Grain Corn	1 CP	56.70	5.75	4.72	1.03
Cereals, dry, Nutri-Grain Nuggets	1 CP	113.40	15.62	13.43	2.18
Cereals, dry, Nutri-Grain Wheat	1 CP	42.50	4.31	3.54	0.77
Cereals, dry, Nutri-Grain Wheat & Raisins	1 CP	59.54	5.54	4.58	0.95
Cereals, dry, Nutrific	1 CP	36.86	5.31	4.76	0.55
Cereals, dry, Oat Bran Flakes (Health Valley)	1 CP	56.70	5.31	3.66	1.67
Cereals, dry, Oat Bran O's	1 CP	37.80	4.51	2.48	2.07
Cereals, dry, Oat Bran Options	1 CP	41.20	3.31	2.00	1.33
Cereals, dry, Oat Squares	1 CP	56.70	5.45	3.12	2.33
Cereals, dry, Oatmeal Raisin Crisp	1 CP	56.70	3.07	2.14	0.92

Cereals, dry, Pebbles Cocoa	1 CP	32.40	0.52	0.08
Cereals, dry, Post Toasties (corn)	1 CP	22.68	0.37	0.08
Cereals, dry, Pro Grain	1 CP	37.80	4.93	2.13
Cereals, dry, Pro Stars	1 CP	28.35	0.37	0.11
Cereals, dry, Product 19	1 CP	28.35	1.24	0.30
Cereals, dry, Puffed Kashi	1 CP	21.26	1.36	0.19
Cereals, dry, Puffed Rice	1 CP	14.00	0.18	0.05
Cereals, dry, Puffed Rice (Malt-O-Meal)	1 CP	14.18	0.19	0.05
Cereals, dry, Puffed Wheat	1 CP	12.00	0.86	0.41
Cereals, dry, Puffed Wheat (Malt-O-Meal)	1 CP	14.18	1.52	0.47
Cereals, dry, Rainbow Brite	1 CP	28.35	0.65	0.15
Cereals, dry, Raisin Bran (Kellogg's)	1 CP	52.92	5.03	1.09
Cereals, dry, Raisin Bran (Ralston)	1 CP	50.40	4.71	0.81
Cereals, dry, Raisin Bran (Skinner's)	1 CP	56.70	5.28	0.91
Cereals, dry, Raisin Nut Bran	1 CP	56.70	7.37	1.45
Cereals, dry, Raisin Squares	1 CP	56.70	5.28	0.91
Cereals, dry, Real Granola and Orangeola (all flavors)	1 CP	113.40	12.02	5.49
Cereals, dry, Rice Krispies	1 CP	28.35	0.45	0.10
Cereals, dry, Rice Toasties	1 CP	28.35	0.46	0.10
Cereals, dry, Rocky Road	1 CP	42.50	0.72	0.13
Cereals, dry, Shredded Wheat 'N Bran	1 CP	42.52	5.38	0.73
Cereals, dry, Shredded Wheat Type	1 Large	23.60	2.19	0.38
Cereals, dry, Shreddies, all varieties	1 CP	50.00	4.65	0.80
Cereals, dry, Smurf-Berry Crunch	1 CP	28.35	0.65	0.15
Cereals, dry, Special K	1 CP	28.35	0.90	0.17
Cereals, dry, Sugar Puffs	1 CP	32.40	1.17	0.55
Cereals, dry, Sugar Sparkled Flakes	1 CP	37.80	0.61	0.14
Cereals, dry, Sun Country Granola w Raisins or Raisin Date	1 CP	113.40	6.13	1.85
Cereals, dry, Sunflakes, Multi-Grain	1 CP	28.35	2.45	0.42
Cereals, dry, Super Golden Crisp	1 CP	32.40	0.22	0.06
Cereals, dry, Tasteeos	1 CP	22.68	1.60	0.76
Cereals, dry, Team Flakes	1 CP	42.00	0.68	0.15
Cereals, dry, Teddy Grahams Breakfast Bears, all flavors	1 CP	85.05	4.83	0.81
Cereals, dry, Teenage Mutant Ninja Turtles	1 CP	28.35	0.65	0.15
Cereals, dry, Total	1 CP	33.00	2.94	0.56
Cereals, dry, Total Raisin Bran	1 CP	42.52	4.05	0.88
Cereals, dry, Trix	1 CP	28.35	0.99	0.10
Cereals, dry, Uncle Sam's High Fiber	1 CP	56.70	14.75	1.49

Table 1 (continued)
DIETARY FIBER VALUES FOR COMMON FOODS

Food	Amount	g	Total dietary fiber (g)	Insoluble fiber (g)	Soluble fiber (g)
Cereals, dry, Vita Crunch Granola	1 CP	113.40	6.13	4.29	1.85
Cereals, dry, Wheat & Raisin Chex	1 CP	50.40	4.17	2.90	1.27
Cereals, dry, Wheat Germ & Fiber	1 CP	113.40	18.16	16.07	2.09
Cereals, dry, Wheaties	1 CP	28.40	2.35	1.66	0.69
Cereals, dry, 100% Bran	1 CP	56.70	19.41	18.14	1.27
Cereals, dry, 100% Natural Granola	1 CP	85.05	7.20	3.14	4.07
Cereals, dry, 40% Bran Flakes (Ralston)	1 CP	37.80	5.06	3.96	1.10
Cereals, Roman Meal, ckd w salt	1 CP	241.00	9.64	8.27	1.37
Cereals, Roman Meal, dry	1 CP	94.00	19.74	16.96	2.78
Corn grits, ckd regular or instant	1 CP	242.00	0.82	0.70	0.15
Corn grits, dry	1 CP	156.00	3.43	2.85	0.58
Cornmeal, ckd	1 CP	240.00	1.70	1.68	0.02
Cornmeal, dry	1 CP	138.00	7.18	7.09	0.08
Cornstarch	1 TB	8.00	0.07		
Couscous, ckd	1 CP	179.00	2.09	1.49	0.61
Couscous, dry	1 CP	184.00	7.18	5.12	2.06
Cream of Rice, ckd	1 CP	244.00	0.63	0.51	0.12
Cream of Rice, dry	1 CP	173.00	2.94	2.30	0.64
Cream of Wheat, instant, ckd	1 CP	241.00	0.72	0.55	0.19
Cream of Wheat, instant, dry	1 CP	178.00	3.10	2.30	0.80
Cream of Wheat, quick, ckd	1 CP	239.00	0.72	0.53	0.19
Cream of Wheat, quick, dry	1 CP	175.00	3.52	2.61	0.91
Cream of Wheat, regular, ckd	1 CP	251.00	0.75	0.55	0.20
Cream of Wheat, regular, dry	1 CP	173.00	3.60	2.68	0.92
Flour, all purpose	1 CP	125.00	4.50	2.50	2.00
Flour, amaranth (whole grain)	1 CP	195.00	29.64	20.16	9.48
Flour, cake or pastry	1 CP	109.00	2.50	0.98	1.52
Flour, rice	1 CP	158.00	3.79	2.95	0.84
Flour, rye, medium	1 CP	102.00	14.89	10.82	4.07

Flour, whole wheat	1 CP	120.00	13.12	10.91	2.20
Hominy, cnd	1 CP	160.00	4.00	2.27	1.73
Mix and eat wheat cereal, dry	1 Packet	28.40	0.85	0.38	0.47
Mix and eat wheat cereal, plain or flavored, prepared with water	1 CP	200.00	1.20	0.54	0.66
Oat bran, ckd	1 CP	219.00	5.30	2.76	2.63
Oat bran, dry	1 CP	94.00	13.54	7.07	6.75
Oatmeal, ckd	1 CP	234.00	3.58	1.75	1.85
Oatmeal, dry	1 CP	81.00	7.69	3.73	3.97
Oatmeal, instant Oatmeal Swirlers (all flavors), prepared with water	1 CP	250.00	4.80	2.87	1.92
Oatmeal, instant Total, prepared w water	1 Packet	161.02	3.22	2.03	1.18
Oatmeal, instant, apple cinnamon, prepared with water	1 CP	234.00	4.61	2.76	1.85
Oatmeal, instant, cinnamon spice, prepared with water	1 CP	234.00	4.56	2.74	1.83
Oatmeal, instant, maple & brown sugar, prepared with water	1 CP	234.00	4.21	2.53	1.68
Oatmeal, instant, raisin spice, prepared with water	1 CP	234.00	3.56	2.13	1.43
Oatmeal, instant, regular flavor, prepared with water	1 CP	234.00	3.67	2.20	1.47
Rice bran, dry	1 CP	83.00	18.01	13.51	4.50
Tapioca, dry	1 CP	152.00	1.67	1.50	0.17
Wheat germ	1 CP	113.00	16.16	14.35	1.47
Wheat germ honey crunch	1 CP	113.40	12.18	10.82	1.10
Wheat, rolled, ckd	1 CP	242.00	5.13	4.26	0.85
Wheat, rolled, dry	1 CP	94.00	11.90	9.90	1.98
PASTA AND RICE					
Chow mein noodles	1 CP	45.00	1.75	1.30	0.45
Egg noddles, ckd	1 CP	160.00	2.88	2.08	0.80
Macaroni, white, ckd	1 CP	140.00	1.40	0.70	0.70
Macaroni, whole wheat, ckd	1 CP	140.00	4.20	3.36	0.84
Manicotti noddles, ckd	1 CP	87.30	1.40	0.59	0.80
Ramen noodles, ckd	1 CP	227.00	1.27	0.93	0.32
Rice mixes, seasoned, ckd w fat	1 CP	205.00	0.74	0.57	0.16
Rice noodles, ckd	1 CP	160.00	0.62	0.48	0.14
Rice, brown, ckd	1 CP	195.00	3.31	3.08	0.23

Table 1 (continued)
DIETARY FIBER VALUES FOR COMMON FOODS

Food	Amount	g	Total dietary fiber (g)	Insoluble fiber (g)	Soluble fiber (g)
Rice, white, ckd	1 CP	205.00	1.02	0.80	0.23
Wild rice, ckd	1 CP	164.00	1.15	0.82	0.33
SNACKS, CRACKERS, AND CHIPS					
Bagel chips (crisps)	1 CP	46.00	1.34	0.78	0.27
Chips, snack type with cheese	1 CP	35.00	1.13	1.12	0.01
Corn chips	1 CP	26.00	0.93	0.92	0.01
Cornnuts	1 CP	92.40	6.38	3.62	2.75
Cracker crumbs, graham	1 CP	85.04	2.72	1.45	1.23
Crackers, cheese	1 OZ	28.35	0.81	0.40	0.40
Crackers, cracked wheat	1 OZ	28.35	2.84	2.27	0.49
Crackers, graham	1 OZ	28.35	1.05	0.89	0.08
Crackers, Japanese rice	1 OZ	28.35	0.24	0.16	0.08
Crackers, matzo	1 OZ	28.35	0.81	0.40	0.40
Crackers, melba toast	1 OZ	28.35	0.97	0.73	0.24
Crackers, oyster	1 OZ	28.35	0.81	0.65	0.24
Crackers, saltine	1 OZ	28.35	0.89	0.65	0.24
Crackers, wheat w cheese filling	1 OZ	28.35	0.97	0.73	0.24
Crackers, zwieback	1 OZ	28.35	0.81	0.49	0.16
Granola bar with fruit, high fiber, 9% fat	1 Bar	28.35	4.20	3.52	0.69
Granola bar, 18% fat	1 Bar	28.35	1.25	0.75	0.50
Granola bar, 25% fat	1 Bar	23.60	1.00	0.50	0.50
Granola bar, 32% fat	1 Bar	36.80	1.41	1.10	0.29
Granola bar, high fiber, 16% fat	1 Bar	34.02	3.39	2.65	0.74
Granola bar, oat bran, 10% fat	1 Bar	42.50	4.19	2.40	1.72
Onion flavored rings	1 CP	13.00	0.53	0.53	0.01
Party mix: cereal, pretzel, and nut combination, homemade	1 CP	58.51	3.19	1.97	0.70
Party mix: cereal, pretzel and nut	1 CP	42.50	2.71	1.69	1.01
Party mix: cereal, pretzel, cracker, and nut	1 CP	56.70	2.30	1.71	0.58

Party mix: cereal, pretzel, and cracker	1 CP	42.50	1.67	1.22	0.44
Popcorn, caramel	1 CP	35.00	1.25	0.63	0.62
Popcorn, cheese flavored	1 CP	11.00	1.13	0.49	0.64
Popcorn, popped w fat	1 CP	11.00	1.21	1.17	0.04
Popcorn, popped w/o fat	1 CP	8.00	1.21	1.17	0.04
Potato chips	1 CP	20.00	0.83	0.64	0.19
Potatoes, shoestring or stixs, fried	1 CP	36.00	1.22	0.95	0.28
Pretzel, cheese filled, hard type	1 CP	84.90	1.90	1.41	0.49
Pretzel, hard type	1 CP	43.50	1.22	0.90	0.31
Rice cakes, plain	1 Cake	9.30	0.08	0.05	0.04
Tortilla chips	1 CP	26.00	1.08	1.07	0.01
Trail mix (peanuts, sunflower seeds, carob chips, raisins)	1 CP	150.00	9.84	4.98	4.88
Wheat cakes, plain	1 Cake	9.00	0.98	0.82	0.16

SOUPS

Bean soup, cnd, diluted	1 CP	250.00	3.85	2.37	1.47
Chowder, clam, Manhattan, cnd, undiluted	1 CP	251.00	2.18	1.46	0.43
Chowder, clam, New England, cnd, undiluted,	1 CP	251.00	0.90	0.55	0.33
Chowder, corn	1 CP	248.00	2.46	1.39	1.07
Cream of asparagus soup, cnd, undiluted	1 CP	251.00	1.36	1.05	0.30
Cream of celery soup, cnd, undiluted	1 CP	251.00	2.18	0.30	0.15
Cream of mushroom soup, cnd, undiluted	1 CP	251.00	0.93	0.63	0.30
Cream of pea soup, cnd, undiluted	1 CP	263.00	5.97	2.71	3.26
Cream of potato soup, cnd, undiluted	1 CP	251.00	1.38	1.10	0.33
Soup, cnd, ready to serve chunky and similar; meat or poultry varieties w veg or noodles	1 CP	240.00	1.82	1.44	0.41
Soup, cnd, ready to serve chunky and similar; vegetable varieties, meatless	1 CP	240.00	2.02	1.63	0.43
Tomato soup, cnd, undiluted	1 CP	251.00	2.84	2.28	0.58

CANDY AND SWEETS

Candy bar or chips, chocolate, sweet or semisweet	1 OZ	28.35	2.52	1.98	0.54
Candy bar, chocolate covered caramel & peanuts	1 OZ	28.35	0.80	0.62	0.17
Candy bar, chocolate covered coconut	1 OZ	28.35	1.92	1.72	0.20
Candy bar, chocolate covered English toffee	1 OZ	28.35	0.51	0.43	0.09
Candy bar, chocolate covered honeycomb & peanut butter	1 OZ	28.35	0.79	0.71	0.09
Candy bar, chocolate covered nougat & caramel	1 OZ	28.35	0.26	0.21	0.04
Candy bar, chocolate covered nougat, caramel & peanuts	1 OZ	28.35	0.91	0.60	0.31

Table 1 (continued)
DIETARY FIBER VALUES FOR COMMON FOODS

Food	Amount	g	Total dietary fiber (g)	Insoluble fiber (g)	Soluble fiber (g)
Candy bar, chocolate covered peanut butter	1 OZ	28.35	1.26	1.12	0.15
Candy bar, chocolate covered rice krispies	1 OZ	28.35	0.77	0.60	0.16
Candy bar, chocolate w almonds, dietetic	1 OZ	28.35	1.13	1.06	0.07
Candy bar, milk chocolate w almonds	1 OZ	28.35	1.40	0.91	0.49
Candy bar, milk chocolate w peanuts	1 OZ	28.35	1.55	1.08	0.47
Candy bar, milk chocolate w/o nuts	1 OZ	28.35	0.79	0.62	0.17
Candy bar, peanut butter coated w toasted coconut	1 OZ	28.35	1.35	1.24	0.11
Candy bar, salted nut rolls	1 OZ	28.35	1.35	0.80	0.55
Candy bar, white chocolate w almonds	1 OZ	28.35	0.48	0.43	0.05
Candy coated almonds	1 OZ	28.35	1.21	0.40	0.81
Candy coated chocolate discs	1 OZ	28.35	0.88	0.69	0.19
Candy coated chocolate peanuts	1 OZ	28.35	1.15	0.77	0.38
Candy coated peanuts	1 OZ	28.35	1.02	0.60	0.42
Candy, bridge mix	1 CP	189.60	4.95	3.92	1.00
Candy, caramel pecan roll	1 OZ	28.35	0.18	0.00	0.00
Candy, caramel, plain	1 OZ	28.35	0.00	0.00	0.00
Candy, carob coated	1 OZ	28.35	0.35	0.15	0.20
Candy, carob covered peanuts	1 CP	170.00	11.32	7.39	3.93
Candy, carob covered raisins	1 CP	190.00	9.90	3.55	6.35
Candy, carob stars or chips	1 CP	130.00	5.12	1.65	3.46
Candy, chocolate covered almonds	1 OZ	28.35	2.12	1.87	0.25
Candy, chocolate covered caramels	1 OZ	28.35	0.40	0.31	0.09
Candy, chocolate covered cherry	1 OZ	28.35	0.61	0.33	0.27
Candy, chocolate covered creams	1 OZ	28.35	0.51	0.43	0.09
Candy, chocolate covered marshmallow egg	1 Medium	11.00	0.17	0.13	0.04
Candy, chocolate covered peanuts	1 OZ	28.35	1.89	1.23	0.65
Candy, chocolate covered peppermints	1 OZ	28.35	0.51	0.43	0.09
Candy, chocolate covered raisins	1 OZ	28.35	1.45	0.68	0.86
Candy, chocolate roll	1 OZ	28.35	0.51	0.47	0.04

Food	Unit	Weight (g)		
Candy, Fruit roll-ups	1 OZ	28.35	1.02	0.58	0.42
Candy, fudge w/o nuts	1 OZ	28.35	0.44	0.42	0.02
Candy, Fun Fruits, Fruit Wrinkles, Shark-Bites, and similar	1 Package	25.52	0.91	0.53	0.37
Candy, halavah	1 OZ	28.35	1.64		
Candy, licorice	1 Piece	10.00	0.07	0.03	0.04
Candy, malted milk balls	1 OZ	28.35	0.72	0.58	0.14
Candy, nut brittle	1 OZ	28.35	1.17	0.73	0.44
Candy, rockyroad (chocolate, peanuts, & marshmallows)	1 OZ	28.35	1.45	1.07	0.38
Candy, trifles (chocolate w nuts & chow mein noodles)	1 Piece	15.33	1.51	1.18	0.33
Candy, truffles	1 Piece	13.00	0.27	0.21	0.06
Candy, yogurt covered peanuts	1 CP	170.00	5.68	3.55	2.12
Candy, yogurt covered raisins	1 CP	176.19	3.59	0.90	3.07
Chocolate, bitter-baking	1 OZ	28.35	4.37	4.19	0.18

SPICES, CONDIMENTS, AND MISCELLANEOUS

Food	Unit	Weight (g)			
Allspice, ground	1 TS	1.90	0.61		
Baking chocolate	1 OZ	28.35	4.37	4.19	0.18
Basil, ground	1 TS	1.40	0.30		
Carob powder	1 TS	2.92	0.95	0.31	0.65
Catsup	1 TB	15.00	0.18	0.12	0.06
Cayenne, red pepper	1 TS	1.80	0.45		
Celery seed	1 TS	2.00	0.37		
Chili powder	1 TS	2.60	0.89		
Cinnamon, ground	1 TS	2.30	0.95		
Cloves, ground	1 TS	2.10	0.22		
Cocoa powder	1 TS	1.80	0.54	0.50	0.04
Cumin seed	1 TS	2.10	0.39		
Curry powder	1 TS	2.00	0.66		
Dill weed	1 TS	1.00	0.15	0.09	0.06
Garlic powder	1 TS	2.80	0.28		
Garlic salt	1 TS	5.70	0.02		
Ginger, ground	1 TS	1.80	0.48		
Jelly	1 TS	6.67	0.08	0.05	0.03
Mustard powder	1 TS	1.50	0.02		
Nutmeg, ground	1 TS	2.20	0.12		
Onion powder	1 TS	2.10	0.25	0.16	0.10
Onion salt	1 TS	5.30	0.16	0.10	0.06
Oregano, ground	1 TS	1.50	0.33		

Table 1 (continued)
DIETARY FIBER VALUES FOR COMMON FOODS

Food	Amount	g	Total dietary fiber (g)	Insoluble fiber (g)	Soluble fiber (g)
Paprika	1 TS	2.10	0.44		
Parsley, dried	1 TS	0.30	0.10	0.09	0.01
Pepper, black	1 TS	2.10	0.52		
Pickle, dill	1 CP	155.00	2.37	1.98	0.39
Pickles, sweet, bread & butter	1 CP	160.00	2.45	2.05	0.40
Pimiento, canned, solids & liquids	1 TB	12.00	0.11		
Sage, ground	1 TS	0.70	0.15		
Thyme, ground	1 TS	1.40	0.29		
Turmeric, ground	1 TS	2.20	0.06		
Yeast, active dry	1 TB	7.00	2.21		
Yeast, brewers	1 TB	8.00	1.30		

REFERENCES

1. **Aalto, T., Lehtonen, M., and Varo, P.,** Dietary fiber content of barley grown in Finland, *Cereal Chem.,* 65, 284, 1988.
2. **Alaoui, L. and Essatara, M.,** Dietary fiber and phytic acid levels in the major food items consumed in Morocco, *Nutr. Rep. Int.,* 31, 469, 1985.
3. **Anderson, J. W. and Bridges, S. R.,** Dietary fiber content of selected foods, *Am. J. Clin. Nutr.,* 47, 440, 1988.
4. **Anderson, J. W., Bridges, S. R., Tietyen, J., and Gustafson, N. J.,** Dietary fiber content of simulated American diet and selected research diets, *Am. J. Clin. Nutr.,* 49, 352, 1989.
5. **Anderson, J. W., Gustafson, N. J., Byrant, C. A., and Tietyen-Clark, J.,** Dietary fiber and diabetes: A comprehensive review and practical application, *J. Am. Dietet. Assoc.,* 87, 1189, 1987.
6. **Anderson, J. W. and Ward, K.,** Long-term effects of high-carbohydrate, high-fiber diets on glucose and lipid metabolism: A preliminary report on patients with diabetes, *Diabetes Care,* 1, 77, 1978.
7. **Anderson, N. E. and Clydesdale, F. M.,** Effects of processing on the dietary fiber content of wheat bran, pureed green beans, and carrots, *J. Food Sci.,* 45, 1533, 1980.
8. **Angus, R., Sutherland, T. M., and Farrell, D. J.,** Insoluble dietary fibre content of some local foods, *Proc. Nutr. Soc. Aust.,* 6, 161, 1981.
9. **Asp, N.-G., Johansson, C.-G., Hallmer, H., and Siljestrom, M.,** Rapid enzymatic assay of insoluble and soluble dietary fiber, *J. Agric. Food Chem.,* 31, 476, 1983.
10. **Babcock, D.,** Rice bran as a source of dietary fiber, *Cereal Foods World,* 32, 538, 1987.
11. **Baker, D.,** The determination of fiber in processed cereal foods by near-infrared reflectance spectroscopy, *Cereal Chem.,* 60, 217, 1983.
12. **Baker, D.,** Fiber in wheat foods, *Cereal Foods World.,* 23, 557, 1978.
13. **Baker, D. and Holden, J. M.,** Fiber in breakfast cereals, *J. Food Sci.,* 46, 396, 1981.
14. **Balasubramaniam, K.,** Polysaccharides of the kernel of maturing and matured coconuts, *J. Food Sci.,* 41, 1370, 1976.
15. **Bell, B. M.,** A rapid method of dietary fibre estimation in wheat products, *J. Sci. Food Agric.,* 36, 815, 1985.
16. **Belo, P. S. and de Lumen, B. O.,** Pectic substance content of detergent-extracted dietary fibers, *J. Agric. Food Chem.,* 29, 373, 1981.
17. **Best, D.,** Building fiber into foods, *Prep. Foods,* July, 112, 1987.
18. **Bittner, A. S., Burritt, E. A., Moser, J., and Street, J. C.,** Composition of dietary fiber: Neutral and acidic sugar composition of the alcohol insoluble residue from human foods, *J. Food Sci.,* 47, 1469, 1982.
19. **Boothby, D.,** Pectic substances in developing and ripening plum fruits, *J. Sci. Food Agric.,* 34, 1117, 1983.
20. **Brandt, L. M., Jeltema, M. A., Zabik, M. E., and Jeltema, B. D.,** Effects of cooking in solutions of varying pH on the dietary fiber components of vegetables, *J. Food Sci.,* 49, 900, 1984.
21. **Brillouet, J.-M., Rouau, X., Hoebler, C., Barry, J.-L., Carre, B., and Lorta, E.,** A new method for determination of insoluble cell walls and soluble nonstarchy polysaccharides from plant materials, *J. Agric. Food Chem.,* 36, 969, 1988.
22. **Candlish, J. K., Gourley, L., and Lee, H. P.,** Dietary fiber and starch in some Southeast Asian fruits, *J. Food Comp. Anal.,* 1, 81, 1987.
23. **Cardozo, M. S. and Eitenmiller, R. R.,** Total dietary fiber analysis of selected baked and cereal products, *Cereal Foods World,* 33, 414, 1988.
24. **Chen, H., Rubenthaler, G. L., Leung, H. K., and Baranowski, J. D.,** Chemical, physical, and baking properties of apple fiber compared with wheat and oat bran, *Cereal Chem.,* 65, 244, 1988.
25. **Chen, M. L., Chang, S. C., and Guoo, J. Y.,** Fiber contents of some Chinese vegetables and their in vitro binding capacity of bile acids, *Nutr. Rep. Int.,* 26, 1053, 1982.
26. **Chen, W.-J. L. and Anderson, J. W.,** Soluble and insoluble plant fiber in selected cereals and vegetables, *Am. J. Clin. Nutr.,* 34, 1077, 1981.
27. *Composition of Foods: Breakfast Cereals,* Agriculture Handbook No. 8-8, Human Nutrition Information Service, U.S. Department of Agriculture, Washington, D.C., 1982.
28. *Composition of Foods: Cereal Grains and Pasta,* Agriculture Handbook No. 8-20, Human Nutrition Information Service, U.S. Department of Agriculture, Washington, D.C., 1989.
29. *Composition of Foods: 1989 Supplement,* Agriculture Handbook No. 8 1989 Supplement, Human Nutrition Information Service, U.S. Department of Agriculture, Washington, D.C., 1989.
30. **Dong, F. M. and Rasco, B. A.,** The neutral detergent fiber, acid detergent fiber, crude fiber, and lignin contents of distillers' dried grains with solubles, *J. Food Sci.,* 52, 403, 1987.

31. **Dreher, M. L., Breedon, C., and Orr, P. H.,** Percent starch hydrolysis and dietary fiber content of chipped and baked potatoes, *Nutr. Rep. Int.,* 28, 687, 1983.
32. **Englyst, H.,** Determination of carbohydrate and its composition in plant materials, in *The Analysis of Dietary Fibers in Food,* James, W. P. T. and Theander, O., Eds., 1981.
33. **Englyst, H. N., Anderson, V., and Cummings, J. H.,** Starch and non-starch polysaccharides in some cereal foods, *J. Sci. Food Agric.,* 34, 1434, 1983.
34. **Englyst, H. N. and Cummings, J. H.,** Improved method for measurement of dietary fiber as non-starch polysaccharides in plant foods, *J. Assoc. Off. Anal. Chem.,* 71, 808, 1988.
35. **Faulks, R. M. and Timms, S. B.,** A rapid method for determining the carbohydrate component of dietary fibre, *Food Chem.,* 17, 273, 1985.
36. **Fleming, S. E.,** A study of relationships between flatus potential and carbohydrate distribution in legume seeds, *J. Food Sci.,* 46, 794, 1981.
37. **Foy, W. L., Evans, J. L., and Wohlt, J. E.,** Detergent fiber analyses on thirty foodstuffs ingested by man, *Nutr. Rep. Int.,* 24, 575, 1981.
38. **Frolich, W. and Asp, N.-G.,** Dietary fiber content in cereals in Norway, *Cereal Chem.,* 58, 524, 1981.
39. **Frolich, W. and Hestangen, B.,** Dietary fiber content of different cereal products in Norway, *Cereal Chem.,* 60, 82, 1983.
40. **Garcia-Lopez, S. and Wyatt, C. J.,** Effect of fiber in corn tortillas and cooked beans on iron availability, *J. Agric. Food Chem.,* 30, 724, 1982.
41. **Graham, H., Rydberg, M.-B. G., and Aman, P.,** Extraction of soluble dietary fiber, *J. Agric. Food Chem.,* 36, 494, 1988.
42. **Harada, T., Tirtohusodo, H., and Paulus, K.,** Influence of the composition of potatoes on their cooking kinetics, *J. Food Sci.,* 50, 463, 1985.
43. **Hardinge, M. G., Swarner, J. B., and Crooks, H.,** Carbohydrates in foods, *J. Am. Dietet. Assoc.,* 46, 197, 1965.
44. **Heckman, M. M. and Lane, S. A.,** Comparison of dietary fiber methods for foods, *J. Assoc. Off. Anal. Chem.,* 64, 1339, 1981.
45. **Hellendoorn, E. W., Noordhoff, M. G., and Slagman, J.,** Enzymatic determination of the indigestible residue (dietary fibre) content of human food, *J. Sci. Food Agric.,* 26, 1461, 1975.
46. **Herranz, J., Vidal-Valverde, C., and Rojas-Hidalgo, E.,** Cellulose, hemicellulose and lignin content of raw and cooked processed vegetables, *J. Food Sci.,* 48, 274, 1983.
47. **Herranz, J., Vidal-Valverde, C., and Rojas-Hidalgo, E.,** Cellulose, hemicellulose and lignin content of raw and cooked Spanish vegetables, *J. Food Sci.,* 46, 1927, 1981.
48. **Holloway, W. D.,** Composition of fruit, vegetable and cereal dietary fibre, *J. Sci. Food Agric.,* 34, 1236, 1983.
49. **Holloway, W. D., Monro, J. A., Gurnsey, J. C., Pomare, E. W., and Stace, N. H.,** Dietary fiber and other constituents of some Tongan foods, *J. Food Sci.,* 50, 1756, 1985.
50. **Holloway, W. D., Tasman-Jones, C., and Maher, K.,** Towards an accurate measurement of dietary fibre, *NZ Med. J.,* 85, 420, 1977.
51. **Horvath, P. J.,** The measurement of dietary fiber and the effects of fermentation, Thesis, Cornell University, 1984.
52. **Jeltema, M. A. and Zabik, M. E.,** Revised method for quantitating dietary fibre components, *J. Sci. Food Agric.,* 31, 820, 1980.
53. **Jeraci, J. L., Lewis, B. A., Van Soest, P. J., and Robertson, J. B.,** Urea enzymatic dialysis procedure for determination of total dietary fiber, *J. Assoc. Off. Anal. Chem.,* 72, 677, 1989.
54. **Johnston, D. E., Kelly, D., and Dorrian, P. P.,** Losses of pectic substances during cooking and the effect of water hardness, *J. Sci. Food Agric.,* 34, 733, 1983.
55. **Johnston, D. E. and Oliver, W. T.,** The influence of cooking technique on dietary fibre of boiled potato, *J. Food Technol.,* 17, 99, 1982.
56. **Jones, G. P., Briggs, D. R., Wahlqvist, M. L., and Flentje, L. M.,** Dietary fibre content of Australian foods. 1. Potatoes, *Food Technol. Aust.,* 37, 81, 1985.
57. **Jwuang, J. W.-L. and Zabik, M. E.,** Enzyme neutral detergent fiber analysis of selected commercial and home-prepared foods, *J. Food Sci.,* 44, 924, 1979.
58. **Kamath, M. V. and Belavady, B.,** Unavailable carbohydrates of commonly consumed Indian foods, *J. Sci. Food Agric.,* 31, 194, 1980.
59. **Katan, M. B. and Van de Bovenkamp, P.,** Analyse van het totale voedingsvezlgehalte en van het pectine-aandeel hierin in Nederlandse voedingsmillelen, *Voeding,* 5, 153, 1982.
60. **Kayisu, K., Hood, L. F., and VanSoest, P. J.,** Characterization of starch and fiber of banana fruit, *J. Food Sci.,* 46, 1885, 1981.
61. **Kunerth, W. H. and Youngs, V. L.,** Effect of variety and growing year on the constituents of durum bran fiber, *Cereal Chem.,* 61, 350, 1984.

62. **Lanza, E. and Butrum, R. R.**, A critical review of food fiber analysis and data, *J. Am. Dietet. Assoc.*, 86, 732, 1986.
63. **Lanza, E., Jones, D. Y., Block, G., and Kessler, L.**, Dietary fiber intake in the U.S. population, *Am. J. Clin. Nutr.*, 46, 790, 1987.
64. **Longe, O. G.**, Effect of boiling on the carbohydrate constituents of some non-leafy vegetables, *Food Chem.*, 6, 1, 1981.
65. **Longe, O. G., Fetuga, B. L., and Akenova, M. E.**, Changes in the composition and carbohydrate constituents of okra (Abelmoschus esculentus, Linn) with age, *Food Chem.*, 8, 27, 1982.
66. **Luh, B. S., Sarhan, M. A., and Wang, Z.**, Pectins and fibres in processing tomatoes, *Food Technol. Aust.*, 36, 70, 1984.
67. **Lund, E. D. and Smoot, J. M.**, Dietary fiber content of some tropical fruits and vegetables, *J. Agric. Food Chem.*, 30, 1123, 1982.
68. **Lund, E. D., Smoot, J. M., and Hall, N. T.**, Dietary fiber content of eleven tropical fruits and vegetables, *J. Agric. Food Chem.*, 31, 1013, 1983.
69. **Marlett, J. A. and Chesters, J. G.**, Measuring dietary fiber in human foods, *J. Food Sci.*, 50, 410, 1985.
70. **Marlett, J. A. and Lee, S. C.**, Dietary fiber, lignocellulose and hemicellulose contents of selected foods determined by modified and unmodified Van Soest procedures, *J. Food Sci.*, 45, 1688, 1980.
71. **Marlett, J. A. and Navis, D.**, Comparison of gravimetric and chemical analyses of total dietary fiber in human foods, *J. Agric. Food Chem.*, 36, 311, 1988.
72. **Matthee, V. and Appledorf, H.**, Effect of cooking on vegetable fiber, *J. Food Sci.*, 43, 1344, 1978.
73. **Matthews, R. H. and Pehrsson, P. R.**, Provisional table on the dietary fiber content of selected foods, Human Nutrition Information Service, U.S. Department of Agriculture, Washington, D.C., 1988.
74. **McCormick, R.**, Function and nutrition guide fiber ingredient selections, *Prep. Foods*, November, 83, 1988.
75. **McQueen, R. E. and Nicholson, J. W. G.**, Modification of the neutral-detergent fiber procedure for cereals and vegetables by using a-amylase, *J. Assoc. Off. Anal. Chem.*, 62, 676, 1979.
76. **Mongeau, R. and Brassard, R.**, A rapid method for the determination of soluble and insoluble dietary fiber: Comparison with AOAC total dietary fiber procedure and Englyst's method, *J. Food Sci.*, 51, 1333, 1986.
77. **Mongeau, R. and Brassard, R.**, Determination of neutral detergent fiber in breakfast cereals: Pentose, hemicellulose, cellulose and lignin content, *J. Food Sci.*, 47, 550, 1982.
78. **Monro, J. A., Harding, W. R., and Russell, C. E.**, Dietary fibre of coconuts from a Pacific atoll: Soluble and insoluble components in relation to maturity, *J. Sci. Food Agric.*, 36, 1013, 1985.
79. **Mori, B.**, Contents of dietary fiber in some Japanese foods and the amount ingested through Japanese meals, *Nutr. Rep. Int.*, 26, 159, 1982.
80. **Neilson, M. J. and Marlett, J. A.**, A comparison between detergent and nondetergent analyses of dietary fiber in human foodstuffs, using high-performance liquid chromatography to measure neutral sugar composition, *J. Agric. Food Chem.*, 31, 1342, 1983.
81. **Park, G. L., Byers, J. L., Pritz, C. M., Nelson, D. B., Navarro, J. L., Smolensky, D. C., and Vandercook, C. E.**, Characteristics of California navel orange juice and pulpwash, *J. Food Sci.*, 48, 627, 1983.
82. **Patrow, C. J. and Marlett, J. A.**, Variability in the dietary fiber content of wheat and mixed-grain commercial breads, *J. Am. Dietet. Assoc.*, 86, 794, 1986.
83. **Paul, A. A. and Southgate, D. A. T.**, McCance and Widdowson's "The Composition of Foods": dietary fibre in egg, meat and fish dishes, *J. Hum. Nutr.*, 33, 335, 1979.
84. **Prosky, L., Asp, N.-G., Furda, I., Devries, J. W., Schweizer, T. F., and Harland, B. F.**, Determination of total dietary fiber in foods, food products, and total diets: interlaboratory study, *J. Assoc. Off. Anal. Chem.*, 67, 1044, 1984.
85. **Prosky, L., Asp, N.-G., Furda, I., Devries, J. W., Schweizer, T. F., and Harland, B. F.**, Determination of total dietary fiber in foods and food products: collaborative study, *J. Assoc. Off. Anal. Chem.*, 68, 677, 1985.
86. **Prosky, L., Asp, N.-G., Schweizer, T. F., Devries, J. W., and Furda, I.**, Determination of insoluble, soluble, and total dietary fiber in foods and food products: interlaboratory study, *J. Assoc. Off. Anal. Chem.*, 71, 1017, 1988.
87. **Przybyla, A. E.**, Formulating fiber into foods, *Food Eng.*, October, 77, 1988.
88. **Ranhotra, G. and Gelroth, J.**, Soluble and insoluble fiber in soda crackers, *Cereal Chem.*, 65, 159, 1988.
89. **Ranhotra, G. and Gelroth, J.**, Soluble and total dietary fiber in white bread, *Cereal Chem.*, 65, 155, 1988.
90. **Reddy, N. N. and Sistrunk, W. A.**, Effect of cultivar size, storage, and cooking method on carbohydrates and some nutrients of sweet potatoes, *J. Food Sci.*, 45, 682, 1980.

91. **Reinhold, J. G. and Garcia, L. J. S.**, Fiber of the maize tortilla, *Am. J. Clin. Nutr.*, 32, 1326, 1979.
92. **Reistad, R., Andelic, I., Steen, M., and Rogeberg, E. S.**, Dietary fibre in some Norwegian plant foods during storage, *Food Chem.*, 17, 265, 1985.
93. **Reistad, R. and Hagen, B. F.**, Dietary fibre in raw and cooked potatoes, *Food Chem.*, 19, 189, 1986.
94. **Ross, J. K., English, C., and Perlmutter, C. A.**, Dietary fiber constituents of selected fruits and vegetables, *J. Am. Dietet. Assoc.*, 85, 1111, 1985.
95. **San Buenaventura, M. L., Dong, F. M., and Rasco, B. A.**, The total dietary fiber content of wheat, corn, barley, sorghum, and distillers' dried grain with solubles, *Cereal Chem.*, 64, 135, 1987.
96. **Schaller, D.**, Fiber content and structure in foods, *Am. J. Clin. Nutr.*, 31, S99, 1978.
97. **Schneeman, B. O.**, Dietary fiber: physical and chemical properties, methods of analysis and physiological effects, *Food Technol.*, February, 104, 1986.
98. **Schweizer, T. F. and Wursch, P.**, Analysis of dietary fibre, *J. Sci. Food Agric.*, 30, 613, 1979.
99. **Seibert, S. E.**, Oat bran as a source of soluble dietary fiber, *Cereal Foods World*, 32, 552, 1987.
100. **Selvendran, R. R.**, The plant cell wall as a source of dietary fiber: chemistry and structure, *Am. J. Clin. Nutr.*, 39, 320, 1984.
101. **Selvendran, R. R. and DuPont, M. S.**, Simplified methods for the preparation and analysis of dietary fibre, *J. Sci. Food Agric.*, 31, 1173, 1980.
102. **Siddiqui, I. R.**, Studies on vegetables: Fiber content and chemical composition of ethanol-insoluble and -soluble residues, *J. Agric. Food Chem.*, 37, 647, 1989.
103. **Skurray, G. R., Wooldridge, D. A., and Nguyen, M.**, Rice bran as a source of dietary fibre in bread, *J. Food Technol.*, 21, 727, 1986.
104. **Slavin, J. L.**, Dietary fiber: Classification, chemical analysis and food sources, *J. Am. Dietet. Assoc.*, 87, 1164, 1987.
105. **Somogyi, L. P.**, Prunes, a fiber-rich ingredient, *Cereal Foods World*, 32, 541, 1987.
106. **Southgate, D. A. T.**, Dietary fiber: Analysis and food sources, *Am. J. Clin. Nutr.*, 31, S107, 1978.
107. **Southgate, D. A. T., Bailey, B., Collinson, E., and Walker, A. F.**, A guide to calculating intakes of dietary fibre, *J. Hum. Nutr.*, 30, 303, 1976.
108. **Southgate, D. A. T., Hudson, G. J., and Englyst, H.**, The analysis of dietary fibre — the choices for the analyst, *J. Sci. Food Agric.*, 29, 979, 1978.
109. **Theander, O. and Aman, P.**, Studies on dietary fibres. I. Analysis and chemical characterization of water-soluble and water-insoluble dietary fibres, *Swed. J. Agric. Res.*, 9, 97, 1979.
110. **Theander, O. and Aman, P.**, Studies on dietary fibre. A method for the analysis and chemical characterisation of total dietary fibre, *J. Sci. Food Agric.*, 33, 340, 1982.
111. **Theander, O. and Westerlund, E. A.**, Studies on dietary fiber. III. Improved procedures for analysis of dietary fiber, *J. Agric. Food Chem.*, 34, 330, 1986.
112. **Torp, J.**, Variation in the concentration of major carbohydrates in the grain of some spring barleys, *J. Sci. Food Agric.*, 31, 1354, 1980.
113. **Varo, P., Laine, R., Veijalainen, K., Pero, K., and Koivistoinen, P.**, Dietary fibre and available carbohydrates in Finnish cereal products, *J. Agric. Sci. Fin.*, 56, 39, 1984.
114. **Varo, P., Veijalainen, K., and Koivistoinen, P.**, Effect of heat treatment on the dietary fibre contents of potato and tomato, *J. Food Technol.*, 19, 485, 1984.
115. **Vidal-Valverde, C., Blanco, I., and Rojas-Hidalgo, E.**, Pectic substances in fresh, dried, desiccated and oleaginous Spanish fruits, *J. Agric. Food Chem.*, 30, 832, 1982.
116. **Vidal-Valverde, C., Herranz, J., Blanco, I., and Rojas-Hidalgo, E.**, Dietary fiber in Spanish fruits, *J. Food Sci.*, 47, 1840, 1982.
117. **Vidal-Valverde, C., Lopez, M. P., and Rojas-Hidalgo, E.**, Pectic substances in raw and cooked, fresh or processed Spanish vegetables, *J. Agric. Food Chem.*, 31, 949, 1983.
118. **Visser, F. R. and Gurnsey, C.**, Inconsistent differences between neutral detergent fiber and total dietary fiber values of fruits and vegetables, *J. Assoc. Off. Anal. Chem.*, 69, 565, 1986.
119. **Waslien, C.**, What is dietary fiber and what is starch?, *Cereal Foods World*, 33, 312, 1988.
120. **Wenlock, R. W., Sivell, L. M., and Agater, I. B.**, Dietary fibre fractions in cereal and cereal-containing products in Britain, *J. Sci. Food Agric.*, 36, 113, 1985.
121. **Wills, R. B. H.**, Composition of Australian fresh fruit and vegetables, *Food Technol. Aust.*, 39, 523, 1987.
122. **Wills, R. B. H., Evans, T. J., Lim, J. S. K., Scriven, F M., and Greenfield, H.**, Composition of Australian foods. XXV. Peas and beans, *Food Technol. Aust.*, 36, 512, 1984.
123. **Wills, R. B. H., Lim, J. S. K., and Greenfield, H.**, Composition of Australian foods. XXIII. Brassica vegetables, *Food Technol. Aust.*, 36, 176, 1984.
124. **Wills, R. B. H., Lim, J. S. K., and Greenfield, H.**, Composition of Australian foods. XXXVIII. Tuber, root and bulb vegetables, *Food Technol. Aust.*, 39, 384, 1987.

125. **Wills, R. B. H., Lim, J. S. K., and Greenfield, H.**, Composition of Australian foods. XXXIX. Vegetable fruits, *Food Technol. Aust.*, 39, 488, 1987.
126. **Wills, R. B. H., Lim, J. S. K., and Greenfield, H.**, Composition of Australian foods. XXXXII. Canned fruits, *Food Technol. Aust.*, 40, 223, 1988.
127. **Wills, R. B. H., Wong, A. W. K., Scriven, F. M., and Greenfield, H.**, Nutrient composition of Chinese vegetables, *J. Agric. Food Chem.*, 32, 413, 1984.
128. **Zyren, J., Elkins, E. R., Dudek, J. A., and Hagen, R. E.**, Fiber contents of selected raw and processed vegetables, fruits and fruit juices as served, *J. Food Sci.*, 48, 600, 1983.

APPENDIX I

Table 2

DRY MATTER, ASH, CRUDE PROTEIN, TOTAL DIETARY FIBER, SOLUBLE FIBER, NEUTRAL DETERGENT RESIDUE, HEMICELLULOSES, CELLULOSE, AND LIGNIN CONTENT OF SELECTED FOODS

James B. Robertson

Description	Maker	%DM	ASH	CP	TDF	SF	NDR	HC	CE	Ls
BREADS, CRACKERS, etc.										
Apple honey wheat, toasted	Brownberry	76.64	ND	13.23	5.50	−0.54	8.19	4.06	2.52	1.61
Apple honey wheat	Brownberry	64.82	ND	12.64	5.76	−0.08	6.43	4.10	1.22	1.10
Bagel		69.89	2.17	16.32	4.41	ND	2.63	1.39	0.58	0.66
Bagel, plain	Cornell	67.37	2.24	16.11	4.35	1.83	3.25	2.17	0.50	0.57
Biscuit mix, buttermilk	Quaker	89.53	5.21	ND	5.67	ND	1.14	1.00	0.28	−0.13
Biscuits, reg. recipe, baked		92.96	4.84	9.20	4.22	−1.60	7.51	5.72	0.58	1.21
Bread mix, corn, white	Quaker	88.79	5.95	ND	10.76	ND	7.55	5.20	1.98	0.38
Bread mix, corn yellow	Quaker	88.41	5.41	ND	6.02	ND	4.06	2.68	1.13	0.25
Bread, corn	Homemade	62.39	2.85	9.99	5.43	−0.25	6.05	3.33	1.37	1.35
Bread, French		64.34	3.17	14.52	4.99	−0.37	5.96	3.87	0.92	1.18
Bread, wheat	Less	51.22	3.67	18.71	19.42	3.30	17.65	3.79	12.85	1.00
Bread, white	Millbrook	59.65	2.82	14.33	5.29	3.41	2.64	1.69	0.49	0.46
Bread, white	Less	52.63	3.74	20.21	19.07	1.80	18.22	3.11	13.66	1.46
Bread, white		62.13	3.40	14.06	5.48	4.81	1.15	0.87	0.03	0.25
Bread, whole wheat	Pepperidge Farm	57.30	3.90	17.13	13.99	1.89	14.32	8.73	2.25	3.35
Cake, yellow	Homemade	72.01	2.09	7.40	3.36	2.97	0.68	0.46	0.06	0.16
Cookie, plain		95.62	1.56	6.29	2.99	1.99	1.53	1.08	0.07	0.38
Cookies, ginger snaps		95.77	1.94	6.18	4.31	1.01	3.97	2.47	0.31	1.19
Cookies, Oreo		93.89	2.11	5.09	14.72	ND	3.33	0.61	0.72	2.01
Cookies, shortbread		92.81	1.52	6.26	9.76	ND	2.22	1.55	0.24	0.46
Fibre Goodness Bread	Stroehmann	56.01	2.98	20.21	11.19	3.31	8.70	2.28	5.77	0.65

595

Table 2 (continued)
DRY MATTER, ASH, CRUDE PROTEIN, TOTAL DIETARY FIBER, SOLUBLE FIBER, NEUTRAL DETERGENT RESIDUE, HEMICELLULOSES, CELLULOSE, AND LIGNIN CONTENT OF SELECTED FOODS

Description	Maker	%DM	ASH	CP	TDF	SF	NDR	HC	CE	Ls
Fibread	Dr. Olindo	52.08	4.39	19.99	26.24	6.13	27.52	18.33	19.03	3.07
Flour, enriched, self-rising	Quaker	89.21	4.50	ND	3.46	ND	1.17	0.98	0.06	0.13
Flour, white		90.20	0.69	12.70	3.70	2.76	1.31	0.98	0.19	0.14
Graham crackers		94.31	2.35	7.15	3.52	3.94	2.69	1.26	1.29	0.13
Muffin mix, blueberry	Quaker	91.78	2.63	ND	4.12	ND	0.57	0.42	0.19	−0.04
Muffin mix, corn	Quaker	91.06	3.17	ND	5.19	ND	2.33	1.56	0.54	0.22
Muffins, plain		70.23	2.49	8.39	3.75	−0.33	4.94	3.05	0.71	1.18
Natural bran	Brownberry	63.19	0.00	13.51	10.09	−0.97	11.60	8.44	1.95	1.20
Natural bran, toasted	Brownberry	73.72	0.00	13.96	9.47	−1.05	12.24	8.13	2.34	1.77
Norwegian flatbread	Kavli	91.99	2.44	9.33	15.32	5.16	11.71	8.17	1.26	2.28
Oatmeal bread	Pepperidge Farm	61.25	3.62	14.22	9.39	7.30	3.25	2.17	0.50	0.57
Pancake mix		90.39	6.40	10.10	4.36	0.70	3.95	2.24	0.52	1.18
Pancake mix, buckwheat	Quaker	90.57	6.64	ND	11.64	ND	9.45	3.39	3.46	2.61
Pancake mix, whole wheat	Quaker	90.78	6.81	ND	9.55	ND	6.89	4.79	1.48	0.62
Premium saltines	Nabisco	96.71	3.53	9.40	5.55	3.88	2.63	1.69	0.06	0.88
Pretzels, hard	Wege	95.79	4.79	10.91	4.58	2.94	3.49	2.55	0.30	0.64
Pretzels, whole wheat	Wege	96.04	1.12	10.50	8.11	4.06	7.20	4.87	1.18	1.15
Prograin bread	Friehofer	63.92	4.03	18.96	13.10	5.92	8.92	4.96	2.35	1.61
Rice cakes	Quaker	93.77	0.00	9.67	4.05	−0.98	5.53	4.04	1.17	0.32
Rolls, sweet, cinnamon		69.96	1.92	10.72	5.76	1.57	4.66	2.88	0.66	1.12
Rye cakes	Quaker	94.61	0.00	16.09	12.21	5.45	7.37	5.14	1.78	0.47
Saltine crackers		96.84	3.36	10.05	3.77	2.11	1.66	0.78	0.92	−0.04
Sesame crackers	Ak-Mak	95.60	3.50	16.36	12.64	2.25	13.74	8.90	2.27	2.57
Snackbread	Ryvita	92.44	1.71	11.25	5.61	2.16	3.82	3.30	0.35	0.17
Snackbread, whole wheat	Ryvita	95.26	2.46	12.67	12.18	3.28	10.10	7.85	1.57	0.68
Swedish rye crispbread	Siljans	90.78	2.27	10.03	17.86	5.46	15.29	12.15	2.00	1.14

Item	Brand								
Taco shells	Old El Paso	93.76	2.78	6.55	12.42	2.51	11.30	8.14	1.67	1.49
Taco shells		94.42	1.85	6.61	7.49	2.07	6.73	3.63	2.73	0.37
Triscuit	Nabisco	97.19	2.69	8.28	12.43	2.49	10.84	8.70	1.86	0.28
Wheat cakes	Quaker	94.88	0.00	16.41	9.77	3.31	7.07	5.29	1.33	0.50
Wheat thins	Nabisco	97.92	2.57	7.54	8.12	3.69	5.16	3.42	0.50	1.24
White extra fiber, toasted	Arnold's	73.86	0.00	15.50	6.15	−1.03	8.55	2.80	4.56	1.20
White extra fiber	Arnold's	60.92	0.00	15.40	7.33	0.60	7.01	2.54	3.92	0.57

PASTA

Item	Brand								
Macaroni		97.01	0.59	15.54	5.07	1.47	4.32	1.44	2.25	0.63
Macaroni, Cooked		28.18	0.42	16.80	4.41	2.50	2.35	1.84	0.37	0.13
Noodles, egg, cooked		30.94	1.22	19.45	3.41	1.72	1.87	1.17	0.53	0.18
Spaghetti		90.02	0.87	16.68	3.47	1.27	2.47	1.57	0.53	0.37
Spaghetti, cooked		37.12	0.74	15.67	4.34	2.57	2.07	1.62	0.31	0.14
Spaghetti w/sauce, cooked	Goia	26.38	3.95	13.96	6.88	ND	3.49	1.77	1.26	0.46
Spaghetti, whole wheat	Goia	91.33	1.80	15.87	10.44	1.07	9.82	7.36	1.70	0.76

CEREALS

Item	Brand								
100% Bran	Nabisco	95.42	6.45	12.30	35.67	5.90	33.16	24.16	6.55	2.45
100% Bran	Nabisco	96.60	6.19	12.42	34.16	5.87	32.63	22.18	7.21	3.24
100% Bran	Nabisco	95.79	6.75	13.45	36.89	5.36	32.67	22.50	6.05	3.64
100% Natural	Quaker	96.41	2.01	12.93	9.78	5.58	4.55	2.70	0.93	0.69
40% Bran Flakes		95.53	4.79	12.02	19.75	9.76	11.76	7.21	2.89	1.41
Bran Flakes		95.93	4.60	11.87	19.90	4.26	21.44	11.76	5.20	4.48
All Bran	Kellogg	96.86	7.18	12.75	38.13	5.40	37.65	27.63	7.30	2.72
All Bran	Kellogg	94.98	6.74	12.78	37.76	6.28	35.41	22.28	8.55	4.59
All Bran	Kellogg	98.39	7.29	13.47	40.26	10.34	38.10	25.09	8.72	4.30
All Bran w/Extra Fiber	Kellogg	95.84	6.03	10.80	50.46	7.00	47.46	34.14	10.76	2.56
All Bran w/Extra Fiber	Kellogg	96.20	6.09	11.82	49.61	6.57	47.45	33.26	11.30	2.90
Bran Flakes	Kellogg	96.66	4.65	12.00	16.93	6.40	15.18	8.74	4.08	2.36
Cap'n Crunch	Quaker	96.35	2.45	ND	2.79	ND	3.67	2.27	1.22	0.19
Cheerios	General Mills	94.48	5.04	14.38	11.04	ND	6.46	4.33	0.95	1.19
Cheerios	General Mills	94.47	4.40	16.63	13.03	8.95	5.06	3.25	0.71	0.94
Cheerios		93.59	4.21	12.78	11.35	6.54	12.76	7.03	2.69	3.04
Choco Crunch	Quaker	95.59	1.94	ND	3.59	ND	4.69	2.99	0.71	0.78
Corn Bran	Quaker	97.73	3.07	ND	18.03	ND	20.35	15.66	3.88	0.82
Corn Flakes	Kellogg	94.63	3.37	7.60	3.30	3.38	0.81	0.43	0.19	0.14

Table 2 (continued)
DRY MATTER, ASH, CRUDE PROTEIN, TOTAL DIETARY FIBER, SOLUBLE FIBER, NEUTRAL DETERGENT RESIDUE, HEMICELLULOSES, CELLULOSE, AND LIGNIN CONTENT OF SELECTED FOODS

Description	Maker	%DM	ASH	CP	TDF	SF	NDR	HC	CE	Ls
Corn Flakes	Kellogg	94.24	2.90	6.87	3.62	3.60	1.59	0.78	0.35	0.47
Corn Flakes	Kellogg	95.45	3.04	7.24	3.68	ND	2.74	1.19	0.46	1.09
Corn Flakes	Kellogg	96.19	3.15	6.73	3.24	2.21	4.97	2.12	1.34	1.52
Corn Flakes	General Mills	95.39	5.94	6.59	2.69	0.44	2.73	1.10	0.39	1.24
Cream of Wheat, cooked		11.33	1.74	11.96	6.30	−2.65	9.50	6.70	1.66	1.14
Creamy Wheat, quick	Quaker	87.42	0.49	ND	3.47	ND	4.49	3.87	−0.09	0.71
Crunchberries	Quaker	96.82	2.23	ND	3.17	ND	4.33	2.78	0.72	0.83
Crunchy Nut Oh's	Quaker	97.15	1.70	ND	5.72	ND	4.65	2.99	0.84	0.82
Double Chex	Ralston Purina	97.36	0.00	7.62	5.08	2.54	3.74	1.91	1.35	0.48
Fibre One	General Mills	95.38	6.56	11.66	48.42	7.39	44.76	33.22	9.50	2.04
Fibre One	General Mills	96.09	6.58	12.92	48.12	6.91	45.94	33.18	10.08	2.68
Grits		89.97	0.43	8.30	7.32	3.54	4.56	2.39	1.95	0.21
Grits, instant	Quaker	90.43	4.25	ND	9.12	ND	6.55	5.21	1.06	0.27
Honey Graham Oh's	Quaker	97.40	2.22	ND	3.34	ND	5.14	2.47	0.46	2.22
King Vitamin	Quaker	95.93	2.75	ND	4.99	ND	4.98	3.41	0.64	0.93
Life	Quaker	95.82	4.13	21.59	10.10	8.07	2.47	1.28	0.46	0.50
Life	Quaker	94.61	4.14	ND	9.77	ND	4.98	3.32	0.87	0.79
Life, Cinnamon	Quaker	95.07	4.14	ND	9.76	ND	5.75	3.87	0.95	0.82
Natural Cereal	Quaker	96.93	1.97	ND	10.78	ND	6.98	4.61	1.25	1.11
Natural Cereal, Apple Cinnamon	Quaker	95.44	1.76	ND	10.30	ND	7.32	4.81	1.51	1.01
Natural Cereal, Raisin Date	Quaker	94.83	1.93	ND	9.31	ND	8.08	4.78	1.39	1.91
Natural Cereal, Whole Wheat	Quaker	88.81	1.79	ND	12.39	ND	12.59	7.35	2.56	1.08
Nature Valley Granola	General Mills	94.35	1.73	9.86	10.47	6.04	7.18	5.56	0.83	0.79
Nature's Harvest Granola		96.12	2.24	16.28	22.08	14.40	8.51	4.57	1.50	1.80
Nutrigrain	Kellogg	96.45	2.74	8.97	10.71	2.16	11.30	7.62	1.77	1.91
Oat Bran	Kellogg	97.83	3.61	10.32	17.30	2.28	17.87	11.34	3.45	3.08

Oat Bran Creamy Hot Cereal	Quaker	91.22	3.39	ND	19.64	ND	16.29	12.77	1.82	1.84
Oats, Instant	Quaker	90.57	5.38	ND	11.81	ND	6.64	4.64	1.00	1.00
Oats, Instant, Apple Cinnamon	Quaker	92.30	4.26	ND	9.41	ND	5.77	3.61	1.28	0.88
Oats, Instant, Apple Raisin	Quaker	92.86	2.40	ND	9.98	ND	6.04	3.13	2.05	0.85
Oats, Instant, Blueberries and Cream	Quaker	93.65	3.21	ND	6.87	ND	5.80	3.76	0.66	1.38
Oats, Instant, Peaches and Cream	Quaker	91.62	3.21	ND	9.45	ND	5.76	3.98	1.12	0.66
Oats, Instant, Raisin Date Walnut	Quaker	92.36	3.71	ND	10.82	ND	6.42	3.67	1.10	1.66
Oats, Instant, Raisin Walnut	Quaker	91.12	3.50	ND	9.75	ND	4.66	3.13	0.90	0.63
Oats, Instant, Strawberries and Cream	Quaker	92.41	3.49	ND	8.25	ND	4.07	2.98	0.78	0.31
Oats, Old Fashioned	Quaker	90.02	2.17	ND	11.90	ND	7.50	5.60	0.89	1.00
Oats, One-Minute, Apple Raisin Spice	Quaker	90.25	1.88	ND	9.24	ND	5.10	3.35	1.04	0.71
Oats, One-Minute, Raisin Cinnamon	Quaker	89.41	1.88	ND	7.80	ND	6.12	3.28	0.54	2.30
Peanut Butter Crunch	Quaker	97.08	2.50	ND	4.56	ND	5.11	2.82	0.93	1.36
Popeye Sweet Puffs	Quaker	97.79	1.23	ND	4.14	ND	4.79	2.47	1.39	0.93
Post Toasties	General Foods	94.12	2.76	8.08	3.75	3.61	1.88	1.16	0.25	0.37
Product 19	Kellogg	95.43	3.81	9.42	6.08	6.38	1.73	1.23	0.25	0.12
Product 19	Kellogg	95.83	3.48	8.12	4.27	0.81	7.09	2.79	1.39	2.91
Puffed Rice	Quaker	95.10	0.48	ND	1.23	ND	4.68	3.86	0.66	0.17
Puffed Rice	Quaker	93.19	0.39	ND	2.13	ND	0.80	0.47	0.13	0.16
Puffed Wheat	Quaker	95.17	1.57	ND	9.50	ND	9.99	5.56	1.26	3.15
Puffed Wheat	Quaker	93.94	0.88	ND	12.24	ND	5.71	3.16	1.35	0.97
Rice Krispies	Kellogg	95.37	3.42	6.82	1.90	2.20	3.31	2.05	0.38	0.89
Rice Krispies	Kellogg	95.28	3.26	7.35	2.01	ND	5.74	3.45	0.76	1.52
Rice Krispies	Kellogg	94.95	3.38	6.64	2.02	1.50	2.21	1.50	0.23	0.35
Shredded Wheat	Nabisco	91.85	1.69	10.43	13.21	1.21	13.51	10.91	2.23	0.37
Shredded Wheat	Nabisco	92.21	1.71	13.80	12.96	2.62	13.65	8.72	4.01	0.93
Shredded Wheat N' Bran	Nabisco	94.70	1.72	13.13	13.49	5.70	10.02	6.81	1.69	0.97
Special K	Kellogg	95.30	0.00	12.10	14.38	4.81	10.61	6.36	0.15	1.21
Sweet Crunch	Quaker	93.74	2.54	20.30	3.15	2.91	2.35	1.78	0.18	0.38
Team	Nabisco	96.20	2.33	ND	3.20	ND	2.92	2.01	0.68	0.24
Total	General Mills	95.45	2.10	7.43	4.17	3.28	2.04	1.22	0.35	0.35
Wheat Germ	Kretschmer	95.28	4.82	12.35	10.66	4.35	7.64	5.25	1.24	0.69
		96.27	4.80	30.35	18.10	7.81	10.73	6.49	2.56	1.35

Table 2 (continued)
DRY MATTER, ASH, CRUDE PROTEIN, TOTAL DIETARY FIBER, SOLUBLE FIBER, NEUTRAL DETERGENT RESIDUE, HEMICELLULOSES, CELLULOSE, AND LIGNIN CONTENT OF SELECTED FOODS

Description		Maker	%DM	ASH	CP	TDF	SF	NDR	HC	CE	Ls
Wheat Germ			95.77	5.11	32.58	17.70	3.37	15.91	9.87	3.38	2.66
Wheaties		General Mills	94.77	5.06	11.82	10.79	7.10	6.04	3.86	1.38	0.71
FRUITS											
Apple Juice		Cornell	10.85	2.25	0.50	2.14	ND	1.27	0.14	0.38	0.75
Apple Sauce			18.13	0.95	0.63	8.36	ND	4.90	1.53	2.54	0.83
Apple, Red Delicious, cored			14.79	3.41	1.19	14.72	7.84	7.06	1.63	4.46	0.97
Apple, Red Delicious, cored & peeled			13.90	2.11	0.32	11.40	4.49	6.91	2.03	4.15	0.73
Avocado, California			21.73	7.92	10.65	25.60	−1.78	27.66	7.25	10.79	9.63
Banana			22.56	3.24	5.14	8.54	3.37	5.83	1.25	1.83	2.75
Blueberries			13.71	1.27	3.25	20.12	ND	17.75	5.24	5.54	6.98
Blueberries	Fresh		11.83	1.51	2.68	22.15	7.12	15.43	3.27	8.06	4.10
Canteloupe	Fresh		9.82	11.33	8.79	9.22	4.55	4.74	0.66	3.31	0.77
Cherries, tart	Canned		7.70	2.96	8.62	13.26	8.25	5.67	1.19	2.53	1.96
Grapes, Thomson	Fresh		17.98	5.64	5.00	6.02	2.20	4.29	0.43	2.35	1.52
Orange juice		Cornell	10.81	13.97	5.22	4.57	ND	1.32	0.02	0.61	0.70
Orange, Florida, peeled	Fresh		11.72	3.69	4.68	17.95	11.76	6.25	1.15	4.19	0.91
Orange, navel, peeled	Fresh		12.76	3.48	7.21	16.39	10.88	5.51	0.88	3.63	1.01
Oranges, mandarin	Canned		11.96	1.85	3.63	4.85	ND	2.26	0.31	0.83	1.12
Peaches	Canned		12.77	1.85	3.68	8.75	ND	4.91	0.94	2.51	1.46
Pear, Bartlett, cored	Fresh		13.74	1.87	1.81	26.28	13.25	13.16	2.20	8.35	2.61
Pears	Canned		9.73	1.16	2.07	17.59	5.78	12.00	2.32	7.80	1.88
Pineapple	Canned		14.83	1.92	2.93	5.05	0.54	4.73	1.99	2.33	0.41
Plum, friar	Fresh		10.97	5.78	4.32	15.59	10.13	5.98	1.05	3.02	1.91
Raisins, seedless	Fresh	Wegmans	85.78	2.13	3.88	ND	ND	4.32	1.06	1.09	2.17

Strawberries	Fresh		26.11	0.95	1.63	6.32	ND	4.25	0.94	1.83	1.47
Strawberries	Fresh		8.76	4.45	7.53	19.50	7.16	13.53	2.01	6.27	5.25
Tangerine, peeled	Fresh		13.30	4.14	6.17	15.21	9.68	5.59	1.05	3.67	0.86
Watermelon	Fresh		8.69	17.19	6.40	4.32	1.59	2.79	0.61	1.58	0.60
VEGETABLES											
Artichoke hearts, frozen		General Foods	12.10	ND	20.40	48.98	ND	12.50	3.10	8.10	1.50
Asparagus, frozen		General Foods	8.50	ND	36.10	25.17	ND	12.60	2.40	9.10	1.10
Asparagus spears, canned			6.14	17.93	36.08	23.31	10.17	17.51	3.22	10.81	3.48
Bean sprouts, canned			3.49	5.01	32.20	30.83	9.26	29.64	6.63	16.65	6.36
Beans, green, cooked			8.83	5.91	15.22	32.42	19.73	18.43	6.52	9.95	1.96
Beans, green, canned			5.29	14.93	16.18	34.69	19.73	22.69	4.29	14.52	3.88
Beans, green, frozen			10.79	ND	ND	32.41	ND	18.76	7.68	10.08	1.01
Beans, green, frozen		General Foods	7.70	ND	18.10	30.09	ND	17.60	3.30	11.20	3.10
Beans, green, boiled			9.24	ND	ND	34.11	ND	24.69	10.78	12.42	1.49
Beans, kidney, canned			21.93	5.64	23.41	23.91	10.40	17.22	4.18	11.12	1.93
Beans, kidney, boiled			39.58	ND	ND	28.86	ND	54.83	43.08	9.50	2.24
Beans, lima, boiled			40.36	ND	ND	27.12	ND	43.97	35.78	7.57	0.62
Beans, lima, canned			24.30	5.31	20.71	18.85	3.94	15.66	3.58	10.83	1.25
Beans, lima, frozen		General Foods	33.20	ND	19.30	20.32	ND	11.90	3.70	7.40	0.80
Beans, navy, microwaved			47.08	ND	ND	35.10	ND	45.62	37.07	8.21	0.34
Beans, pork, canned			23.62	7.01	18.49	22.22	12.36	14.50	0.77	10.49	3.25
Beans, wax, frozen		General Foods	8.50	ND	18.90	37.66	ND	18.70	2.30	14.30	2.10
Beans, wax, microwaved			9.31	ND	ND	37.73	ND	24.27	7.57	14.85	1.85
Beet root, canned			7.17	11.62	10.92	25.26	10.29	15.99	6.92	8.83	0.24
Broccoli, frozen		General Foods	7.30	ND	33.60	35.60	ND	18.40	2.00	13.60	2.70
Broccoli, cooked			9.12	6.74	39.61	36.30	15.68	22.20	4.89	13.43	3.88
Broccoli, cooked			9.18	7.10	29.91	34.84	ND	18.53	5.37	11.38	1.78
Brussels sprouts, frozen			12.41	ND	ND	33.86	ND	28.35	12.19	14.61	1.54
Brussels sprouts, frozen		General Foods	10.20	ND	23.90	35.23	ND	21.90	7.40	13.00	1.80
Cabbage, boiled			20.91	ND	ND	28.98	ND	18.33	5.74	11.42	1.16
Cabbage			6.01	10.82	20.89	28.70	15.26	13.77	2.05	11.18	0.54
Cabbage, red, microwaved			12.87	ND	ND	30.19	ND	15.89	3.80	11.51	0.58
Carrots, peeled			11.64	6.75	9.17	24.25	14.18	10.31	1.47	8.48	0.36
Carrots, boiled			11.70	ND	ND	27.53	ND	10.15	1.96	7.67	0.52
Carrots, cooked			11.63	4.66	6.46	34.18	11.64	11.64	2.13	9.01	0.50
Cauliflower, cooked			5.43	6.59	27.34	36.49	16.37	21.75	4.76	15.34	1.64
Cauliflower, cooked			5.43	6.59	27.34	36.49	16.37	21.75	4.76	15.34	1.64

Table 2 (continued)
DRY MATTER, ASH, CRUDE PROTEIN, TOTAL DIETARY FIBER, SOLUBLE FIBER, NEUTRAL DETERGENT RESIDUE, HEMICELLULOSES, CELLULOSE, AND LIGNIN CONTENT OF SELECTED FOODS

Description	Maker	%DM	ASH	CP	TDF	SF	NDR	HC	CE	Ls
Cauliflower, frozen	General Foods	6.20	ND	24.70	27.67	ND	16.00	4.10	10.80	1.50
Cauliflower		8.03	ND	ND	34.89	ND	23.89	8.07	13.47	2.35
Celery		5.17	16.96	11.24	40.12	19.55	21.04	1.80	17.95	1.29
Collards greens, frozen	General Foods	9.60	ND	27.80	32.83	ND	18.60	3.20	12.10	3.10
Corn, canned		21.96	3.98	10.94	7.87	1.43	7.58	5.00	2.01	0.58
Corn, frozen	General Foods	20.40	ND	13.80	11.65	ND	7.90	3.40	2.60	1.90
Cucumber, with skin		3.66	10.74	18.43	27.21	10.14	17.83	2.09	11.57	4.17
Cucumber, peeled		3.36	10.31	16.13	19.49	7.17	12.44	2.56	9.09	0.79
Kale, frozen	General Foods	8.40	ND	27.70	34.91	ND	16.50	2.00	12.30	2.30
Lentils, boiled		40.28	ND	ND	32.95	ND	43.90	33.93	7.69	2.28
Mushrooms		9.85	ND	ND	20.83	ND	21.65	12.10	9.31	0.24
Mustard greens, frozen	General Foods	7.60	ND	31.20	36.21	ND	21.70	4.10	14.40	3.10
Okra, frozen		9.07	ND	ND	40.08	ND	24.51	7.22	9.74	7.55
Okra, frozen	General Foods	7.50	ND	20.60	40.91	ND	14.10	3.30	9.20	1.60
Olives, black		18.88	10.52	5.50	14.68	−6.93	26.00	7.90	5.16	12.95
Olives, green, stuffed		23.24	25.16	3.67	13.30	−5.18	20.96	6.98	4.88	9.15
Onions, boiled		8.96	ND	ND	19.48	ND	11.05	3.09	7.02	0.93
Onions, frozen	General Foods	6.60	ND	9.20	18.65	ND	7.60	0.90	6.20	0.60
Onions, peeled		9.05	4.39	8.96	16.35	8.84	7.64	1.93	5.47	0.24
Onions, green		6.69	11.00	20.24	28.58	12.86	15.72	3.29	10.65	1.78
Peas, black-eyed, canned		20.75	6.23	26.86	18.86	−2.20	27.65	18.91	7.02	1.73
Peas, black-eyed, frozen	General Foods	35.00	ND	27.00	19.34	ND	9.00	0.90	6.30	1.80
Peas, black-eyed, boiled		41.71	ND	ND	32.54	ND	19.10	13.66	4.07	1.36
Peas, green, microwaved		44.26	ND	ND	31.75	ND	11.71	6.77	4.00	0.94
Peas, green, canned		17.58	5.00	23.34	26.49	8.17	19.28	4.25	14.87	0.16
Peas, green, frozen	General Foods	20.70	ND	30.90	20.51	ND	13.30	2.80	10.00	0.50

Food	Brand									
Pepper, green seeded		5.58		11.68	29.36	8.97	20.39	2.09	11.63	6.67
Pickles, dill		4.95	6.03	6.39	23.09	8.88	14.21	1.10	11.10	2.01
Potatoes, french fries	Ore-Ida	30.62	61.05	7.83	7.11	2.90	4.40	1.41	2.37	0.62
Potatoes, boiled, mashed		18.84	3.21	7.61	13.73	ND	4.89	2.21	1.97	0.71
Potatoes, peeled, boiled		19.38	3.07	10.91	9.61	5.69	3.92	0.88	2.99	0.06
Potatoes, w/skins, baked		25.23	3.40	11.74	9.29	3.17	6.41	1.43	4.18	0.79
Radishes		5.32	4.55	14.86	25.32	12.26	13.06	1.35	10.93	0.79
Rice, cooked		27.40	12.96	7.49	1.49	1.08	1.25	0.69	0.31	0.25
Rice, boiled		26.85	0.68	7.32	7.09	ND	3.75	1.80	1.11	0.83
Rutabaga, boiled		11.14	0.95	ND	28.67	ND	14.11	2.91	10.60	0.60
Spinach, microwaved		9.70	ND	ND	29.27	ND	26.56	12.93	9.93	3.70
Squash, frozen	General Foods	11.20	ND	ND	21.48	ND	15.14	3.58	11.43	0.13
Squash, cooked		9.80	ND	20.60	19.28	ND	13.60	2.40	10.50	0.70
Squash, summer, frozen	General Foods	5.00	ND	20.60	21.41	ND	11.40	1.60	8.10	1.70
Squash, summer, microwaved		14.86	ND	ND	20.83	ND	13.82	4.15	8.21	1.46
Squash, summer, zucchini		4.89	11.77	19.43	22.42	11.96	10.46	1.87	7.77	0.82
Squash, zucchini, frozen	General Foods	4.60	ND	18.90	23.51	ND	12.50	2.10	8.80	1.60
Sweet potatoes		23.36	2.12	4.81	7.85	1.82	7.91	1.46	4.47	1.99
Sweet potatoes, baked		21.86	ND	ND	14.48	ND	8.16	2.67	4.59	0.90
Tomato catsup		27.96	11.90	4.32	5.09	2.32	2.98	0.38	2.11	0.49
Tomatoes, canned		5.46	21.63	16.48	13.63	4.58	10.33	1.74	6.28	2.32
Turnip		8.28	ND	ND	29.24	ND	15.23	2.02	12.52	0.69
Turnip greens, frozen		6.65	13.47	29.47	37.39	17.93	21.12	3.34	15.15	2.63
Turnip greens, frozen	General Foods	6.60	ND	34.90	35.51	ND	19.40	1.40	15.20	2.80
Vegetable soup, canned		16.53	13.33	12.48	12.27	0.94	14.29	8.19	5.05	1.05
Yams		26.15	ND	ND	11.36	ND	11.09	7.21	3.48	0.40
NUTS										
Peanuts		95.50	3.40	29.57	9.18	3.88	10.27	4.16	4.35	1.76
Walnuts		99.05	1.64	16.72	6.30	2.27	4.30	1.47	2.35	0.48
OTHER										
Fruit Wrinkles (Fruit Punch)	Fresh	95.64	0.00	0.00	1.27	1.27	0.00	0.00	0.00	0.00
Fruit Wrinkles (Strawberry)	Fresh	93.15	0.00	0.00	1.15	0.99	0.16	0.00	0.00	0.16
FIBER SUPPLEMENTS										
Fiber 88	Natrol	94.88	8.38	6.32	48.80	1.12	48.28	21.12	21.36	5.80

Table 2 (continued)
DRY MATTER, ASH, CRUDE PROTEIN, TOTAL DIETARY FIBER, SOLUBLE FIBER, NEUTRAL DETERGENT RESIDUE, HEMICELLULOSES, CELLULOSE, AND LIGNIN CONTENT OF SELECTED FOODS

Description	Maker	%DM	ASH	CP	TDF	SF	NDR	HC	CE	Ls
Fiber Diet	Puritan's Pride	95.45	5.92	6.94	54.12	10.54	47.27	6.57	39.47	1.23
Fiber Diet	Vitamin World	94.10	6.52	9.31	52.73	9.63	45.55	8.08	35.77	1.70
Fiber Diet	BQE Vit. & Suppl.	96.16	28.91	17.86	53.57	2.45	51.12	14.95	33.27	2.90
Fiber Filler	Your Life	94.70	2.08	1.45	83.39	3.47	80.80	3.49	74.90	2.42
Fiber Full	Solar Nutrition	93.63	6.84	9.96	64.34	8.73	58.77	20.36	31.04	7.37
Fiber-Off	Nutrition Headquarters	95.18	5.60	13.00	47.86	8.00	41.00	6.34	33.93	0.73
Fiberall Orange Sugarfree	Rydelle Laboratories	89.07	3.06	6.99	65.57	52.82	12.75	8.48	3.87	0.40
Fiberall Regular Sugarfree	Rydelle Laboratories	89.59	2.91	8.24	84.53	72.28	12.25	7.70	4.23	0.32
Fiberall Wafers	Rydelle Laboratories	93.49	1.62	6.41	28.37	24.10	6.72	4.65	1.51	0.55
Fiberguard	Ayerst	91.79	14.33	14.41	62.74	32.43	33.70	12.99	19.34	1.37
Fiberguard	Ayerst	92.13	15.21	13.53	59.04	23.36	40.43	18.33	19.03	3.07
Fibermed Wafers	Purdue Fredrick	92.86	3.57	9.76	30.69	6.45	28.34	21.39	6.20	0.75
Fibretrim	Schering	90.86	5.03	24.86	44.88	8.80	42.71	21.41	15.26	6.03
Fibretrim	Schering	92.71	6.11	23.85	46.00	9.07	48.22	25.18	16.51	6.53
Fibretrim w/Calcium	Schering	92.99	23.26	19.58	41.97	6.85	44.93	25.02	14.77	5.14
Full of Fiber	Jameson Nutritional	95.80	42.27	6.43	14.58	3.36	12.01	2.41	9.08	0.52
Grain 'N Citrus	Hilstone	94.66	38.18	4.18	49.70	16.20	35.72	12.19	17.51	6.02
Hi-Fiber	Walgreen Laboratories	93.83	5.32	9.04	51.96	8.34	45.89	8.40	36.09	1.40
Metamucil Regular	Searle	90.47	1.40	17.40	52.59	44.31	8.28	6.55	1.68	0.05
Metamucil Regular Sugarfree	Searle	89.80	2.76	16.16	98.51	84.51	14.00	10.20	3.92	−0.12
Serutan, Regular	J. W. Williams Co	94.10	1.91	4.66	52.98	44.48	8.50	5.88	2.26	0.36
Serutan, Toasted	J. W. Williams Co	97.05	3.65	11.31	46.82	35.32	11.50	8.85	2.25	0.40
Slim with Fiber	Nature's Bounty	95.18	9.14	10.07	49.65	8.72	43.25	6.58	34.09	2.58
Ultra Plan	Hi-Health	93.10	6.83	12.54	16.95	4.04	13.64	4.54	5.25	3.85

Notes: 1. DM = Dry matter; CP = Crude protein (N × 6.25); TDF = Total dietary fiber; SF = Soluble fiber; NDR = Neutral detergent residue (insoluble fiber); HC = Hemicellulose; CE = Cellulose; Ls = Klason lignin.

2. METHODS: (A) Total dietary fibre values obtained by the methods of: Prosky, L., Asp, N.-G., Furda, I., DeVries, J. W., Schweizer, T. F., and Harland, B., Determination of total dietary fiber in foods, food products and total diets: interlaboratory study, *J. AOAC*, 67, 1044, 1984. Prosky, L., Asp, N.-G., Schweizer, T. F., DeVries, J. W., and Furda, I., Determination of insoluble, soluble, and total dietary fiber in foods and food products. Interlaboratory study, *J. AOAC*, 71, 1017, 1988. (B) Neutral detergent residue and its components by the methods of Van Soest: Robertson, J. B. and Van Soest, P. J., The detergent system of analysis and its application to human foods, in *The Analysis of Dietary Fiber in Food*. James, W. P. T. and Theander, O., Eds., Marcel Deckker, New York, 1981. 123. Jeraci, J. L., Hernandez, T. M., Robertson, J. B., and Van Soest, P. J., New and improved procedure for neutral-detergent fiber, *J. Anim. Sci.*, 66 (Suppl.) 1, 351, 1988. (C) Soluble fiber determined directly or by the difference (TDF-NDF corrected for residual protein).

3. Samples provided mainly by J. A. Marllett, B. A. Lewis, D. H. Hurt, and P. J. Van Soest.

4. The majority of these analyses were supported by the National Cancer Institute Contract N01-CN-45182.

APPENDIX I

Table 3

DIETARY FIBER CONTENT OF SELECTED FOODS BY THE SOUTHGATE METHODS (GRAMS PER 100 G EDIBLE PART)

David A. T. Southgate

	Total dietary fiber	Noncellulosic polysaccharides[a]	Cellulose[b]	Lignin[c]
Flours				
White, bread-making	3.15	2.52	0.60	0.03
Brown	7.87	5.70	1.42	0.75
Whole meal	9.51	6.25	2.46	0.80
Breads				
White	2.72	2.01	0.71	Tr
Brown	5.11	3.63	1.33	0.15
Hovis	4.54	3.19	1.04	0.32
Whole meal	8.50	5.95	1.31	1.24
Breakfast cereals				
All Bran	26.70	17.82	6.01	2.88
Cornflakes	11.00	7.26	2.42	1.32
Grapenuts	7.00	5.14	1.28	0.58
Readibreak	7.60	5.39	0.99	1.22
Rice Krispies	4.47	3.47	0.78	0.22
Puffed Wheat	15.41	10.35	2.59	2.47
Sugar Puffs	6.08	4.00	0.99	1.09
Shredded Wheat	12.26	8.79	2.63	0.84
Special K	5.45	3.68	0.72	1.05
Swiss breakfast (mixed brands)	7.41	5.31	1.36	0.74
Weetabix	12.72	9.18	2.35	1.19
Cookies and crispbreads				
Chocolate digestive (half-coated)	3.50	2.13	0.59	0.78
Chocolate (fully coated)	3.09	1.36	0.42	1.31
Crispbread, rye	11.73	8.33	1.66	1.74
Crispbread, wheat	4.83	3.34	0.94	0.55
Ginger biscuits	1.99	1.45	0.30	0.24
Matzo	3.85	2.72	0.70	0.43
Oatcakes	4.00	3.16	0.40	0.44
Semisweet	2.31	1.76	0.33	0.22
Short-sweet	1.66	1.42	0.11	0.13
Wafers (filled)	1.62	1.08	0.47	0.07
Leafy vegetables				
Broccoli tops (boiled)	4.10	2.92	1.15	0.03
Brussels sprouts (boiled)	2.86	1.99	0.80	0.07
Cabbage (boiled)	2.83	1.76	0.69	0.38
Cauliflower (boiled)	1.80	0.67	1.13	Tr
Lettuce (raw)	1.53	0.47	1.06	Tr
Onions (raw)	2.10	1.55	0.55	Tr
Legumes				
Beans, baked (canned)	7.27	5.67	1.41	0.19
Beans, runner (boiled)	3.35	1.85	1.29	0.21
Peas, frozen (raw)	7.75	5.48	2.09	0.18
garden (canned)[d]	6.28	3.80	2.47	0.01
processed (canned)[d]	7.85	5.20	2.30	0.35

Table 3 (continued)

DIETARY FIBER CONTENT OF SELECTED FOODS BY THE SOUTHGATE METHODS (GRAMS PER 100 G EDIBLE PART)

	Total dietary fiber	Noncellulosic polysaccharides[a]	Cellulose[b]	Lignin[c]
Peanuts	9.30	6.40	1.69	1.21
Root vegetables				
Carrots, young (boiled)	3.70	2.22	1.48	Tr
Parsnips (raw)	4.90	3.77	1.13	Tr
Swedes (raw)	2.40	1.61	0.79	Tr
Turnips (raw)	2.20	1.50	0.70	Tr
Potato				
Main crop (raw)	3.51	2.49	1.02	Tr
Chips (fries)	3.20	2.05	1.12	0.03
Crisps	11.90	10.60	1.07	0.32
Canned	2.51	2.23	0.28	Tr
Peppers (cooked)	0.93	0.59	0.34	Tr
Tomato				
(fresh)	1.40	0.65	0.45	0.30
(canned)[d]	0.85	0.45	0.37	0.03
Sweet corn				
(cooked)	4.74	4.31	0.31	0.12
(canned)[d]	5.69	4.97	0.64	0.08
Fruits				
Apples				
(flesh only)	1.42	0.94	0.48	0.01
(peel only)	3.71	2.21	1.01	0.49
Bananas	1.75	1.12	0.37	0.26
Cherries (flesh and skin)	1.24	0.92	0.25	0.07
Grapefruit (canned)[d]	0.44	0.34	0.04	0.06
Guavas (canned)[d]	3.64	1.67	1.17	0.80
Mandarin oranges (canned)[d]	0.29	0.22	0.04	0.03
Mangoes (canned)[d]	1.00	0.65	0.32	0.03
Peaches (flesh and skin)	2.28	1.46	0.20	0.62
Pears				
(flesh only)	2.44	1.32	0.67	0.45
(peel only)	8.59	3.72	2.18	2.67
Plums (flesh and skin)	1.52	0.99	0.23	0.30
Rhubarb (raw)	1.78	0.93	0.70	0.15
Strawberries				
(raw)	2.12	0.98	0.33	0.81
(canned)[d]	1.00	0.48	0.20	0.33
Sultanas	4.40	2.40	0.83	1.17
Nuts				
Brazils	7.73	3.60	2.17	1.96
Preserves				
Jam				
Plum	0.96	0.80	0.14	0.03
Strawberry	1.12	0.85	0.11	0.15
Lemon curd	0.20	0.18	0.02	Tr
Marmalade	0.71	0.64	0.05	0.01
Fruit mincemeat	3.19	2.09	0.60	0.50
Peanut butter	7.55	5.64	1.91	Tr
Pickle	1.53	0.91	0.50	0.12

Table 3 (continued)

DIETARY FIBER CONTENT OF SELECTED FOODS BY THE SOUTHGATE METHODS (GRAMS PER 100 G EDIBLE PART)

	Total dietary fiber	Noncellulosic polysaccharides[a]	Cellulose[b]	Lignin[c]
Dried soups (as purchased)				
Minestrone	6.61	4.60	1.91	0.10
Oxtail	3.84	2.89	0.94	0.01
Tomato	3.32	1.95	1.33	0.04
Beverages (concentrated)				
Cocoa	43.27	11.25	4.13	27.90
Drinking chocolate	8.20	2.61	1.16	4.43
Coffee and chicory essence	0.79	0.73	0.02	0.04
Instant coffee	16.41	15.55	0.53	0.33
Extracts				
Bovril (beef extract)	0.91	0.85	0.03	0.03
Marmite (yeast extract)	2.69	2.60	0.03	0.06

[a] Expressed as the sum of the component monosaccharides.
[b] Expressed as glucose.
[c] This value includes heat-induced artefacts analyzing as lignin.
[d] Drained material.

REFERENCE

Southgate, D. A. T., Bailey, B., Collinson, E., and Walker, A. F., A guide to calculating intakes of dietary fiber, *J. Hum. Nutr.,* 30, 303, 1976.

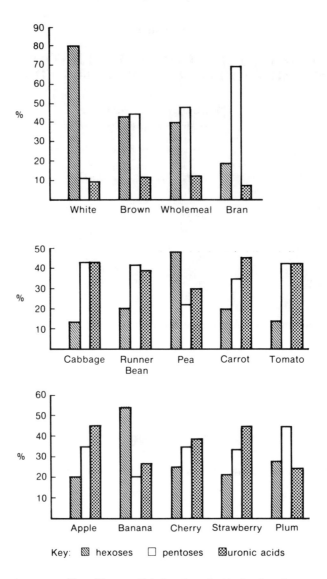

FIGURE 1. Percentage composition of the noncellulosic polysaccharides in wheat flours, vegetables, and fruits.

APPENDIX I

Table 4

DIETARY FIBER CONTENT OF CEREALS IN NORWAY

Wenche Frølich

	Dietary fiber (wet weight %)	Moisture (%)	Dietary fiber (dry weight %)
White wheat flour (78 to 80% extraction)	3.1	11.2	3.5
Whole grain flour	12.1	11.4	13.6
Rye flour (mixed with 15% white wheat flour)	6.9	10.9	7.7
Whole grain flour, rye	14.1	11.4	15.9
Barley flour (50% extraction)	10.8	10.7	12.1
Barley flour (70% extraction)	13.6	10.4	15.2
Whole grain, barley	21.5	8.5	25.3
Oat flakes	10.7	8.6	11.7
Bran of wheat	50.7	11.4	57.2
Bran-germ of wheat	22.1	8.1	24.0
Germ of wheat	18.4	9.1	20.2
Semolina	2.3	11.7	2.6
Triticale	13.9	7.4	15.0
Everyday breakfast cereal	9.8	6.1	10.2
4-Grain breakfast	10.0	8.0	10.9
Bran-cracker type I	45.8	4.4	47.9
Bran-cracker type II	34.9	2.9	35.9
Bran-cracker type III	42.0	3.5	43.5
Bran-cracker, health shop	36.6	4.9	38.5
Kavli flatbread	17.9	3.4	18.5
Kavli breakfast flatbread	18.6	3.0	19.2
Kavli flatbread with bran	22.0	4.2	23.0
Kavli thin crispbread	21.9	4.8	23.0
Ideal flatbread	7.6	3.0	7.8
Ideal homemade	10.7	3.2	11.1
Ideal fiber flatbread	15.7	3.7	16.2
Spaghetti, wheat flour	4.1	9.6	4.5
Macaroni, wheat flour	4.5	8.9	5.0
Spaghetti, whole wheat flour	9.7	8.7	10.7
Macaroni, whole wheat flour	10.8	8.1	11.0
Rice, porridge	3.0	10.0	3.3
Rice, parboiled	3.1	7.8	3.4
Rice, precooked	3.3	8.9	3.6
Rice, quick rice	2.5	9.0	2.7
Rice, nature rice	4.6	10.7	5.1
Rice, brown rice	9.1	10.2	10.1
Unpolished, round grain rice (health shop)	3.4	6.8	3.7
Unpolished, long grain rice (health shop)	4.2	11.6	4.7
Nature, biodynamic-grown rice (health shop)	4.5	10.2	5.0

REFERENCE

Asp, N.-G., Johansson, C.-G., Hallner, H., and Siljeström, M., Rapid enzymatic assay of insoluble and soluble dietary fiber, *Agric. Food Chem.*, 31, 476, 1983.
This method is also mentioned in Chapter 3.1.

APPENDIX I

Table 5

CRUDE FIBER VALUES OF TYPICAL SAMPLES[a]

Ivan Furda

Sample	Crude fiber (g/100 g)	Moisture (%)	Crude fiber (moisture-free basis) (%)
Avocados, raw	1.6	74.0	6.2
Artichokes, raw	2.4	85.5	16.5
Apples, fresh, raw	1.0	84.4	6.4
Almonds, dried	2.6	4.7	2.7
Bean flour, lima	2.0	10.5	2.2
Beans, lima, raw	1.0	90.1	10.0
Bananas	1.8	67.5	5.5
Breads			
White	0.2	35.6	0.31
Rye	0.4	35.5	0.6
French	0.2	30.6	0.3
Pumpernickel	1.1	34.0	1.7
Whole wheat	1.6	36.4	2.5
Broccoli, raw	1.5	89.1	13.6
Cabbage, raw	0.8	92.4	10.5
Carob flour	7.7	11.2	8.7
Chocolate, bitter	2.5	2.3	2.6
Cocoa, dry powder	4.3	3.0	4.4
Corn grits, dry	0.4	12.0	0.5
Corn flour	0.7	12.0	0.8
Corn, field, whole grain, raw	2.0	13.8	2.3
Carrots			
Raw	1.0	88.2	8.5
Dehydrated	9.3	4.0	9.7
Cauliflower, raw	1.0	91.0	11.1
Cornmeal, whole-ground	1.6	12.0	1.8
Grapefruit, raw	0.2	88.4	1.7
Grapes, raw	0.6	81.6	3.2
Horseradish, raw	2.4	74.6	9.4
Macadamia nuts	2.5	3.0	2.6
Malt, dry	5.2	5.7	5.5
Mushrooms, raw	0.8	90.4	8.3
Oatmeal, dry	1.2	8.3	1.3
Okra, raw	1.0	88.9	9.0
Olives, green	1.3	78.2	6.0
Onions, raw	0.6	89.1	5.5
Onions, dehydrated	4.4	4.0	4.6
Oranges, raw peeled fruit	0.5	86.0	3.6
Peaches	0.6	89.1	5.4
Peanuts, raw without skins	1.9	5.4	2.0
Peanut flour, defatted	2.7	7.3	2.9
Pears, raw (including skin)	1.4	83.2	8.3
Peas, edible-podded, raw	1.2	83.3	7.2
Peppers, sweet, immature, green, raw	1.4	93.4	21.2
Pineapple, raw	0.4	85.3	2.7
Plums, raw prune type	0.4	78.7	1.9

APPENDIX I

Table 5 (continued)

CRUDE FIBER VALUES OF TYPICAL SAMPLES[a]

Sample	Crude fiber (g/100 g)	Moisture (%)	Crude fiber (moisture-free basis) (%)
Popcorn, popped, plain	2.2	4.0	2.3
Potatoes, raw	0.5	79.8	2.5
Potato flour	1.6	7.6	1.7
Pumpkin, raw	1.1	91.6	13.1
Rice, white (milled or polished), enriched, raw	0.3	12.0	0.3
Rice, brown, raw	0.9	12.0	1.0
Rice bran	11.5	9.7	12.7
Rye (whole grain)	2.0	11.0	2.2
Rye flour (light)	0.4	11.0	0.4
Rye flour (dark)	2.4	11.0	2.7
Rye wafers (whole grain)	2.2	6.0	2.3
Soybeans (mature seeds), dry, raw	4.9	10.0	5.5
Soybean flour			
(full fat)	2.4	8.0	2.6
(defatted)	2.3	8.0	2.5
Spinach, raw	0.1	90.7	6.5
Squash, raw	0.6	94.0	10.0
Strawberries, raw	1.3	89.9	12.9
Sweet potatoes, raw	0.7	70.6	2.4
Tomatoes, ripe, raw	0.5	93.5	7.7
Turnips, raw	0.9	91.5	10.6
Walnuts, black	1.7	3.1	1.8
Wheat, whole grain			
Hard Red Spring	2.3	13.0	2.6
White	1.9	11.5	2.1
Wheat flours			
Whole (from hard wheats)			
80% extraction	0.5	12.0	0.6
Straight, soft wheat	0.4	12.0	0.45
Bread flour (enriched)	0.3	12.0	0.3
Wheat bran (crude, commercially milled)	9.1	11.5	10.3
Wheat germ (crude, commercially milled)	2.5	11.5	2.8
Yeast (brewer's, debittered)	1.7	5.0	1.8
Yam, tuber, raw	0.9	73.5	3.4

[a] Adapted from *Composition of Foods,* Agriculture Handbook No. 8, Watt, B. K. and Merrill, A. L., Eds., Agricultural Research Service, U.S. Department of Agriculture, Washington, D.C., 1963.

APPENDIX I

Table 6

COMPARISON OF ANALYSES OF DIETARY FIBER AND CRUDE FIBER

Gene A. Spiller

Foods	Crude fiber[1] (%)	Total dietary fiber[2] (%)
Vegetables		
Beans, baked	1.50	7.27
Beans, green	1.00	3.35
Carrots, cooked	1.00	3.70
Corn, sweet, cooked	0.70	4.74
Lettuce, raw	0.60	1.53
Onions, raw	0.60	2.10
Parsnips, raw	2.00	4.90
Peas, frozen, raw	1.90	7.75
Peas, canned	1.40	7.07
Potatoes, raw	0.50	3.51
Tomatoes, fresh	0.50	1.40
Fruits		
Apples, flesh only	0.60	1.42
Bananas	0.50	1.75
Cherries, flesh and skin	0.40	1.24
Peaches, flesh and skin	0.60	2.28
Pears, flesh only	1.40	2.44
Plums, flesh and skin	0.50	1.52
Strawberries, raw	1.30	2.12
Nut-like products		
Peanut butter	1.90	7.55
Grains and grain products		
Flour, white	0.30	3.15
Flour, whole wheat	2.30	9.15
Bran	9.41	44.00
Bread, white	0.20	2.72
Bread, whole wheat	1.60	8.50
All Bran cereal	7.80	26.70
Corn Flakes	0.70	11.00

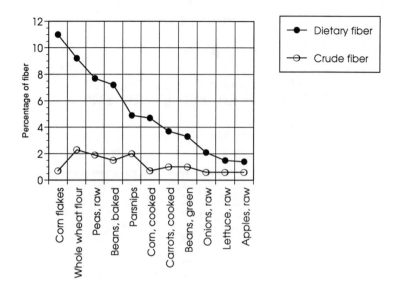

FIGURE 1. Data for dietary fiber (Southgate method, Chapter 3.4) and crude fiber for various foods showing lack of correlation between the two measurements.

REFERENCES

1. Crude fiber data from *Composition of Foods,* Handbook Number 8, U.S. Department of Agriculture, Washington, D.C., 1963.
2. Dietary fiber data from Southgate, D. A. T., Bailey, B., Collinson, E., and Walker, A. F., A guide to calculating intakes of dietary fiber, *J. Hum. Nutr.,* 30, 303, 1976.

APPENDIX I

Table 7

PHYTATE CONTENTS OF FOODS[a]

Barbara F. Harland

Food	Moisture[b] %	Serving U[c]	Size g	Phytate per serving mg	EP[d], mg	100 g dry wt, mg
Almonds (Taylor's Sunshine Colony)	5.0	1/2 c	71	909	1280	347 ± 17[c]
Apples, raw, not pared	84.4	1	150	94	63	404
Artichoke, Jerusalem, boiled	80.2	1 bud	380	110	29	146
Artichoke, Jerusalem, flour	10.9	1 Tbsp	15	70	468	525 ± 24[f]
Artichoke hearts, whole (S & W)	90.0	1	120	11	9	88 ± 2[c]
Avocado	66.1	1	201	2	1	3 ± 2[c]
Bacon chips, imitation (Bacos, Betty Crocker)	5.0	1 Tbsp	15	196	1310	1379 ± 9[e]
Baking mix, buttermilk (Bimix, Martha White)	7.5	1 Tbsp	15	27	180	195 ± 14[e]
Baking mix, buttermilk (Bisquick)	7.5	1 Tbsp	15	11	73	79 ± 7[e]
Barley, infant cereal, instant cooking, dry (Gerber)	10.3	1 oz	28	251	897	1000
Barley, pearl, boiled	69.6	1/2 c	120	197	164	539
Beans, broad, boiled	83.7	1/2 c	120	22	18	110
Beans,[g] green, casserole with cheddar cheese	70.0	1 c	124	112	90	300
Beans, kidney, canned, drained	69.0	1/2 c	92	282	307	990 ± 2[h]
Beans, lima immature, raw	67.5	1/2 c	55	124	226	695 ± 9[f]
Beans, lima, mature, dry, raw	10.3	1/4 c	40	404	1010	1126
Beans, navy, mature, dry, boiled, drained	69.0	1/2 c	85	294	346	1116
Beans, navy, mature, dry, raw	10.9	1/2 c	62	564	910	1021 ± 18[e]
Beans, pinto, raw	67.5	1/2 c	55	122	222	684 ± 5[f]
Beans, snap, green, canned, drained	91.9	1/2 c	62	56	91	1123
Beets, canned sliced (Del Monte)	90.7	1/2 c	85	2	3	30 ± 7[e]
Blackberries	82.0	1/2 c	72	7	10	56
Blueberries sweetened, canned, drained	72.3	1/2 c	115	3	3	11 ± 4[h]
Boullion cubes, beef-flavored (Wyler's)	4.0	2 cubes	8	7	88	92 ± 2[c]

Table 7 (continued)
PHYTATE CONTENTS OF FOODS[a]

Food	Moisture[b] %	Serving U[c]	Size g	Phytate per serving mg	EP[d], mg	100 g dry wt, mg
Boullion cubes, chicken-flavored (Wyler's)	4.0	2 cubes	8	3	32	33 ± 2[e]
Brazil nuts	8.5	1/2 c	70	1259	1799	1966
Bread, French	30.6	1 sl	35	6	17	24
Bread, high fiber, wheat (Fresh Horizons)	36.4	1 sl	28	65	232	365 ± 2[h]
Bread, high fiber, white (Fresh Horizons)	35.8	1 sl	27	21	79	123 ± 1[h]
Bread, Norwegian flat (Kauli)	4.3	1	10	65	654	683 ± 3[h]
Bread, pita (Giant)	25.0	1	35	43	123	164 ± 2[h]
Bread, pumper-nickel (Giant)	34.0	1 sl	32	34	107	162
Bread, raisin (Giant)	35.3	1 sl	25	14	58	89
Bread, rye, American (Giant)	35.5	1 sl	25	39	155	240
Bread, wheat (Melba Toast, Borden)	6.0	2 sl	10	18	183	195 ± 5[e]
Bread, white, enriched (Giant)	35.8	1 sl	27	18	69	107
Bread, whole wheat (Giant)	36.4	1 sl	28	109	390	613
Bread, whole wheat (Oroweat)	36.9	1 sl	24	80	334	529 ± 2[e]
Breading mix (Shake n' Bake)	8.0	1 oz	28	102	365	397 ± 2[e]
Broccoli, fresh	88.8	1 bud	44	8	18	164 ± 0[e]
Bun, plain, hamburger (United Premium Quality)	33.3	1	52	43	82	124 ± 0[e]
Cake, chocolate, without icing (Duncan Hines Swiss Choc. Mix)	24.2	1 sl	120	637	531	701 ± 6[h]
Cake, white, lightly iced (Duncan Hines Mix)	20.0	1 sl	104	18	17	21
Candy, milk chocolate (Hershey)	0.9	1 oz	28	36	127	128 ± 12[h]
Caraway seeds	5.5	1 Tbsp	8	81	1019	1078 ± 11[h]
Carrots, raw	88.2	1	81	8	9	76
Cashew nuts	5.2	1/2 c	70	1306	1866	1968 ± 31[h]
Cashew nuts, honey roasted (Eagle Snacks)	5.0	1/2 c	70	665	950	1000 ± 20[e]
Chestnuts	51.7	1/2 c	80	38	47	97
Chickpeas, (garbanzos) dry, raw	10.7	1/2 c	100	730	730	817 ± 9[h]
Chickpeas or garbanzos, mature seeds, dry, boiled, drained	69.0	1/2 c	62	129	208	670
Chili con carne, no beans (Wolf)	70.7	1 c	225	187	83	284 ± 10[e]

Food						
Chili con carne, w/beans (Wolf)	73.1	1 c	225	169	75	280 ± 3[e]
Cocoa, dry powder (Hershey)	4.1	1 Tbsp	5	94	1880	1960
Coconut meat, dried, sweetened, shredded	3.3	1 oz	28	65	230	237
Coffee cake (Butter Streusel, Sara Lee)	22.0	1 sl	42	21	50	64 ± 6[h]
Coffee, brewed (Folgers Flaked)	98.1	6 oz c	180	12	7	368
Coffee, instant (Tasters Choice 100% Freeze-Dried)	98.1	6 oz c	180	1	0.7	37
Coffee substitute, grain and spice (Celestial Seasonings)	98.1	6 oz c	180	18	10	526
Collard greens, raw	88.9	1 c	80	10	12	112 ± 9[f]
Cookie, chocolate chip (Chips Ahoy, Nabisco)	8.0	4	60	89	148	161 ± 3[e]
Cookie, chocolate sandwich cream-filled (Oreos, Nabisco)	2.2	4	40	74	186	190 ± 6[h]
Cookie, coconut bar (Rippin Good)	3.8	10	90	294	327	340 ± 10[h]
Cookie, fig bar (Fig Newtons, Nabisco)	12.7	4	56	20	35	40 ± 6[h]
Cookie (Nilla Wafers, Nabisco)	2.8	2	20	7	37	38 ± 3[e]
Cookie, oatmeal and raisin (Pepperidge Farm)	2.8	4	52	101	194	200 ± 6[h]
Cookie (Peanut Butter Nut, Duncan Hines)	11.0	2	28	92	328	368 ± 10[e]
Cookie (Toddler Biter Biscuits, Gerber)	4.0	2	38	38	100	104 ± 3[e]
Cookie mix, brownie, baked (Duncan Hines)	11.0	1	20	31	153	161 ± 3[e]
Cookie mix, peanut butter (Duncan Hines)	10.0	1 oz	28	55	197	219 ± 7[e]
Cornbread, whole ground corn meal (Washington Cornbread Mix)	53.9	1 sl	78	489	627	1360
Corn, canned, whole kernel, yellow, drained solids	75.9	1/2 c	82	26	31	129
Corn cereal, ready-to-eat (Corn Bran, Quaker)	3.5	1 oz	28	65	232	240 ± 16[h]
Corn cereal, ready-to-eat (Corn Flakes, Kellogg's)	2.6	1 oz	28	20	70	72 ± 3[e]
Corn cereal, ready-to-eat (Corn Pops, Kellogg's)	3.4	1 oz	28	26	94	97 ± 10[e]
Corn chips (Cheetos)	6.0	1 oz	28	20	73	78 ± 3[e]
Corn chips (Cornquistos, Snack Master)	5.0	1 oz	28	65	232	244 ± 18[e]
Corn chips (Doritos)	3.8	1 oz	28	178	635	660
Corn chips (Fritos)	6.0	1 oz	28	142	506	538 ± 2[e]
Corn chips (Nacho Dorritos)	6.0	1 oz	28	142	507	570 ± 3[e]
Corn germ flour (Quaker)	11.0	1 c	120	2048	1707	1940 ± 6[h]
Corn meal (Quaker)	12.0	1 c	80	754	943	1072 ± 6[h]
Cornmeal, unbolted, stoneground (Stone Mountain)	12.0	1/2 c	15	107	711	808 ± 0[e]
Corn pudding[i]	34.0	1 Tbsp	122	20	16	24
Cracker, animal (Barnum's, Nabisco)	6.0	4	10	8	84	89 ± 3[e]
Cracker, graham (Honey Maid, Nabisco)	6.0	4	28	50	179	190 ± 5[e]
Cracker (Ritz, Nabisco)	4.0	4	11	11	103	107 ± 3[e]
Cracker, saltines (Nabisco)	4.3	4	11	19	172	180

Table 7 (continued)
PHYTATE CONTENTS OF FOODS[a]

Food	Moisture[b] %	Serving U[c]	Size g	Phytate per serving mg	EP[d], mg	100 g dry wt, mg
Cracker (Wheat Thins, Nabisco)	6.0	2	30	95	317	337 ± 3[e]
Croutons, toasted (Brownberry)	7.0	2 oz	56	79	141	152 ± 2[e]
Cucumber, raw	54.1	1/2 c	52	15	28	62 ± 5[e]
Doughnut, cake, sugar-coated (Mrs. Baird's)	24.0	1	32	117	366	481 ± 15[e]
Farina, regular, cooked (Cream of Wheat)	89.5	1/2 c	122	5	4	38
Figs, dried, uncooked	23.0	1/2 c	89	343	385	500 ± 57[h]
Filberts (hazelnuts), shelled, chopped	5.8	1/2 c	59	956	1620	1720
Granola, coconut, assorted nuts, and raisins (Nature Valley)	3.8	1 oz	28	175	625	650
Hickory nuts	3.3	1/2 c	78	1260	1615	1670
High-protein infant cereal, instant dry form (Gerber)	10.3	1 oz	28	311	1112	1240
Hominy, cooked (corn grits), degermed, enriched	87.1	1/2 c	122	344	282	2186 ± 38[h]
Hot chocolate, instant (Swiss Miss Hot Cocoa Mix)	98.1	6 oz c	180	2	1	53
Kale, raw	88.7	1 c	80	11	14	128 ± 7[f]
Ketchup, tomato (Heinz)	65.9	1 Tbsp	15	1	7	20 ± 3[e]
Lentils, raw	12.2	1/2 c	95	412	434	494
Macaroni, elbow, enriched (Kroger)	10.4	1/2 c	43	112	260	290 ± 5[e]
Millet, dry	11.8	1/4 c	25	124	494	560 ± 8[h]
Mixed grain cereal, ready-to-eat (Alpha Bits, Post)	1.3	1 oz	28	143	510	517 ± 7[e]
Mixed grain cereal, ready-to-eat (Apple Jacks, Kellogg's)	2.3	1 oz	28	50	177	181 ± 0[e]
Mixed grain cereal, ready-to-eat (Froot Loops, Kellogg's)	2.5	1 oz	28	45	162	166 ± 5[e]
Mixed grain cereal, ready-to-eat (Product 19, Kellogg's)	3.2	1 oz	28	76	272	281 ± 2[e]
Mixed grain cereal, ready-to-eat (Special K, Kellogg's)	2.2	1 oz	28	76	272	278 ± 8[e]
Mixed grain cereal, ready-to-eat (Team, Nabisco)	3.2	1 oz	28	65	232	240
Mixed grain cereal, infant, instant, dry form (Gerber)	10.3	1 oz	28	203	726	809
Muffin, English (Thomas)	39.0	1	66	48	73	120 ± 6[h]
Muffin, wheat bran (Duncan Hines Mix)	35.1	1	40	199	498	767 ± 8[h]
Noodles, chow mein (La Choy)	1.0	1 oz	28	114	409	413 ± 2[e]
Oatmeal or rolled oats, cooked (Quaker)	86.5	1/2 c	120	133	111	822

Food					
Oatmeal, dry (Quaker)	8.9	1 oz	28	264	943	1035
Oatmeal, infant cereal, instant, dry form (Gerber)	10.3	1 oz	28	251	897	1000
Okra, cooked (Trappey's)	94.8	1/2 c	80	4	5	88 ± 2[e]
Okra, raw	88.9	1/2 c	48	15	32	286 ± 4[e]
Olives, green, Spanish w/pimiento	74.9	2	40	1	3	11 ± 3[e]
Olives, ripe, sliced	85.1	2	48	1	2	15 ± 2[e]
Pancakes, wheat germ (Aunt Jemima Mix plus 1 teaspoon of wheat germ/pancake)	50.6	1	28	244	871	1763
Parsnips, raw	76.9	1 c	67	21	32	137 ± 3[e]
Peach pie (Giant)	47.5	1 sl	118	4	3	6
Peanuts, toasted, salted (Tom's)	6.6	1 oz	28	261	933	999 ± 22[e]
Peanut butter (Jif, extra crunchy)	2.2	1 Tbsp	16	200	1252	1280
Peas, blackeyed, dried, raw	10.5	1/2 c	100	815	815	911 ± 7[h]
Peas, dried, raw	13.3	1/2 c	100	851	851	982
Peas, green, immature, canned, drained solids	81.5	1/2 c	85	24	28	151
Peas, split, dry	11.7	1/2 c	100	664	664	752 ± 2[h]
Pecans, shelled	3.4	1/2 c	54	793	1468	1519
Piecrust stick (Betty Crocker)	19.0	1/6	53	62	117	144 ± 3[e]
Plantain, raw	66.4	1/2 c	50	16	32	95 ± 16[f]
Popcorn, popped, plain	4.0	1 c	6	37	614	640
Popcorn, unpopped (Orville Redenbacher's Gourmet)	9.8	1/8 c	6	34	561	622 ± 13[e]
Poppy seeds	5.5	1 Tbsp	8	175	2189	2316 ± 13[h]
Potato chips	1.8	1 oz	28	55	196	200 ± 15[h]
Potatoes, boiled in skin, drained, pared	79.8	1/2 c	78	63	81	401
Potatoes, French fries	44.7	10	50	50	100	181 ± 1[h]
Potato salad w/egg (Giant, Deli)	82.8	1/2 c	75	63	84	488
Pretzels, butter (Seyferts)	5.0	10	60	63	105	111 ± 6[e]
Pumpkin seeds	5.5	1 oz	28	529	1889	1998 ± 15[h]
Radish, fresh	94.4	1	45	3	6	108 ± 15[e]
Rice, brown, dry	10.3	1/4 c	25	130	518	577 ± 22[h]
Rice, long grain, uncooked (Minute, General Foods)	9.6	1/4 c	45	65	144	159 ± 7[e]
Rice, white, regular, dry form, fully milled or polished	10.3	1/4 c	25	64	255	284
Rice, wild	12.0	1/2 c	100	1936	1936	2200
Rice cereal, ready-to-eat (Cocoa Krispies, Kellogg's)	2.5	1 oz	28	38	136	139 ± 2[e]
Rice cereal, ready-to-eat (Cocoa Pebbles, Post)	2.1	1 oz	28	53	189	193 ± 2[e]
Rice cereal, ready-to-eat (Fruity Pebbles, Post)	2.9	1 oz	28	41	146	150 ± 2[e]

Table 7 (continued)
PHYTATE CONTENTS OF FOODS[a]

Food	Moisture[b] %	Serving U[c]	Size g	Phytate per serving mg	100 g EP[d], mg	100 g dry wt, mg
Rice cereal, ready-to-eat (Rice Krispies, Kellogg's)	2.3	1 oz	28	58	207	212 ± 10[e]
Rice cereal, infant, instant dry form (Gerber)	10.3	1 oz	28	246	879	980
Roll, ready-to-serve, plain (Giant)	31.4	1	28	18	64	93
Rye flour (Pillsbury)	15.0	1 c	128	1176	919	1081
Sesame seeds	5.5	1 Tbsp	8	129	1616	1710 ± 14[h]
Soy-based chicken analog (General Mills)	7.0	1 oz	28	70	251	270
Soy-based ham analog (General Mills)	7.0	1 oz	28	31	112	120
Soy-based infant formula (Advance, Concentrate)	87.0	4 oz	120	10	8	62 ± 2[h]
Soy-based TVP bacon (Archer Daniels Midlands)	7.0	1 oz	28	248	884	951
Soy-based TVP bacon and vitamins (Archer Daniels Midlands)	7.0	1 oz	28	300	1070	1151
Soy-based TVP, beef (Archer Daniels Midlands)	7.0	1 oz	28	354	1265	1360
Soy-based TVP ham (Archer Daniels Midlands)	7.0	1 oz	28	328	1172	1260
Soy-based TVP pork (Archer Daniels Midlands)	7.0	1 oz	28	370	1321	1420
Soy-based TVP unflavored and vitamins (Archer Daniels Midlands)	7.0	1 oz	28	424	1516	1630
Soybeans, mature seeds, dry, raw Elton variety	10.0	1/2 c	105	2438	2322	2580
Soy flour (Ralston Purina)	8.0	1 c	137	1915	1398	1520 ± 11[h]
Soy isolate (Ralston Purina)	8.0	1 c	137	1689	1233	1340 ± 11[h]
Soy, textured concentrate (Patti Pro, General Mills)	5.0	1 oz	28	399	1425	1500
Strawberries, frozen, sweetened, drained	71.3	1/2 c	128	8	6	21 ± 2[h]
Sunflower seeds	5.5	1 Tbsp	8	128	1606	1699 ± 4[h]
Sweet potato, raw	70.0	1	180	9	5	17
Taco shells (Paco's)	4.0	1	20	110	549	572 ± 8[e]
Tea, brewed (Kaffree, dried leaves)	99.4	6 oz c	180	3	2	333
Tea, instant (Nestea 100% Instant)	99.4	6 oz c	180	2	1	167
Tomato seeds	5.5	1 Tbsp	8	148	1847	1955 ± 8[h]
Tomato soup (Campbell's)	87.8	1/2 c	122	8	6	49
Tomatoes, canned solids and liquid	93.7	1/2 c	120	8	6	95

Food	Amount	g	mg/portion	mg/100 g
Triticale flour	11.0			670 ± 0[f]
Turnips, raw	87.2	1 Tbsp	15	597
Walnuts, black, shelled	3.1	1/2 c	65	6	47 ± 3[e]
Walnuts, English, shelled	23.5	1/2 c	62	1977	2040
Wheat bran, crude AACC ref.[j]	10.4	1/2 c	50	760	993
Wheat cereal, ready-to-eat (40% Bran, Post)	3.0	1 oz	28	843	3011	3360
Wheat cereal, ready-to-eat 100% bran (All Bran, Kellogg's)	3.6	1 oz	28	305	1088	1122 ± 10[e]
Wheat cereal, ready-to-eat, Bran Chex (Ralston Purina)	3.5	1 oz	28	887	3168	3286 ± 2[h]
Wheat cereal, ready-to-eat (Bran Flakes, Kellogg's)	3.0	1 oz	28	375	1341	1390 ± 22[h]
Wheat cereal, ready-to-eat (Frosted Flakes, Kellogg's)	2.5	1 oz	28	298	1066	1099 ± 2[e]
Wheat cereal, ready-to-eat (Grape Nuts Flakes, Post)	3.4	1 oz	28	16	58	60 ± 2[e]
Wheat cereal, ready-to-eat (Honey Smacks, Kellogg's)	3.2	1 oz	28	151	541	560 ± 3[e]
Wheat cereal, ready-to-eat (Post Toasties)	3.0	1 oz	28	51	182	188 ± 8[e]
Wheat cereal, ready-to-eat (Raisin Bran, Kellogg's)	8.3	1 oz	28	22	80	83 ± 0[e]
Wheat cereal, ready-to-eat (Shredded, Nabisco)	3.2	1 oz	28	184	659	719 ± 2[e]
Wheat cereal, ready-to-eat fortified (Special K, Kellogg's)	3.5	1 oz	28	415	1481	1530
Wheat cereal, ready-to-eat (Super Sugar Crisps, Post)	1.5	1 oz	28	186	666	690 ± 10[h]
Wheat cereal, ready-to-eat (Wheaties, General Mills)	3.5	1 oz	28	77	274	278 ± 7[e]
Wheat flour, all-purpose (General Mills)	12.0	1 c	137	411	1467	1520
Wheat flour, enriched, unbleached (Gold Medal, General Mills)	12.0	1 Tbsp	15	386	282	320
Wheat flour, whole wheat (Pillsbury)	12.0	1 c	120	20	136	154 ± 2[e]
Wheat germ (Kretchmer)	11.5	1 Tbsp	6	1014	845	960
Wheat gluten flour	8.5	1 Tbsp	15	244	4071	4600
Yam, raw	73.0	1	180	38	252	276 ± 4[f]
Yeast, baker's dry	5.0	1/4 oz	7	94	52	193
			35	495	521 ± 7[f]

a Table 1 is taken in part from Harland, B. F. and Oberleas, D., *Phytate in Foods*, World Review of Nutrition and Dietetics, Vol. 52, S. Karger, Basel, 1987, 235.
b If no value was given, a "best estimate" was calculated from existing data.
c c = 8 oz cup, oz = ounce, Tbsp = tablespoon, and sl = slice.
d Edible portion.
e Mean ± SE of triplicate determinations by Oberleas and Roy (1985).
f Mean ± SE of triplicate determinations by Harland et al. (1986).
g Two c snap green beans, drained, 1 can Campbell's Cream of Mushroom Soup, 1/2 c grated cheddar cheese. Mix and heat.
h Mean ± SE of triplicate determinations by Harland and Oberlease (1986).
i One c whole kernel corn, 2 c cream-style corn, 1/2 c melted butter, 2 beaten eggs, 1 c sour cream, 1 pkg Jiffy cornbread mix. Mix ingredients, bake at 350°F for 30 min.
j AACC Certified Food Grade Wheat Bran (10-4-77) used as a reference material during phytate analyses (American Association of Cereal Chemists, 3340 Pilot Knob Road, St. Paul, MN 55121). This food has been certified to contain 3 ± 0.2% or 3348 ± 223 mg phytate/100 g (dry weight).

APPENDIX I

Table 8

PLANT FOODS THAT CONTAIN SIGNIFICANT LEVELS OF SAPONINS AND THEIR ESTIMATED SAPONIN CONTENT

David Oakenfull and John D. Potter

Plant	Saponin content (g/Kg dry weight)
Alfalfa sprouts *(Medicago sativa)*	80
Asparagus *(Asparagus officinalis)*	15
Broad bean *(Vicia faba)*	3.5
Chickpea *(Cicer arietinum)*	2.3–60
Green pea *(Pisum sativum)*	1.8–11
Kidney bean *(Phaseolus vulgaris)*	2–16
Lentil *(Lens culinaris)*	1.1–5.1
Mung bean *(Phaseolus mungo)*	0.5–6
Navy bean *(Phaseolus vulgaris)*	4.5–21
Oats *(Avena sativa)*	1–13
Peanut *(Arachis hypogaea)*	0.05–16
Sesame seed *(Sesamum indicum)*	3
Silver beet *(Beta vulgaris)*	58
Soy bean *(Glycine max)*	5.6–56
Spinach *(Spinacea oleracia)*	47

Appendix II

APPENDIX II

REPORT OF THE RECOMMENDATIONS ON FIBER CLASSIFICATION OF THE FIBER SUPPLEMENT WORKSHOP AT THE XIII INTERNATIONAL CONGRESS OF NUTRITION, BRIGHTON, U.K.*

Gene A. Spiller and David J. A. Jenkins

DIETARY FIBER SUPPLEMENTS, PHYSIOLOGICAL AND PHARMACOLOGICAL ASPECTS: A WORKSHOP REPORT

Participants and contributors

N.-G. Asp (Lund, Sweden); C. Bonfield (Washington, D.C., U.S.); A. Frew (Kent, U.K.); I. Furda (Minneapolis, MN, U.S.); K. Heaton (Bristol, U.K.); H. Kasper (Wester Germany); Helen Klisser (Auckland, New Zealand); D. Kritchevsky (Philadelphia, PA, U.S.); A. Leeds (London, U.K.); J. de Nadon (Paris, France); and R. Taylor (London, U.K.)

Introduction

Dietary fiber supplements are today being researched and/or produced in many countries. The workshop participants, from both industry and academic institutions, agreed that various points need clarification and better definition. It was also agreed that we are ready for some preliminary suggestions on what is a supplement as compared to a high fiber food.

Purpose of fiber supplements

Fiber supplements have two main purposes: (1) to add fiber to the diet of seemingly healthy people who habitually consume too little fiber and (2) to act as a pharmacological agent in the diets of constipated, hyperlipidemic, diabetic, and other patients.

Classification of fiber foods and supplements

(1) *High-fiber foods:* natural foods in which the dietary fiber portion has not been removed or to which additional fiber has not been added. Examples are typical unrefined whole grain product, beans, whole vegetables, and fruits. (2) *Fiber-enriched foods:* products that are typical foods, such as bread, to which fiber concentrates have been added to increase fiber beyond the natural level. Example: a whole grain bread with extra wheat bran added. (3) *Fiber supplements for healthy individuals.* These could be called physiological supplements, and have the general function of increasing the fiber content of the diet but are not intended to have a medical or pharmacological effect. They are intended for people who are unable or unwilling to consume enough fiber in the diet. Some participants felt that these should supply a wide spectrum of fiber polymers and should contain both water soluble and insoluble components. (4) *Fiber supplements for medical use.* These are supplements with a pharmacological goal, to be recommended or prescribed by a physician to achieve a definite improvement in a pathological state, such as lowering serum cholesterol or reducing urine glucose losses in diabetic patients. Guar gum is an example of such supplements.

---

* From Taylor, T.G. and Jenkins, N.K., Eds., *Proceedings of the XIII International Congress of Nutrition,* John Libbey & Co., Ltd., London, 1986.

Need to define type of fiber

There seems to be agreement that the source and type of fiber should be precisely defined, and that it should be clearly stated on the label whether the fiber is an isolate or a natural concentrate.

Labels for fiber supplements

Statements as to amount of total dietary fiber should be mandatory on the label. Listing of individual polymers would be highly desirable (polymeric pattern of the fiber). Some of the workshop participants felt the polymeric pattern should be mandatory on a supplement label. In addition, water-soluble and insoluble fractions should be listed. The basic thrust was that labeling of supplements should be much more detailed than that of foods.

Special isolated fibers

The use of fiber products not normally used as part of the diet, such as sugar beet fiber, was discussed and the consensus was that they may fill a needed gap in supplementation, but that they should be carefully studied in a clinical setting.

Diet versus supplements

Supplement manufacturers have the responsibility to emphasize that diets high in high fiber foods are different from fiber supplemented diets. Diets high in unrefined carbohydrate not only increase fiber intake, as supplements do, but usually supply higher levels of energy from starchy foods and less from fat. Nevertheless, fiber supplements fill an important need in the modern world.

Summary

The key results of the workshop were as follows. (1) A proposed classification covering fiber foods and fiber supplements, including supplements for general or medical use; (2) A strong recommendation for specific details of fiber composition on the label, including water-soluble and insoluble fiber or fiber polymers; (3) The need to continue studies on isolated fibers for special uses. All participants agreed that fiber supplements, when properly formulated and when they supply sufficient fiber, have a place in countries where the diet is typically low in fiber.

Appendix III

APPENDIX III

BEYOND DIETARY FIBER*

Gene A. Spiller

ABSTRACT

The complexity of plant foods high in dietary fiber poses new challenges to clinical investigators and leads to many study-design dilemmas. There are basic differences in studying purified polymers, highly concentrated but not purified fibers, and diets high in high fiber whole foods. The fibrils of the plant cell wall are most likely altered when prepared as a pure chemical entity and when fiber concentrates (e.g., wheat bran) are used; the method of preparation may alter the composition of the final product. Whole-plant, high fiber foods are complex storehouses of a diversity of polymers, including resistant starch, and of bioactive compounds. Furthermore, the addition of a reasonable amount of high fiber food to the diet not only adds dietary fiber but many digestible, caloric macronutrients that alter the entire diet composition. These problems and dilemmas are reviewed.

INTRODUCTION

The complexity of plant foods high in dietary fiber poses new challenges to the investigator of the effects of dietary fiber on health and physiological function. Study-design dilemmas are many, and in this short perspective I hope to convey some concepts that may help to avoid some of the often conflicting results we read in the medical literature when studies on fiber are published.

In studying dietary fiber we have three options: (1) to use purified polymers (e.g., pectin, cellulose); (2) to use highly concentrated but unpurified fibers (e.g., wheat bran, guar gum, psyllium-seed husk); and (3) to use whole natural foods high in fiber that result in a high-fiber diet (e.g., whole grain breads, beans, vegetables).

FIBER POLYMERS DEFY ISOLATION

The complex polymeric structure of the fibrils of the plant cell wall is inevitably altered when attempts are made to purify and isolate a polymer as a pure chemical entity. These intricate and beautiful interwoven fibrils defy isolation without modification. Pectin and cellulose are typical examples of such plant-cell-wall polymers.

The dream of the researcher, which is to take a pure substance, test it in humans (or animals), and extrapolate the results to whole foods, is in fact an impossible dream when it comes to purified-fiber polymers. Let me say, before this statement is misunderstood, that we should study isolated polymers if they are available, that the basic knowledge derived from these studies is important, and that some of them may have an important place in medicine. But we must be extremely careful in extrapolating the results obtained with such polymers to whole foods and to concentrated portions of whole foods where these polymers are in their native physicochemical form and combined with a host of other compounds.

---

*Reproduced with permission of the *American Journal of Clinical Nutrition*, 54, 615, 1991.

FIBER CONCENTRATES

Some plant seeds and portions of seeds (as well as other plant products) are often extremely high in fiber of a very specific type. Wheat and oat bran, psyllium-seed husk, some seed gums such as guar and locust bean, and some tree exudates such as acacia gum are examples of such fiber concentrates. In this category we may include the fibrous portion of foods (e.g., apples or sugar beets) that have been extracted without resorting to any physical or chemical process that could alter the original physical or chemical description of the fiber during its separation from the digestible portion of the food. However, there is sometimes extreme variability in the extent to which the separation from the digestible portion of the food is made. For example, the bran of grains can have widely varying amounts of germ, aleurone layer, and endosperm present. These layers contain many physiologically active substances. Many conflicting results in the literature are most likely due to differences in the product used. The work of the American Association of Cereal Chemists in defining oat and wheat bran can help only if clinical researchers publish their results as those for a specifically described fiber concentrate.

HIGH-FIBER DIETS: A STUDY IN COMPLEXITY

The research picture is yet more complex when we deal with whole foods. A high-fiber food is a complex storehouse of not only a diversity of polymers but of an array of possibly bioactive compounds, and the addition of a reasonable amount of high fiber food to the diet not only adds digestible carbohydrates and plant proteins but also more often than not it adds some lipids.[1] It usually displaces other foods, often of a different nature — a problem investigators have attempted to solve with variable success.

BIOACTIVE COMPOUNDS IN HIGH FIBER PLANT FOODS

Not only are high fiber plant foods high in well-known essential compounds such as β-carotene, but they also supply many bioactive, nonessential substances that we often tend to overlook. The list of such bioactive, nonessential compounds includes plant sterols, tocotrienols, saponins, ω-3 fatty acids, and, less studied for their physiological activity, plant waxes.

The hypocholesterolemic effect of plant sterols has been extensively studied in humans. We find them in almost every unrefined plant food used by humans, not only in foods containing reasonable amount of lipids such as almonds, walnuts, sesame and sunflower seeds, wheat and corn germ, peanuts, and soybeans, but even in very low fat beans such as kidney beans, in roots such as carrots, in many commonly eaten green leaves, and in fruits from apples to apricots and oranges.[2-4]

Tocotrienols found in the lipid fractions of barley, oats, wheat, and other grains have been found to be hypocholesterolemic as well.[5-7] Saponins, known to affect bile-acid excretion and sometimes serum lipids, are present in just about any plant food we eat from beans to spinach and from oats to sesame seeds and peanuts.[8]

Many green leaves are forgotten as a source of fatty acids (ω-3 as α-linolenic acid), which are known to affect blood coagulation and cell-membrane composition.[9] Some Mediterranean salad greens such as purslane *(Portulaca oleracea)* are extremely rich in these fatty acids. They are also present in English walnuts, wheat germ, and other common seeds as well.

Not yet well studied for their physiological functions are the many waxy substances found on just about all leaves and on the peel of fruits. In this group we find the cutins (polymers containing hydroxyaliphatic acids), suberins (polymers of long chain acids and alcohols), and other plant waxes. Theoretically, their composition could have an effect on people consuming high fiber unrefined diets and hopefully someone will decide to do some clinical studies with these waxes.[1]

In addition, many plant foods contain compounds such as flavonoids, indoles, and phenols, which have been found to reduce the incidence of some chemically induced cancers in experimental animals.[10]

RESISTANT STARCH

An additional difference between purified fiber polymers or highly concentrated fiber products and whole foods high in fiber is the presence of resistant starch in whole-plant foods.[11] Because resistant starch is, by definition, resistant to digestion by human digestive enzymes, a substantial amount reaches the colon undigested and is available for fermentation by the colonic microflora.[12] In populations consuming a high plant-food diet, the amount of resistant starch consumed may be far greater than the total dietary fiber. The protective effect of some of these high fiber diets may well be due to the sum of the effects of the resistant starch and the dietary fiber.

A typical example of the effect of resistant starch is the increased production of volatile fatty acids and possibly of other metabolites when the resistant starch reaches the colon. The sum of the volatile fatty acids produced by fiber polymers and the ones produced by the resistant starch when metabolized by colonic microorganisms could lead to much greater changes in the colonic environment than the changes caused by fiber polymers alone.[12]

CHANGES INDUCED IN THE INTAKE OF OTHER FOODS

When high fiber foods are added to a diet, they alter the intake of other foods in a more drastic way than do purified fibers. A complex set of exchanges takes place by which more plant proteins and fats and less animal proteins and fats are consumed. Often, in addition, more calories come from carbohydrates when whole grains and plant foods are a predominant part of the diet than when animal products are its major component.

It is intrinsic to high fiber plant foods to displace other foods and sources of energy, protein, and fat. How to design studies when such foods are investigated has been the cause of innumerable debates in scientific meetings and many contradictions in publications.

On the contrary, when a concentrated or purified fiber product is added to an otherwise low fiber diet, no other major change needs to take place. The fiber in this case works as a supplement and may have major physiological effects (e.g., guar gum on serum cholesterol or wheat bran on fecal output), but the diet does not need to be altered to a large extent to accommodate the supplement, i.e., it can still be a diet in which most of the calories are derived from animal products rather than from plant products, which have all the differences we have just seen.

THE BRIGHTON CLASSIFICATION

In 1985 a classification for dietary fiber products and foods was suggested at the XIII International Congress of Nutrition in Brighton, U.K.[13] Following is an expanded version of that classification: (1) high fiber whole foods; (2) high fiber fraction of whole foods produced with no special processing that could alter their physicochemical structure (e.g., wheat bran); (3) highly concentrated fiber polymers that have undergone fairly drastic purification and inevitable alteration (pectins, cellulose); and (4) fiber-enriched foods, i.e., foods to which a purified fiber has been added (e.g., white bread with added fiber concentrate).

CONCLUSION

Unless researchers and reviewers demand as full a description as possible of the dietary fiber used and a careful assessment of the study design, the confusion will not be limited to the world of scientific meetings and medical journals read by trained people but will cause a great deal of skepticism and confusion when the popular media report studies in this field. Something as simple as the title of a paper, if not properly stated, can lead to a sequence of both scientific and popular misunderstandings that can lead the general public to cynicism rather than enlightenment.

In our minds, let us keep the effects of high fiber whole foods separate from those of fiber concentrates and let us find the proper role, if any, for each in disease prevention and treatment.

REFERENCES

1. **Spiller, G. A., Ed.**, *CRC Handbook of Dietary Fiber in Human Nutrition*, CRC Press, Boca Raton, FL, 1986.
2. **Mattson, F. H., Grundy, S. M., and Crouse, J. R.**, Optimizing the effect of plant sterols on cholesterol absorption in man, *Am. J. Clin. Nutr.*, 35, 697, 1982.
3. **Lees, R. S. and Lees, A. M.**, Effects of sitosterol therapy on plasma lipids and lipoprotein concentrations, in *Lipoprotein Metabolism*, Greten, H., Ed., Springer-Verlag, Berlin, 1976, 119.
4. **Weihrauch, J. L. and Gardner, J. M.**, Sterol content of foods of plant origin, *J. Am. Diet. Assoc.*, 73, 39, 1978.
5. **Morrison, W. R. and Barnes, P. J.**, Distribution of acyl lipids and tocols into millstreams, in *Lipids in Cereal Technology*, Barnes, P. J., Ed., Academic Press, London, 1983, 149.
6. **Morrison, W. R.**, Lipids, in *Wheat Chemistry and Technology*, Pomerarans, Y., Ed., American Association of Cereal Chemists, Saint Paul, MN, 1988.
7. **Qureshi, A. A., Burger, W. C., Peterson, D. M., and Elson, C. E.**, The structure of an inhibitor of cholesterol biosynthesis isolated from barley, *J. Biol. Chem.*, 261, 10544, 1986.
8. **Oakenfull, D. and Potter, J. D.**, Saponin content of food plants and some prepared foods, in *CRC Handbook of Dietary Fiber in Human Nutrition*, Spiller, G. A., Ed., CRC Press, Boca Raton, FL, 1986, 459.
9. **Simopolous, A. P. and Salem, N.**, Purslane: a terrestrial source of omega-3 fatty acids, *N. Engl. J. Med.*, 315, 833 (letter), 1986.
10. **Wattenberg, L. W.**, Inhibition of carcinogenesis by minor anutrient constituents of the diet, *Proc. Nutr. Soc.*, 49, 173, 1990.
11. **Englyst, H. N. and Cummings, J. H.**, Resistant starch, a 'new' food component: a classification of starch for nutritional purposes, in *Cereals in a European Context*, Morton, I. D., Ed., Ellis Horwood, Chichester, U.K., 1987, 221.
12. **Bingham, S. A.**, Mechanisms and experimental and epidemiological evidence relating dietary fibre (non-starch polysaccharides) and starch to protection against large bowel cancer, *Proc. Nutr. Soc.*, 49, 153, 1990.
13. **Spiller, G. and Jenkins, D. J. A.**, Dietary fiber supplements, physiological and pharmacological aspects: a workshop report, in *Proceedings of the XIII International Congress of Nutrition 1985*, Taylor, T. G. and Jenkins, N. K., Eds., John Libbey, London, 1986, 184.

Index

INDEX

A

AAOC total dietary fiber analysis, 42–47
Acid detergent fiber, 29
  nitrogen excretion and (wheat bran), 191–192
  protein digestibility and, 181
  protein utilization and, 199
Acid detergent system, 49–51
African diet studies, 364
African fiber consumption, 517–518
Agar, 29
  antitoxicity/anticarcinogenicity, 502
  nitrogen excretion and, 193
  protein digestibility and, 183
Agar-agar
  enzyme activity and, 378
  fecal composition and, 296–300
Alfalfa
  antitoxicity/anticarcinogenicity, 504
  bacterial interactions, 372, 373
  enzyme activity and, 378
  fecal excretion studies, 407
  saponin content, 624
  short chain fatty acid metabolism and, 404
Alfalfa meal, 305, 502
Algae: dietary fiber content, 19–20
Algal gum, 372
Algal polysaccharides, 28–29
Algin, 200
Alginate, 29, 183, 193, see also Na-alginate
Alginic acid, 29
All Bran, 365, 367
  crude vs. dietary fiber, 615
  dietary fiber values, 577–578
  dry matter analysis, 597
  fecal composition and, 328
  fecal excretion, 277, 279, see also Bran
  Southgate analysis, 607
American Diabetes Association, 440
Analytic methods
  component analysis, 77–78
  detergent analysis of foods, 49–51
  dietary fiber
    Englyst GLC procedure, 55–67
    lignin excluded, 68–70
    as nonstarch polysaccharide, 54–55
    selection of method, 53–54
  enzymatic gravimetric
    for insoluble and soluble fiber, 37–39
    for insoluble fiber, 37
    interlaboratory methods, 42–43
    steps in process, 40–42
    total dietary fiber (AAOC) method, 43–47
  phytate determination, 101–103
  saponin determination, 105–106
  Southgate method, 73–74, see also Southgate analysis
  starch: resistant, 67–68
  Uppsala method, 78–80
    applications, 91–95
    fractional analysis, 83–91
    steps compared, 80–83
Animal vs. human studies, 211
Apple fiber in diabetes mellitus, 451
Apple powder, 502
Apples, see Fruits
Arabinans, 29
Arabinogalactans, 29, 372
Arabinoxylans, 29
Ascorbic acid, see Vitamins: C
Ash content of selected foods, 595–606
Australasian fiber consumption, 518
Australian fiber intake, 535–539
Autoimmune factors in diabetes mellitus, 440

B

Bacteria/fibrous substrate interactions, 371–375
Bacterial gums, 28
Bagasse, 306, 367
Bananas, 312, 367, see also Fruits
Barley
  in vitro binding studies, 233–234
  in vitro hydrolysis, 380
  dietary fiber values, 577
  mineral bioavailability, 219, 226, 228
Barley hulls
  protein digestibility and, 186
  protein utilization and, 202
Barley husk
  mineral bioavailability, 226
  protein digestibility and, 187
  protein utilization and, 202
Basari, 278, 293
Bean cell wall: protein digestibility and, 187–188
Beans, see Legumes
Beet fiber: in diabetes mellitus, 453
Beverages
  phytate content, 619, 622
  Southgate analysis, 609
Bile acid metabolic studies, 153–165, see also Lipid metabolism
Blood glucose response, see Diabetes mellitus; Glucose metabolism
Bran, 186, 188, see also specific types
  antitoxicity/anticarcinogenicity, 504, 505
  casein digestibility inhibition, 379
  crude vs. dietary fiber, 615
  in diabetes mellitus, 444–446, 449–455
  in diverticular disease, 323–325
  dry matter analysis, 597
  fecal composition and, 301–304, 326–330
  fecal excretion and, 273–285, 407–409, see also Fecal excretion

fecal microflora studies, 365–370
in gallstone therapy, 473–474
in hyperlipidemia, 427, 428–430
in vitro binding studies, 231–234
lipid metabolism and, 382
mineral bioavailability, 215–217, 219, 221–236, see also specific minerals
mineral/trace element utilization studies, 246–249
nitrogen excretion and, 191, 195
pancreatic enzyme activity and, 381
particle size and fecal composition, 320–322
phytate content, 619, 623
protein utilization and, 199, 202
short chain fatty acid metabolism and, 403–406
Bran Buds, 276, 578, see also Bran; Cereals/cereal grains
Bran cell wall fiber: protein utilization and, 203
Bran tablets, 325
Breads
dietary fiber values, 575–577
dry matter analysis, 595–597
fecal composition and, 326–327
fecal excretion, 277–278, 283–285
glycemic index, 126
in vitro binding studies, 231–234
mineral bioavailability, 214–218, 221–229, 235
mineral/trace element utilization studies, 246–249
particle size and fecal composition, 320–322
phytate content, 618
Southgate analysis, 607
Breakfast cereals, see Cereals/cereal grains
Brighton classification system, 635–636
British diet studies, 364, 365; World War II and diabetes mellitus, 439–440
Brush border enzymes, 379–380, 383
Burne, John, 263

C

Ca
bioavailability, 224–229
from cereals, 214, 215, 218, 220–222
tabulation of studies, 213
in vitro binding studies, 231, 232
utilization studies, 246
Cabbage, 305, 306, 309, 366, 372, 601, see also Vegetables
fecal excretion studies, 408
nitrogen excretion and, 196
Calcium, see Ca
Cancer
carcinogenesis animal studies, 502–504
colon, see Colon cancer
Italian fiber consumption and, 561
South African patterns, 492
Candy and sweets: dietary fiber values, 585–587
Canoia hulls, 187
Canola cell wall, 188
Carbohydrate metabolism, see also Diabetes mellitus; Glucose metabolism
in vitro hydrolysis, 380
long-term effects

in diabetes mellitus, 113–114, 128–132
in normal subjects, 112–113
single test meals, 111–112
Carob bean, 378
Carob bean gum, 183, 193
Carob flour, 381
Carotene, 253
Carrageenan, 29–30
enzyme activity and, 378
nitrogen excretion and, 193
pancreatic enzyme activity and, 381
protein digestibility and, 183
Carrots, 305, 307, 313, 365, 505, 601, see also Vegetables
Casein digestibility, 379
Cellulose, 20, 30
antitoxicity/anticarcinogenicity, 502, 505
bacterial interactions, 372
casein digestibility inhibition, 379
content in selected foods, 595–606
in diabetes mellitus, 444, 445, 449, 452
enzyme activity and, 378
as food additives, 28
fecal composition and, 291–295, 318
fecal excretion studies, 407, 408
fecal microflora studies, 368
in hyperlipidemia, 420–422
lipid metabolism and, 382
mineral bioavailability, 218, 227, 229
mineral/trace element utilization studies, 246–249
nitrogen excretion and, 190–191
pancreatic enzyme activity and, 381
protein digestibility and, 180–181, 183
protein utilization and, 197–198
short chain fatty acid metabolism and, 403–405, 406
Cell wall fraction: *in vitro* mineral binding studies, 231
Cereal gums, 372
Cereals/cereal grains, see also Bran
Chinese consumption, 544, 545
crude vs. dietary fiber, 615
dietary fiber values, 577–583
dry matter analysis, 597–600
fecal composition and, 326–330
French consumption, 548–549
glycemic index, 126
in vitro mineral binding studies, 231–232
mineral bioavailability, 214–224, 235
Norwegian fiber study, 611
pancreatic lipase inhibition *in vivo*, 379
phytate content, 620
Southgate analysis, 607
Chapathi, see Breads
Chelating properties of fiber, 209–210, 245
Chinese consumption of fiber-rich foods, 543–545
Chitosan, 382
Chloride, see Cl
Cholelithiasis, 471–475, see also Gallstones
Cholesterol, see also Hyperlipidemia
bile salt-fiber interactions, 168–173
blood and liver, 163–168

Index

current research status, 9–10
deoxycholic acid and bile saturation, 472–473
fecal composition and, 317
fecal excretion, 172–178, 419
intestinal absorption, 153–155
  animal studies, 156–159
  human studies, 159–160
treatment options, 634–635
Citric acid and mineral bioavailability, 236
Citrus fiber antitoxicity/anticarcinogenicity, 504
Cl bioavailability, 220
Colon cancer
  antitoxicity/anticarcinogenicity studies, 501–505
  current research status, 9
  Danish diet studies, 364
  epidemiological studies in humans, 477–480
  fecal-luminal mutagenesis, 413–414
  fiber hypothesis history, 477
  Finnish studies, 364, 413–414
  Scandinavian study, 351–352
  South African patterns, 491–494
Colonic diverticular disease, see Diverticular disease
Colorometric measurements, 64–67
Constipation, see also Fecal excretion; current research status, 7–8
Consumption patterns, see also Epidemiological studies
  Australian fiber intake, 535–539
  Chinese consumption of fiber-rich foods, 543–545
  France, 547–554
    cereals, 548–549
    fiber, 553–554
    fruits and vegetables, 548, 550–552
  human fiber consumption
    Africa, 517–518
    Australasia, 518, 535–539
    Europe, 512–517
    India, 518
    Japan, 364, 497–500, 518–520, 528–529
    methods of study, 509–510
    Middle East, 521
    nonstarch polysaccharides, 510–512
    North America, 520
    South America, 521
  Italy, 557–563
  Seventh Day Adventists vs. general nonvegetarian population, 530–532
  vegetarian vs. nonvegetarian crude fiber intake, 525–529
Cookies and crispbreads: Southgate analysis, 607
Copper, see Cu
Corn, 379
  fecal composition and, 329
  in vitro hydrolysis, 380
  in vitro mineral binding studies, 233–234
  mineral bioavailability, 214, 217, 219, 224, 225, 228, 229, 235
  mineral/trace element utilization studies, 246–249
Corn bran, 368
  antitoxicity/anticarcinogenicity, 504
  in diabetes mellitus, 451
dry matter analysis, 597
fecal composition and, 301–304
fecal excretion studies, 408
mineral bioavailability, 224, 227
phytate content, 619
protein digestibility and, 186
protein utilization and, 202
Corn germ: mineral bioavailability, 236
Corn hay and short chain fatty acid metabolism, 404
Corn hulls: protein digestibility and, 187
Corn meal: mineral bioavailability, 224
Corn oil and short chain fatty acid metabolism, 405
Corn products
  fecal composition and, 301–304
  mineral bioavailability, 226
Corn soy: and short chain fatty acid metabolism, 404
Cottonseed fiber in diabetes mellitus, 453
Cottonseed hulls, 305, 407
Crackers: phytate content, 619
Critical fecal weight, 351
Crohn's disease, 487–488
Crude fiber, 30, see also Dietary fiber
  dietary fiber comparative analysis, 615
  in particular samples, 613–614
  in selected foods, 595–604
Cu
  bioavailability, 224, 227–229
    from cereals, 215, 217
    tabulation of studies, 213
  in vitro binding studies, 231, 232
  mineral/trace element utilization studies, 248
Cutin, 24, 25, 30

D

Dairy products: glycemic index, 127
Detergent analysis of foods, 49–51
Diabetes mellitus
  autonomic neuropathy in, 444
  "chemical," 444, 445
  fiber hypothesis history, 439–440
  fiber supplementation studies, 113–115
  gestational, 445
  glycemic index in, 122–132
  South African patterns, 492
  treatment
    fiber supplementation, 120–121
      diet response, 448–453
      single-meal response, 443–447
    high carbohydrate, high fiber diets, 128–132, 138–141
    high carbohydrate, low fiber diets, 136–137
    high fiber diet response, 448, 456–461
    IDDM vs. NIDDM, 448
    long-term effects, 141
    mechanism, 448
    safety, 452
Dietary fiber
  defined and classified, 30, 267, 629–630, 635–636
  definitions and alternative terms, 15–17

food components behaving as, 21–22
plant and algae content, 19–20
Dietary fiber values
 breads, 575–577
 candy and sweets, 585–587
 cereals, 577–583
 fruit juices, 568
 fruits
  dried, 570–571
  fresh or unsweetened, 569
  sweetened, 570
 grains, 577–583
 legumes, 574–575
 meat substitutes, 574–575
 nuts and seeds, 567–568
 pasta and rice, 583–584
 pastries, 577
 snack foods, 584–585
 soups, 585
 spices and condiments, 587–588
 vegetables
  cooked or canned, 572–574
  raw, 571
Dietary recommendations, 351–354
Dietary regimens
 in diabetes mellitus, 444–461, see also Diabetes mellitus: treatment
 in diverticular disease, 324–330
 fecal composition and
  formula, 301, 313
  fruit/vegetable combinations, 311–312, 314, 315
  Guatemalan, 313
  high cholesterol, 317
  high fat, high fiber, 311
  high fat, low fiber, 311
  high fiber, 314, 315, 319, 324–325, 337–339
  high protein, 280
  high protein + fiber, 280
  increased fiber, 313
  low cholesterol, 317
  low fat, high fiber, 311
  low fiber, 273, 313–315, 319, 323, 337–339
  mixed fiber sources, 317–319
  vegetarian, 337
  very low fiber, 273
 fecal microflora and, 364, 365–370
 fiber supplementation studies, 365–370
 in gallstone therapy, 473–474
 high fiber, 634; in diabetes mellitus, 456–461
 low residue, 365
 recommended fiber intake, 351–354
 vegetarian, 364
 vs. supplements, 630
 Western and non-Western fecal flora compared, 364
Digestibility: proteins
 fiber-rich food animal studies, 186–189
 purified fiber animal studies, 180–184
Diverticular disease, 483–485, 492
 current research status, 8
 fecal composition in, 324–330

Doss: mineral bioavailability, 225
Dry matter content of selected foods, 595–606, see also individual foods and fiber components
Duodenal juice viscosity, 383
Duration of feeding: short chain fatty acid metabolism and, 393–395

E

Edible fiber, see Dietary fiber
EEC/IARC interlaboratory comparison study, 42–43
Endosperm: mineral bioavailability, 226
Englyst GLC procedure
 breaks, 64
 procedure, 58–64
 reagents, 55–58
 troubleshooting, 64–67
 vs. Uppsala method, 77
Enrichment studies: of mineral bioavailability, 210
Enteral vitamin synthesis, 257–258
Enzymatic gravimetric assays, 37–47, see also Analytic methods
Enzyme activity, 377–383
Epidemiological studies, see also Cancer; Colon cancer; Consumption patterns
 colon cancer, 477–480
 gallstones, 471
 Japanese disease patterns and fiber intake, 497–500
 Scandinavian colon cancer study, 351–352
 South African disease patterns and fiber intake, 491–494
European fiber consumption, 512–517
Extracts: Southgate analysis, 609

F

Fats, see Lipid metabolism
Fat-soluble vitamins: absorption, 253–255
Fatty acid metabolism, 387–410, see also Short chain fatty acids
Fava beans, see Legume protein; Legumes
Fe
 bioavailability, 224, 225–228
  from cereals, 214–216, 222
  food additive effects, 235–236
  tabulation of studies, 213
 in vitro binding studies, 231, 232
 utilization studies, 247
Fecal excretion
 average increase per gram of fiber fed, 264
 cellulose/cellulose derivatives and, 291–295
 cereal products and composition, 326–330
 of cholesterol, 172–178
 in diverticular disease, 323–325
 fiber-containing foods and, 310–316
 gums, mucilages, and other purified sources and, 333–336
 historical aspects, 263–264
 legumes and composition, 331–332
 mechanisms of fiber action, 266
 modern studies, 264–266, 268–272

mutagenesis and, 413–414
oats and corn products, 301–304
particle size and composition, 320–322
plant gums, mucilages, and polysaccharides and composition, 296–300
purified fiber forms and composition, 305–309
purified pectin and composition, 286–290
of short chain fatty acids, 407–409
of sterols, 419
transit time and weight, 351–352
wheat fiber effects, 273–285
Fecal microflora, see also Intestinal microflora, 363–368
Fenugreek seeds in diabetes mellitus, 453
Fiber, see Dietary fiber
Fiber concentrates, 634
Fiber intake, see Consumption patterns
Fiber One, 328, 579, 598, see also Cereals/cereal grains
Fiber polymers, 633–634
Fiber supplements
　dry matter analysis, 603–605
　vs. diets, 630
Fiber Supplement Workshop Report of International Congress of Nutrition, 629–630
Finnish colon cancer studies, 413–414
Fish and mineral bioavailability, 235
Fish oil and short chain fatty acid metabolism, 404, 405
Flours, see Breads
Folic acid, 257–258
Foods
　components associated with dietery fiber, 23–24
　components behaving as dietary fiber, 21–22
　dietary fiber content, 19–20
Free sugar removal, 80–81
French studies of consumption patterns, 547–554
Fruit juices: dietary fiber values, 568, see also Fruits
Fruits
　Chinese consumption patterns, 547–554
　crude fiber values, 613–614
　crude vs. dietary fiber, 615
　dietary fiber values, 569–571
　dry matter analysis, 600–601
　fecal composition and, 310–316, 337
　French consumption, 548, 550–552
　glycemic index, 127
　mineral bioavailibility, 225, 228
　nitrogen excretion and, 196
　phytate content, 617–623
　protein digestibility and, 188
　Southgate analysis, 608
Future prospects, 633–636

G

Galactans, 30
Galactomannans, 28, 30
Gallstones
　animal experiments, 473–474
　associated diseases/metabolic disturbances, 471–472
　current dietary theories, 471
　deoxycholic acid and cholesterol saturation of bile, 472–473
　epidemiologic studies, 471
　wheat bran/fiber rich diet in, 473–474
Gastric viscosity, 383
Gastrointestinal tract, 355–356
Gelling agents and insulin response, 114
Gender effects: short chain fatty acid metabolism, 390–391
Genetic factors
　in diabetes mellitus, 440
　in hyperlipidemia, 420
Glossary of fiber components, 29–33
Glucofructans, 30
Glucomannan, 30, 449
Glucoronoxylans, 30
Glucose metabolism, see also Diabetes mellitus
　current research status, 9
　fiber-free glucose tolerance tests, 117
　gelling agents and, 114
　glycemic index of foods, 114–122
　psyllium and, 116
　purified fiber and, 116
　refining (fiber removal) and, 115
　single test meals, 112–115
Glycan, 30
Glycemic index, see also Diabetes mellitus
　clinical applications, 122–132
　digestibility and, 118–121
　long-term effect of low index diets, 141
　predictive value, 133–135
Glycuronans, 30
Grains, see also Cereals/cereal grains and individual types
　dietary fiber values, 577–583
　mineral bioavailability, 219
Grinding and metabolic response, 131
Guar/guar gum, 30–31
　bacterial interactions, 372
　in carbohydrate metabolism, 112
　in diabetes mellitus, 118–119, 444–446, 449–455
　enzyme activity and, 378
　fecal composition and, 296–300, 333–335, 335
　fecal microflora studies, 365, 367
　in hyperlipidemia, 422, 424–426
　lipid metabolism and, 382
　mineral bioavailability, 227
　mineral/trace element utilization studies, 246–249
　nitrogen excretion and, 193
　pancreatic enzyme activity and, 381
　protein digestibility and, 183
　protein utilization and, 200
　short chain fatty acid metabolism and, 406
Guatemalan diet
　fecal composition and, 313
　protein digestibility and, 188
Gum arabic, 300, 367
　fecal excretion studies, 407–409
　short chain fatty acid metabolism and, 403–405, 406

Gums, 20, 28, 31, see also Guar/guar gum
Guran, see Guar/guar gum

H

Haricot beans, 316
Hawaiian diet studies, 364
Hemicelluloses, 19–20, 31
   bacterial interactions, 372
   in carbohydrate metabolism, 112
   content in selected foods, 595–606
   in diabetes mellitus, 444
   mineral bioavailability, 218
   nitrogen excretion and, 191
   protein utilization and, 198
Hertz (Hurst), Sir Arthur, 263
Heteroglycans, 31
Hexoses, 31
High fiber diet, see Dietary regimens
Historical aspects
   of fiber consumption, 3–8
   of fiber research, 7–10
Homoglycan, 31
HPLC in saponin determination, 106
Human vs. animal studies, 211
Hyperlipidemia, see also Cholesterol; Short chain fatty acid metabolism
   conclusions, 431
   current research status, 9–10
   genetic factors, 420
   mechanisms of fiber action, 419–420
   specific fibers in, 420–434
      dosage, 431
      dried legumes, 426, 431
      fiber-rich whole foods, 428–430
      guar, 422
      legume protein, 431–433
      lignin and cellulose, 420–422
      locust bean gum, 422, 427
      oat bran, 426
      pectin, 422
      purified soluble, 423–426
   treatment, 634–635

I

Imbicoli, 296
Indian (Asia) fiber consumption, 518
Inflammatory bowel disease
   Crohn's disease, 487–488
   short chain fatty acids and, 489–490
   South African patterns, 492
   ulcerative colitis, 488–489
Inorganics associated with fiber, 24, 25
Inoxalol, 234
Insoluble fiber:enzymatic gravimetric analysis, 37–39
Insulin metabolism, 112–115, see also Diabetes mellitus; Glucose metabolism; and hyperlipidemia, 420
Intake of fiber, see Consumption patterns

International Congress of Nutrition Fiber Supplement Workshop Report, 629–630
Intestinal absorption of lipids
   animal studies, 156–159
   human studies, 159–160
Intestinal brush border enzymes, 379–380, 383
Intestinal microflora, 361–363
   anaerobic bacteria found in human intestine, 372
   fecal
      in different human populations, 363
      fiber effects, 364–368
   fiber substrate interactions, 371–375
   short chain fatty acid metabolism and, 388–389
Intestinal viscosity, 383
Intestinal vitamin synthesis, 257–258
In vitro vs. *in vivo* studies, 211
Iron, see Fe
Isphagula, 183, 298–299, 325, 333
Italian consumption patterns
   cancer, 561
   cardiovascular disease, 561
   EEC study, 558, 560
   INN study, 558, 560
   Trento study, 557, 559
   Verona vegetarian study, 559, 563

J

Japanese diet studies, 364, 497–500, 518–520, 528–529
Junk food dry matter analysis, 603

K

K (potassium)
   bioavailability, 227, 230
   from cereals, 220
   in vitro binding studies, 232
Karaya, 296, 299, 379, 502
Klason lignin values, 90–92
Konjac and seaweed, 188
Konjac mannan, 382
Konsil, 297
Kylan, 300

L

Laboratory techniques, see Analytic methods
Lactulose, 325, 333
Laminarin, 365
Laxative properties, 263–266, see also Fecal excretion
Legume protein: in hyperlipidemia, 431–433
Legumes, 305, 379
   antitoxicity/anticarcinogenicity, 504, 505
   Chinese consumption, 544, 545
   crude fiber values, 613
   in diabetes mellitus, 444–447
   dietary fiber values, 574–575
   dry matter analysis, 601–603
   fecal composition and, 331–332
   fecal excretion studies, 407, 408

glycemic index, 127
in hyperlipidemia, 427–428, 429–430
in vitro hydrolysis, 380
phytate content, 617–623
saponin content, 624
short chain fatty acid metabolism and, 404
Southgate analysis, 607–608
Lignins, 20, 23, 25, 31
antitoxicity/anticarcinogenicity, 505
bacterial interactions, 372
casein digestibility inhibition, 379
content in selected foods, 595–606
enzyme activity and, 378
exclusion from NSP measurements, 68–70
fecal composition and, 308
fractional analysis, 89–91
in hyperlipidemia, 420–422
nitrogen excretion and, 191
protein digestibility and, 181
protein utilization and, 198
Lipid metabolism, 153–155, see also Hyperlipidemia
animal studies, 382
bile salt-fiber interactions, 168–173
blood and liver lipid effects, 163–168
enzyme activity and, 378–379
fecal steroid excretion, 172–178
human studies, 382
intestinal absorption, 156–160
short chain fatty acids, 387–410, see also Short chain fatty acid metabolism
Lipid removal, 81–82
Locust bean gum
antitoxicity/anticarcinogenicity, 502
bacterial interactions, 372
in diabetes mellitus, 444
in hyperlipidemia, 422, 426, 427
nitrogen excretion and, 195
pancreatic enzyme activity and, 381
Low cholesterol diet, see Dietary regimens
Low-density lipoproteins (LDLs), see Cholesterol
Low fat diets, see Dietary regimens
Lupin hulls, 187
Lymphatic system: cholesterol absorption and fiber supplementation, 157

M

Magnesium, see Mg
Maillard polymer: bacterial interactions, 372
Maize, see Corn
Manganese, see Mn
Mannans, 31
Measurement, see Analytic methods
Meat substitutes
dietary fiber values, 574–575
phytate content, 622
Metamucil, see Psyllium
Mg
bioavailability, 224–225, 227–229
from cereals, 214–217, 220–222
tabulation of studies, 213
in vitro binding studies, 231, 232
utilization studies, 246
Microflora
fecal, 364–368
intestinal, 361–363, 371–375
Middle Eastern fiber consumption, 521
Middle lamella, 31
Milk and mineral bioavailability, 235, 236
Minerals, see also Trace elements and individual minerals
additives and utilization, 245–249
bioavailability, 210–211, 231–234
Mn, 213, 224, 227, 228, 232
Mucilages, 20, 31; fecal composition and, 296–300
Mucin: effects of fiber feeding, 156
Mucin glycoprotein, 372
Mucopolysaccharide, 372
Muffins, see Breads
Mutagenesis: fecal-luminal activity, 413–414, see also Colon cancer

N

Na (sodium), 220, 227, 230, 232
Na-alginate
enzyme activity and, 378
nitrogen excretion and, 193
pancreatic enzyme activity and, 381
protein digestibility and, 183
Native Americans: diabetes mellitus in, 447
Neutral detergent polysaccharide, 31–32, 49–51, 84–88, see also Dietary fiber
nitrogen excretion and, 191
protein utilization and, 199
of selected foods, 595–606
Nicotinic acid, 257
Nitrogen excretion
fiber-rich food animal studies, 195–196
purified fiber animal studies, 190–194
Noncellulosic polysaccharides, 19, 32
Nonstarch polysaccharides, 32, 55–67, 355, see also Dietary fiber
Nopal leaves, 451
North American fiber consumption, 520
Nuts
crude vs. dietary fiber, 615
dry matter analysis, 603
phytate content, 617–623
saponin content, 624
Southgate analysis, 608
Nuts and seeds: dietary fiber values, 567–568

O

Oat bran, see also Bran
antitoxicity/anticarcinogenicity, 502
dietary fiber values, 583
dry matter analysis, 598–599
enzyme activity and, 378
fecal composition and, 303
in hyperlipidemia, 427–430
mineral bioavailability, 227

nitrogen excretion and, 195
protein digestibility and, 186
short chain fatty acid metabolism and, 403, 406
Oat hulls, 187
Oat husk, 227
Oatmeal, 226, 232
Oats
  in vitro binding studies, 233–234
  in vitro hydrolysis, 380
  fecal composition and, 301–304
  mineral bioavailability, 228
  saponin content, 624
Oat straw, 196
Oligosaccharides, 32
Orange juice, 235, 236, see also Fruit juices

P

P (phosphorus)
  bioavailability, 225–230
    from cereals, 217, 220–222
    tabulation of studies, 213
  in vitro binding studies, 232
  utilization studies, 249
Pancreatic enzymes, 379, 381, see also Enzyme activity
Particle size: fecal composition and, 320–322
Pasta, see also Cereals/cereal grains
  dietary fiber values, 583–584
  dry matter analysis, 597
  glycemic index, 126
  Norwegian fiber study, 611
Pastries: dietary fiber values, 577
Pea hulls, 187
Peas, see Legumes
Pectic substances, 20, 32
Pectin, 32
  antitoxicity/anticarcinogenicity, 505
  bacterial interactions, 372, 374
  in carbohydrate metabolism, 112, 113
  casein digestibility inhibition, 379
  in diabetes mellitus, 444, 445, 449, 451
  enzyme activity and, 378
  fecal composition and, 286–290, 318, 336
  fecal excretion studies, 408
  fecal microflora studies, 367
  as food additive, 28
  in hyperlipidemia, 422–424
  lipid metabolism and, 382
  mineral/trace element utilization studies, 246–249
  nitrogen excretion and, 192
  pancreatic enzyme activity and, 381
  protein digestibility and, 182–183
  protein utilization and, 199–200
  short chain fatty acid metabolism and, 403–406
Pectinic acid, 32
Pentoses, 32
Phosphorus, see P
Phytate, 24
  determination of, 101–103
  food content chart, 617–623
  mineral bioavailability, 224
  mineral/trace element utilization studies, 246–249

Phytic acid, 504; and mineral bioavailability, 209–210
Plantago, 334
Plantain, 312, 367
Plant foods: dietary fiber content, 19–20, 56–57, see also Cereals/cereal grains; Fruits; Legumes; Vegetables
Planti, 15, 16
Plantix, 32
Plant waxes, 24, 25
Polysaccharides
  algal, 28, 29
  determination of neutral, 84–88
  as food additives, 27–28
  noncellulosic, 19, 32
  non-glucan, 22
  nonstarch, see Dietary fiber; Nonstarch polysaccharides
  soy and protein digestibility, 188
Potassium, see K
Potatoes, 307, 312, 313, 446, see also Vegetables
Preserves: Southgate analysis, 608
Primary plant cell wall, 32
Propionate and antihyperlipidemic action, 419–420
Prosky (AAOC) total dietary fiber analysis, 42–47
Protein, 23–25; and mineral bioavailability, 235
Protein metabolism, 129–130, 179
  digestibility
    fiber-rich sources and, 186–189
    purified fiber and, 180–184
  enzyme activity, 377–383
  nitrogen excretion and balance, 190–194
  utilization
    fiber-rich food animal studies, 202–203
    purified fiber animal studies, 197–201
Protopectin, 32
Psyllium
  antitoxicity/anticarcinogenicity, 502
  in diabetes mellitus, 445, 453
  dry matter analysis, 604
  enzyme activity and, 378
  fecal composition and, 296–300, 333–335
  fecal excretion studies, 407
  fecal microflora studies, 365
  lipid metabolism and, 382
  nitrogen excretion and, 196
  short chain fatty acid metabolism and, 405
Purified fiber
  fecal composition and, 286–290, 305–309, 333–336
  glucose metabolism and, 116
  nitrogen excretion and, 190–194
  protein metabolism and
    digestion, 180–184
    utilization, 197–201

R

Raffinose, 181, 183
Reagents for Englyst GLC procedure, 55–58

Index

Recommended intake, 351–354; see also Dietary regimens
Red kidney beans, see Legumes
Research: current status, 7–10
Resistant starch, see Dietary fiber
Rice
  brown
    nitrogen excretion and, 196
    protein digestibility and, 188
  casein digestibility inhibition, 379
  Chinese consumption, 544
  dietary fiber values, 583–584
  fecal composition and, 329
  French consumption, 549
  in vitro binding studies, 231–234
  in vitro hydrolysis, 380
  mineral bioavailability, 214, 217, 219, 225, 227, 229, 230, 235, 236
  Norwegian fiber study, 611
  phytate content, 621–622
Rice bran, see also Bran
  antitoxicity/anticarcinogenicity, 504
  dietary fiber values, 583
  enzyme activity and, 378
  in vitro mineral binding studies, 231, 232
Rice hulls, 195
Rolls, see Breads
Rye, see also Breads
  in diabetes mellitus, 446
  in vitro binding studies, 233–234
  in vitro hydrolysis, 380
  mineral bioavailability, 226
Rye bran in diabetes mellitus, 452

S

Safflower meal, 378
Saponins, 24
  determination, 105–106
  plant foods containing significant levels, 624
Sclerenchyma, 32
Se (selenium), 226, 228, 213
Secondary cell wall, 32
Selenium, see Se
Seventh Day Adventist studies, 364, 413–414, 530–532
Short chain fatty acid metabolism, 387, see also Hyperlipidemia
  dietary fiber concentration and, 396–398
  dietary fiber presence/absence and, 399–402
  dietary fiber source and, 403–405
  duration of feeding and, 393–395
  gender effects, 390–391
  in inflammatory bowel disease, 489–490
  microfloral effects, 388–389
Siblin, 297
Silica, 32
Slippery elm, 195
Small intestinal effects of fiber, 356
Snack foods: dietary fiber values, 584–585
Sodium, see Na
Solka floc, 371–375
Soluble fiber: enzymatic gravimetric analysis, 38–39
Sorghum, 225, 227, 326
Sorghum fiber, 195
Sorghum meal, 186
Soups
  dietary fiber values, 585
  Southgate analysis, 609
South African disease patterns and fiber intake, 491–494
South American fiber consumption, 521
Southgate analysis
  method, 73–74
  of selected foods, 607–609
Soybean products, 187–188, 196, 224, 227, 308–309, 451, 502, 504, 622, see also Legume protein; Legumes
Spices and condiments, 587–588, 609
Starch
  analytic procedures Englyst GLC method, 67–68
  removal/analysis methods compared, 81–83
  resistant, 32, 635
Stomach effects of fiber, 355
Suberin, 24, 25, 32
Sugar beet fiber, 195, 283
Sugars: glycemic index, 127
Supplementation studies, see Dietary regimens

T

Tea and mineral bioavailability, 235
Total dietary fiber analysis (AAOC) method, 42–47
Total dietary fiber of selected foods, 595–606
Toxicity modification, 501–504, see also Cancer
Trace elements: additives and utilization, 245–249, see also Minerals
Transit time and fecal weight, 351–352
A Treatise on the Causes and Consequences of Habitual Constipation (Burne), 263
Triticale, 226, 229, 611

U

Ugandan diet studies, 364
U.K. Ministry of Agriculture classification guidelines, 70, 77–78
Ulcerative colitis, 488–489, 492
Unavailable carbohydrate, see Dietary fiber
Upper gastrointestinal tract effects, 355–356
Uppsala method, 77–80
Uronic acid, 32, 88–89
Utilization: proteins, 197–203

V

Vegetables, see also individual vegetables; Legumes
  casein digestibility inhibition, 379
  Chinese consumption, 544
  crude fiber values, 613–614
  crude vs. dietary fiber, 615
  dietary fiber values, 571–574
  dry matter analysis, 601–603

fecal composition and, 310–316
French consumption, 548, 550–552
glycemic index, 127
mineral bioavailability, 225, 228
nitrogen excretion and, 193, 196
phytate content, 617–623
protein digestibility and, 188
saponin content, 624
Southgate analysis, 607–608
Vegetarians, 364, see also Dietary regimens; Seventh Day Adventist studies
consumption studies, 525–529
fecal composition, 337
Verona study, 559, 563
Very high-density lipoproteins (VLDLs), see Cholesterol
Vitamin metabolism, 253–258
Vitamins
A, 253
B complex, 255–258
C (ascorbic acid), 235, 236, 257
D, 254
E, 255
folic acid, 257–258
K, 255, 257–258
PP (nicotinic acid), 257
Vivonex low residue diet, 365
Volatile fatty acids, see Short chain fatty acid metabolism

W

Water-holding capacity, 33
Water-insoluble fraction, 91–92
Water-soluble fraction, 33, 91–92
Water-soluble vitamin absorption, 255–257
Waxes, 24, 25
Wheat, see also Breads; Cereals/cereal grains
Chinese consumption, 544
crude fiber values, 614
dietary fiber values, 583
fecal composition and, 326
French consumption, 549
in vitro binding studies, 231–234
in vitro hydrolysis, 380
mineral bioavailability, 214, 217, 226, 228, 229, 235
Wheat bran, see also Bran; Wheat fiber
antitoxicity/anticarcinogenicity, 504–505
bacterial interactions, 372–373
casein digestibility inhibition, 379
in diabetes mellitus, 118–119, 444–446, 449–455
enzyme activity and, 378
fecal excretion studies, 407–409
fecal microflora studies, 366, 367
in gallstone therapy, 473–474
in hyperlipidemia, 427, 428–430
in vitro binding studies, 231–234
lipid metabolism and, 382
mineral bioavailability studies, 215, 218–230, 236
mineral/trace element utilization studies, 246–249
nitrogen excretion and, 191–192, 195
Norwegian fiber study, 611
pancreatic enzyme activity and, 381
phytate content, 623
protein digestibility and, 186
protein utilization and, 199, 202
short chain fatty acid metabolism and, 403–406
Wheat fiber
fecal excretion, 273–285, 408
mineral bioavailability, 222, 225
nitrogen excretion and, 195
Wheat flakes, 218
Wheat flour, see Breads
Wheat fractions and short chain fatty acid metabolism, 403
Wheat germ, 382, 611, 623
Wheat straw, 374
Whole wheat bread, see Breads
Whole wheat flour, see Breads; Cereals/cereal grains
World War II British diet studies, 439–440

X

Xanthan, 333, 335, 381, 452
Xylan, 33, 365, 368
enzyme activity and, 378
fecal excretion studies, 408
protein digestibility and, 181, 183
protein utilization and, 198

Z

Zn (zinc)
bioavailability, 224–229
from cereals, 215, 217–222
food additive effects, 235–236
tabulation of studies, 213
in vitro binding studies, 231, 232
utilization studies, 248